This book is the ~~property~~

Do. ☟

W9-CDY-285

Stedman's

ABBREV.

ABBREVIATIONS,
ACRONYMS & SYMBOLS

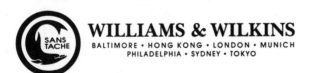

WILLIAMS & WILKINS
BALTIMORE · HONG KONG · LONDON · MUNICH
PHILADELPHIA · SYDNEY · TOKYO

Editor: William R. Hensyl
Database Manager: Harriet Felscher
Production Coordinator: Jennifer Dandy
Cover Design: Carla Frank

Copyright © 1992
Willliams & Wilkins
428 East Preston Street
Baltimore, Maryland 21202, USA

All rights reserved. This book is protected by copyright. No part of this book may be reproduced in any form or by any means, including photocopying, or utilized by any information storage and retrieval system without written permission from the copyright owner.

Accurate indications, adverse reactions, and dosage schedules for drugs are provided in this book, but it is possible that they may change. The reader is urged to review the package information data of the manufacturers of the medications mentioned.

Printed in the United States of America

Library of Congress Cataloging-in-Publication Data

Stedman's abbreviations, acronyms, & symbols.
    p.   cm.
  ISBN 0-683-07926-3
    1. Medicine—Abbreviations—Dictionaries. 2. Medicine—Acronyms—Dictionaries. I. Williams & Wilkins. II. Title: Stedman's abbreviations, acronyms, and symbols. III. title: Abbreviations, acronyms, & symbols. IV. Title: Abbreviations, acronyms and symbols.
    [DNLM: 1. Medicine—abbreviations. 2. Medicine—acronums. W 13 S8119]
R123.S69 1992
610'.148—dc20
DNLM/DLC
for Library of Congress   91-30701
                                                                                  CIP

92 93 94 95
1 2 3 4 5 6 7 8 9 10

CONTENTS

EXPLANATORY NOTES

This reference is a primary resource for anyone involved in transcribing, recording, copyediting, or reading records, reports, and other material generated by health care professionals. Its development originated from an ongoing review of medical and allied health professional literature to enhance the coverage in *Stedman's Medical Dictionary*. An expanded review of existing dictionaries, style manuals, "approved lists" from teaching hospitals, nomenclatures, glossaries, and other compendia produced this compilation of over 20,000 clinically relevant abbreviations, acronyms, and symbols. Each abbreviation and its usage(s) has been verified in at least two sources.

The concept of "user-friendly" was a major focus of this book from design specifications to construction of individual entries so that sought-after information could be efficiently located, easily read, and quickly understood. Novices as well as seasoned professionals are encouraged to read the following descriptions of this reference's organization, format, and style to enhance pragmatic application of its features.

To keep this book in managable proportions, the *Stedman's* staff had to make some difficult decisions to restrict or exclude coverage of certain cateogories of abbreviations not directly related to the practice of health care professionals. Some of these categories are professional, specialty, and honorary associations; undergraduate, honorary, and non-certification or -licensure degrees; titles of publications; chemical formulas and expressions; and spurious and ad hoc coinages.

The form of an abbreviation as well as its meaning often varies from institution to institution and specialty to specialty. "Official" abbreviations issued by nomenclatural groups often are slow to become universally accepted. For these reasons, preferred forms or preferred usages have not been cited. Instead, any variants of form and/or usage are given at all of the variant entries.

Creation of new abbreviations and the variety of usages outpaces any compilation of them. New editions of this reference will be published as often as justified by worthwhile new entries and revisions. Users are encouraged to submit their recommendations to the Reference Division at Williams & Wilkins. We also welcome all suggestions for improving this *Stedman's* product.

Alphabetical Organization

Entries are alphabetized letter by letter as written or spoken, in the following order: capital letters precede lower-case letters, italics follow non-italics, roman numerals precede arabic numbers. Numbers, diacritics, punctuation, spaces, etc. are not considered in alphabetization except when they are the only difference between entries having the same letters. For example:

A	A250
Å	a
A_1	$\bar{a}$
A_2	*a*
AI	(a)

In some instances the alphabetical order is arbitrary out of necessity, but such listings are brief and consistent throughout the vocabulary. For example:

AA	A–a
$\overline{AA}$	a–A
A–A	a/A
A/A	aa
A&A	$\overline{aa}$

Entries beginning with a Greek letter are located where the name of the letter would be found alphabetically; thus: A and α are located at "alpha," B and β at "beta," Γ and γ at "gamma." A table of the Greek alphabet is located between the end of this section and the beginning of the A section.

Symbols that are composed of characters other than letters, and therefore cannot be logically alphabetized, are located in a special Symbols section following the Z section. Here, symbols are organized according to similarities of form and construction in a format similar to that of the A—Z abbreviations.

Format and Style

Each entry consists of a boldface abbreviation, acronym, or symbol and its "definition" or meaning(s) in lightface. When there is more than one meaning, each meaning is listed in alphabetical order and separated by a bullet (•). Bracketed derivations and parenthetical explanatory material are not considered in the alphabetization of meanings.

Periods are used in abbreviations only when the abbreviation or a part of it could be confused with a word. For example:

add.   **addict.**   **all.**

Brackets contain derivations of abbreviations originating from a foreign word. Each derivation consists of the abbreviation of the language of origin (L., Latin; G., Greek; Ger., German; Fr., French; Sp., Spanish; It., Italian) and the foreign word in italics. A derivation immediately precedes the meaning of the abbreviation to which it pertains. For example:

> **b i d** [L. *bis in die*] twice a day

> **ad** [L. *adde*] add •
> axiodistal • [L. *addetur*] let
> there be added *also* add. •
> [L. *auris dextra*] right ear
> *also* AD

Parentheses enclose explanatory material to complete an abbreviated term or phrase:

> **A** absolute (temperature) •
> (start of) anesthesia

to clarify usage that otherwise might be ambiguous:

> **BEPTI** bionomics,
> environment, *Plasmodium,*
> treatment, and immunity
> (malaria epidemiology)

to provide a mini-definition:

> **Gy** gray (unit of absorbed dose
> of ionizing radiation)

or to identify the generic name of a trade name:

> **CAM** cyclophosphamide,
> Adriamycin (doxorubicin),
> and methotrexate

Virgules (*slashes*) replace "or" in definitions where unnecessary repetition of multiple-word descriptors has been eliminated and where the meaning of an abbreviation can be any variant of a word. For example:

> **DAT** differential agglutination
> test/titer

> **GYN, gyn** gynecologic/
> gynecologist/gynecology

"*Also*" is used to highlight variant forms of an abbreviation that have the same meaning. For example:

> **g** gram *also* gm   **gm** gram *also* g

GREEK ALPHABET

Name of Greek Letters	Small	Capital	English Transcription
alpha	α	A	A
beta	β	B	B
chi	χ	X	CH
delta	δ	Δ	D
episilon	ε	E	E
eta	η	H	Ē
gamma	γ	Γ	G
iota	ι	I	I
kappa	κ	K	K, C (Latin)
lambda	λ	Λ	L
mu	μ	M	M
nu	ν	N	N
omega	ω	Ω	Ō
omicron	o	O	O
phi	φ	Φ	PH
pi	π	Π	P
psi	ψ	Ψ	PS
rho	ρ	P	R, RH
sigma	σ	Σ	S
tau	τ	T	T
theta	θ	Θ	TH
upsilon	υ	Y	Y
xi	ξ	Ξ	X
zeta	ζ	Z	Z

Small or lower case Greek letters are used primarily as symbols. Those used as symbols, along with their meanings, will be found at the alphabetical locations of their spelled-out forms. For example:

A or α at **alpha**   B or β at **beta**   Γ or γ at **gamma**

A abnormal *also* AB, ABN, Abn, abn, abnor, abnorm • abortion *also* AB, Ab, ab, Abor • absolute (temperature) • absorbance *also* abs • acceptor • accommodation *also* a, ACC, acc, accom • acetum (vinegar) • acid *also* a, AC • acidophil/ acidophilic • actin • activity (radiation) • adenine • adenoma • adenosine • admittance • adrenalin(e) • adult • age • akinetic • alanine • albumin (5%, followed by amount in mL) *also* AL, ALB, Alb, alb • alive • allergy *also* ALL, all. • alpha (cell) alternate • alveolar gas (subscript) • ambulatory • ampere *also* a • amphetamine • ampicillin *also* AM, AMP • anaphylaxis • andros- terone • (start of) anesthesia/anesthetic • angioplasty • angle *also* ang • angstrom • Ångström unit *also* Å • anisotropic (band in striated muscle) • anode *also* a, AN, An • anterior *also* a, AN, ANT, ant. • apical • aqueous • area *also* A • argon • [L. *arteria*] artery *also* a, ART, art. • assessment • atomic weight • atrium *also* At • atropine *also* ATRO • auricle • axial *also* a, ax. • axillary (temperature) *also* (a) • blood group in the ABO system • [L. *auris*] ear • mass number • subspinale (point A in cephalometrics) • total acidity *also* a • [L. *aqua*]

water *also* a, aq • [L. *annum*] year

Å angstrom/Ångström unit *also* A, antinuclear antibody • cumulated activity

A₁ aortic first sound

A₂ aortic second sound

AI, AII, AIII ngiotensin I, II, III

A250 5% albumin, 250 mL

A1000 5% albumin, 1000 mL

a absorptivity • acceleration *also* acc, accel • accommodation *also* A, ACC, acc, accom • acid/ acidity *also* A, AC • agar • alpha • ampere *also* A • annum • anode *also* A, AN, An • anterior *also* A, ANT, ant. • area *also* A • [L. *arteria*] arterial/artery *also* A, ART, art. • arterial blood (subscript) • asymmetric • atto– • axial *also* A, ax. • [L. *ante*] before *also* ā • thermodynamic activity • total acidity *also* A • [L. *aqua*] water *also* A, aq. [L. *ante*] before *also* a

(a) axillary temperature *also* A

AA acetic acid • achievement age • active alcoholic • active–assistive (range of motion) *also* AAROM • active avoidance • acupuncture analgesia • acute asthma • adenine arabinoside • adenylic acid • adjuvant arthritis • adrenal androgen •

adrenocortical autoantibody • aggregated albumin • agranulocytic angina • alcohol abuse • Alcoholics Anonymous • alopecia areata • alveolar–arterial (gradient) also A–a • aminoacetone • amino acid • aminoacyl • amyloid A • antiarrhythmic agent • anticipatory avoidance • antigen aerosol • aortic amplitude • aortic aneurysm • aortic arch • aplastic anemia • arabinosylcytosine (cytarabine) and Adriamycin (doxorubicin) • arachidonic acid • arm–ankle (pulse ratio) • [L. *arteriae*] arteries also aa • ascaris antigen • ascending aorta also Asc–A • atomic absorption • audiologic assessment • Australia antigen (radioimmunossay) also AU, Au Ag • authorized absence • autoanalyzer • axonal arborization • [G. *ana*] (so much of) each also $\overline{\text{AA}}$, aa, $\overline{\text{aa}}$, ana

$\overline{\text{AA}}$ [G. *ana*] (so much of) each also AA, aa, $\overline{\text{aa}}$, ana

A–A atlantoaxial

A/A automobile accident

A&A aid and attendance • arthroscopy and arthrotomy • awake and aware

A–a alveolar–arterial (gradient) also AA

aA abampere • azure A

a/A arterial to alveolar (oxygen ratio)

aa [L. *arteriae*] arteries also AA • [G. *ana*] (so much of) each also AA, $\overline{\text{AA}}$, $\overline{\text{aa}}$, ana

$\overline{\text{aa}}$ [G. *ana*] (so much of) each also AA, $\overline{\text{AA}}$, aa, ana

AAA abdominal aortic aneurysm/aneurysmectomy • acquired aplastic anemia • acute anxiety attack • addiction, autoimmune diseases, and aging • amalgam also aaa • androgenic anabolic agent • aneurysm of ascending aorta • aromatic amino acid

aaa amalgam also AAA

AAAAA aphasia, agnosia, apraxia, agraphia, and alexia

AAAE amino acid–activating enzymes

AA–AMP amino acid adenylate (adenomonophosphate)

AAB action against burns • aminoazobenzene

AABB American Association of Blood Banks

AABCC alertness (consciousness), airway, breathing, circulation, and cervical spine

AAC antibiotic–associated colitis • antimicrobial agent–induced colitis • antimicrobial agents and chemotherapy

AACA acylamino-cephalosporanic acid

AACE antigen–antibody crossed electrophoresis

AACG acute angle closure

AACSH adrenal androgen corticotropic stimulating hormone

AAD acid–ash diet • alloxazine adenine dinucleotide • α–1–antitrypsin deficiency • antibiotic–associated diarrhea • aromatic acid decarboxylase

AADC amino acid decarboxylase

AAdC anterior adductor of the coxa

(A–a)D$_{N2}$ difference in nitrogen tension between mixed alveolar gas and mixed arterial blood

(A–a)D$_{O2}$ difference in partial pressures of oxygen in mixed alveolar gas and mixed arterial blood

AAE active assistive exercise *also* A/AEX • acute allergic encephalitis • annuloaortic ectasia

A/AEX active assistive exercise *also* AAE

AAF acetic acid–alcohol–formalin (fixative) • acetylaminofluorene • ascorbic acid factor

AAG α_1–acid glycoprotein *also* AGP

AaG alveolar arterial gradient

AAGS adult adrenogenital syndrome

A:AGT antiglobulin test

AAI acute alveolar injury • arm–ankle indices • atrial inhibited (pacemaker)

AAIA acquired artery immune augmentation

AAIB α_1–aminoisobutyrate

AAIN acute allergic intestinal nephritis

AAL anterior axillary line

AAME acetylarginine methyl ester

AAMRS automated ambulatory medical record system

AAMS acute aseptic meningitis syndrome

AAMT American Association for Medical Transcription

AAN α–amino nitrogen • amino acid nitrogen • analgesic abuse nephropathy • analgesic–associated nephropathy • attending's admission notes

AAO amino acid oxidase • awake to alert and oriented

(A–a)O$_2$ alveolar–arterial oxygen gradient

AAOx3 awake and oriented to time, place, and person

AAP air at atmospheric pressure • α_1–anti-protease • assessment adjustment pass

AAPC antibiotic–associated pseudomembranous colitis *also* AAPMC

A–aP$_{CO2}$ alveolar–arterial carbon dioxide difference

AAPF anti–arteriosclerosis polysaccharide factor

AAPMC antibiotic–associated pseudomembranous colitis *also* AAPC

AAR active avoidance reaction · acute articular rheumatism · antigen–antiglobulin reaction · Australia antigen radioimmunoassay

AAROM active–assistive range of motion *also* AA

AAS acute abdominal series · aneurysm of atrial septum · anthrax antiserum · aortic arch syndrome · atlantoaxial subluxation · atomic absorption spectrophotometry · atypical absence seizure

AASCRN amino acid screen

Aase asparaginase

AASH adrenal androgen stimulating hormone

AASP acute atrophic spinal paralysis · ascending aorta synchronized pulsation

AAT Aachen aphasia test · academic aptitude test · acute abdominal tympany · alanine aminotransferase · alkylating agent therapy · α–1–antitrypsin *also* A1AT · amino-azotoluene · atrial triggered (pacemaker) · auditory apperception test

A1AT α–1–antitrypsin *also* AAT

AAU acute anterior uveitis

AAV adeno–associated virus

AAVV accumulated alveolar ventilatory volume

AAW anterior aortic wall

AB abdominal · abnormal *also* A, ABN, Abn, abn, abnor, abnorm · abortion *also* A, Ab, ab, Abor · Ace bandage · aid to the blind · air bleed · Alcian blue · antibiotic · antibody *also* Ab, ab · apex beat · asbestos body · asthmatic bronchitis · axiobuccal *also* ab · blood group in ABO system

A/B acid–base ratio · apnea and bradycardia *also* A&B · apnea/bradycardia moderate stimulation

A&B apnea and bradycardia *also* A/B

A>B air greater than bone (conduction)

Ab abortion *also* A, AB, ab, Abor · antibody *also* AB, ab

aB azure B

ab abortion *also* A, AB, Ab, Abor · about · antibody *also* AB, Ab · axiobuccal *also* AB · [L.] from

ABA abscissic acid · allergic bronchopulmonary aspergillosis · antibacterial activity

AbAP antibody–against–panel

ABB Albright–Butler–Bloomberg (syndrome)

abbr, abbrev abbreviated/abbreviation

ABC abbreviated blood count · absolute band count · absolute basophil count · absolute bone conduction · acalculous biliary colic • acid balance control • aconite–belladonna–chloroform • airway, breathing, and circulation • alternative birth center • antigen–binding capacity • apnea, bradycardia, and cyanosis • applesauce, bananas, and cereal (diet) • artificial beta cells • aspiration biopsy cytology • avidin–biotin complex • axiobuccocervical

ABC and C&C airway, breathing, circulation, cervical spine, and consciousness level

ABCD asymmetry, border, color, and diameter (of melanoma)

ABCDE botulism toxin pentavalent

ABCIL antibody–mediated cell–dependent immunolympholysis

ABCM Adriamycin (doxorubicin), bleomycin, cyclophosphamide, and mitomycin C

ABCX Adriamycin (doxorubicin), bleomycin, cisplatin, and radiation therapy

ABD after bronchodilator • aged, blind, and disabled • aggressive behavioral disturbance • average body dose

ABd (type of) plain gauze dressing

Abd, abd abdomen/abdominal *also* abdom • abduction

also abduc • abductor (muscle)

ABDCT atrial bolus dynamic computer tomography

abdom abdomen/abdominal *also* Abd, abd

abd poll abductor pollicis (muscle)

abduc abduction *also* Abd

ABDV Adriamycin (doxorubicin), bleomycin, vinblastine, and dacarbazine

ABE acute bacterial endocarditis • adult basic education • botulism equine trivalent antitoxin

ABEP auditory brainstem–evoked potentials

ABF aortobifemoral (bypass)

ABG aortoiliac bypass graft • arterial blood gas • axiobuccogingival

abg addictive behavior group

ABI ankle–brachial index • atherothrombotic brain infarction

ABID antibody identification

ABIG absence of immunoglobulin G

ABK aphakic bullous keratopathy

ABL abetalipoproteinemia • African Burkitt lymphoma • Albright–Butler–Lightwood (syndrome) • allograft–bound lymphocyte • angioblastic lymph-adenopathy • antigen–binding lymphocyte • axiobuccolingual

ABLB alternate binaural loudness balance

ABM adjusted body mass • alveolar basement membrane • autologous bone marrow

A/B MS apnea/bradycardia mild stimulation

ABMT autologous bone marrow transplantation

ABN, Abn, abn abnormal *also* A, abnor, abnorm • abnormality

ABNC abnormal curve

ABN F% abnormal forms percent (sperm count)

ABNG AB negative (blood type)

abnor, abnorm abnormal *also* A, ABN, Abn, abn

ABO absent bed occupancy • blood group system of groups A, AB, B, and O

ABO–HD ABO hemolytic disease

Abor abortion *also* A, AB, Ab, ab

ABP Adriamycin (doxorubicin), bleomycin, and prednisone • antigen–binding protein • arterial blood pressure

ABPA acute bronchopulmonary asthma • allergic bronchopulmonary aspergillosis

ABPC antibody–producing cell

ABPE acute bovine pulmonary edema

ABR abortus–Bang–ring (test) • absolute bedrest • auditory brainstem response

ABr agglutination test for brucellosis

Abras, abras abrasion

ABS abdominal surgery • abnormal brainstem • absent *also* abs • absorbed/absorption *also* absorb • acrylonitrile–butadiene–styrene • acute brain syndrome • Adaptive Behavior Scale • admitting blood sugar • adult bovine serum • alkylbenzene sulfonate • aloin, belladonna, and strychnine (laxative) • amniotic band sequence • anti–B serum • at bedside

1:5 ABS 1:5 Absorption–Reiter–Strain (cerebrospinal fluid test)

abs absent *also* ABS • absolute • absorbance *also* A

absc abscissa

ABSe ascending bladder septum

abs feb [L. *absente febre*] while fever is absent

absorb. absorption *also* ABS

A/B ss apnea/bradycardia self–stimulation

abst, abstr abstract

ABT aminopyrine breath test

abt about

ABTX α–bungarotoxin

ABU aminobutyrate • asymptomatic bacteriuria

ABV actinomycin D, bleomycin, and vincristine • arthropod–borne virus

ABVD Adriamycin (doxorubicin), bleomycin, vinblastine, and dacarbazine

ABW actual body weight

ABx, abx antibiotics

ABY acid bismuth yeast (medium)

AC abdominal circumference • abdominal compression • absorption coefficient • absorptive cell • abuse case • acetate • acetylcholine *also* AcCh, ACH, ACh • acetylcysteine • acid *also* A, a • acidified complement • aconitine • acromioclavicular • activated charcoal • acupuncture clinic • acute *also* ac • acute cholecystitis • adenocarcinoma *also* ACA • adenylate cyclase • adherent cell • adrenal cortex • Adriamycin (doxorubicin) and cyclophosphamide • air changes • air conduction • all culture (broth) • alternating current • ambulatory care • ambulatory controls • anchored catheter • anesthesia circuit • anodal closure • antecubital • anterior chamber (of eye) *also* A/C • anterior column • anterior commissure • anterior cruciate • antibiotic concentrate • anticoagulant •

anticomplement • anti–inflammatory corticoid • antiphlogistic corticoid • aortic closure • aortocoronary • arterial capillary • ascending colon • atriocarotid • auriculocarotid • axiocervical

5–AC 5–azacytidine

A–C adult–versus–child

A/C albumin–coagulin ratio • anterior chamber (of eye) *also* AC • assist/control • assisted control ventilation

A2C apical two–chamber

Ac accelerator (globulin) • acetyl *also* ac • actinium

aC abcoulomb • arabinosylcytosine • azure C

ac acetyl *also* Ac • acute *also* AC • assisted control • [L. *ante cibum*] before meals

ACA acute cerebellar ataxia • acyclovir • adenine–cytosine–adenine • adenocarcinoma *also* AC • adenylate cyclase activity • aminocaproic acid • aminocephalosporanic acid • ammonia, copper, and arsenic • anomalous coronary artery • anterior cerebral artery • anterior communicating aneurysm • anterior communicating artery • anticardiolipin antibody • anticentromere antibody • anticollagen autoantibody • anticomplement activity • anticytoplasmic antibody • automatic clinical analyzer

AC/A accommodation convergence–accommodation (ratio)

AcAcOH acetoacetic acid

A–CAH autoimmune chronic active hepatitis

ACAN, ACANTH acan-throcyte

ACAO acylcoenzyme A oxidase

ACAT acylcholesterol acyltransferase

ACB alveolar–capillary block • antibody–coated bacteria • aortocoronary bypass • arterialized capillary blood • asymptomatic carotid bruit

AC&BC air conduction and bone conduction

ACBE air contrast barium enema

ACBG aortocoronary bypass graft

ACC accident *also* Acc, acc, accid • acetylcoenzyme A carboxylase • acinar cell carcinoma • accommodation *also* A, a, acc, accom • acute care center • adenoid cystic carcinoma • administrative control center • adrenocortical carcinoma • alveolar cell carcinoma • ambulatory care center • amylase creatinine clearance • anodal closure contraction *also* AnCC • antitoxin–containing cell • aplasia cutis congenita • articular chondrocalcinosis

Acc acceleration • accident

also ACC, acc, accid • adenoid cystic carcinoma *also* ACC

acc acceleration *also* a, accel • accident *also* ACC, Acc, accid • accommodation *also* A, a, ACC, accom • according

accel acceleration *also* a, acc

AcCh acetylcholine *also* AC, ACH, ACh

AcChR acetylcholine receptor

AcCHS acetylcholinesterase

accid accident *also* ACC, Acc, acc

ACCL, Accl anodal closure contraction

AcCoA acetylcoenzyme A *also* acetyl–CoA

accom accommodation *also* A, a, ACC, acc

ACCR amylase creatinine clearance ratio

accum accumulated/ accumulation

accur [L. *accuratissime*] accurately • most carefully

ACD absolute cardiac dullness • (citric) acid–citrate (trisodium)–dextrose (solution) • actinomycin D (dactimomycin) • adult celiac disease • allergic contact dermatitis • alpha–chain disease • anterior chamber diameter • anterior chest diameter • anticonvulsant drug *also* AED • area of cardiac disease/dullness

AcD alive with disease

AC–DC, ac/dc alternating current or direct current • bisexual (slang)

ACE acetonitrile • actinium emanation • adrenocortical extract • Adriamycin (doxorubicin), cyclophosphamide, and etopside • aerobic chair exercises • alcohol, chloroform, and ether (mixture) • angiotensin–converting enzyme

ace. acentric

ACED anhydrotic congenital ectodermal dysplasia

ACEH acid cholesterol ester hydrolase

ACEI angiotensin–converting enzyme inhibitor

AcEst acetyl esterase

acetyl–CoA acetylcoenzyme A *also* AcCoA

ACF accessory clinical findings • acute care facility • advanced communications function • area correction factor

ACFn additional cost of false negatives

ACFp additional cost of false positives

ACFUCY actinomycin D, 5–fluorouracil, and cyclophosphamide

ACG accelerator globulin *also* AC–G, AcG, ac–G • angiocardiogram/ angiocardiography • aortocoronary graft • apexcardiogram

AC–G, AcG, ac–G accelerator globulin (factor V) *also* ACG

ACH acetylcholine *also* AC, AcCh, ACh • achalasia • active chronic hepatitis • adrenocortical hormone • aftercoming head • amyotropic cerebellar hypoplasia • arm, chest, height • arm girth, chest depth, and hip width (nutritional index)

ACh acetylcholine *also* AC, AcCh, ACH

AChE acetylcholinesterase

AChR acetylcholine receptor

AChRAb acetylcholine receptor antibody

AC&HS [L. *antecibum* + *hora somni*] before meals and at bedtime

ACI acoustic comfort index • acute coronary infarction/ insufficiency • adenylate cyclase inhibitor • adrenocortical insufficiency • aftercare instructions • anticlonus index • average cost of illness

ACID Arithmetic, Coding, Information, and Digit Span

ACIDS acquired cellular immunodeficiency syndrome

ACIP acute canine idiopathic polyneuropathy

ACJ acromioclavicular joint

AcK actinium K • francium

ACL anterior cruciate ligament

ACl aspiryl chloride

ACLC Assessment of Children Language Comprehension

ACLR anterior cruciate ligament repair

ACLS advanced cardiac life support

ACM aclacinomycin (aclarubicin) • acute cerebrospinal meningitis • Adriamycin (doxorubicin), cyclophosphamide, and methotrexate • albumin–calcium–magnesium • alveolar capillary membrane • anticardiac myosin • Arnold–Chiari malformation

ACME aphatic cystoid macular edema

ACMF arachnoid cyst of the middle fossa

ACMP alveolar–capillary membrane permeability

ACMT artificial circus movement tachycardia

ACMV assist–controlled mechanical ventilation

ACN acute conditioned neurosis

ACO acute coronary occlusion

ACOA adult child of alcholic

ACoA anterior communicating artery

ACOAP Adriamycin (doxorubicin), cyclophosphamide, Oncovin (vincristine), cytosine arabinoside, and prednisone

A–comm anterior communicating (artery)

ACOP Adriamycin (doxorubicin), cyclophosphamide, Oncovin (vincristine), and prednisone

ACOPP Adriamycin (doxorubicin), cyclophosphamide, Oncovin (vincristine), prednisone, and procarbazine

acous acoustic/acoustics

ACP accessory conduction pathway • acid phosphatase *also* AcP, AC–PH, ac phos • acyl carrier protein • anodal closure picture • aspirin–caffeine–phenacetin

AcP acid phosphatase *also* ACP, AC–PH, ac phos

ACPA anticytoplasmic antibodies

AC–PH, ac phos acid phosphatase *also* ACP, AcP

ACPP adrenocortical polypeptide

ACPP–PF acid phosphatase prostatic fluid

ACPS acrocephalo-polysyndactyly *also* ACS

acq acquired • acquisition

ACR abnormally contracting regions • absolute catabolic rate • acriflavine *also* Acr • adenomatosis of colon and rectum • anticonstipation regimen • axillary count rate

Acr acriflavine *also* ACR • acrylic

ACRF ambulatory care research facility

ACS acetyl strophanthidin • acrocephalosyndactyly *also* ACPS • acute confusional state • acute mountain sickness • ambulatory care services • anodal closure sound • antireticular cytotoxic serum • aperture current setting • arterial cannulation support

ACSV aortocoronary–saphenous vein (graft)

ACSVBG aortocoronary–saphenous vein bypass graft

ACT achievement through counseling and treatment • actinomycin • activated coagulation time • advanced coronary treatment • allergen challenge test • antichromotrypsin • anticoagulant therapy • antrocolic transposition • anxiety control training • asthma care training • atropine coma therapy

act. active • activity *also* activ

ACTA automatic computed transverse axial (scanning)

ACTC, Act–C actinomycin C

ACTD, Act–D actinomycin D (dactinomycin)

ACTe anodal closure tetanus

Act Ex active exercise

ACTH adrenocorticotropic hormone (corticotropin)

ACTH–RF adrenocorticotropic hormone–releasing factor

activ activity *also* act

ACTN adrenocorticotropin

ACTP adrenocorticotropic polypeptide

ACTSEB anterior chamber tube shunt encircling band

ACU acute care unit • ambulatory care unit

ACUTENS acupuncture and transcutaneous electrical nerve stimulation

ACV acyclovir • atrial/carotid/ventricular

ACVB aortocoronary venous bypass

ACVD acute cardiovascular disease

ACVRD arteriosclerotic cardiovascular renal disease

AC/W acetone in water

acyl–CoA acylcoenzyme A

AD abdominal diameter • accident dispensary • acetate dialysis • achievement drive • active disease • acute dermatomyositis • addict • addiction *also* addict. • adenoid degeneration (agent) • admitting diagnosis • aerosol deposition • after discharge • alcohol dehydrogenase • Aleutian disease (of mink) *also* AMD • alveolar duct • Alzheimer dementia/disease • analgesic dose • anodal duration • anterior division • antigenic determinant • appropriate disability • arthritic dose • atopic dermatitis • attentional disturbance •

autonomic dysreflexia • average day • average deviation • axiodistal • axis deviation • cytosine arabinoside and daunomycin *also* DA • [L. *atrium dextrum*] right atrium • [L. *auris dextra*] right ear *also* ad

A/D analog–to–digital (converter)

A&D admission and discharge • alcohol and drugs • ascending and descending • vitamins A and D

Ad adipocyte • adrenal

ad [L. *adde*] add • axiodistal • [L. *addetur*] let there be added *also* add. • [L. *auris dextra*] right ear *also* AD

a.d. [L. *alternis diebus*] alternating days (every other day)

ADA adenosine deaminase • anterior descending artery • antideoxyribonucleic acid antibody

ADA # American Diabetes Association diet number

ADase adenosine deaminase

ADAU adolescent drug abuse unit

ADB accidental death benefit

ADC affective disorders clinic • Aid to Dependent Children • albumin, dextrose, and catalase (medium) • ambulance design criteria • analog–to–digital converter • anodal duration

contraction • antral diverticulum of the colon • anxiety disorder clinic • average daily census • axiodistocervical

AdC adenylate cyclase • adrenal cortex

ADCC antibody–dependent cell–mediated cytotoxicity

ADCONFU Adriamycin (doxorubicin), cyclophosphamide, Oncovin (vincristine), and 5–fluorouracil

ADD adduction • adenosine deaminase • alcohol and drug dependency (unit) • attentional deficit disorder • average daily dose

add. addition • adduction/adductor • [L. *addatur*] let there be added *also* ad

add. c trit [L. *adde cum tritu*] add with trituration

ad def an. [L. *ad defectionem animi*] to the point of fainting

ad deliq. [L. *ad deliquium*] to fainting

addend. [L. *addendus*] to be added

ADDH, ADD/H, ADD–HA attention deficit disorder with hyperactivity

addict. addiction *also* AD • addictive

ADDU alcohol and drug dependence unit

ADE acute disseminated encephalitis • antibody–dependent enhancement • apparent digestible energy

Ade adenine

AdeCbl adenosyl cobalamine

ADEE age–dependent epileptic encephalopathy

ad effect. [L. *ad effectum*] until effective

ADEM acute disseminated encephalomyelitis

adeq adequate

ad feb [L. *adstante febre*] fever being present

ADFU agar diffusion for fungus

ADG atrial diastolic gallop • axiodistogingival

ad gr acid. [L. *ad gratum aciditatem*] to an agreeable acidity

ad gr gust. [L. *ad gratum gustum*] to an agreeable taste

ADH adhesion • alcohol dehydrogenase • antidiuretic hormone

adhib. [L. *adhibendus*] to be administered

ad hoc for this (purpose) • temporary

ADI acceptable/allowable daily intake • antral diverticulum of the ileum • autosomal–dominant ichthyosis • axiodistoincisal

ADIC Adriamycin (doxorubicin) and dimethyltriazenylimidazole carboxamide (dacarbazine)

ad int [L. *ad interium*] meanwhile

adj adjoining/adjunct

ADK adenosine kinase

ADKC atopic dermatitis with keratoconjunctivitis

ADL activities of daily living

ADLC antibody–dependent lymphocyte–mediated cytotoxicity

ad lib [L. *ad libitum*] as desired

ADM administrative medicine • administrator • admission • Adriamycin *also* ADR, ADRIA, Adria • apparent distribution mass

AdM adrenal medulla

adm administration *also* Admin • admission

ADME absorption, distribution, metabolism, and excretion

Admin administration *also* adm

admov [L. *admove, admoveatur*] let there be applied

ADN antideoxyribonuclease *also* ADNase • aortic depressor nerve • Associate Degree in Nursing

ADNase antideoxyribonuclease *also* ADN

ad naus [L. *ad nauseam*] to the point of producing nausea

ADN–B antideoxyribonuclease B

ad neut [L. *ad neutralizandum*] to neutralization

ADO adolescent medicine • axiodisto–occlusal

Ado adenosine

ADOAP Adriamycin (doxorubicin), Oncovin (vincristine), arabinosylcytosine, and prednisone

ADOD arthrodentosteo-dysplasia

AdoDABA adenosyl-diaminobutyric acid

ADODM adult–onset diabetes mellitus

AdoHcy *S*–adenosyl-homocysteine

adol adolescent

AdoMet *S*–adenosyl-methionine

Adox oxidized adenosine

ADP acute dermatomyositis and polymyositis • adenosine 5′–diphosphate • administrative psychiatry • advanced pancreatitis • ammonium dihydrogen phosphate • approved drug product • area diastolic pressure • arterial demand pacing • automatic data processing

ad part. dolent [L. *ad partes dolentes*] to the painful parts

ADPase adenosine 5′–diphos-phatase

ADPKD autosomal–dominant polycystic kidney disease

ADPL average daily patient load

ad pond. om [L. *ad pondus omnium*] to the weight of the whole

ADPR adenosine diphosphate ribose

ADQ abductor digiti quinti (muscles) • adequate

ADR acceptable dental remedies • acute dystonic reaction • Adriamycin *also* ADM, ADRIA, Adria • adverse drug reaction • airway dilation reflex

Adr adrenaline

adr adrenal

Adrenex . adrenalectomy

ADRIA, Adria Adriamycin *also* ADM, ADR

ADS acute diarrheal syndrome • alternative delivery system • anatomical dead space • anonymous donor's sperm • anterior drawer sign • antibody deficiency syndrome • antidiuretic substance

ad sat [L. *ad saturandum*] to saturation

adst feb [L. *adstante febre*] while fever is present

ADT accepted dental therapeutics • adenosine triphosphate • admission, discharge, transfer • agar–gel diffusion test • alternate day therapy • anticipate discharge tomorrow • any desired thing placebo • Auditory Discrimination Test • automated dithionite test

ADTe anodal duration tetanus

ADTP adolescent day treatment program • alcohol dependence treatment program

ADU acute duodenal ulcer

ad us. [L. *ad usum*] according to custom

ad us. ext [L. *ad usum externum*] for external application

ADV, Adv adenovirus • adventitia

A–DV arterial–deep venous difference

adv advice • advise • [L. *adversum*] against

ad 2 vic [L. *ad duas vices*] at two times • for two doses

ADVIRC autosomal–dominant vitreoretinochoroidopathy

A5D5W 5% alcohol and 5% dextrose in water

ADX adrenalectomized (jargon)

AE above elbow (amputation) • accident and emergency (department) *also* A&E • acrodermatitis enteropathica • activation energy • adrenal epinephrine • adult erythrocyte • aftereffect • agarose electrophoresis • air embolism • air entry • alcoholic embryopathy • androstanediol • anoxic encephalopathy • [Ger. *Antitoxineinheit*] antitoxic unit • apoenzyme • aryepiglottic (fold)

A&E accident and emergency (department) *also* AE

AEA above elbow amputation • alcohol, ether, and acetone (solution)

AEB as evidenced by • avian erythroblastosis

AEC ankyloblepharon, ectodermal defects, and cleft lip (syndrome) • aortic ejection click • at earliest convenience

AED antiepileptic (anticonvulsant) drug *also* ACD • automated external defibrillator

AEDP automated external defibrillator pacemaker

AEEU admission, entrance, and evaluation unit

AEF allogenic effect factor • amyloid enhancing factor • aryepiglottic fold

AEG air encephalogram/ encephalography

aeg [L. *aeger, aegra*] patient

AEI atrial emptying index

AEL acute erythroleukemia

AEM ambulatory electrogram monitor • analytical electron microscopy • avian encephalomyelitis

AEN aseptic epiphyseal necrosis

AEP acute edematous pancreatitis • appropriateness evaluation protocol • artificial endocrine pancreas • auditory evoked potential • average evoked potential

AEq age equivalent

aeq [L. *aequales*] equal

AER acoustic evoked response • agranular endoplasmic reticulum • aided equalization response • albumin excretion rate • aldosterone excretion rate • apical ectodermal ridge • auditory evoked response • average electroencephalic response • average evoked response

aer aerosol

AERA average evoked response audiometry

AerM aerosol mask

AERP atrial effective refractory period

AerT aerosol tent

AES acetone–extracted serum • antiembolic stockings • antieosinophilic sera • antral ethmoidal sphenoidectomy • Auger electron spectroscopy

AEST aeromedical evacuation support team

AET absorption–equivalent thickness • atrial ectopic tachycardia

aet [L. *aetas*] age

aetat [L. *aetatis*] aged

AEV avian erythroblastosis virus

AEVS automated eligibility verification system

AF abnormal frequency • acid–fast • aflatoxin *also* AFT • albumose–free (tuberculin) • aldehyde fuchsin • alleged father • amaurosis fugax • aminophylline • amniotic fluid • anchoring fibril • angiogenesis factor • anteflexed/anteflexion • anterior fontanel • anterofrontal • antibody forming • antifibrinogen • aortic flow • aortofemoral • artificially fed • ascitic fluid • atrial fibrillation *also* AFib, At Fib, at. fib., ATR FIB, atr fib. • atrial flutter *also* AFL • atrial fusion • attenuation factor • attributable fraction • audiofrequency *also* af • auricular fibrillation *also* AUR FIB, aur fib.

A–F ankle–foot (orthosis) • antifibrinogen

A/F air fluid (level)

aF abfarad

af audio frequency *also* AF

AFA alcohol–formaldehyde–acetic (fixative or solution)

AFB acid–fast bacillus • aflatoxin B • aortofemoral bypass • aspirated foreign body

AFBG aortofemoral bypass graft

AFC adult foster care • air–filled cushions • antibody–forming cell

AFCI acute focal cerebral ischemia

AFD accelerated freeze–drying

AFDC Aid to Families with Dependent Children

AFE amniotic fluid embolization

AFEB afebrile

AFF atrial filling fraction

AF/F atrial fibrillation and/or flutter

aff afferent • [L. *affinis*] having an affinity with but not identical with

AFG aflatoxin G • alpha fetal globulin • amniotic fluid glucose • auditory figure–ground

AFH anterior facial height

AFI amaurotic familial idiocy • amniotic fluid index

AFIb atrial fibrillation *also* AF, At Fib, at. fib., ATR FIB, atr fib.

AFL air/fluid level • antifatty liver (factor) • atrial flutter *also* AF

AFLNH angiofollicular lymph node hyperplasia

AFLP acute fatty liver of pregnancy

AFM aflatoxin M

AFN afunctional neutrophil

AFND acute febrile neutrophilic dermatosis

AFO ankle–foot orthrosis

AFP α–fetoprotein also aFP • anterior faucial pillar • atrial filling pressure • atypical facial pain

aFP α–fetoprotein also AFP

AFPP acute fibropurulent pneumonia

AFQ aflatoxin Q

AFR aqueous flare response • ascorbic free radical

AFRD acute febrile respiratory disease

AFRI acute febrile respiratory illness

AFS acid–fast smear • antifibroblast serum

AFSP acute fibrinoserous pneumonia

AFT aflatoxin *also* AF • agglutination–flocculation test

AFT$_3$ absolute free triiodothyronine

AFT$_4$ absolute free thyroxine

AFTC apparent free testosterone concentration

AFV amniotic fluid volume

AFVSS afebrile, vital signs stable

AFX air–fluid exchange • atypical fibroxanthoma

AG abdominal girth • agarose • aminoglutethimide *also* AGL • aminoglycoside • analytical grade • anion gap • antigen *also* Ag, ag, AGN • antiglobulin • antigravity • atrial gallop *also* ag • attached gingiva • axiogingival • azurophilic granule

AG, A/G, A:G albumin–globulin (ratio) *also* ALB/GLOB

Ag antigen *also* AG, ag, AGN • [L. *argentum*] silver *also* arg

ag antigen *also* AG, Ag, AGN • atrial gallop *also* AG

AGA accelerated growth area • acetylglutamate • acute gonococcal arthritis • antiglomerular antibody • appropriate for gestational age • average for gestational age

Ag–Ab antigen–antibody complex

AGAG acidic glycosaminoglycans

AGAS acetylglutamate synthetase

AGC absolute granulocyte count • automatic gain control

AGD agar/agarose–gel diffusion (method)

AGDD agar–agarose–gel double diffusion (method)

AGE acrylamide gel electrophoresis • acute gastroenteritis • angle of greatest extension

AGED automated general experimental device

AGF angle of greatest flexion

ag feb [L. *aggrediente febre*] when the fever is coming on *also* aggred feb

AGG agammaglobulinemia

agg agglutinate/agglutination *also* aggl, agglut • aggravation • aggregation *also* aggreg

aggl, agglut agglutinate/agglutination *also* agg

aggred feb [L. *aggrediente febre*] while the fever is coming on *also* ag feb

aggreg aggregation *also* agg

AGGS anti–gas gangrene serum

agit [L. *agita*] shake

agit ante sum . [L. *agita ante sumendum*] shake before taking

agit ante us. [L. *agita ante usum*] shake before using

agit bene [L. *agita bene*] shake well

agit vas [L. *agitato vase*] the vial being shaken

AGL acute glomerular nephritis • acute granulocytic leukemia • aminoglutethimide *also* AG

A–GLACTO–LK α–galacto-side leukocytes

AGMK, AGMk African green monkey kidney (cell)

AGML acute gastric mucosal lesion

AGN acute glomerulo-nephritis • agnosia *also* agn • antigen *also* AG, Ag, ag

agn agnosia *also* AGN

AgNOR silver–staining nucleolar organizer region

AGP agar–gel precipitation (test) • α₁–acid glycoprotein *also* AAG

AGPT agar–gel precipitation test

AGR aniridia, genitourinary abnormalities, and mental retardation • anticipatory goal response

AGS adrenogenital syndrome • antiglucagon • audiogenic seizures

AGT abnormal glucose tolerance • activity group therapy • acute generalized tuberculosis • adrenoglomerulotropin *also* AGTr • antiglobulin test

AGTH adrenoglomerulotropic hormone

AGTr adrenoglomerulotropin *also* AGT

AGTT abnormal glucose tolerance test

AGU aspartylglycosaminuria

AGV aniline gentian violet

AH abdominal hysterectomy • absorptive hypercalciuria • accidental hypothermia • acetohexamide • acid hydrolysis • acute hepatitis • after–hyperpolarization *also* AHP • alcoholic hepatitis • amenorrhea and hirsutism • amenorrhea and hyperprolactinemia *also* A/H • aminohippurate • anterior hypothalamus • antihyaluronidase • arcuate hypothalamus • arterial hypertension • artificial heart • ascites hepatoma • astigmatic hypermetropia • autonomic hyperreflexia • axillary hair

A/H amenorrhea and hyperprolactinemia *also* AH

A&H accident and health (policy)

A–h ampere–hour

aH abhenry

AHA acetohydroxamic acid • acquired hemolytic anemia • acute hemolytic anemia • anterior hypothalamic area • antiheart antibody • antihistone antibody • area health authority • aspartylhydroxamic acid • autoimmune hemolytic anemia

AHB α–hydroxybutyric dehydrogenase

AHBC hepatitis B core antibody

AHC acute hemorrhagic conjunctivitis • acute hemorrhagic cystitis

AHCy S–adenosyl-homocysteine

AHD antihypertensive drug • arteriosclerotic/ atherosclerotic heart disease • autoimmune hemolytic disease

AHDMS automated hospital data management system

AHDP azacycloheptane diphosphonate

AHE acute hemorrhagic encephalomyelitis

AHEC area health education center

AHES artificial heart energy system

AHF acute heart failure • antihemolytic factor (factor VIII) • antihemophilic factor • Argentinian hemorrhagic fever

AHFS American Hospital Formulary Service

AHFS–DI American Hospital Formulary Service–Drug Information

AHG aggregated human globulin • antihemolytic/ antihemophilic globulin • anti–human globulin

AHGG aggregated human gamma globulin • anti– human gamma globulin

AHGS acute herpetic gingival stomatitis

AHH α–hydrazine analog of histidine • anosmia and hypogonadotropic hypogonadism (syndrome) • arylhydrocarbon hydroxylase

AHI active hostility index • apnea–plus–hypopnea index

AHIP assisted health insurance plan

AHIS automated hospital information system

AHL apparent half–life

AHLE acute hemorrhagic leukoencephalitis

AHLG anti–human lymphocyte globulin

AHLS anti–human lymphocyte serum

AHM ambulatory Holter monitor

AHN adenomatous hyperplastic nodule • Army head nurse • assistant head nurse

AHO Albright hereditary osteodystrophy

AHP acute hemorrhagic pancreatitis • after– hyperpolarization *also* AH • air at high pressure • Assistant House Physician

AHPO anterior hypothalamic preoptic (area)

AHR autonomic hyperreflexia

AHS adaptive hand skills • African horse sickness • alveolar hypoventilation syndrome • Assistant House Surgeon

AHSDF area health service development fund

AHT aggregation half–time • antihyaluronidase titer • augmented histamine test • autoantibodies to human thyroglobulin

AHTG anti–human thymocyte globulin

AHTP anti–human thymocyte plasma

AHU acute hemolytic uremic (syndrome) • arginine, hypoxanthine, and uracil

AHV avian herpesvirus

AI accidental injury • acciden-tally incurred • adiposity index • aggregation index • agiogenesis inhibitor • allergy and immunology *also* A&I •

allergy index • angiotensin I • anxiety index • aortic incompetence/insufficiency • apical impulse • articulation index • artificial insemination • artificial intelligence • atherogenic index • atrial insufficiency • autoimmune • axioincisal

A–I aortoiliac

A&I allergy and immunology *also* AI

AIA allylisopropylacetamide • amylase inhibitor activity • anti–insulin antibody *also* AI–Ab • aspirin–induced asthma • automated image analysis

AI–Ab anti–insulin antibody *also* AIA

AIB aminoisobutyric acid *also* AIBA • avian infectious bronchitis

AIBA aminoisobutyric acid *also* AIB

AIBF anterior interbody fusion

AIC aminoimidazole carboxamide

AICA anterior inferior cerebellar artery

AICAR aminoimidazole carboxamide ribonucleotide

AICC anti–inhibitor coagulant complex

AICD automatic implantable cardioverter–defibrillator

AICE angiotensin I–converting enzyme

AICF autoimmune complement fixation

AID acquired immunodeficiency disease • acute infectious disease • acute ionization detector • anti–inflammatory drug • argon ionization detector • artificial insemination donor • autoimmune deficiency/disease • automatic implantable defibrillator • average interocular difference

AIDH artificial insemination donor, husband

AIDS acquired immunodeficiency syndrome • acute infectious disease series

AIDS–KS acquired immunodeficiency syndrome with Kaposi sarcoma

AIE acute inclusion body encephalitis • acute infectious encephalitis • acute infectious endocarditis

AIEP amount of insulin extractable from pancreas

AIF anemia–inducing factor • anti–inflammatory • anti–invasion factor • aortic-iliac–femoral

AIG anti–immunoglobulin

AIgA absence of immunoglobulin A

AIgM absence of immunoglobulin M

A–IGP activity–interview group psychotherapy

AIH artificial insemination by husband • artificial insemination, homologous

AIHA autoimmune hemolytic anemia

AIHD acquired immune hemolytic disease

AIIS anterior inferior iliac spine

AIL acute infectious lymphocytosis • angiocentric immunoproliferative lesion • angio-immunoblastic lymphadenopathy

AILD alveolar–interstitial lung disease • angio-immunoblastic lymphadenopathy with dysproteinemia

AILT amiloride–inhibitable lithium transport

AIM artificial intelligence in medicine

AIMD abnormal involuntary movement disorder

AIMS abnormal involuntary movement scale • arthritis impact measurement scale

AIN acute interstitial nephritis • anal intraepithelial neoplasia

AINS anti–inflammatory nonsteroidal (agent)

A Insuf aortic insufficiency

AIO amyloid of immunoglobulin origin

AION anterior ischemic optic neuropathy

AIP acute idiopathic pericarditis • acute infectious polyneuritis • acute inflammatory

polyneuropathy • acute intermittent porphyria • aldosterone–induced protein • annual implementation plan • automated immuno-precipitation • average intravascular pressure

AIR accelerated idioventricular rhythm *also* AIVR • aminoimidazole ribonucleotide • average impairment rating

AIRA anti–insulin receptor antibody

AIRF alteration in respiratory function

AIS Abbreviated Injury Score • androgen insensitivity syndrome • anterior interosseous nerve syndrome • anti–insulin serum

AISA acquired idiopathic sideroblastic anemia

AIS/ISS Abbreviated Injury Score/Injury Severity Score

AIS/MR Alternative Intermediate Services for the Mentally Retarded

AIT administrator–in–training

AITP autoimmune thrombocytopenia purpura

AITT arginine insulin tolerance test

AIU absolute iodine uptake • antigen–inducing unit

AIVR accelerated idioventricular rhythm *also* AIR

AIVV anterior internal vertebral vein

AJ, A/J ankle jerk

AJR abnormal jugular reflex

AK above knee (amputation) *also* A/K, AKA, AK amp • actinic keratosis • adenosine kinase • adenylate kinase • artificial kidney

A/K above knee (amputation) *also* AK, AKA, AK amp

AKA above knee amputation *also* AK, A/K, AK amp • alcoholic ketoacidosis • all known allergies • α–allokainic acid • also known as *also* aka • antikeratin antibody

aka also known as *also* aka

AK amp above knee amputation *also* AK, A/K, AKA

AKE acrokeratoelastoidosis

A/kg amperes per kilogram

AKP alkaline phosphatase *also* ALK-P, alk phos, alk p'tase, ALP, AP, KA

AKS auditory and kinesthetic sensation

AL absolute latency • acinar lumina • acute leukemia • adaptation level • albumin *also* A, ALB, Alb, alb • alcoholism • alignment mark • amyloidosis • annoyance level • anti–human lymphocytic (globulin) • argininsuccinate lysate • argon laser • arterial line *also* A–line • avian leukosis • axial length • axiolingual • [L. *auris laeva*] left ear *also* al • lethal antigen

Al allantoic • aluminum

al [L. *auris laeva*] left ear *also* AL

ALA aminolevulinic acid • anterior lip of the acetabulum • axiolabial *also* ALa

ALa axiolabial *also* ALA

Ala alanine

AL–Ab antilymphocyte antibody

ALAC antibiotic–loaded acrylic cement

ALAD abnormal left axis deviation • aminolevulinic acid dehydrase *also* ALA–D

ALA–D aminolevulinic acid dehydrase *also* ALAD

ALAG, ALaG axiolabiogingival

ALAL, ALaL axiolabiolingual

ALARA as low as reasonably achievable (radiation exposure)

ALAS aminolevulinic acid synthetase

ALAT alanine aminotransferase

ALAX apical long axis

ALB albumin *also* A, AL, Alb, alb • avian lymphoblastosis

Alb albumin *also* A, AL, ALB, alb

alb albumin *also* A, AL, ALB, Alb • [L. *albus*] white

ALB/GLOB albumin–globulin (ratio) *also* AG, A/G, A:G

ALC absolute lymphocyte

count • acute lethal
catatonia • alcohol *also*
alc • allogeneic
lymphocyte cytoxicity •
alternate level of care •
Alternative Lifestyle
Checklist • approximate
lethal concentration • avian
leukosis complex •
axiolinguocervical

alc alcohol *also* ALC •
alcoholic/alcoholism

ALCA anomalous left coronary
artery

ALCAPA anomalous origin of
left coronary artery from
pulmonary artery

ALCR, AlcR alcohol rub

AlCr aluminum crown

ALD adrenoleukodystrophy •
alcoholic liver disease •
aldolase *also* Ald •
aldosterone *also* Aldo,
ALDOST • anterior
latissimus dorsi •
Appraisal of Language
Disturbances

Ald aldolase *also* ALD

ALDH aldehyde
dehydrogenase

Aldo, ALDOST aldosterone
also ALD

ALE allowable limits of error

ALEP atypical
lymphoepithelioid cell
proliferation

ALF acute liver failure •
anterior long fiber

ALFT abnormal liver function
test

ALG Annapolis lymphoblast

globulin • antilympho-
blastic globulin •
antilymphocytic globulin •
axiolinguogingival

ALGOL algorithm–oriented
language

ALH anterior lobe hormone •
anterior lobe of hypophysis

ALI argon laser iridotomy

A–line arterial catheter •
arterial line *also* AL

ALIP abnormal localized
immature myeloid precursor

ALK, alk alkaline • alkylating
(agent)

ALK–P, alk phos, alk p'tase
alkaline phosphatase *also*
AKP, ALP, AP, KA

ALL acute lymphatic
leukemia • acute
lymphoblastic/lymphocytic
leukemia • allergy *also* A,
all. • anterior longitudinal
ligament

all. allergic/allergy *also* A,
ALL

ALLA acute lymphocytic
leukemia antigen

ALLO atypical *Legionella*–like
organism

ALM acral lentiginous
melanoma • alveolar living
material

ALME acetyl–lysine methyl
ester

ALMI anterior lateral
myocardial infarction

ALMV anterior leaflet of the
mitral valve

ALN anterior lymph node

ALO average lymphocyte output • axiolinguo–occlusal

ALOMAD Adriamycin (doxorubicin), Leukeran (chlorambucil), Oncovin (vincristine), methotrexate, actinomycin D, and dacarbazine

ALOS average length of stay

ALP acute lupus pericarditis • alkaline phosphatase *also* AKP, ALK–P, alk phos, alk p'tase, AP, KA • Alupent • anterior lobe of pituitary • antilymphocytic plasma • argon laser photocoagulation

alpha (A, α) first letter of Greek alphabet

α angular acceleration • constituent of alpha plasma protein fraction • first in a series or group • heavy chain of immunoglobulin A • optical rotation (chemistry) • probability of type I error (statistics) • (Bunsen's) solubility coefficient

α–GLUC α–glucosidase

α–KG α–ketoglutarate

α–LP α–lipoprotein

α₂M α_2–macroglobulin

ALPI alkaline phosphatase isoenzymes

ALPS angiolympho-proliferative syndrome • Aphasia Language Performance Scales

ALPZ alprazolam

ALRI anterolateral rotational instability

ALS acute lateral sclerosis • advanced life support (system) • afferent loop syndrome • amyotrophic lateral sclerosis • angiotensin–like substance • anticipated life–span • antilymphocyte serum • antiviral lymphocyte serum

ALSD Alzheimer–like senile dementia

ALT alanine amino-transferase • argon laser trabeculoplasty *also* Alt alt • avian laryngotracheitis

Alt, alt alternate • altitude • argon laser trabeculoplasty *also* ALT

ALT/AST ratio of serum alanine aminotransferase to serum aspartate aminotransferase

ALTB acute laryngo-tracheobronchitis

alt dieb [L. *alternis diebus*] every other day

ALTE apparent life–threatening event

ALTEE acetyl–L–tyrosine ethyl ester

alt hor [L. *alternis horis*] every other hour

alt noct [L. *alternis nocta*] every other night

ALU arithmetic and logic unit

ALV adeno–like virus • ascending lumbar vein • avian leukosis virus

Alv, alv alveolar/alveolus

ALVAD abdominal left ventricular assist device

alv adst [L. *alvo adstricta*] when the bowels are constipated

alv deject. [L. *alvi dejectiones*] discharge from the bowels

ALVM alveolar mucosa

ALVT aortic and left ventricular tunnel

Alvx alveolectomy

ALW arch–loop–whorl

ALWMI anterolateral wall myocardial infarct

AM acrylamide • actomyosin • acute myelofibrosis • adult male • adult monocyte • aerospace medicine • alveolar macrophase • alveolar mucosa • amalgam *also* AMAL • ambulatory *also* AMB, amb, ambul • amethopterin • ametropia • ammeter • amperemeter • ampicillin *also* A, AMP • amplitude modulation *also* A–mode • anovular menstruation • arithmetic mean • arousal mechanism • Austin–Moore (prosthesis) • aviation medicine • axiomesial • [L. *ante meridiem*] before noon *also* a.m. • meter angle • mixed astigmatism • myopic astigmatism

Am americium • amnion • amyl

A–m² ampere–square meter

A/m amperes per meter

am. ametropia • amplitude • meter angle • myopic astigmatism

a.m. [L. *ante meridiem*] before noon *also* AM

AMA actual mechanical advantage • against medical advice • antimitochondrial antibody • antimyosin antibody

AMAD morning admission

AMA–DE American Medical Association Drug Evaluation

AMAG adrenal medullary autograft

AMAL amalgam *also* AM

AMAP as much as possible

AMAT anti–malignant antibody test

A–MAT amorphous material

AMB ambulate/ambulatory *also* AM, amb, ambul • amphotericin B • avian myeloblastosis

amb ambient • ambiguous *also* ambig • ambulance • ambulate/ambulatory *also* AM, AMB, ambul

ambig ambiguous *also* amb

AMBL acute myeloblastic leukemia

ambul ambulatory *also* AM, AMB, amb

AMC antibody–mediated cytoxicity • antimalaria campaign • arm muscle circumference •

arthrogryposis multiplex congenita • automated mixture control • axiomesiocervical

AMCHA aminomethylcyclohexane–carboxylic acid

AMCN anteromedial caudate nucleus

AM /CR amylase to creatinine ratio

AMD acid maltase deficiency • acromandibular dysplasia • actinomycin D • adrenomyelodystrophy • age–related macular degeneration • Aleutian mink disease *also* AD • α-methyldopa • axiomesiodistal

AME aseptic meningo-encephalitis

AMEGL, AMegL acute megakaryoblastic leukemia

Amerind American Indian sign language

Ameslan American sign language *also* ASL

AMet adenosyl–l–methionine

AMF antimuscle factor • autocrine motility factor

AMG acoustic myography • aminoglycoside • amyloglucosidase/amyloglucoside • antimacrophage globulin • axiomesiogingival

AMH automated medical history

Amh mixed astigmatism with myopia predominating

AMHT automated multiphasic health testing

AMI acquired monosaccharide intolerance • acute myocardial infarction • amitriptyline • anterior myocardial infarction • axiomesioincisal

AML acute monocytic/myeloblastic/myelocytic/myelogenous/myeloid leukemia • anterior mitral leaflet

AMLB alternate monaural loudness balance (test)

AMLC adherent macrophage–like cell • autologous mixed lymphocyte culture

AMLR autologous mixed lymphocyte reaction

AMLS anti–mouse lymphocyte serum

AMM agnogenic myeloid metaplasia • ammonia *also* ammon • antibody to murine cardiac myosin

AMML, AMMOL, AMMoL acute myelomonocytic leukemia

ammon. ammonia *also* AMM

AMN adrenomyelo-neuropathy • alloxazine mononucleotide • anterior median nucleus

amnio amniocentesis

AMN SC amniotic fluid scan

AMO Assistant Medical Officer • axiomesio-occlusal

A–mode amplitude mode • amplitude modulation *also* AM

AMOL acute monoblastic/ monocytic leukemia

AMOR, amor, AMORP, amorp amorphous (sediment)

AMP accelerated mental processes • acid mucopolysaccharide • adenosine monophosphate (adenylic acid) • amphetamine • ampicillin *also* A, AM • ampule *also* amp • amputation *also* amp • average mean pressure

amp ampere • amplification • ampule *also* AMP • amputation *also* AMP • amputee

AMP–c cyclic adenosine monophosphate *also* cAMP

AMPH amphetamine

amph amphoric (respiratory sound)

amp–hr ampere–hour

ampl [L. *amplus*] large

A–M pr Austin–Moore prosthesis

AMPS abnormal mucopolysacchariduria • acid mucopolysaccharide

AMP–S adenylosuccinic acid

AMPT α–methyl–*p*–tyrosine (antihypertensive in pheochromocytoma)

AMR acoustic muscle reflex • activity metabolic rate • alternate motion rate • alternating motion reflex

AMRA American Medical Record Association

AMRI anteromedial rotatory instability

AMRS automated medical record system

AMS acute mountain sickness • aggravated in military service • altered mental status • amylase • antimacrophage serum • atypical measles syndrome • auditory memory span • automated multiphastic screening • automicrobic system

AMSA amsacrine

AMSIT appearance, mood, sensorium, intelligence, and thought process (portion of mental status examination)

AMT acute miliary tuberculosis • α– methyltyrosine • amethopterin • amitriptyline • amphetamine

amt amount

AMTP α–methyltryptophan

amu atomic mass unit

AmuLV Abelson murine leukemia virus

AMV assisted mechanical ventilation • avian myeloblastosis virus

AMVI acute mesenteric vascular insufficiency

AMX amoxicillin

AMY amylase

AMY–SP amylase urine spot (test)

AN acanthosis nigricans • acne neonatorum •

acoustic neuroma • administratively necessary • aminonucleoside • amyl nitrate • adult, normal • aneurysm • anisometropia *also* An • anode *also* A, a, An • anorexia nervosa • antenatal • anterior *also* A, a, ANT, ant. • antineuraminidase • aseptic necrosis • atrionodal • autonomic neuropathy • avascular necrosis

A/N artery and/or nerve • as needed

An actinon • anatomy response • aniridia • anisometropia *also* AN • anodal/anode *also* A, a, AN

A$_n$ normal atmosphere

ANA acetylneuraminic acid • anesthesia *also* anes, anesth • antibody to nuclear antigens • antinuclear antibody • aspartyl naphthylamide

ana [G. *ana*] (so much of) each *also* AA, $\overline{\text{AA}}$, aa, $\overline{\text{aa}}$

ANAD anorexia nervosa and associated disorders • antinicotinamide adenine dinucleotidase

ANA–FL antinuclear antibody fluid

anal analgesia/analgesic • analysis/analyst/analytic

ANAP agglutination negative, absorption positive (reaction)

anast anastomosis

Anat, anat anatomical/anatomist/anatomy

ANC absolute neutrophil count • acid neutralization capacity • antigen–neutralizing capacity

ANCA antineutrophil cytoplasmic antibodies

AnCC anodal closure contraction *also* ACC

anch anchored

ANCOVA analysis of covariance

AND administratively necessary days • algoneurodystrophy • anterior nasal discharge

And androgen

ANDA Abbreviated New Drug Application

Andro, Andros androsterone

ANDTE, AnDTe anodal duration tetanus

anes anesthesia/anesthesiology/anesthetic *also* An, anesth

ANESR apparent norepinephrine secretion rate

anesth anesthesia/anesthesiology/anesthetic *also* An, anes

AnEx, an ex anodal excitation

ANF α–naphthoflavone • antineuritic factor • antinuclear factor • atrial natriuretic factor

ANG angiogram/angiography *also* ang

ang angiogram/angiography *also* ANG • angle *also* A • angular

Ang GR angiotensin generation rate

anh anhydrous

ANIS, ANISO anisocytosis

ANIT α–naphthyl-isothiocyanate

ank ankle

ANL, ANLL acute nonlymphoblastic/nonlymphocytic leukemia

ANLL acute nonlymphocytic leukemia

ANM auxiliary nurse midwife

Ann annual

ann fib annulus fibrosus

annot. annotation

ANoA antinucleolar antibody

AnOC anodal opening contraction *also* AOC

ANOVA analysis of variance

ANP acute necrotizing pancreatitis • Adult Nurse Practitioner • Advanced Nurse Practitioner • A–norprogesterone • atrial natriuretic peptide

A–NPP absorbed normal pooled plasma

ANRL antihypertensive neural renomedullary lipids

ANS anterior nasal spine • antineutrophilic serum • arterionephrosclerosis • autonomic nervous system

ANSCII American National Standard Code for Information Interchange

ANSI American National Standards Institute

ANT acoustic noise test • aminoglycoside 2′–0–nucleotidyltransferase • aminonitrothiazole • anterior *also* A, a, AN, ant. • antimycin *also* ant.

ant antenna • anterior *also* A, a, AN, ANT • antimycin *also* ANT

AntA antimycin A

antag antagonist

ant ax line anterior axillary line

ante [L. *ante*] before

anti antidote

ANTI A:AGT anti–blood group A antiglobulin test

Anti bx antibiotic

anticoag anticoagulant

anti–HA antihepatitis antigen

anti–HAA antibody to hepatitis–associated antigen

anti–HAV antibody to hepatitis A virus

anti–HB$_c$ antibody to hepatitis B core antigen

anti–HB$_s$ antibody to hepatitis B surface antigen

anti–log antilogarithm

anti–PNM Ab anti–peripheral nerve myelin antibody

anti–S anti–sulfanilic acid

anti–Sm anti–Smith (antibody)

ant. jentac [L. *ante jentaculum*] before breakfast

ant. pit. anterior pituitary

ant. prand [L. *ante prandium*] before dinner *also* AP, ap

ANTR apparent net transfer rate

ant. sag D anterior sagittal diameter

ant. sup. spine anterior superior spine

ANuA antinuclear antibody

ANUG acute necrotizing ulcerative gingivitis

ANX, anx anxiety/anxious

anx neur anxiety neurosis

anx react anxiety reaction

AO abdominal aorta • achievement orientation • acid output • acridine orange (dye or test) • anodal opening • anterior oblique • aorta *also* Ao • aortic opening • ascending aorta • atomic orbital • atrioventricular valve opening • auriculo-ventricular valve opening • average optical density • avoidance of others • axio-occlusal

A–O acoustic–optic

A/O analog to digital

A&O alert and oriented

Ao aorta *also* AO

A&Ox3 alert and oriented to person, place, and time

A&Ox4 alert and oriented to person, place, time, and date

AOA abnormal oxygen affinity • average orifice area

AOAA amino–oxyacetic acid

AOAP as often as possible

AOB accessory olfactory bulb • alcohol on breath

AOBS acute organic brain syndrome

AOC abridged ocular chart • amyloxycarbonyl • anodal opening contraction *also* AnOC • antacid of choice • aortic opening click • area of concern

AOCD anemia of chronic disease

AOCl anodal opening clonus

AOD adult–onset diabetes *also* AODM • alleged onset date • arterial occlusive disease • arterial oxygen desaturation • auriculo-osteodysplasia

AODA alcohol and other drug abuse

AODM adult–onset diabetes mellitus *also* AOD

ao–Il aorta–iliac

AOIVM angiographically occult intracranial vascular malformation

AOL acro–osteolysis

AOM acute otitis media • azoxymethane

AoMP aortic mean pressure

AOP anodal opening picture • aortic pressure

AoP left ventricle to aorta pressure gradient

AoPW aortic posterior wall

AOR auditory oculogyric reflex

aor regurg aortic regurgitation *also* AR

aort sten aortic stenosis *also* AS

AOS acridine orange staining • anodal opening sound • anterior (o)esophageal sensor

AOSD adult–onset Still disease

AOT accessory optic tract • antiovotransferrin

AOTe anodal opening tetanus

AOU apparent oxygen utilization

AOV aortic valve

AP abdominoperineal (resection) *also* A–P • accessory pathway • acid phosphatase • acinar parenchyma • action potential • active pepsin • acute pancreatitis • acute phase • acute pneumonia • acute proliferative • adolescent psychiatry • after parturition • alkaline phosphatase *also* AKP, ALK-P, alk p'tase, ALP, KA • alum–precipitated (vaccine) • amino-peptidase • aminopyrine • angina pectoris • [L. *ante partum*] antepartum • anterior pituitary • anteroposterior • antidromic potential • antiparkinsonian *also* APK • antipyrine • antral peristalsis • aortic pressure • aortic pulmonary • apical pulse • apothecary • appendectomy • appendicitis • appendix •

area postrema • arithmetic progression • arterial pressure • artificial pneumothorax • aspiration pneumonitis • assessment and plans *also* A&P • association period • atherosclerotic plaque • atrial pacing • atrioventricular pathway • attending physician • axiopulpal • [L. *ante prandium*] before dinner *also* ant. prand, ap • [L. *ante partum*] before parturition

A–P anterior–posterior (radiologic projection)

3–AP 3–acetylpyridine (nicotinic antagonist)

4–AP 4–aminopyridine

A–P abdominoperineal (resection) *also* AP • analytic–psychologic

A/P ascites–plasma (ratio)

A&P active and present • anatomy and physiology • anterior and posterior • assessment and plans *also* AP • auscultation and palpation • auscultation and percussion

A$_2$P$_2$ aortic second sound, pulmonary second sound

A$_2$ > P$_2$ second aortic sound greater than second pulmonic sound

A$_2$ = P$_2$ second aortic sound equals second pulmonic sound

A$_2$ < P$_2$ second aortic sound less than second pulmonic sound

Ap apex

ap apothecary • [L. *ante prandium*] before dinner • [L. *a priori*] prior to

APA aldosterone–producing adenoma • aminopenicillanic acid • antiparietal antibody • antipernicious anemia (factor)

6–APA 6–aminopenicillanic acid

APACHE acute physiology and chronic health evaluation (system)

APAD anterior–posterior abdominal diameter

APAF antipernicious anemia factor

APB abductor pollicis brevis (muscle) • atrial premature beat • auricular premature beat

APC acetylsalicylic acid, phenacetin, and caffeine • acute pharyngoconjunctival (fever) • adenoidal–pharngeal–conjunctival (agent or virus) • adenomatous polyposis coli • all–purpose capsule (jargon for aspirin–phenacetin–caffeine) • alternative patterns of complement • amsacrine, prednisone, and chlorambucil • antigen–presenting cell • antiphlogistic corticoid • aperture current • apneustic center (of brain) • aspirin–phenacetin–caffeine • atrial premature contraction

APCA antiparietal cell antibody

APCC, APC–C aspirin–phenacetin–caffeine–codeine

APCD adult polycystic kidney disease *also* APKD

APCF acute pharyngo-conjunctival fever

APCG apex cardiogram

APD action potential duration • acute polycystic disease • adult polycystic disease • afferent pupillary defect • aminohydro-xypropylidene diphos-phate • anteroposterior diameter *also* A–PD • atrial premature depolarization • autoimmune progesterone dermatitis • automated peritoneal dialysis

A–PD anteroposterior diameter *also* APD

APDC anxiety and panic disorder clinic

APE acetone powder extract • acute polioencephalitis • acute psychotic episode • acute pulmonary edema • airway pressure excursion • aminophylline, phenobarbital, and ephedrine • anterior pituitary extract • avian pneumoencephalitis

APECED autoimmune polyendocrinopathy–candidosis–ectodermal dystrophy

APF acidulated phosphofluoride •

anabolism–promoting factor • animal protein factor • antiperinuclear factor

APG acid–precipated globulin • animal pituitary gonadotropin • Apgar (score)

APGAR adaptability, partnership, growth, affection, and resolve (family screening, not Apgar score of newborn physical status)

APGL alkaline phosphatase activity of granular leukocytes

APH adult psychiatric hospital • alcohol–positive history • antepartum hemorrhage • anterior pituitary hormone

aph aphasia

AP/HC accreditation program/ hospice care

AP/HHC accreditation program/home health care

APHP anti–*Pseudomonas* human plasma

API alkaline protease inhibitor • analytical profile index • ankle–arm pressure index

APIE assessment plan, implementation, and evaluation

APIP additional personal injury protection

APIVR artificial pacemaker–induced ventricular rhythm

APK antiparkinsonian *also* AP

APKD adult polycystic kidney disease *also* APCD

APL abductor pollicis longus (muscle) • accelerated painless labor • acute promyelocytic leukemia • animal placenta lactogen • anterior pituitary–like (hormone)

AP&L, AP&Lat anteroposterior and lateral (radiologic view)

AP/LTC accreditation program/long–term care

APM acid–precipitable material • alternating pressure mattress • anterior papillary muscle • anteroposterior movement • aspartame

APN acute pyelonephritis • average peak noise

APO adductor pollicis obliquus (muscle) • Adriamycin (doxorubicin), prednisone, and Oncovin (vincristine) • adverse patient occurrences • aphoxide *also* TEPA • apomorphine

Apo apolipoprotein

APORF acute postoperative renal failure

apoth apothecary

APP acute phase protein • alum–precipitated pyridine • amino–pyrazolopyrimidine • antiplatelet plasma • appendix *also* app, Appx • aqueous procaine peni-cillin • automated physi-

ologic profile · avian
pancreatic polypeptide

app appendix *also* APP,
Appx · applied ·
approximate *also* appr,
approx

appar apparatus · apparent

APPG aqueous procaine
penicillin G

appl appliance · applicable/
application/applied

applan [L. *applanatus*]
flattened

applicand [L. *applicandus*] to
be applied

appoint. appointment *also*
appt

appr, approx approximate
also app · approximately/
approximation

appt appointment *also* appoint.

Appx appendix *also* App, app

Appy, appy appendectomy

APR abdominoperineal
resection · absolute
proximal reabsorption ·
accelerator–produced
radiopharmaceuticals ·
acute phase reactant ·
amebic prevalence rate ·
anatomic porous
replacement · anterior
pituitary resection ·
auropalpebral reflex

aprax apraxia

APRO aprobarbital

AProL acute promyelocytic
leukemia

APRP acidic proline–rich
protein · acute–phase
reactant protein

APRT adenine phosphoribosyltransferase

APS acute physiology score ·
adenosine phosphosulfate ·
Adult Protective Services ·
Adult Psychiatric Service

APSAC anisoylated
plasminogen streptokinase
activator complex

APSD Alzheimer presenile
dementia

APSGN acute
poststreptococcal
glomerulonephritis

APSQ Abbreviated Parent
Symptom Questionnaire

APT alum–precipitated toxoid

APTA aneurysm of persistent
trigeminal artery

APTD Aid to Permanently and
Totally Disabled

APTT, aPTT activated partial
thromboplastin time

APTX acute parathyroidectomy

APUD amine precursor uptake
and decarboxylation (cell)

APVD anomalous pulmonary
venous drainage

APVR aortic pulmonary valve

AQ achievement quotient ·
any quantity

aq aqueous *also* aqu · [L.
aqua] water *also* A, a

aq ad [L. *aquam ad*] add water

aq astr [L. *aqua astrieta*]
frozen water (ice)

aq bull. [L. *aqua bulliens*]
boiling water

aq cal [L. *aqua calida*] hot water

aq com [L. *aqua communis*] common water

aq dest [L. *aqua destillata*] distilled water

aq ferv [L. *aqua fervens*] hot water

aq font. [L. *aqua fontana*] spring water

aq frig [L. *aqua frigata*] cold water

aq mar. [L. *aqua marina*] sea water

aq pluv [L. *aqua pluvialis*] rain water

aq pur [L. *aqua pura*] pure water

AQS additional qualifying symptoms

aq tep [L. *aqua tepida*] tepid water

aqu aqueous *also* aq

AR abnormal record • achievement ratio • actinic reticuloid (syndrome) • active resistance • acute rejection • adherence ratio • airway resistance • alarm reaction • alcohol related • allergic rhinitis • alloy restoration • amplitude ratio • analytical reagent • androgen receptor • anterior root • aortic regurgitation *also* aor regurg • apical–radial (pulse) *also* A–R, A/R • Argyll Robertson (pupil) • arsphenamine • articulare (craniometric point) *also* Ar • artificial respiration •

artifically ruptured • assisted respiration • atrial regurgitation • at risk • atrophic rhinitis • attack rate • aural rehabilitation • autoradiography • autorefractor • autosomal recessive

A–R apical–radial (pulse) *also* AR, A/R

A/R accounts receivable • apical/radial (pulse) *also* AR, A–R

A&R adenoidectomy with radium • advised and released

Ar argon • articulare (craniometric point) *also* AR

ARA acetylene reduction activity • antireticulin antibody

Ara arabinose

Ara–A, araA arabinosyladenine (vidarabine)

Ara–C, araC arabinosylcytosine (cytarabine)

araC–Hu arabinosylcytosine (cytarabine) and hydroxyurea

ARAS ascending reticular activating system

ARB adrenergic receptor binder • any reliable brand

arb arbitrary unit

ARBOR arthropod–borne (virus)

ARBOW artificial rupture of bag of waters

ARC accelerating rate calorimetry • acquired immunodeficiency syndrome–related complex • active renin concentration • alcohol rehabilitation center • American Red Cross • anomalous retinal correspondence • antigen–reactive cell • arcuate nucleus (of brain) • average response computer

ARCA acquired red–cell aplasia

ARCBS American Red Cross Blood Services

Arch. archives

ARCO antigen–reactive cell opsonization

ARD absolute reaction of degeneration • acute respiratory disease/distress • adult respiratory disease/distress • anorectal dressing • antibiotic/antimicrobial removal device • aphakic retinal detachment • arthritis and rheumatic diseases • atopic respiratory disease

ARDS adult respiratory distress syndrome

ARE active–resistive exercises

AREDYLD acrorenal field defect, ectodermal dysplasia, and lipoatrophic diabetes

ARF acute renal/respiratory failure • acute rheumatic fever • area resource file

ARFC active rosette–forming T cell

ARF/CRF acute renal failure and chronic renal failure

ARG, Arg arginine

arg [L. *argentum*] silver *also* Ag

ARI acute respiratory infection • airway reactivity index • aldose reductase inhibitor

ARIA automated radioimmunoassay

ARL average remaining lifetime

ARLD alcohol–related liver disease

ARM adrenergic receptor material • aerosol rebreathing method • allergy relief medicine • alternating rate of motion • anorectal manometry • anxiety reaction, mild • artificial rupture of membranes *also* AROM • atomic resolution microscopy

ARMS amplification refractory mutation system

ARN acute renal/retinal necrosis

ARNP Advanced Registered Nurse Practitioner

AROM active range of motion • artificial rupture of membranes *also* ARM

ARP absolute refractory period • alcohol rehabilitation program • assay reference plasma • assimilation regulatory protein • at–risk period • automaticity recovery phase

ARPES angular resolved photoelectron spectroscopy

Arry arrhythmia

ARS acquiescent response scale • adult recovery services • AIDS–related syndrome • alizarin red S (dye) • antirabies serum

Ars arsphenamine • arylsulfatase

Ars–A arylsulfatase A *also* AsA

ARS–B arylsulfatase B *also* AsB

ARS–C arylsulfatase C *also* AsC

ARSM acute respiratory system malfunction

ART absolute retention time • Accredited Record Technician • Achilles (tendon) reflex text • acoustic reflex threshold(s) • algebraic reconstruction technique • arterial (line) • artery *also* A, a, art. • autologous reactive T cell • automated reagin test • automaticity recovery time

art. arterial/artery *also* A, a, ART • articulation *also* artic • artificial *also* artif

arthro arthroscopy

ARTI acute respiratory tract illness

artic articulated/articulation *also* art.

artif artificial *also* art.

Art T art therapy

ARV AIDS–associated retrovirus • AIDS–related virus • anterior right ventricular (wall)

ARVD arrhythmogenic right ventricular dysplasia

ARW accredited rehabilitation worker

ARWY airway

AS above scale • acetyl-strophanthidin • acidified serum • acoustic stimulation • active sarcoidosis • active sleep • acute salpingitis • Adams–Stokes (disease or syndrome) • adolescent suicide • aerosol steroid • affective style • Alport syndrome • alveolar sac/space • amyloid substance • anal sphincter • andros-terone sulfate • ankylosing spondylitis *also* ASP • annulospiral • anovulatory syndrome • (doctor called through) answering service • antiserum • antisocial • antistreptolysin • antral spasm • anxiety state • aortic sac • aortic stenosis *also* aort sten • aqueous solution/suspension • arteriosclerosis • artificial sweetener • asthma astrocyte • astigmatism *also* As, AST, Ast, ASTIG • asymmetric • atherosclerosis • atrial sense • atrial septum • atrial stenosis • atropine sulfate • audiogenic seizure • [L. *auris sinistra*] left ear *also* a.s. • sickle-cell trait (heterozygous genotype for hemoglobin) *also* A/S

A–S Adams–Stokes (disease or syndrome) • ascendance–submission

A/S sickle–cell trait (heterozygous genotype for hemoglobin) *also* AS

As arsenic • astigmatism *also* AS, AST, Ast, ASTIG • atmosphere, standard

A·s ampere–second

Axs ampere per second

aS absiemens

a.s. [L. *auris sinistra*] left ear *also* AS

ASA acetylsalicylic acid • active systemic anaphylaxis • Adams–Stokes attack • argininosuccinic acid • aspirin–sensitive asthma

ASA I—V American Society of Anesthesiologists' patient classifications I to V, followed by "E" for emergency operations

ASA I healthy patient with localized pathologic process

ASA II patient with mild to moderate systemic disease

ASA III patient with severe systemic disease limiting activity but not incapacitating

ASA IV patient with incapacitating systemic disease

ASA V moribund patient not expected to live

AsA arylsulfatase A *also* Ars-A

Asa arsenate

ASAA acquired severe aplastic anemia

ASAC acidified serum, acidified complement

ASACL American Society of Anesthesiologists' classification

ASA–G guaiacolic acid ester of acetylsalicylic acid

ASAI aortic stenosis and aortic insufficiency (murmurs)

ASAL argininosuccinic acid lyase

ASAP as soon as possible

ASAS argininosuccinate synthetase

ASAT aspartate aminotransferase *also* AST

ASB anesthesia standby • asymptomatic bacteriuria

AsB arylsulfatase B *also* Ars-B

ASBS arteriosclerotic brain syndrome

ASC acetylsulfanilyl chloride • adenosine–coupled spleen cell • altered state of consciousness • ambulatory surgery center • anterior subscapular cataract • antigen–sensitive cell • antimony–sulfur colloid • ascorbic acid

AsC arylsulfatase C *also* Ars-C

Asc–A ascending aorta *also* AA

ASCAD arteriosclerotic/atherosclerotic coronary artery disease

ASCII American Standard Code for Information Interchange

ASCL anteriosclerosis

ascr [L. *ascriptum*] ascribed to

ASCT autologous stem–cell transplantation

ASCVD arteriosclerotic/atherosclerotic cardiovascular disease

ASD aldosterone secretion defect • Alzheimer senile dementia • anterior sagittal diameter • antisiphon device • arthritis syphilitica deformans • atrial septal defect

ASDH acute subdural hematoma

ASE acute stress erosion • axilla, shoulder, elbow (bandage)

ASES Adult Self–Expression Scale

ASF African swine fever • aniline–sulfur–formaldehyde (resin) • asialofetium

ASFR age–specific fertility rate

ASG advanced stage group

AS/GP antiserum, guinea pig

ASH aldosterone–stimulating hormone • ankylosing spinal hyperostosis • antistreptococcal hyaluronidase • asymmetric septal hypertrophy • hypermetropic astigmatism • hyperopic astigmatism *also* AsH

AsH hyperopic astigmatism *also* ASH

ASHD arteriosclerotic/atherosclerotic heart disease • atrial septal heart disease

ASHN acute sclerosing hyaline necrosis

AS/Ho antiserum, horse

ASI addiction severity index • Anxiety Status Inventory

ASIS anterior superior iliac spine

ASK antistreptokinase

ASKA antiskeletal antibody

ASL American sign language *also* Ameslan • ankylosing spondylitis, lung • antistreptolysin

ASLC acute self–limited colitis

ASLO, ASL–O anti-streptolysin–O *also* ASO, ASTO

ASLT antistreptolysin test

ASM airway smooth muscle • anterior scalenus muscle • myopic astigmatism *also* AsM

AsM myopic astigmatism *also* ASM

ASMA anti–smooth muscle antibody

ASMD atonic sclerotic muscle dystrophy

ASMI anteroseptal myocardial infarction

As/Mk antiserum, monkey

ASMR age–standardized mortality ratio

asmt assessment

ASN alkali–soluble nitrogen • arteriosclerotic nephritis • asparagine *also* Asn

Asn asparagine *also* ASN

ASO aldicarb sulfoxide • antistreptolysin–O *also* ASLO, ASL–O, ASTO • arteriosclerosis obliterans • automatic stop order

ASOR asialo–orosomucoid

ASOT antistreptolysin–O titer

ASP acute suppurative parotitis • acute symmetric polyarthritis • African swine pox • aged substrate plasma • alkali–stable pepsin • ankylosing spondylitis *also* AS • antisocial personality • aortic systolic pressure • area systolic pressure • asparaginase *also* Asp • aspartic acid *also* Asp • aspiration

Asp asparaginase *also* ASP • aspartic acid *also* ASP

asp. aspirate

ASPAT antistreptococcal polysaccharide A test

Asper aspergillosis

ASPG antispleen globulin

ASPVD arteriosclerotic peripheral vascular disease

ASQ abbreviated symptom questionnaire • anxiety scale questionnaire

ASR aldosterone secretion rate • atrial septal resection

AS/Rab antiserum, rabbit

ASS acute serum sickness • anterior superior spine • argininosuccinate synthetase

ASSC acute splenic sequestration crisis

AS–SCORE assessing severity: age of patient, systems involved, stage of disease, complications, response to therapy

Assn, assn association *also* Assoc

Assoc, assoc associate/ association *also* Assn, assn

assocd associated (with)

asst assistant

AST angiotensin sensitivity test • anterior spinothalamic tract • antistreoptolysin titer • aspartate aminotransferase *also* ASAT • astemizole • astigmatism *also* AS, As, Ast, ASTIG • atrial overdrive stimulation rate • audiometry sweep test

Ast, ASTIG astigmatism *also* AS, As, AST

ASTA anti–α–staphylolysin

A sten aortic stenosis

Asth asthenopia

ASTI antispasticity index

ASTO anti–streptolysin O *also* ASLO, ASL–O, ASO

AS TOL, as tol as tolerated

ASTZ antistreptozyme (test)

ASU acute stroke unit • ambulatory surgical unit

ASV, AS–V, A/SV anodic stripping voltametry • antisiphon valve • antisnake venom • arteriosuperficial venous difference • avian sarcoma virus

ASVD arteriosclerotic vascular disease

ASVIP atrial–synchronous ventricular–inhibited pacemaker

ASW artificial seawater

asw artificially sweetened

Asx amino acid that gives aspartic acid after hydrolysis • asymptomatic

ASYM, asym asymmetric/ asymmetry

AT abdominal tympany • achievement test • Achilles tendon • activity therapy • adaptive thermogenesis • adjunctive therapy • air temperature • air trapping • aminotransferase • aminotriazole • amitriptyline • anaerobic threshold • anionic trypsinogen • antithrombin • antitrypsin • antral transplantation • applanation tonometry • ataxia–telangiectasia *also* A–T • atraumatic • atrial tachycardia • atropine • autoimmune thrombocytopenia • axonal terminal • [Ger. *alt Tuberkulin*] old tuberculin

A–T ataxia–telangiectasia *also* AT

AT$_7$ hexachlorophene

AT$_{10}$ dihydrotachysterol

AT I angiotensin I

AT III antithrombin III

At astatine • atrial *also* ATR • atrium *also* A

at. atom/atomic

a.t. air tight • ampere turn

ATA alimentary toxic aleukia • aminotriazole • antithymic activity • antithyroglobulin antibody • antithyroid antibody • anti–*Toxoplasma* antibody • atmosphere absolute *also* ata • aurin tricarboxylic acid

ata atmosphere absolute *also* ATA

ATB antibiotic • atrial tachycardia with block • atypical tuberculosis

ATC activated thymus cell • alcoholism therapy classes • around the clock

ATCS active trabecular calcification surface • anterior tibial compartment syndrome

ATD Alzheimer–type dementia • androstatrienedione • anthropomorphic test dummy • antithyroid drugs • asphyxiating thoracic dystrophy • autoimmune thyroid disease

ATE acute toxic encephalopathy • adipose tissue extract • autologous tumor extract

ATEE, ATEe *N*–acetyl–l–tyrosine ethyl ester

ATEM analytic transmission electron microscope

ATEN atenolol

A tetra P adenosine tetraphosphate

ATF ascites tumor fluid

ATFC alternative temporal forced choice

At Fib, at. fib. atrial fibrillation *also* AF, AFib, ATR FIB, atr fib.

AT III FUN antithrombin III functional

ATG adenine–thymine–guanine • anti–human thymocyte globulin • antithrombocyte/ antithymocyte globulin • antithyroglobulin

ATGAM antithymocyte gamma–globulin

AT/GC adenine–thymine/ guanine–cytosine (ratio)

ATH acetyltyrosine hydrazide

ATHC allotetrahydrocortisol

ATHR angina threshold heart rate

Athsc atherosclerosis

ATL Achilles tendon lengthening • adult T–cell leukemia • anterior tricuspid leaflet • antitension line • atypical lymphocytes

ATLA adult T–cell leukemia antigen

ATLL adult T–cell leukemia/ lymphoma

ATLS advanced trauma life support

ATLV adult T–cell leukemia virus

ATM abnormal tubular myelin • acute transverse myelitis/myelopathy

atm (standard) atmosphere

ATMA antithyroid plasma membrane antibody

At ma atrial milliampere

atmos atmospheric

ATN acute tubular necrosis • augmented transition network

ATNC, AT/NC atraumatic normocephalic

aTNM (at) autopsy tumor, nodes, and metastases (staging of cancer)

at. no. atomic number

ATNR asymmetric tonic neck reflex

ATP addiction treatment program • adenosine triphosphate • ambient temperature and pressure • autoimmune thrombocytopenic purpura

A–TP absorbed test plasma

ATPase adenosine triphosphatase

ATPD ambient temperature and pressure, dry

ATP–2Na adenosine triphosphate disodium

ATPS ambient temperature and pressure, saturated (with water vapor)

ATPTX acute thyroparathyroidectomy

ATR Achilles tendon reflex • atrial *also* At • attenuated total reflection

atr atrophy

ATR FIB, atr fib. atrial fibrillation *also* AF, AFib

ATRO atropine *also* A

ATS Achard–Thiers syndrome • acid test solution • adjustable thigh antiembolism stockings • anti–rat thymocyte serum • antitetanic/antitetanus serum • antithymocyte serum • anxiety tension state • arteriosclerosis • atherosclerosis

ATT arginine tolerance test • aspirin tolerance time

att attending

ATTR attached report

ATU alcohol treatment unit • allylthiourea

ATV avian tumor virus

AtV arteriovenous *also* AV, A-V • assisted ventilation *also* AV • atrioventricular *also* AV, A–V

at. vol atomic volume

at. wt atomic weight *also* AW

AU [L. *ad usum*] according to custom • allergenic unit • Ångström unit • antitoxin unit • arbitrary unit • atomic unit • Australia (antigen) *also* AA, Au Ag • azauridine *also* AZU, AZUR, AzUr • [L. *aures unitas*] both ears together *also* a u • [L. *auris uterque*] each ear *also* a u

Au [L. *aurum*] gold

198Au colloidal gold • radioactive gold

a u [L. *aures unitas*] both ears together *also* AU • [L. *auris utergue*] each ear *also* AU

Au Ag Australia antigen *also* AA, AU

AUB abnormal uterine bleeding

AUC area under the curve

AUD, aud arthritis of unknown diagnosis • auditory

aud–vis audiovisual *also* AV

AUFS absorbance units, full scale

AUG acute ulcerative gingivitis • adenine, uracil, guanine • adenine, uridine, guanosine

aug [L. *augere*] increase

AUGIB acute upper gastrointestinal bleeding

AUHAA Australia hepatitis–associated antigen

AUI alcohol use inventory

AUL acute undifferentiated leukemia

AUM asymmetric unit membrane

AUO amyloid of unknown origin

AuP Australia antigen protein

AUR acute urinary retention

aur, auric auricle/auricular

AUR FIB, aur fib. auricular fibrillation *also* AF

AUS acute urethral syndrome • ascultation *also* aus, ausc, auscul

aus, ausc, auscul ascultation *also* AUS

AuSH Australia serum hepatitis (antigen)

aux auxiliary

AV Adriamycin (doxorubicin) and vincristine alveolar duct • anteroventral • anteversion/anteverted *also* Av, av • anticipatory vomiting • aortic valve • arteriovenous *also* AtV, A–V • artificial ventilation • assisted ventilation *also* AtV • atrioventricular *also* AtV, A–V • audiovisual *also* aud–vis • auditory-visual • augmented vector • auriculoventricular *also* A–V • average *also* Av, av, avg • aviation medicine • avoirdupois *also* Av, av, AVDP, avdp

A–V arteriovenous *also* AtV, AV • atrioventricular *also* AtV, AV • auriculoventricular *also* AV

A/V ampere/volt • arterial/venous • atrial/ventricular • auricular/ventricular

A:V arterial–venous (ratio in fundi)

Av, av anteverted *also* AV • average *also* AV, avg • avoirdupois *also* AV, AVDP, avdp

aV abvolt

AVA antiviral antibody • aortic valve area • aortic valve atresia • arteriovenous anastomosis • availability

AV/AF anteverted, anteflexed

AVB atrioventricular block

AVBR automated ventricular brain ratio

AVC aberrant ventricular conduction • allantoin vaginal cream • associative visual cortex • atrioventricular canal • automatic volume control

AvCDO$_2$ arteriovenous oxygen content difference *also* AVDO$_2$

AVCS atrioventricular conduction system

AVD aortic valvular disease • apparent volume of distribution • arteriovenous difference • atrioventricular dissociation

AVDO$_2$ arteriovenous oxygen content difference *also* AvCDO$_2$

AVDP, avdp asparaginase, vincristine, daunorubicin, and prednisone • avoirdupois *also* AV, Av, av

AvDP average diastolic pressure

AVE aortic valve echocardiogram

AVF antiviral factor • arteriovenous fistula

aVF augmented voltage unipolar left foot lead (electrocardiography)

avg average *also* AV, Av, av

AVG ambulatory visit groups (patient classification)

AVH acute viral hepatitis

AVHB atrioventricular heart block

AVHD acquired valvular heart disease

AVI air velocity index

A–V IMA arteriovenous internal mammary (fistula)

AVJR atrioventricular junctional rhythm

AVJT atrioventricular functional tachycardia

AVL anterior vein of the leg

aVL augmented voltage unipolar left arm lead (electrocardiography)

AVLINE audiovisuals on–line

AVM Adriamycin (doxorubicin), vinblastine, and methotrexate • arteriovenous malformation • atrioventricular malformation • aviation medicine *also* AM

AVN acute varomotor nephropathy • arbitrary valve unit • arteriovenous nicking • atrioventricular nodal (conduction) • atrioventricular node • avascular necrosis

AVNFRP atrioventricular node functional refractory period

AVNR atrioventricular nodal re–entry

AVNRT atrioventricular nodal re–entry tachycardia

AVO atrioventricular opening

A–VO$_2$ arteriovenous oxygen difference

AVP Adriamycin (doxorubicin), vincristine, and procarbazine • ambulatory venous pressure • antiviral protein • aqueous vasopressin • arginine vasopressin

AVR accelerated ventricular rhythm • aortic valve replacement

aVR augmented voltage unipolar right arm lead (electrocardiography)

AVr antiviral regulator

AVRB added viscous resistance to breathing

AVRI acute viral respiratory infection

AVRP atrioventricular refractory period

AVRT atrioventricular re–entrant tachycardia

AVS aneurysm of membranous ventricular septum • aortic valve stenosis • arteriovenous shunt • auditory vocal sequencing

AVSC aortic valve cusp separation

AVSD atrioventricular septal defect

AVSS afebrile, vital signs stable

AVSV aortic valve stroke volume

AVT Allen vision test • arginine oxytocin • arginine vasotocin • atrioventricular tachycardia • atypical ventricular tachycardia

AVTB absolute volume of trabecular bone

Av3V anteroventral third ventricle

AVZ avascular zone

AW abdominal wall • abnormal wave • above waist • abrupt withdrawal • alcohol withdrawal • aluminum wafer • alveolar wall • alveolar wash • anterior wall • atomic warfare • atomic weight *also* at. wt

A/W able to work

A&W alive and well

A3W crystalline amino–acid solution

aw airways

AWA as well as • away without authorization

AWBM alveolar wall basement membrane

AWF adrenal weight factor

AWG American wire gauge

AWI anterior wall infarction • authorized walk–in (patient)

AWMI anterior wall myocardial infarction

AWO airway obstruction

AWOL absent without leave

AWP airway pressure

AWRS anti–whole rabbit serum

AWRU active wrist rotation unit

AWS alcohol withdrawal syndrome

AWTA aniridia–Wilms tumor association

awu atomic weight unit

AX alloxan

Ax axilla/axillary *also* ax.

ax. axilla/axillary *also* Ax • axis • axial *also* A, a • axon

AXF advanced x–ray facility

ax. grad axial gradient

AXL axillary lymphoscintigraphy

AXM acetoxycyclohexamide

AXR abdominal x–ray

AXT alternating exotropia

AYA acute yellow atrophy

AYF antiyeast factor

AYP autolyzed yeast protein

AZ acetazolamide • Aschheim–Zondek (test) • azathioprine *also* AZA

Az [Fr. *azote*] nitrogen

AZA azathioprine *also* AZ

5–AZA 5–azacytidine

AZG, azg azaguanine

AZO, azo indicates presence of the group –N:N–

AZS automatic zero set

AZT Aschheim–Zondek test • azidothymidine (zidovudine)

AZU, AZUR, AzUr azauridine *also* AU

B bacitracin • bands • barometric *also* BAR, bar. • base (chemistry, of a prism) *also* b • baseline • basophil *also* ba, bas, baso • basophilic • [L. *balneum*] bath *also* BAL, bal • Baumé scale • behavior • bel • Benoist scale • benzoate • beta • bicuspid • bilateral *also* BIL, bil, bilat • black *also* Bl, blk • blood *also* bl, bld • bloody • blue *also* bl • body • boils at *also* b • Bolton point • bone marrow–derived (cell or lymphocyte) • born *also* b • boron • both • bound *also* BD • bovine • bregma • brother *also* br, BRO, bro • buccal • Bucky (film in cassette in Potter–Bucky diaphragm) • bursa cells • corticosterone (compound B) • gauss (unit of magnetic induction) • magnetic induction • supramentale (craniometric point) *also* b • tomogram with oscillating Bucky • [L. *bis*] twice *also* b • whole blood

b barn (unit of area for atomic nuclei) • base *also* B • boils at *also* B • born *also* B • brain • supramentale (point) *also* B • [L. *bis*] twice *also* B

B$_0$ constant magnetic field in nuclear magnetic resonance

B$_1$ radiofrequency magnetic field in nuclear magnetic resonance • thiamin

B$_2$ riboflavin

B$_6$ pyridoxine

B$_7$ biotin

B$_8$ adenosine phosphate

B$_{12}$ cyanocobalamin

BI Billroth I (operation)

BII Billroth II (operation)

BA backache *also* B/A • background activity • bacterial agglutination • basilar artery • basion *also* Ba, ba • basket axon • benzanthracene • benzyladenine • benzyl alcohol • benzylamine • best amplitude • betamethasone acetate • bilateral asymmetric • bile acid • biliary atresia • biologic activity • blocking antibody • blood agar • blood alcohol • bone age • boric acid • Bourns assist • bovine albumin • brachial artery (pressure) • breathing apparatus • bronchial asthma • bronchoalveolar • buccoaxial • buffered acetone • butyric acid • [L. *baleum arenae*] sand bath *also* bal are.

B/A backache *also* BA

B&A brisk and active

B>A bone greater than air (conduction) *also* BC > AC

B<A bone less than air (conduction) *also* BC < AC

Ba barium • basion *also* BA, ba

ba basion *also* BA, Ba •
basophil *also* B, baso

BAA benzoylarginine amide •
branched–chain amino acid

BAB blood agar base

Bab Babinski (reflex, sign)

BabK baboon kidney

BAC bacterial adherent
colony • bacterial antigen
complex • benzalkonium
chloride • blood alcohol
concentration •
bronchoalveolar cells •
buccoaxiocervical

Bac, bac [L. *Bacillus*]
bacillary • *Bacillus*

BaClr barium chloride

BACO bleomycin, Adriamycin
(doxorubicin), CCNU
(lomustine), and Oncovin
(vincristine)

BACON bleomycin,
Adriamycin (doxorubicin),
CCNU (lomustine),
Oncovin (vincristine), and
nitrogen mustard
(mechlorethamine)

BACOP bleomycin,
Adriamycin (doxorubicin),
cyclophosphamide, Oncovin
(vincristine), and
prednisone

BACT bischloroethyl-
nitrosourea, arabinosyl-
cytosine, Cytoxan
(cyclophosphamide), and 6–
thioguanine • bleomycin,
Adriamycin (doxorubicin),
Cytoxan (cyclophospha-
mide), and tamoxifen citrate

Bact, bact [L. *Bacterium*]

bacteria/bacterial •
bacteriologist/bacteriology

BAD biologic aerosol
detection • dipolar
affective disorder

BAE bovine aortic
endothelium • bronchial
artery embolization

BaE barium enema *also* BaEn,
BE

BAEE benzoylarginine ethyl
ester

BaEn barium enema *also* BaE,
BE

BAEP brainstem auditory
evoked potential

BAER brainstem auditory
evoked response

BAG buccoaxiogingival

BAGG buffered azide glucose
glycerol

BAI basilar artery insufficiency

BAIB β–aminoisobutyric (acid)

BAIF bile acid independent
flow/fraction

BAIT bacterial automated
identification technique

BAL balance • [L. *balneum*]
bath *also* B, bal • blood
alcohol level • British
antilewisite (dimercaprol) •
bronchoalveolar lavage

bal balance • balsam *also*
bals • [L. *balneum*] bath
also B, BAL

bal are. [L. *balneum arenae*]
sand bath *also* BA

BALB binaural alternate
loudness balance

bal cal [L. *balneum calidum*] hot bath

bal coen [L. *balneum coenosum*] mud bath

BALF bronchoalveolar lavage fluid

bal frig [L. *balneum frigidum*] cold bath

B ALL B–cell acute lymphoblastic leukemia

bal lact [L. *balneum lacteum*] milk bath

bal mar [L. *balneum maris*] salt–water or sea–water bath *also* bm

bal pneu [L. *balneum pneumaticum*] air bath

bals balsam *also* bal

BALT bronchus–associated lymphoid tissue

bal tep [L. *balneum tepidum*] warm bath

bal vap [L. *balneum vapor*] steam or vapor bath

BAM bronchoalveolar macrophage

BAm mean brachial artery (pressure)

BaM barium meal

Bam benzamide

BAME benzoylarginine methyl ester

BAN British approved name

BAND band neutrophil (stab)

BANS back, arm, neck, and scalp

BAO basal acid output • brachial artery output

BAO/MAO ratio of basal acid output to maximal acid output

BAP bacterial alkaline phosphatase • basic adaptive process • Behavior Activity Profile • bleomycin, Adriamycin (doxorubicin), and prednisone • blood agar plate • bovine albumin in phosphate buffer • brachial artery pressure

BaP benzo[*a*]pyrene

BAPI barley alkaline protease inhibitor

BAPN β–aminoproprionitrile fumarate

BAPS bovine albumin phosphate saline

BAPV bovine alimentary papilloma virus

BAQ brain–age quotient

BAR, bar . bariatrics • barometer/barometric *also* B

Barb, barb barbiturate

BARN bilateral acute retinal necrosis

BART blood–activated recalcification time

BAS balloon atrial septostomy • benzyl antiserotonin • bioanalytical systems • boric acid solution

BaS barium swallow *also* BS

bas basilar • basophil *also* B, ba, baso

BASH body acceleration synchronous with heart rate

BASK basket cell *also* BC

baso basophil *also* B, ba, bas

BASO STIP basophilic stippling

BAT Basic Aid Training • basic assurance test • benzilic acid 3α–tropanyl ester • best available technology • brown adipose tissue

batt battery

BAV bicuspid aortic valve

BAVFO bradycardia after arteriovenous fistula occlusion

BAVIP bleomycin, Adriamycin (doxorubicin), vinblastine, imidazole carboxamide (dacarbazine), and prednisone

BAVP balloon aortic valvuloplasty

BAW bronchoalveolar washing

BB baby boy • backboard • bad breath • bath blanket • bed bath • bed board • beta blockade • beta–blocker • BioBreeding (rat) • blanket bath • blood bank *also* BLBK • blood buffer (base) • blow bottle • blue bloater (emphysema) • body belts • both bones (fractures) • bowel and bladder (function) *also* B&B • breakthrough bleeding • breast biopsy *also* B Bx • brush border • buffer base • bundle–branch • isoenzyme of creatine kinase containing two B subunits

B/B backward bending

B&B bowel and bladder *also* BB

bb Bolton point

BBA born before arrival

BBB blood–brain barrier • blood buffer base • bundle–branch block

BBBB bilateral bundle–branch block

BBC bromobenzylcyanide

BBD before bronchodilator • benign breast disease

BBE *Bacteroides* bile esculin (agar)

BBEP brush border endopeptidase

BBF bronchial blood flow

BBG big big gastrin

BBI Bowman–Birk soybean inhibitor

BBM banked breast milk • brush border membrane

BBMV brush border membrane vesicle

BBN broad band noise

BBOW bulging bag of water

BBP butylbenzyl phthalate

BBPRL big big prolactin

BBS bashful bladder syndrome • benign breast syndrome • bilateral breath sounds • bombesin

BBT basal body temperature

BB to MM belly button to medial malleolus

BB/W BioBreeding/Worcester (rat)

B Bx breast biopsy *also* BB

BC back care *also* bc • backcross • background counts • bactericidal concentration • basal cell • basket cell *also* BASK • battle casualty • bed and chair *also* B&C • bicarbonate • biliary colic • biotin carboxylase • bipolar cell • birth control • blastic crisis • blood cardioplegia • blood center • blood culture *also* BlC, BL CULT, bl cult • Blue Cross (plan) *also* BX • board certified • bone conduction • Bourn control • Bowman capsule • brachiocephalic • bronchial carcinoma • buccal cartilage • buccocervical • buffy coat • bulbus chordae

B/C because • blood urea nitrogen/creatinine (ratio)

B&C bed and chair *also* BC • biopsy and curettage • board and care • breathed and cried

bc back care *also* BC

b/c benefit/cost (ratio)

BCA balloon catheter angioplasty • basal–cell atypia • blood color analyzer • Blue Cross Association • brachiocephalic artery • branchial cleft anomaly • breast cancer antigen

BCAA branched chain amino acid

BC > AC bone conduction

greater than air conduction *also* B > A

BC < AC bone conduction less than air conduction *also* B < A

BCAC Breast Cancer Advisory Center

B–CAVE bleomycin, CCNU (lomustine), Adriamycin (doxorubicin), and Velban (vinblastine)

BCB brilliant cresyl blue (stain)

BCBR bilateral carotid body resection

BC/BS Blue Cross/Blue Shield (plan) *also* BX/BS, BX BS

BCC basal cell carcinoma *also* BCCa • biliary cholesterol concentration • birth control clinic

bcc body–centered–cubic

BCCa basal cell carcinoma *also* BCC

BCCG British Cooperative Clinical Group

BCCP biotin carboxyl carrier protein

BCD basal cell dysplasia • binary–coded decimal • bleomycin, cyclophosphamide, and dactinomycin

BCDDP Breast Cancer Detection Demonstration Project

BCDSP Boston Collaborative Drug Surveillance Program

BCE basal cell epithelioma • B–cell enriched • bubble chamber equipment

BCF basophil chemotactic factor • bioconcentration factor • breast cyst fluid

BCFP breast cyst fluid protein

BCG Bacille bilié de Calmette–Guérin (vaccine) • ballistocardiogram • ballistocardiography • bicolor guaiac (test) • bilateral cystogram • bromcresol green

BCH basal–cell hyperplasia/ hypoplasia

bChl, Bchl bacterial chlorophyll

BCHS Bureau of Community Health Services

BCIC Birth Control Investigation Committee

BCKA branched–chain keto acids

BCL basic cycle length

BCLL B–cell chronic lymphocytic leukemia

BCLP bilateral cleft of lip and palate

BCLS basic cardiac life support (system)

BCM birth control medication • body cell mass

BCME bischloromethyl ether

BCNP board–certified nuclear pharmacist

BCNS basal cell nevus syndrome

BCNU bischloroethyl- nitrosourea (carmustine)

BCO biliary cholesterol output

BCOC bowel care of choice

BCP birth control pill • blood cell profile • Blue Cross Plan • bromcresol purple • bischloroethylnitrosourea (carmustine), cyclophosphamide, and prednisone

BCP–D bromocresol purple desoxycholate (agar)

BCPS battery–charging power supply

BCPV bovine cutaneous papilloma virus

BCR B–cell reactivity • bromocriptine • bulbocavernosus reflex

bcr breakpoint cluster region

BCS battered child syndrome • blood cell separator • Budd–Chiari syndrome

BCSI breast cancer screening indicator

BCT brachiocephalic trunk

BCTF Breast Cancer Task Force

BCtg bovine chymotrypsinogen

BCtr bovine chymotrypsin

BCU burn care unit

BCW biologic and chemical warfare

BCYE buffered charcoal yeast extract

BD band neutrophil • barbital–dependent • barbiturate dependence • base deficit • base (of

prism) down • basophilic
degeneration • Batten
disease • beclomethasone
dipropionate • Becton–
Dickinson (spinal needle) •
behavioral disorder •
Beh(et disease • bella-
donna • below diaphragm •
benzidine • benzo-
diazepine • bicarbonate
dialysis • bile duct •
binocular deprivation •
birth date • birth defect •
black death • block design
(test) • blood donor • blue
diaper (syndrome) • board
also Bd • borderline dull •
bound *also* B • brain
death • bronchial
drainage • bronchodilator •
buccodistal • [L. *bis die*]
twice a day *also* bd, BID,
b.i.d.

B&D bondage and discipline

Bd board *also* BD

bd [L. *bis die*] twice a day *also*
BD, BID, b.i.d.

BDAC Bureau of Drug Abuse
Control

BDAE Boston Diagnostic
Aphasia Examination

BDBS Bonnet–Delchaume–
Blanc syndrome

BDC burn–dressing change

BDE bile duct examination/
exploration

BDF black divorced female

BDG bilirubin diglucuronide •
buccal developmental
groove • buffered
desoxycholate glucose

BDI Beck Depression Index •
burn depth indicator

BDIBS Boston Diagnostic
Inventory of Basic Skills

BDID bystander dominates
initial dominant
(psychology)

BDI SF Beck Depression
Index—Short Form

BDL below detectable limits •
bile duct ligation

BDLS Brachmann–de Lange
syndrome

BDM benzphetamine
demethylase • black
divorced male • border
detection method

BDMP Birth Defects
Monitoring Program

B–DOPA bleomycin,
dacarbazine, Oncovin
(vincristine), prednisone,
and Adriamycin
(doxorubicin)

BDP beclomethasone
diproprionate • bilateral
diaphragm paralysis

BDR background diabetic
retinopathy

BDS biologic detection system

bds [L. *bid in die summendus*]
to be taken twice a day

BDTVMI Beery Developmental
Test of Visual–Motor
Integration

BDUR bromodeoxyuridine

BE bacillary emulsion •
bacterial endocarditis •
barium enema *also* BaE,
BaEn • Barrett
esophagus • base excess •
below–elbow (amputation)
also B/E • bile esculin

(test) • board eligible •
bovine enteritis • brain
edema • bread equivalent •
breast examination •
bronchoesophagology

B/E below–elbow (amputation)
also BE

Be Baumé (scale) • beryllium

B&E brisk and equal

B↑E both upper extremities

B↓E both lower extremities

BEA below–elbow
amputation •
bromoethylamine

BEAM brain electrical activity
mapping/monitoring

BEAR Biologic Effects of
Atomic Radiation
(Committee)

BEC bacterial endocarditis •
blood ethanol content •
bromoergocryptine

BEE basal energy expenditure

BEEP both end–expiratory
pressures

BEF bronchoesophageal fistula

bef before

beg. begin/beginning

beh behavior/behavioral

Beh Sp behavior specialist

BEI back–scattered electron
imaging • butanol–
extractable iodine

BEIR biologic effects of
ionizing radiation

BEK bovine embryonic kidney
(cell)

BEL blood ethanol level •
bovine embryonic lung

ben [L. *bene*] well

Benz benzidine

BEP bleomycin, etoposide, and
Platinol (cisplatin) •
brainstem evoked potential

BEPI β–endorphin
immunoreactivity

bepti bionomics, environment,
Plasmodium, treatment, and
immunity (malaria
epidemiology)

BER basic electrical rhythm

BERA brainstem electric
response audiometry

BES balanced electrolyte
solution

BESM bovine embryo skeletal
muscle

BESP bovine embryonic
spleen (cells)

BET benign epithelial tumor •
Brunauer–Emmet–Teller
(method)

bet. between

beta (B, β) second letter of
Greek alphabet

β anomer of carbohydrate •
buffer capacity • carbon
separated from carboxyl by
one other carbon in aliphatic
compounds • constituent of
plasma protein fraction •
probability of type II error •
second in series or group •
substituent group of steroid
that projects above plane of
ring

β$_2$m β$_2$–microglobulin

BETS benign epileptiform
transients of sleep

BEV baboon endogenous virus • billion electron volts *also* BeV, Bev, bev • bleeding esophageal varices

BeV, Bev, bev billion electron volts *also* BEV

Bex base excess

BF betonite flocculation (test) • bile flow • black female *also* B/F • blastogenic factor • blister fluid • blocking factor • blood flow • body fat • Bolivian hemorrhagic fever • bone fragment • bouillon filtrate (tuberculin) *also* bf • boyfriend • breakfast fed • breast fed • buccofacial • buffered • burning feet (syndrome) • butter fat

B/F black female *also* BF • bound/free (antigen ratio)

bf bouillon filtrate (tuberculin) *also* BF

BFA baby for adoption • bifemoral arteriogram

BFB biologic feedback

BFC benign febrile convulsion

BFD bias flow down

BFDI bronchodilation following deep inspiration

BFDT Bekesy Functionality Detection Test

BFH benign familial hematuria

BFL bird fancier's lung • breast firm and lactating

BFLS Börjeson–Forssman–Lehmann syndrome

BFM bendroflumethiazide • black married female

BFO balanced/ball–bearing forearm orthesis • blood–forming organ • buccofacial obturator

BFP biologic false–positive

BFPR biologic false–positive reaction

BFR blood filtration/flow rate • bone formation rate • buffered Ringer (solution) *also* BFR sol

BFR sol buffered Ringer solution *also* BFR

BFS blood fasting sugar

BFT bentonite flocculation test • biofeedback training • bladder flap tube

BFU burst–forming unit

BFU–E burst–forming unit, erythroid

BG baby girl • background *also* BKg • basal ganglion • basic gastrin • β–galactosidase • β–glucuronidase • bicolor guaiac (test) • big gastrin • blood glucose *also* BGlu • bone graft • Bordet–Gengou (agar, bacillus, phenomenon) *also* B–G • brilliant green • buccogingival

B–G Bender–Gestalt (test) • Bordet–Gengou (agar, bacillus, phenomenon) *also* BG

BGA blue–green algae

BGAg blood group antigen

B–GALACTO β–galacto-sidase

BGAV blue–green algae virus

BGC basal–ganglion calcification • blood group class

BGCA bronchogenic carcinoma

BG–corr background corrected

BGD blood group degrading (enzyme)

BGDC Bartholin gland duct cyst

BGE butyl glycidyl ether

BGG bovine gamma–globulin

bGH bovine growth hormone

Bg^J beige (mouse)

BGL blood glucose level

BGLB brilliant green lactose broth

BGlu blood glucose *also* BG

BGO bismuth germinate

BGP β–glycerophosphatase

BGRS blood glucose reagent strip

BGS blood group substance

BGSA blood granulocyte–specific activity

BGT basophil granulation test • Bender–Gestalt test • bungarotoxin

BGTT borderline glucose tolerance test

BH base hospital • benzalkonium and eparin • bill of health • board of health • Bolton–Hunter (reagent) • borderline hypertensive • both hands • brain hormone • Braxton–Hicks (contraction) • breath holding • bronchial hyperactivity/hyperreactivity • Bryan high titer • bundle of His

BH$_4$ tetrahydrobiopterin

BHA benign/bilateral hilar adenopathy • bound hepatitis antibody • butylated hydroxyanisole

BHAT beta–blocker heart attack trial

BHB β–hydroxybutyrate

bHb bovine hemoglobin

BHBA β–hydroxybutyric acid

BHC benzene hexachloride

BHD BCNU (carmustine), hydroxyurea, and dacarbazine

BHD–V BCNU (carmustine), hydroxyurea, dacarbazine, and vincristine

B–HEXOS–A–LK β–hexosaminidase A leukocytes

BHF Bolivian hemorrhagic fever

BHI beef heart infusion (broth) • biosynthetic human insulin • brain–heart infusion (broth) • Bureau of Health Insurance

BHIA brain–heart infusion agar

BHI–ac brain–heart infusion broth with acetone

BHIB brain–heart infusion broth

BHIBA brain–heart infusion blood agar

BHIRS brain–heart infusion and rabbit serum

BHIS beef heart infusion–supplemented (broth)

BHK baby hamster kidney (cells) • type B Hong Kong (influenza virus)

BHL bilateral hilar lymphadenopathy • biologic half–life

BHM Bureau of Health Manpower

BHN bephenium hydroxynaphthoate • bridging hepatic necrosis • Brinell hardness number

BHP basic health profile • Bureau of Health Professions

BHR basal heart rate

BHS β–hemolytic streptococcus • breath–holding spell

BHT β–hydroxytheophylline • breath hydrogen test • butylated hydroxytoluene

BHU basic health unit

BHV bovine herpes virus

BH/VH body hematocrit–venous hematocrit (ratio)

BI background interval • bacterial/bactericidal/bacteriologic index • base (of prism) in • basilar impression • bifocal *also* BIF, bif • biologic indicator • bodily/bone injury • bowel impaction • brain injured/injury • burn index

Bi bismuth

bi between • bilateral

BIB, bib brought in by • [L. *bibe*] drink

biblio bibliography

BIC blood isotope clearance • brain injury center

Bic biceps

Bicarb, bicarb bicarbonate

BICROS bilateral contralateral routing of signals

BID bibliographic information and documentation • brought in dead • [L. *bis in die*] twice a day *also* BD, bd, b.i.d.

b.i.d. [L. *bis in die*] twice a day *also* BD, bd, BID

BIDLB block in posteroinferior division of left branch

BIDS bedtime insulin, daytime sulfonylurea (therapy)

BIF, bif bifocal *also* BI

BIGGY bismuth glycine glucose yeast (agar)

BIH benign intracranial hypertension • bilateral inguinal hernia

Bi Isch, bi isch between ischial tuberosities

BIL, bil basal insulin level • bilateral *also* B, bilat • bilirubin • brother–in–law

BIL/ALB bilirubin to albumin (ratio)

bilat bilateral *also* B, BIL, bil

BILAT SLC bilateral short–leg cane

BILAT SXO, bilat sxo bilateral salpingo-oophorectomy

bili bilirubin *also* BIL, bil, bilirub

bili–c conjugated bilirubin

bilirub bilirubin *also* BIL, bil, bili

BIMA bilateral internal mammary arteries

BIN benign introdermal nerves

b.i.n. [L. *bis in noctus*] twice a night

biochem biochemistry/ biochemical

BIOETHICSLINE Bioethical Information On–Line

BIOF biofeedback

biol biologic/biology

biophys biophysical/ biophysics

BIOSIS BioScience Information Service

BIP Background Interference Procedure • bacterial intravenous protein • biparietal (diameter) • bismuth iodoform paraffin • Blue Cross interim payment • brief infertile period

BIPD biparietal diameter (fetal skull)

BIPLED bilateral, independent, periodic, lateralized epileptiform discharge

BIPM [Fr. *Bureau International des Poids et Mesures*] International Bureau of Weights and Measures

BIPP bismuth iodoform paraffin/petrolatum paste

BIR backward internal rotation • basic incidence rate

BIS, bis Brain Information Service • sodium bicarbonate in invert sugar • [Latin] twice

BISP, BiSP between ischial spines

Bisp, bisp bispinous or interspinous diameter

BIT, BIT between great trochanters

BITU benzylthiourea

BIU barrier isolation unit

BIW, biw, bi wk biweekly

BIZ–PLT bizarre platelets

BJ Bence Jones (protein, proteinuria) • biceps jerk • Bielschowsky–Jansky (syndrome) • bones and joints *also* B&J

B&J bones and joints *also* BJ

BJE bone and joint examination

BJM bones, joints, and muscles

BJP Bence Jones protein/ proteinuria

BK bekanamycin • below–knee (amputation) *also* B/K • bovine kidney (cells) • bradykinin • bullous keratopathy

B–K initials of two patients after whom a multiple cutaneous nevus (mole) was named

B/K below–knee (amputation) *also* BK

Bk berkelium

bk back

BKA below–knee amputation

BK–A basophil kallikrein of anaphylaxis

BKC blepharokerato-conjunctivitis

bkf, bkfst, bkft breakfast *also* Brkf

Bkg background *also* BG

bkly back lying

BKS beekeeper serum

BKTT below–knee to toe (cast)

BKU base up

BKWC below–knee walking cast

BKWP below–knee walking plaster

BL bacterial levan • baralyme • basal lamina • baseline (fetal heart rate) • Bessey–Lowry (unit) • black light • bland *also* bl • blast cells • bleeding *also* bl • blind loop • blood level/loss • bone marrow lymphocyte • borderline lepromatous • bronchial lavage • buccolingual • Burkitt lymphoma • butyrolactone

B–L bursa–equivalent lymphocyte

Bl black *also* B, blk

bl bland *also* BL • bleeding *also* BL, bldg • blood *also* B, bld • blue *also* B

BLa buccolabial

BLAD borderline left axis deviation

blad bladder

BLB Bessey–Lowry–Brock (method or unit) • Boothby–Lovelace–Bulbulian (oxygen mask)

BLBK blood bank *also* BB

BL=BS bilateral equal breath sounds

BLC beef liver catalase

BlC blood culture *also* BC, BL CULT, bl cult

BLCL Burkitt lymphoma cell line

BL CULT, bl cult blood culture *also* BC, BlC

BLD basal–cell liquefactive degeneration • benign lymphoepithelial disease • beryllium lung disease

bld blood *also* B, bl

bldg bleeding *also* BL, bl

bld tm bleeding time *also* BT

BLE both lower extremities

BLEO bleomycin *also* BLM

BLEO–MOPP bleomycin, mechlorethamine, Oncovin (vincristine), and prednisone

BLEP Breast Lesion Evaluation Project

bleph blepharoplasty

BLESS bath, laxative, enema, shampoo, and shower

BLFD buccolinguofacial dyskinesia

BLFG bilateral firm (hand) grips

BL–FST blood–fasting (glucose tolerance test)

BLG β–lactoglobulin

BLI bombesin–like immunoreactivity

blk black *also* B, Bl

BLL below lower limit • bilateral lower lobe • brows, lids, and lashes

BLLS bilateral leg strength

BLM basolateral membrane • bilayer lipid membrane • bimolecular liquid membrane • black lipid membrane • bleomycin *also* BLEO

BLN bronchial lymph node

BlObs bladder obstruction

BLP β–lipoprotein

BlP blood pressure *also* BL PR, bl pr, BP, B/P

BLPO β–lactamase–producing organism

BL PR, bl pr blood pressure *also* BlP, BP, B/P

BLQ both lower quadrants

BLRA β–lactamase–resistant antimicrobial

BLS basic life support • blind loop syndrome • blood and lymphatic system • Bloom syndrome *also* BS

BlS blood sugar *also* BS

BLSD bovine lumpy skin disease

BLST Bankson Language Screening Test

BLT, BlT blood–clot lysis time • blood test • blood type/typing

BLU, B.L. unit Bessey–Lowry unit

BLV blood volume • bovine leukemia virus

BM basal medium • basal metabolism • basement membrane • basilar membrane • Bergersen medium • betamethasone • biomedical • black male *also* B/M • blood monocyte • body mass • Bohr magneton • bone marrow • bowel movement • breast milk • buccal mass • buccomesial

B/M black male *also* BM

bm [L. *balneum maris*] salt–water bath *also* bal mar

BMA bone marrow arrest • bone marrow aspirate

BmA *Brugia malayi* adult antigen

BMAP bone marrow acid phosphatase

BMB biomedical belt • bone marrow biopsy

BMBL benign monoclonal B–cell lymphocytosis

BMC bone marrow cells • bone mineral content • blood mononuclear cell

BMD Becker muscular dystrophy • Boehringer Mannheim Diagnostics • bone marrow depression • bone mineral density • bovine mucosal disease • Bureau of Medical Devices

BMDC Biomedical Documentation Center

BME basal medium, Eagle • brief maximal effort • biundulant meningoencephalitis

BMET biomedical equipment technician

BMG benign monoclonal gammopathy

BMI bicuculline methiodide • body mass index

BMJ bones, muscles, joints

BMK, bmk birthmark

BML bone marrow lymphocytosis

BMLM basement membrane–like material

BMLS billowing mitral leaflet syndrome

BMM black married male

BMMP benign mucous membrane pemphigoid

BMN bone marrow necrosis

BMNR bone marrow neutrophil reserve

BMOC Brinster medium for ovum culture

Bmod behavior modification

B–mode brightness modulation

BMP behavior management plan • bone marrow pressure • bone morphogenetic protein • BCNU, methotrexate, and procarbazine

BMPI bronchial mucous proteinase inhibitor

BMPP benign mucous membrane pemphigus

BMR basal metabolic rate • best motor response

BMS betamethasone • biomedical monitoring system • bleomycin sulfate

BMST Bruce maximal stress test

BMT basement membrane thickness • benign mesenchymal tumor • bilateral myringotomy and tubes • bone marrow transplantation

BMTU bone marrow transplant unit

BMU basic multicellular unit

BMZ basement membrane zone

BN bladder neck • brachial neuritis • bronchial nodes • brown Norway (rat) • bucconasal

BNB blood–nerve barrier

BNC bladder neck contracture

BNCT boron neutron capture therapy

BNDD Bureau of Narcotics and Dangerous Drugs

BNEG B negative (blood type)

BNG bromonaphthyl–β–galactoside

BNGase bromonaphthyl–β–glactosidase

BNGF β–nerve growth factor

BNIST [Fr. *Bureau National d'Information Scientifique*] National Bureau of Scientific Information

BNL breast needle location

BNO bladder neck

obstruction • bowels not opened

BNPA binasal pharyngeal airway

BNR bladder neck resection/retraction

BNS benign nephrosclerosis

BNSME Brief Neuropsychologic Mental Status Examination

BNT brain neurotransmitter

BO base (of prism) out • behavior objective • body odor • bowel *also* bo • bowel obstruction • bowels open • bucco–occlusal

B/O because of

B&O belladonna and opium

Bo Bolton point

bo bowel *also* BO

BOA behavioral observation audiometry • born on arrival • born out of asepsis

BOB ball on back

BOBA β–oxybutyric acid

BOC blood oxygen capacity • butyloxycarbonyl

BOCG Brudzinski, Oppenheim, Chaddock, and Gullaird (reflexes or signs)

BOD bilateral orbital decompression • biochemical/biologic oxygen demand • borderline *also* BORD • Bureau of Drugs

Bod units Bodansky units

BOE bilateral otitis externa

BOEA ethyl biscoumacetate

BOFA β–oncofecal antigen

BOH Board of Health

bol [L. *bolus*] pill

BOLD bleomycin, Oncovin (vincristine), lomustine, and dacarbazine

BOM bilateral otitis media

BOMA bilateral otitis media, acute

BOO bladder outlet obstruction

BOOP bronchiolitis obliterans–organizing pneumonia

BOP bleomycin, Oncovin (vincristine), and prednisone • bromo–oxyprogesterone • Buffalo orphan prototype (virus)

BOPAM bleomycin, Oncovin (vincristine), prednisone, Adriamycin (doxorubicin), and methotrexate

BOR basal optic root • before time of operation • bowels open regularly • branchio–otorenal (syndrome)

BORD borderline *also* BOD

BORR blood oxygen release rate

B–O₂S blood oxygen saturation

BOT base of tongue • botulinum toxin

bot botany • bottle

BOW bag of waters

BOWI bag of waters intact

BP back pressure • barometric

pressure • basic protein • bathroom privileges • bed pan • before present • behavior pattern • Bell palsy • benzoyl peroxide • benzpyrene • bioequivalence problem • biotic potential • biparietal • biphenyl • bipolar • birthplace • blood pressure *also* BlP, BL PR, bl pr, B/P • body part • body plethysmography • boiling point *also* bp • Bolton point • borderline personality • British Pharmacopoeia • bronchopleural • bronchopulmonary • buccopulpal • bullous pemphigoid/pemphigus • bypass

B/P blood pressure *also* BlP, BL PR, bl pr, BP

bp base pair • boiling point *also* BP

BPA Bauhinia purpura agglutinin • blood pressure assembly • bovine plasma albumin • bronchopulmonary aspergillosis • burst–promoting activity

BPB bromphenol blue

BPC Behavior Problem Checklist • bile phospholipid concentration • British Pharmaceutical Codex • bronchial provocation challenge

B–Pco₂ blood partial pressure of carbon dioxide

BPD biparietal diameter • blood pressure decreased • borderline personality

disorder • broncho-pulmonary dysplasia

BPd diastolic blood pressure

BPE bacterial phosphatidylethanolamine

BPEC bipolar electrocoagulation

BPF bradykinin–potentiating factor • bronchopleural fistula • burst–promoting factor

BPG blood pressure gauge • bypass graft

BPH benign prostatic hyperplasia/hypertrophy

BPh buccopharyngeal

B–pH blood pH

Bph bacteriopheophytin

BPI Basic Personality Inventory • beef–pork insulin • bipolar affective disorder, Type 1 • blood pressure increased

BPL benign proliferative lesion • benzylpenicilloyl polylysine *also* BPO • β–propiolactone • bone phosphate of lime

BP lar blood pressure, left arm

BPLN bilateral pelvic lymph nodes

BPLND bilateral pelvic lymph node dissection

BPM, bpm beats per minute • bipiperidyl mustard • births per minute • breaths per minute • brompheni-ramine maleate

BPMS blood plasma measuring system

BPN bacitracin, polymyxin B, and neomycin sulfate • brachial plexus neuropathy

BPO basal pepsin output • benzylpenicilloyl polylysine *also* BPL • bilateral partial oophorectomy • bile phospholipid output

BPP biophysical profile • bovine pancreatic polypeptide • bradykinin potentiating peptide • breast parenchymal pattern

BPPN benign paroxysmal positioning nystagmus

BPPP bilateral pedal pulses present

BP,P,R,T blood pressure, pulse, respiration, and temperature

BPPV benign paroxysmal positional vertigo • bovine paragenital papilloma virus

BPR blood per rectum • blood pressure recorder • blood production rate

BP rar blood pressure, right arm

BPRS brief psychiatric rating scale • brief psychiatric reacting scale

BPS beats per second • bilateral partial salpingectomy • bovine papular stomatitis • brain protein solvent • breaths per second

BPs blood pressure, systolic

BPSD bronchopulmonary segmental drainage

BPT benign paroxysmal torticollis

BPTI basic pancreatic trypsin inhibitor • basic polyvalent trypsin inhibitor

BPV benign paroxysmal vertigo • benign positional vertigo • bioprosthetic valve • bovine papilloma virus

BP(VET) British Pharmacopoeia (Veterinary)

Bq becquerel (SI unit of radionuclide activity)

BQA Bureau of Quality Assurance

BQC sol 2,6–dibromoquinone–4–chlorimide solution

BR barrier–reared (experimental animals) • baseline recovery • bathroom • bed rest • bedside rounds • Benzing retrograde • benzodiazepine receptor • bilirubin • biologic response • blink reflex • bowel rest • brachialis • breathing rate • bronchitis *also* Br • brown *also* br

Br breech • bregma • bridge • bromide • bromine • bronchitis *also* BR

br boiling range • brachial *also* Brach • branch • breath • broiled • brother *also* B, BRO, bro • brown *also* BR

BRA β–resorcylic acid • bilateral renal agenesis • brain

BRAC basic rest–activity cycle

Brach brachial *also* br

BRADY bradycardia

BRAO branch retinal artery occlusion *also* BR RAO

BRAP burst of rapid atrial pacing

BrAP brachial artery pressure

BRAT bananas, rice cereal, applesauce, and toast (diet)

BRATT bananas, rice, applesauce, tea, and toast (diet)

BRB blood–retinal barrier • bright red blood

BRBC bovine red blood cell

BRBNS blue rubber bleb nevus syndrome

BRBPR, BRBR bright red blood per rectum

br bx breast biopsy

BRCM below right costal margin

BRD bladder retraining drill

BrDu, BrdU, BrdUrd bromodeoxyuridine

BRET bretylium tosylate

BRH benign recurrent hematuria • Bureau of Radiological Health

BRI Bio–Research Index

BRIC benign recurrent intrahepatic cholestasis

Brit British

BRJ brachial radialis jerk

Brkf breakfast *also* bkf, bkfst, bkft

BRM biologic response modifiers • biuret–reactive material

BrM breast milk

BRMP Biological Response Modification Program

BRN Board of Registered Nursing

BRO bromocriptine • bronchoscopy *also* bronch • brother *also* B, br, bro

bro brother *also* B, br, BRO

Bron bronchi/bronchial

bronch bronchoscope/ bronchoscopy *also* BRO

BRP bathroom privileges • bilirubin production

Brph bronchophony

BRR baroreceptor reflex response

BR RAO branch retinal artery occlusion *also* BRAO

BR RVO branch retinal vein occlusion *also* BRVO

BR S breath sounds *also* BS

brth breath

BRU bromide urine

BrU bromouracil

BRVO branch retinal vein occlusion *also* BR RVO

BS barium swallow *also* BaS • Bartter syndrome • bedside • before sleep • Beh(et syndrome • Bennett seal • bilateral symmetric • bile salt • bismuth subgallate/ subsalicylate • blood sugar *also* BlS • Bloom syndrome *also* BLS • Blue Shield (plan) • borderline schizophrenia • bowel sounds *also* bs • breaking strength • breath sounds *also* BRS, bs • British Standard • Bureau of Standards

B–S Bjork–Shiley (valve prosthesis) • Binet–Simon (test)

B&S Bartholin and Skene (glands)

bs bowel sounds *also BS* • breath sounds *also* BRS, BS

BSA beef serum albumin • benzenesulfonic acid • bismuth–sulfite agar • bis–trimethylsilylacetamide • Blue Shield Association • body surface area *also* bsa • bovine serum albumin *also* bsa • bowel sounds active

bsa body surface area *also* BSA • bovine serum albumin *also* BSA

BSAB Balthazar Scales of Adaptive Behavior

BSAER brainstem auditory evoked response

BSAG Bristol Social Adjustment Guides

BSAP brief short–action potential • brief, small, abundant potentials

BSB bedside bag • body surface burned

BSBC buffer–soluble binding component

BSC bedside care • bedside commode • bench scale calorimeter • bile salt concentration • Biological Stain Commission • burn scar contracture

BSCIF bile salt independent canalicular fraction

BSCP bovine spinal cord protein

BSD baby soft diet • bedside drainage

BSDLB block in antero-superior division of left branch

BSE bacillus species enzyme • bilateral, symmetrical, and equal • breast self–examination

BSEP brainstem evoked potential

BSepF black separated female

BSepM black separated male

BSER brainstem evoked response (audiometry)

BSF backscatter factor • basal skull fracture • black single female • busulfan

BSG branchioskeletogenital (syndrome)

BSGA β–hemolytic streptococcus group A

BSI body substance isolation • borderline syndrome index • bound serum iron • brainstem injury • British Standards Institution

BSID Bayley Scales of Infant Development

BSIF bile salt independent fraction

BSL benign symmetric lipomatosis • blood sugar level

BS L base breath sounds diminished, left base

BSN bowel sounds normal

BSNA bowel sounds normal and active

BSNT breast soft and nontender

BSO bilateral sagittal osteotomy • bilateral salpingo–oophorectomy • bilateral serous otitis

BSOM bilateral serous otitis media

BSP body segment parameter • Bromsulfophthalein (liver function)

BSp bronchospasm

BSPA bowel sounds present and active

BSPM body surface potential mapping

BSQ Behavior Style Questionnaire

BSR basal skin resistance • blood sedimentation rate • bowel sounds regular • brain stimulation reinforcement

BSRI Bem Sex Role Inventory

BSS balanced salt solution • bedside scale • Bernard–Soulier syndrome *also* B–SS • bismuth subsalicylate • black silk suture • buffered salt solution • buffered single substrate

B–SS Bernard–Soulier syndrome *also* BSS

BSSE bile salt–stimulated esterase

BSSG sitogluside

BSSI Basic School Skills Inventory

BSSL bile salt–stimulated lipase

BSSS benign sporadic sleep spikes

BST Bacteriuria Screening Test • bedside testing • biceps semitendinosus • blood serologic test • breast stimulation test • brief stimulus therapy

BSTFA bis–trimethylsilyl-trifluoroacetamide

BSTP basophilic stippling (on differential)

BSU Bartholin, Skene, and urethral (glands) • British Standard Unit

BSV Batten–Spielmyer–Vogt (syndrome)

BT base of tongue • bedtime • bitemporal (diameter of fetal head) • bituberous • bladder tumor • bleeding time *also* bld tm • blood transfusion • blood type/typing • blue tetrazolium • blue tongue • body temperature • borderline tuberculoid • bovine turbinate (cells) • brain tumor • breast tumor • bulbotruncal

BTA N–benzoyl–1–tyrosine amide • brief tone audiometry

BTB breakthrough bleeding • bromthymol blue

BTBC Boehm Test of Basic Concepts

BTBL bromothymol blue lactose

BTBV beat–to–beat variability

BTC basal temperature chart • bilateral tubal coagulation •

bladder tumor check • by the clock

BTE behind–the–ear (hearing aid) • bovine thymus extract

BTEA Boston Test for Examining Aphasia

BTF blenderized tube feeding

BTFS breast tumor frozen section

BTG β–thromboglobulin

BTg bovine trypsinogen

BThU British thermal unit *also* BTU

BTL bilateral tubal ligation

BTM benign tertian malaria • bilateral tympanic membranes

BTMD Botten–Turner muscular dystrophy

BTMSA bis–trimethyl-silacetylene

BTP biliary tract pain

BTPD body temperature, pressure, dry

BTPS body temperature, ambient pressure, and saturated with water vapor (gas)

BTR Bezold–type reflex • bladder tumor recheck • bovine trypsin

BTS bioptic telescopic spectacle • bithional sulfoxide • blood transfusion service • bradycardia–tachycardia syndrome

BTSH, bTSH beef/bovine thyroid–stimulating hormone

BTU British thermal unit *also* BThU

BTV blue tongue virus

BTX bactrachotoxin • benzene, toluene, and xylene

BTX–B brevetoxin–B

BU base (of prism) up • below the umbilicus • blood urea • Bodansky unit • bromouracil • burn unit

Bu bilirubin • butyl

BUA blood uric acid

Buc, bucc buccal

BUD budesonide

BUDR, BUdR 5–bromode-oxyuridine

BUDS bilateral upper dorsal sympathectomy

BUE both upper extremities • built–up edge

BUF Buffalo (rat)

BUFA baby up for adoption

BUG buccal ganglion

BUI brain uptake index

BULL buccal or upper lingual of lower

bull. bulletin • [L. *bulliat*] let it boil

BUMP Behavioral Regression or Upset in Hospitalized Medical Patients (scale)

BUN blood urea nitrogen • bunion

BUO bilateral ureteral

occlusion • bilirubin/ bleeding/bruising of undetermined origin

BUR back–up rate (ventilator)

Bur bureau

Burd Burdick (suction)

BUS Bartholin, urethral, and Skene (glands) • busulfan

Bus busulfan

BUSEG Bartholin, urethral, and Skene (glands), and external genitalia

BUT break–up time

But, but. [L. *butyrum*] butter • butyrate/butyric

BV bacitracin V • bacterial vaginitis • billion volts • biologic value • blood vessel • blood volume • bronchovesicular • buccoversion • bulboventricular

bv [L. *balneum vaporis*] steam bath

BVAD biventricular assist device

BVAP BCNU (carmustine), vincristine, Adriamycin (doxorubicin), and prednisone

BVAT Binocular Visual Acuity Test

BVC British Veterinary Codex

BVD bovine viral diarrhea • BCNU (carmustine), vincristine, and dacarbazine

BVDT Brief Vestibular Disorientation Test

BVE binocular visual

efficiency • biventricular enlargement • blood vessel endothelium • blood volume expander/expansion

BVH biventricular hypertrophy

BVI Better Vision Institute • blood vessel invasion

BVL bilateral vas ligation

BVM bronchovascular markings • Bureau of Veterinary Medicine

BVMGT Bender Visual–Motor Gestalt Test

BVO branch vein occlusion • brominated vegetable oil

BVP blood vessel prosthesis • blood volume pulse • Bonhoeffer van der Pol • burst of ventricular pacing

BVR baboon virus replication

BVRT–R Benton Visual Retention Test, Revised

BVS blanked ventricular sense

BVU bromoisovalerylurea

BVV bovine vaginitis virus

BW bacteriologic warfare • below waist • bite–wing (radiograph) • biologic weapon • birth weight *also* BWt • bladder washout • blood Wasserman • body water • body weight *also* bw

B&W black and white (milk of magnesia and cascara extract)

bw body weight *also* BW

BWA bed wetter admission

BWCS bagged white–cell study

BWD bacillary white diarrhea

BWFI bacteriostatic water for injection

BWidF black widowed female

BWidM black widowed male

BWS battered woman syndrome • Beckwith–Wiedemann syndrome

BWST black widow spider toxin

BWSV black widow spider venom

BWt birth weight *also* BW

BX bacitracin X • biopsy *also* Bx • Blue Cross (plan) *also* BC

Bx biopsy

BX/BS, BX BS Blue Cross and Blue Shield (plan) *also* BC/BS

BXM B–cell cross–match

BYE Barila–Yaguchi–Eveland (medium)

BZ, bz benzodiazepine *also* BZD, BZDZ • benzoyl

BZA benzylamine

BZD, BZDZ benzodiazepine *also* BZ, bz

Bz–Ty–PABA benzoyltyrosyl–*p*–aminobenzoic acid (test)

BZQ benzquinamide

C ascorbic acid • [L. *contusus*] bruised • calcitonin–forming (cell) • calculus • calorie (large) *also* Cal • canine (tooth) *also* c • capacitance • carbohydrate *also* CHO • carbon • cardiovascular (disease) • carrier • cathode *also* CA, Ca, Cath, cath • Catholic • Caucasian *also* Cau, Cauc, cauc • Celsius *also* CEL, Cel • centigrade *also* CENT, cent. • central *also* CENT, cent. • central electrode placement in electroencephalography • centromeric or constitutive heterochromatic chromosome (banding) • cerebrospinal (fluid) • certified *also* CRT • cervical (spine) • cesarean (section) • chest (precordial lead in electrocardiography) • chloramphenicol *also* chloro, CMC, CP • cholesterol *also* CH, CHO, CHOL, chol • clear • clearance rate (renal) • clonus • closure • clubbing • coarse (bacterial colonies) • cocaine • coefficient • colored (guinea pig) • color sense • complement *also* C′ • compliance • component • [L. *compositus*] compound *also* comp, compd, CP, cpd • concentration *also* c • conditioned/conditioning • condyle • constant • contact *also* c • content • contraction *also* Cx •

control • conventionally reared (experimental animal) • cornea • correct • cortex *also* cort • coulomb • creatinine • cubic *also* c, cu • cup *also* c • curie *also* c, Ci, CU, cu • cuspid (secondary dentition) • cuticular • cyanosis • cylinder • cysteine *also* Cys • cytidine • cytochrome • cytosine • [L. *congius*] gallon • [L. *centum*] hundred *also* c • molar heat capacity • [L. *costa*] rib • velocity of light • [L. *cum*] with *also* c, $\bar{c}$

C₁–C₁₂ [L. *costa*] first through twelfth ribs

C₃ Collins solution

¹⁴C, C14 carbon–14 (isotope)

CI—CXII cranial nerves I through XII *also* C1–C12

C1—C7 cervical vertebrae 1 through 7

C1—C8 cervical nerves 1 through 8

C1—C9 components of complement 1 through 9

C1—C12 cranial nerves I through XII *also* CI–CXII

C–1—C–9 activated components of complement 1 through 9

C–I—C–V DEA controlled substances schedules I through V

C–6 hexamethonium

C–10 decamethonium

c [L. *circa*] about *also* ca • calorie (small) *also* cal • candle *also* ca • canine (tooth) *also* C • capacity *also* cap. • capillary blood (subscript) • carat • centi– (prefix) • concentration *also* C • contact *also* C • cubic *also* C, cu • cup *also* C • curie *also* C, Ci, CU, cu • cuspid (primary dentition) • cycle/cyclic • [L. *centum*] hundred *also* C • [L. *cibus*] meal • specific heat capacity • [L. *cum*] with *also* C, c̄

c̄ [L. *cum*] with *also* C, c

c′ pulmonary end–capillary (blood phase)

CA [L. *commissura anterior*] anterior commissure • calcium antagonist • California (rabbit) • cancer *also* Ca, Can • cancer antigen • caproic acid • carbohydrate antigen • carbonic anhydrase • carcinoma *also* Ca • cardiac–apnea (monitor) • cardiac arrest • cardiac arrhythmia • carotid artery • catecholamine *also* CAT • catechola-minergic • cathode *also* C, Ca, Cath, cath • celiac artery • cellulose acetate • cerebral aqueduct • cervicoaxial • *Chemical Abstracts* (Service) • chemotactic activity *also* CTA • chloroam-phetamine • cholic acid • chronic anovulation • chronologic age • citric

acid • clotting assay • coagglutination (test) • coarctation of the aorta *also* CoA, C of A • Cocaine Anonymous • coefficient of absorption • cold agglutinin • collagen antigen • collagenolytic activity • colloid antigen • commissural associated • common antigen • community acquired • compressed air • con-ceptional age • conditioned abstinence • conditioned air • coronary angioplasty • coronary arrest • coronary artery • corpora allata • corpora amylacea • cortisone acetate • cricoid arch • croup–associated (virus) • cytosine arabino-side • cytotoxic antibody

C/A, c/a Clinitest/Acetest *also* C&A

C&A Clinitest and Acetest *also* C/A, c/a • conscious and alert

Ca calcium • cancer *also* CA • carcinoma *also* CA • carmustine • cathode *also* C, CA, Cath, cath

^{45}Ca calcium–45 (radioisotope)

ca [L. *circa*] about *also* c • candle *also* c

CAA carotid audiofrequency analysis • chloracet-aldehyde • computer–aided assessment • computer-assisted assessment • constitutional aplastic anemia • crystalline amino acids

CAAT computer–assisted axial tomography

CAB captive air bubble •
catheter–associated
bacteriuria • cellulose
acetate butyrate • coronary
artery bypass

CABG coronary artery bypass
graft

CABGS coronary artery
bypass graft surgery

CaBI calcium bone index

CABOP, CA–BOP
cyclophosphamide,
Adriamycin (doxorubicin),
bleomycin, Oncovin
(vincristine), and prednisone

CaBP calcium–binding protein

CABS coronary artery bypass
surgery

CAC cancer (malignant) cell •
cardiac–accelerator center •
cardiac arrest code • carotid
artery canal • circulating
anticoagulant • compre-
hensive ambulatory care

CACB calcium carbonate

CaCC cathodal closure
contraction *also* CCC

CACI computer–assisted
continuous infusion

CACP cisplatin

CaCV *Calicivirus*

CACX cancer of cervix

CAD cadaver *also* Cad • cold
agglutinin disease •
compressed air disease •
computer–assisted design •
computer–assisted
diagnosis • coronary artery
disease • cyclophos-
phamide, Adriamycin
(doxorubicin), and

dacarbazine • cytosine
arabinoside and daunorubicin

Cad cadaver *also* CAD

CADI computer–assisted
diabetic instruction (system)

CADIC cyclophosphamide,
Adriamycin (doxorubicin),
and dacarbazine (DTIC)

CADL Communicative
Abilities in Daily Living

CaDTe cathodal–duration
tetanus

CAE caprine arthritis–
encephalitis • cellulose
acetate electrophoresis •
contingent aftereffects •
coronary artery
embolization •
cyclophosphamide,
Adriamycin (doxorubicin),
and etoposide

CaE calcium excretion

CAEC cardiac arrhythmia
evaluation center

CaEDTA, CaEdTA calcium
disodium edetate •
edathamil calcium
disodium • calcium
disodium ethylenedia-
minetetraacetate

CAER caerulein

CAEV caprine arthritis–
encephalitis virus

CAF cell adhesion factor •
citric acid fermenters •
continuous atrial
fibrillation/flutter •
contract administration
fees • cyclophosphamide,
Adriamycin (doxorubicin),
and fluorouracil

CaF correction of area factor
also ACF

Caf caffeine

CAFP cyclophosphamide, Adriamycin (doxorubicin), fluorouracil, and prednisone

CAFT Clinitron air fluidized therapy

CAFVP cyclophosphamide, Adriamycin (doxorubicin), fluorouracil, vincristine, and prednisone

CAG cholangiogram • chronic atrophic gastritis • continuous ambulatory gamma–globulin (infusion) • coronary angiogram/angiography

CaG calcium gluconate

CAH central alveolar hypoventilation • chronic active hepatitis • chronic aggressive hepatitis • combined atrial hypertrophy • congenital adrenal hyperplasia • congenital adrenogenital hyperplasia • cyanacetic acid hydrazide

CaHA calcium hydroxyapatite

CAHC chronic active hepatitis with cirrhosis

CAHD coronary arteriosclerotic heart disease • coronary atherosclerotic heart disease

CAI complete androgen insensitivity • computer–assisted instruction • confused artificial insemination

CAIS complete androgen insensitivity syndrome

CAL calcium (test) • calculated average life • callus •

calories • chronic airflow limitation • computer–assisted learning

Cal (large) calorie *also* C

cal caliber • (small) calorie *also* c

C_{alb} albumin clearance

Calc calcium

calc calculate/calculated

cal ct calorie count

CALD chronic active liver disease

CALEF, calef [L. *calefac*] make warm • [L. *calefactus*] warmed

CALGB cancer and leukemia group B

calib callibrated

cALL common null cell acute lymphocytic leukemia

CALLA, cALLA common acute lymphocytic leukemia antigen

CAM calf aortic microsome • carminomycin • Caucasian adult male • cell adhesion molecule • cell–associating molecule • chorioallantoic membrane • computer–assisted (or aided) myelography • contralateral axillary metastasis • cyclophosphamide, Adriamycin (doxorubicin), and methotrexate

CaM calmodulin

C_{am} amylase clearance

CAMAC computer–automated measurement and control

CAMB cyclophosphamide, Adriamycin (doxorubicin), methotrexate, and bleomycin

CAMEO cyclophosphamide, Adriamycin (doxorubicin), methotrexate, etoposide, and Oncovin (vincristine)

CAMF cyclophosphamide, Adriamycin (doxorubicin), methotrexate, and fluorouracil

CAMP computer–assisted menu planning • concentration of adenosine monophosphate • cyclophosphamide, Adriamycin (doxorubicin), methotrexate, and procarbazine

cAMP cyclic adenosine monophosphate *also* AMP–c

c amplum [L. *cochleare amplum*] heaping spoonful • tablespoonful

CAMS computer–assisted monitoring system

CAMU cardiac ambulatory monitoring unit • coronary arrhythmia monitoring unit

CaMV cauliflower mosaic virus

CAN cord (umbilical) around neck

CA/N child abuse and neglect

Can cancer *also* CA, Ca

can. cannabis

CANC, canc cancelled

CANCERLIT Cancer Literature

CancerProj Cancer Research Projects

CANP calcium–activated neutral protease

CANS central auditory nervous system

CAO chronic airway obstruction • coronary artery obstruction

Ca$_{O2}$ arterial oxygen concentration

CaOC cathodal opening contraction

CAOD coronary artery occlusive disease

CAOM chronic adhesive otitis media

Ca ox calcium oxalate (crystal)

CAP cancer of prostate • capsule *also* cap., caps. • captopril • catabolite (gene) activator protein • cell attachment protein • cellular acetate propionate • cellulose acetate phthalate • central apical portion • chloramphenicol • chloroacetophenone • cholesteric analysis profile • chronic alcoholic pancreatitis • community– acquired pneumonia • complement–activated plasma • compound action potential • computerized automated psychophysiologic (device) • coupled atrial pacing • cyclic AMP–binding protein • cyclosphosphamide, Adriamycin (doxorubicin), and Platino (cisplatin) • cyclophosphamide, Adriamycin (doxorubicin), and prednisone • cystine aminopeptidase

Ca/P calcium to phosphorus ratio

cap. capacity *also* c • capillary • capsule *also* CAP, caps. • [L. *capiat*] let him take

CAPA caffeine, alcohol, pepper, and aspirin (diet free of) • cancer–associated polypeptide antigen

CAPB central auditory processing battery

CAPD chronic/continuous ambulatory peritoneal dialysis

CAPERS Computer–assisted Psychiatric Evaluation and Review System

capiend [L. *capiendus*] to be taken

cap. moll [L. *capsula mollis*] soft capsule

CAPPS Current and Past Psychopathology Scales

cap. quant vult [L. *capiat quantum vult*] to be taken as much as one wants to

CAPRCA chronic, acquired, pure red cell aplasia

CAPRI Cardiopulmonary Research Institute

CAPS caffeine, alcohol, pepper, and spicy foods (diet free of)

caps. capsule *also* CAP, cap.

CAPYA child and adolescent psychoanalysis

CAR cardiac ambulation routine • chronic articular rheumatism • computer–assisted research • conditioned avoidance response

car. carotid

CARB carbohydrate *also* carb, carbo

carb carbohydrate *also* CARB, carbo • carbonate

CARBAM carbamazepine

carbo carbohydrate *also* CARB, carb

CARD, Card., Cardiol cardiology

CARF Commission on Accreditation of Rehabilitation Facilities

CAROT carotene

CARS childhood autism rating scale • Children's Affective Rating Scale

CART computer–assisted real time transcription

CARTOS computer–assisted reconstruction by tracing of serial sections

CAS calcarine sulcus • calcific aortic stenosis • carbohydrate–active steroid • cardiac adjustment scale • cardiac surgery • carotid artery stenosis • casein • Celite–activated normal serum • Center for Alcohol Studies • cerebral arteriosclerosis • Chemical Abstracts Service • chronic anovulation syndrome • cold agglutinin syndrome • congenital alcoholic syndrome • congenital asplenia syndrome • control adjustment strap • coronary artery spasm

Cas casualty

cas castrated • castration

CASA computer–assisted self–assessment

CASH Commission for Administrative Services in Hospitals

CASHD coronary arteriosclerotic heart disease • coronary atherosclerotic heart disease

CASMD congenital atonic sclerotic muscular dystrophy

CA–SP calcium urine spot (test)

CAS–REGN Chemical Abstracts Service Registry Number

CASRT corrected adjusted sinus (node) recovery time

CASS computer–aided sleep system • Coronary Artery Surgery Study

CAST cardiac arrhythmia suppression trial • Children of Alcoholism Screening Test

C–AST cytoplasmic aspartate aminotransferase

CASTNO cast number (urinalysis)

CAT capillary agglutination test • catalase *also* CAT'ase • cataract *also* cat. • catecholamine *also* CA • cellular atypia •

Children's Apperception Test • chloramphenicol acetyltransferase • chlormerodrin accumulation test • choline acetyltransferase • chronic abdominal tympany • classified anaphylatoxin • computed abdominal tomography • computer–assisted tomography • computed axial tomography • computer of average transients • cytosine arabinoside, Adriamycin (doxorubicin), and thioguanine

cat. catalyst • cataract *also* CAT

CAT–A–KIT Catecholamine Radioenzymatic Assay Kit

CAT'ase catalase *also* CAT

CATCH Community Actions to Control High Blood Pressure

cat c̄ IL cataract with intraocular lens

Cath, cath cathartic • catheterization/catheter/catheterize • cathode *also* C, CA, Ca

CATLINE Catalog On–Line

CAT–S Children's Apperception Test, Supplemental

CATT calcium tolerance test

Cau, Cauc, cauc Caucasian *also* C

caud caudal

CAV computer–assisted ventilation • congenital absence of vagina • congenital adrenal virilism • constant angular velocity • croup–associated virus • cyclophosphamide, Adriamycin (doxorubicin), and vincristine

cav cavity

CAVB complete atrioventricular block

CAVC common arterioventricular canal

CAVD complete atrioventricular dissociation • completion, arithmetic problems, vocabulary, following directions (battery)

C(a–VDO₂) arteriovenous oxygen difference

CAVE CCNU (lomustine), Adriamycin (doxorubicin), and vinblastine

CAVH continuous arteriovenous hemofiltration

CAVHD continuous arterio-venous hemodialysis • continuous arteriovenous hemofiltration (with) dialysis

CA virus croup–associated virus

CAVO common atrioventricular orifice

CAVP cyclosphosphamide, Adriamycin (doxorubicin), vincristine, and prednisone

CAV–P–VP cyclo-phosphamide, Adriamycin (doxorubicin), vincristine, Platino (cisplatin), and VP16–213 (etoposide)

CAW central airways

Cₐw airway conductance

CAWO closing abductory wedge osteotomy

CAZ ceftazidime

CB carbenicillin • carbonated beverage • carotid body • catheterized bladder • ceased breathing • cesarean birth • chair and bed *also* C&B • chest–back • chocolate blood (agar) *also* CB agar • chronic bronchitis • circumflex branch • code blue • color blind • compensated base • conjugated bilirubin • contrast baths • cytochalasin B

C–B, C/B chest–back

C&B chair and bed *also* CB • crown and bridge

CB₁₁ phenadoxone hydrochloride

Cb niobium (columbium)

cb cardboard (or plastic film holder without intensifying screens)

CBA carcinoma–bearing animal • chronic bronchitis and asthma • competitive–binding assay • cost–benefit analysis

CBAB complement–binding antibody

CB agar chocolate blood agar *also* CB

CBAT Coulter battery

CBB Coomassi brilliant blue R–250 (stain)

CBBB complete bundle branch block

CBC carbenicillin *also*

CBCN • cerebrobuccal connective • child behavior characteristics • complete blood (cell) count *also* cbc

cbc complete blood (cell) count *also* CBC

CBCL Child Behavior Checklist

CBCME computer–based continuing medical education

CBCN carbenicillin *also* CBC

CBD cannabidiol • carotid body denervation • closed bladder drainage • common bile duct • community based distribution

CBDC chronic bullous disease of childhood

CBDE common bile duct exploration

CBDL chronic bile duct ligation

CBDS Carcinogenesis Bioassay Data System

CBF capillary blood flow • cerebral blood flow • ciliary beat frequency • coronary blood flow • cortical blood flow

CBFS cerebral blood flow studies

CBFV cerebral blood flow velocity

CBG capillary blood gases • capillary blood glucose • coronary bypass graft • corticosteroid–binding globulin • cortisol–binding globulin

CBG_v corticosteroid–binding globulin variant

CBH chronic benign hepatitis • cutaneous basophilic hypersensitivity

CBI continuous bladder irrigation

CBIL conjugated bilirubin

CBL circulating blood lymphocytes • (umbilical) cord blood leukocytes

Cbl cobalamin

cbl chronic blood loss

CBM capillary basement membrane

CBMMP chronic benign mucous membrane pemphigus

CBMT capillary basement membrane thickness

CBMW capillary basement membrane width

CBN cannibinol • central benign neoplasm • chronic benign neutropenia • Commission on Biological Nomenclature

CBOC completion bed occupancy care

CBP carbohydrate–binding protein • cobalamin– binding protein

CBPPA cyclophosphamide, bleomycin, procarbazine, prednisone, and Adriamycin (doxorubicin)

CBPS coronary bypass surgery

CBR carotid bodies resected • chemical, bacteriologic, and radiologic (warfare) •

chemically bound residue • chronic bed rest • complete bed rest • crude birth rate

C_BR bilirubin clearance

CBRAM controlled partial rebreathing – anesthesia method

CBS chronic brain syndrome • conjugated bile salts • Cruveilhier–Baumgarten syndrome

CBT carotid body tumor • cognitive behavior therapy • computed body tomography

CBV capillary blood (flow) velocity • central blood volume • cerebral blood volume • circulating blood volume • corrected blood volume • Coxsackie B virus • cyclophosphamide, BCNU (carmustine), and VP16–213 (etoposide)

CBVD cerebrovascular disease

CBW chemical and biologic warfare • critical bandwidth (range of frequencies)

CBX computer–based examination

CBZ carbamazepine

Cbz carbobenzoxy chloride

CC calcaneo–cuboid • calcium cyclamate • cardiac catheterization • cardiac cycle • cardio-vascular clinic • carotid–cavernous • case coordinator • caval catheterization • cell culture • cellular compartment • central compartment • cerebral commissure •

cerebral concussion • cervical collar • chest circumference *also* cc • chief complaint • cholecalciferol • chondrocalcinosis • choriocarcinoma *also* CCA • chronic complainer • ciliated cell • circulatory collapse • classical conditioning • clean catch (of urine) • clinical course • closing capacity • coefficient of correlation • colorectal cancer • commission–certified (stain) • complications and comorbidities • compound cathartic • computer calculated • concave *also* Cc, cc • continuing care • contractile component • coracoclavicular • cord compression • coronary collateral • corpus callosum • costochondral • Coulter counter • creatinine clearance *also* C_{cr} • critical care • critical condition • crus cerebri • crus communis • cubic centimeter *also* cc, cm^3, cu cm • cup cell • current complaint • cytochrome C • with correction (with glasses)

C/C chief complaint • cholecystectomy and (operative) cholangiogram • complete upper and lower dentures

C&C cold and clammy • confirmed and compatible

Cc concave *also* CC, cc

cc chest circumference *also* CC • concave *also* CC, Cc • condylocephalic • corrected • cubic centimeter *also* CC, cm^3, cu cm

CCA cephalin cholesterol antigen • chick–cell agglutination (unit) • chimpanzee coryza agent • choriocarcinoma *also* CC • chromated copper arsenak • circumflex coronary artery • colitis colon antigen • common carotid artery • concentrated care area • congenital contractural arachno-dactyly • constitutional chromosome abnormality

CCAP capsule cartilage articular preservation

CCAT conglutinating complement absorption test

CCB calcium channel blocker

CCBV central circulating blood volume

CCC calcium cyanamide (carbimide) citrated • Cancer Care Center • care–cure coordination • cathodal closure contraction *also* CACC, CaCC • central counteradaptive changes • child care clinic • chronic calculous cholecystitis • citrated calcium carbimide • comprehensive cancer center • comprehensive care clinic • consecutive case conference • continuing community care • critical care complex

CC&C colony count and culture

CCCC centrifugal counter-current chromatography

CCCL, CCCl cathodal closure clonus

CCCP carbonyl cyanide *m*–chlorophenyl–hydrazone

CCCR closed–chest cardiac/cardiopulmonary resuscitation

CCCS condom catheter collecting system

CCCT closed craniocerebral trauma

CCCU comprehensive cardiovascular care unit

CCD calibration curve data • charge–coupled device • childhood celiac disease • cortical collecting duct • countercurrent distribution • cumulative cardiotoxic dose

CCDC Canadian Communicable Disease Center

CCDN Central Council for District Nursing

CCE carboline–carboxylic (acid) ester • chamois contagious ecthyma • clubbing, cyanosis, and edema • countercurrent electrophoresis

CCEI Crown–Crisp Experimental Index

CCF carotid–cavernous fistula • centrifuged culture fluid • cephalin–cholesterol flocculation • compound comminuted fracture • congestive cardiac failure • crystal-induced chemotactic factor

CCFA cycloserine–cefoxitin–fructose agar

CCFE cyclophosphamide, cisplatin, fluorouracil, and estramustine

CCG cholecystogram

CCGC capillary column gas chromatography

CCGG cytosine–cytosine–guanine–guanine

CCH chronic cholestatic hepatitis

CCh carbamylcholine

CCHD cyanotic congenital heart disease

CCHP Consumer Choice Health Plan

CCHS congenital central hypoventilation syndrome

CCI chronic coronary insufficiency • corrected count increment

CCJ costochondral junction

CCK cholecystokinin

CCK–8 cholecystokinin octapeptide *also* CCK–OP

CCK–GB cholecystokinin-gallbladder (cholecystogram)

CCKLI cholecystokinin–like immunoreactivity

CCK–OP cholecystokinin octapeptide *also* CCK–8

CCK–PZ cholecystokinin-pancreozymin

CCL carcinoma cell line • cardiac catheterization laboratory • certified cell line • critical carbohydrate level • critical condition list

CCLI composite clinical and laboratory index

CCM cerebrocostomandibular (syndrome) • congestive cardiomyopathy • contralateral competing message • craniocervical malformation • critical care medicine • cyclophosphamide, CCNU (lomustine), and methotrexate

CCMS clean catch midstream (urine) *also* CCMSU • clinical care management system

CCMSU clean–catch midstream urine *also* CCMS

CCMSUA clean–catch midstream urinalysis

CCMT catechol methyltransferase

CCMU critical care medicine unit

CCN caudal central nucleus • coronary care nursing • critical care nursing

CCNS cell–cycle nonspecific (agent)

CCNSC Cancer Chemotherapy National Service Center

CCNU chloroethylcyclo-hexylnitrosourea (lomustine)

CcO$_2$ pulmonary end–capillary blood oxygen concentration

CCOF CCNU, Oncovin (vincristine), and prednisone

CCOF chromosomally competent ovarian failure

C–collar cervical collar

CCP chronic calcifying pancreatitis •

ciliocytophthoria • Crippled Children's Program • cytidine cyclic phosphate

CCPD continuous cycling/cyclical peritoneal dialysis • crystalline calcium pyrophosphate dihydrate

CCPDS Centralized Cancer Patient Data System

CCPR crypt cell production rate

CCR cardiac catheterization recovery • complete continuous remission • continuous complete remission

C$_{cr}$ creatinine clearance *also* CC

CCRC continuing care residential community

CCRN Critical Care Registered Nurse

CCRS carotid chemoreceptor stimulation

CCRU critical care recovery unit

CCS casualty clearing station • cell cycle specific (agent) • cholecystosonography • cloudy cornea syndrome • concentration camp syndrome • costoclavicular syndrome • Crippled Children's Services • Critical Care Services

CC&S cornea, conjunctiva, and sclera

CCSA central chemosensitive area

CCSCS central cervical spinal cord syndrome

CCSG Children's Cancer Study Group

CCT calcitriol • carotid compression tomography • central conduction time • chocolate–coated tablet • closed cerebral trauma • coated compressed tablet • combined cortical thickness • composite cyclic therapy • congenitally corrected transposition (of the great vessels) • controlled cord traction • coronary care team • cranial computed tomography • crude coal tar • cyclocarbothiamine

cct circuit

CCTe cathodal closure tetanus

CCTGA congenitally corrected transposition of the great arteries

CCT in PET crude coal tar in petroleum

CCTV closed circuit television

CCU cardiac care unit • cardiovascular care unit • Cherry–Crandall unit • community care unit • coronary care unit • critical care unit

CCUA clean catch urinalysis

CCUP colpocystourethropexy

CCV CCNU (lomustine), cyclophosphamide, and vincristine • channel catfish virus • conductivity cell volume

CCVB CCNU (lomustine), cyclophosphamide, vincristine, and bleomycine

CCVD chronic cerebrovascular disease

CCVPP CCNU (lomustine), cyclophosphamide, vinblastine, procarbazine, and prednisone

CCW childcare worker • counterclockwise

Ccw chest wall compliance

CCX complications

CD cadaver donor • canine distemper • carbohydrate dehydratase • carbon dioxide • cardiac disease • cardiac dullness • cardiac dysrrhythmia • cardio-vascular deconditioning • cardiovascular disease *also* CVD • Carrel–Dakin (fluid) • caudad/caudal • cefaloridine • celiac disease • cell dissociation • central deposition • cesarean delivered • cesarean delivery • channel down • character disorder • chemical dependency • chemotactic difference • childhood disease • circular dichroism • civil defense • colloid droplet • combination drug • common duct • communicable disease • communication deviance • communication disorders • completely denatured • complicated delivery • conduct disorder • consanguineous donor • contact dermatitis • contagious disease • continuous drainage • control diet • convulsive disorder • convulsive dose • copying drawings • corneal dystrophy • covert dyskinesia • Crohn

disease • crossed diagonal • curative dose • current diagnosis • cutdown • cystic duct • cytarabine and daunorubicin • Czapek–Dox • [L. *conjugata diagonalis*] diagonal conjugate diameter of the pelvis • [L. *colla dextra*] with the right hand

C/D cigarettes per day • cup to disc ratio

C&D curettage and dessication • cystoscopy and dilation

CD$_{50}$ median curative dose

Cd cadmium • caudal *also* cd • coccygeal *also* cd • color denial • condylion

cd candela • caudal *also* Cd • coccygeal *also* Cd • cord

CDA Certified Dental Assistant • chenodeoxycholic acid • ciliary dyskinesia activity • complement–dependent antibody • completely denatured alcohol • congenital dyserythropoietic anemia

CDAA chlorodiallylacetamide (herbicide)

CDAI Crohn Disease Activity Index

CDAK Cordis Dow Artificial Kidney

CDB, C&DB cough and deep breath

CDC calculated date of confinement • cancer detection center • capillary diffusion capacity •

carboplatin, doxorubicin, and cyclophosphamide • cardiac diagnostic center • cell division cycle • Centers for Disease Control • chenodeoxycholate • chenodeoxycholic (acid) *also* CDCA • child development clinic • Communicable Disease Center • complement–dependent cytotoxicity • Crohn disease of the colon

CD–C controlled drinker–control

CDCA chenodeoxycholic acid *also* CDC

CDCF *Clostridium difficile* culture filtrate

CDD certificate of disability for discharge • chronic degenerative disease • chronic disabling dermatosis • critical degree of deformation

CDDP *cis*–diamminedichloroplatinum

CDE canine distemper encephalitis • Certified Diabetes Educator • chlordiazepoxide • common duct exploration

CD–E controlled drinker–experimental

CDF chondrodystrophia foetalis

CDFR cumulative duration of the first remission

CDG central developmental groove

CDGD constitutional delay in growth and development

CDH ceramide dihexoside • chronic daily headache • chronic disease hospital • congenital diaphragmatic hernia • congenital dislocation of hip • congenital dysplasia of hip

CDI cell–directed inhibitor • central diabetes insipidus • Children's Depression Inventory • chronic diabetes insipidus

CDILD chronic diffuse interstitial lung disease

CDK climatic droplet keratopathy

CDL chlordeoxylincomycin • Copying Drawings with Landmarks

CDLE chronic discoid lupus erythematosus

CDLS Cornelia de Lange syndrome

CDM chemically defined medium • clinical decision making

cDNA complementary deoxyribonucleic acid

CDP chlordiazepoxide • chronic destructive periodontitis • collagenase–digestible protein • constant distending pressure • continuous distending pressure • Coronary Drug Project • cytidine diphosphate

CDPC cytidine diphosphate choline

CDPS common duct pigment stones

CDQ corrected development quotient

CDR calcium–dependent regulator • chronologic drinking record • computed digital radiography • continuing disability review

CDR(H) cup–to–disc ratio horizontal

CDRS–R Children's Depression Rating Scale–Revised

CDR(V) cup–to–disc ratio vertical

CDS caudal dysplasia syndrome • Chemical Data System • cul–de–sac • cumulative duration of survival

cd–sr candela–steradian

CDSS clinical decision support system

CDT carbon dioxide therapy • Certified Dental Technician • combined diphtheria tetanus

CDTe cathode duration tetanus

CDU chemical dependency unit • cumulative dose unit

CDV canine distemper virus

CDX chlordiazepoxide *also* CDZ

CDYN, Cdyn, C$_{dyn}$ dynamic compliance (of lung in pulmonary function test)

CDZ chlordiazepoxide *also* CDX

CE California encephalitis • cardiac emergency • cardiac enlargement • cardioesophageal (junction) *also* CED • cataract extraction • cell extract • central episiotomy • chemical energy • chick embryo • chloroform–ether • cholera exotoxin • cholesterol esters • cholinesterase • chromatoelectrophoresis • clinical emphysema • columnar epithelium • community education • conjugated estrogens • constant error • constant estrus • continuing education • contractile element • contrast echocardiology • converting enzyme • crude extract • stroke • cytopathic effect

C–E chloroform–ether

C&E consultation and examination • cough and exercise • curettage and electrodessication

Ce cerium

CEA carcinoembryonic antigen • carotid endarterectomy • cholesterol–esterifying activity • cholinesterase • cost–effectiveness analysis • crystalline egg albumin

CEARP Continuing Education Approval and Recognition Program

CEB cotton elastic bandage

CEBD controlled extrahepatic biliary drainage

CEBV chronic Epstein–Barr virus

CEC ciliated epithelial cell • contractile electrical complex

CECT contrast enhancement computed tomography

CED chondroectodermal dysplasia • chronic enthusiasm disorder • cultural/ethnic diversity

CEE chick embryo extract

CEEC calf esophagus epithelial cell

CEEV Central European encephalitis virus

CEF centrifugation extractable fluid • chick embryo fibroblast • constant electric field

CEG chronic erosive gastritis

CEH cholesterol ester hydrolase

CEHC calf embryonic heart cell

CEI character education inquiry • continuous extravascular infusion • converting enzyme inhibitor • corneal epithelial involvement

CEID crossed electroimmunodiffusion

CEJ cardioesophageal junction *also* CE • cement–enamel junction

CEK chick embryo kidney

CEL cardiac exercise laboratory • Celsius *also* C, Cel

Cel Celsius *also* C, CEL

Cell celluloid

CELOV chick embryonal lethal orphan virus

CEM conventional transmission electron microscope

cemf counterelectromotive force

CEN Certificate for Emergency Nursing

cen central • centromere

CENP centromere protein

CENT, cent. centigrade *also* C • centimeter *also* cm • central *also* C

CEO chick embryo origin • chloroethylene oxide

CEOT calcifying epithelial odontogenic tumor

CEP chronic eosinophilic pneumonia • chronic erythropoietic porphyria • cognitive evoked potential • congenital erythropoietic porphyria • continuing education program • cortical evoked potential • countercurrent electrophoresis • counterelectrophoresis

CEPA chloroethane phosphoric acid

CEPB Carpentier–Edwards porcine bioprosthesis

CEPH cephalic *also* ceph • cephalin *also* ceph • cephalosporin

ceph cephalic *also* CEPH • cephalosporin *also* CEPH

CEPH FLOC, ceph–floc cephalin flocculation (test)

CEPT cyclophosphamide, fluorouracil, prednisone, and tamoxifen

CEQ Council on Environmental Quality

CER capital expenditure

review • ceramide • conditioned emotional response • conditioned escape response • control electrical rhythm • cortical evoked response

CE&R central episiotomy and repair

CERA cardiac evoked response audiometry

CERD chronic end–stage renal disease

CERP Continuing Education Recognition Program

Cert, cert certificate *also* CTF • certified

CERULO ceruloplasmin

cerv cervical • cervix

CES cat's–eye syndrome • central excitatory state • chronic electrophysiologic study • cognitive environmental stimulation

CESD cholesterol ester storage disease

CET capital expenditure threshold • cephalothin • congenital eyelid tetrad • controlled environment treatment

CETE Central European tick–borne encephalitis

CEU congenital ectropion uveae • continuing education unit

CEV cyclophosphamide, etoposide, and vincristine

CEZ cefazolin

CF calcium leucovorin • calf blood flow • calibration factor • cancer–free •

carbol–fuchsin (stain) • cardiac failure • carotid foramen • carrier–free • cascade filtration • case file • Caucasian female • cephalothin • characteristic frequency • chemotactic factor • chest and left leg (lead in electrocardiography) • Chiari–Frommel (syndrome) • chick fibroblast • choroid fissure • Christmas factor • cisplatin and fluorouracil • citrovorum factor • climbing fiber • clotting factor • colicin factor • collected fluid • colonization factor • colony–forming • color and form • [L. *confer*] compare *also* cf, cp • complement fixation *also* com fix • completely follicular • constant frequency • contractile force • coronary flow • cough frequency • count fingers (visual acuity test) *also* C/F, cf • coupling factor • cycling fibroblast • cystic fibrosis *also* C/F

C'F complement fixing

C/F colored female • count fingers (visual acuity test) *also* CF, cf • cystic fibrosis *also* CF

C&F cell and flare • curretage and fulguration

CFII Cohn fraction II

Cf californium • [L. *ferrum*] iron carrier

cf bring together • centrifugal force • [L. *confer*] compare *also* CF, cp • count fingers (visual acuity test) *also* CF, C/F

CFA clofibric acid • colonization factor antigen • colony–forming assay • common femoral artery • complement–fixing antibody • complete Freund adjuvant • cryptogenic fibrosing alveolitis

CFAC complement–fixing antibody consumption

C–factor cleverness factor

CFB central fibrous body

CFC capillary filtration coefficient • chloro-fluorocarbon • colony–forming capacity/cells • continuous flow centrifugation

CFCL continuous flow centrifugation leukapheresis

CFC–S colony–forming cells–spleen

CFD cephalofacial deformity • craniofacial dysostosis

CFF critical flicker frequency • critical flicker fusion (test) *also* cff • critical fusion frequency *also* cff • cystic fibrosis factor • Cystic Fibrosis Foundation

cff critical flicker fusion *also* CFF • critical fusion frequency *also* CFF

CFFA cystic fibrosis factor activity

Cf–Fe carrier–bound iron [L. *ferrum*]

CFH Council on Family Health

CFI cardiac function index • chemotactic–factor inactivator • complement fixation inhibition • confrontation fields intact

CFL cisplatin, fluorouracil, and leucovorin calcium

CFM chlorofluoromethane • close–fitting mask • craniofacial microsomia • cyclophosphamide, fluorouracil, and citoxantrone

cfm cubic feet per minute

CFNS chills, fever, and night sweats

CFO chief financial officer

CFP chronic false positive • Clinical Fellowship Program • cyclophos-phamide, fluorouracil, and prednisone • cystic fibrosis of pancreas • cystic fibrosis patients/protein

CFPD critical frequency of photic driving

CFR case–fatality ratio • citrovorum–factor rescue • complement–fixation reaction • cyclic flow reduction

CFS call for service • cancer family syndrome • chronic fatigue syndrome • contoured femoral stem • craniofaciostenosis • crush fracture syndrome • Cystic Fibrosis Society

cfs cubic feet per second

CFSE crystal field stabilization energy

CFSTI Clearinghouse for

Federal Scientific and Technical Information

CFT cardiolipin flocculation test • clinical full–time • complement fixation test • complement–fixing titer

CFU colony–forming unit • color–forming unit

CFU–C colony–forming unit– culture

CFU–E colony–forming unit– erythrocyte • colony– forming unit–erythroid

CFU$_{EOS}$ colony–forming unit– eosinophil

CFU–F colony–forming unit– fibroblastoid

CFU$_{GM}$ colony–forming unit– granulocyte macrophage

CFU$_L$ colony–forming unit– lymphoid

CFU$_M$, CFU$_{MEG}$ colony– forming unit– megakaryocyte

CFU/mL colony–forming units/ mL

CFU$_{NM}$ colony–forming unit– neutrophil–monocyte

CFU–S, CFU$_S$ colony– forming unit–spleen • colony–forming unit–stem (cell)

CFW cancer–free white (mouse) *also* CFWM • Carworth farm (mouse), Webster strain

CFWM cancer–free white mouse *also* CFW

CFX cefoxitin • circumflex (coronary artery)

CFZ capillary–free zone

CFZC continuous–flow zonal centrifugation

CG calcium gluconate • cardiogreen • center of gravity *also* cg • central gray • choking gas (phosgene) • cholecystogram • cholecystography • choriogenic gynecomastia • chorionic gonadotropin • chronic glomerulo- nephritis • cingulate gyrus • colloidal gold • contact guarding • control group • cryoglobulin • cystine guanine

cg center of gravity *also* CG • centigram • chemoglobulin

CGA catabolite gene activator

CGAS Children's Global Assessment Scale

CGB chronic gastrointestinal (tract) bleeding

CGC Certified Gastrointestinal Clinician

CGD chromosomal gonadal dysgenesis • chronic granulomatous disease

CGDE contact glow discharge electrolysis

CGFH congenital fibrous histiocytoma

CGH chorionic gonadotropic hormone

CGI chronic granulomatous inflammation • Clinical Global Impression (Scale)

CGL chronic granulocytic leukemia • correction with glasses *also* c gl

c gl correction with glasses *also* CGL

CGM central gray matter (spinal cord)

cgm centigram

CGMMV cucumber green mottle mosaic virus

cGMP cyclic guanosine monophosphate

CGN chronic glomerulonephritis • Convalescent Growing Nursery

CGNB composite ganglioneuroblastoma

CG/OQ cerebral glucose-oxygen quotient

CGP chorionic growth hormone prolactin • choline glycerophosphatide • circulating granulocyte pool

CGS cardiogenic shock • catgut suture • centimeter–gram–second (system) *also* cgs

cgs centimeter–gram–second (system) *also* CGS

CGT chorionic gonadotropin • cyclodextrin glucanotransferase

CGTT cortisol/cortisone glucose tolerance test

cGy centigray

CH case history • casein hydrolysate • Chédiak–Higashi (syndrome) • child (children) *also* Ch • Chinese hamster • chloral hydrate • cholesterol *also* Ch, CHO, CHOL, chol • Christchurch chromosome

also Ch^1 • chronic hepatitis • chronic hypertension • Clarke–Hadfield (syndrome) • cluster headache • common hepatic (duct) • communicating hydrocele • complete healing • congenital hypothyroidism • Conradi–HHnermann (syndrome) • continuous heparinization • convalescent hospital • crown–heel (length) • cycloheximide • wheelchair

C$_H$ constant domain of H chain

C&H cocaine and heroin

CH$_{50}$ (total serum) hemolytic complement

Ch chest *also* ch • Chido (antibody) • chief *also* ch • child *also* CH, ch • cholesterol *also* CH, CHO, CHOL, chol • choline *also* ch • chromosome

Ch^1 Christchurch chromosome *also* CH

cH hydrogen ion concentration

ch chest *also* Ch • chief *also* Ch • child *also* CH, Ch • choline *also* Ch • chronic

CHA Catholic Hospital Association • chronic hemolytic anemia • common hepatic artery • congenital hypoplastic anemia • continuous heated aerosols • cyclohexyladenosine • cyclohexylamine

ChA choline acetylase

ChAc, ChAct choline acetyltransferase

CHAD cyclophosphamide, hexamethylmelamine, Adriamycin (doxorubicin), and cisplatin

CHAI continuous hepatic artery infusion

CHAID chi–square automatic interaction detection

CHAL chronic haloperidol

CHAM–OCA cyclophosphamide, hydroxyurea, actinomycin D (dactinomycin), methotrexate, Oncovin (vincristine), citrovorum factor (leucovorin), and Adriamycin (doxorubicin)

CHAMPUS Civilian Health and Medical Programs of Uniformed Services

CHAMPVA Civilian Health and Medical Program of Veterans Administration

Chang C Chang conjunctiva cells

Chang L Chang liver cells

CHAP Certified Hospital Admission Program • Child Health Assessment Program • cyclophospha-mide, hexamethylmelamine, Adriamycin (doxorubicin), and Platino (cisplatin)

CHARGE coloboma, heart disease, atresia choanae, retarded growth and retarded development and/ or CNS anomalies, genital hypoplasia, and ear anomalies and/or deafness (syndrome)

CHAS Center for Health Administration Studies

CHAT, ChaT choline acetyltransferase

CHB complete/congenital heart block

CHBHA congenital Heinz body hemolytic anemia

CHC community health center/ council

CHCP correctional health care program

CHD center hemodialysis • Chediak–Higashi disease • childhood disease(s) • chronic hemodialysis • common hepatic duct • congenital heart disease • congenital hip disease/ dysplasia • congestive heart disease • constitutional hepatic dysfunction • coordinate home care • coronary/ cyanotic heart disease • cyclophosphamide, hexamethylmelamine, cisplatin

CHE, ChE cholesterol ester • cholinesterase

CHEC community hypertension evaluation clinic

CHEF Chinese hamster embryo fibroblast

Chem chemical • chemistry

CHEMLINE Chemical Dictionary On–Line

chemo chemotherapy

CHEP Cuban/Haitian Entrant Program

CHERSS continuous high–amplitude electroenceph-alogram rhythmical synchronous slowing

CHEST Chick Embryotoxicity Screening Test

CHF chick embryo fibroblast • congenital hepatic fibrosis • chronic/congestive heart failure • Crimean hemorrhagic fever • cyclophosphamide, hexamethylmelamine, and 5–fluorouracil

CHFV combined high–frequency ventilation

CHG, chg change • changed

Ch Gn chronic glomerulomephritis

CHH cartilage–hair hypoplasia

CHI closed head injury • creatinine height index

chi (X, χ) 22nd letter of the Greek alphabet

χ_2 chi–squared (distribution, test)

χ_e electric susceptibility

χ_m magnetic susceptibility

CHILD congenital hemidysplasia with ichthyosiform erythroderma and limb defects (syndrome)

CHINA chronic infectious neuropathic/neurotropic agent

CHINS child in need of service (petition)

CHIP comprehensive health insurance plan • comprehensive hospital infections project

Chix chickenpox *also* CHPX, chpx, Cp

CHL Chinese hamster lung • chlorambucil • chloramphenicol

Chl, chl chloroform *also* chlor

CHLA cyclohexyllinoleic acid

Chlb chlorobutanol

CHLD chronic hypoxic lung disease

chlor chloride *also* Cl • chloroform *also* Chl, chl

chloro chloramphenicol *also* C, CMC, CP

CHMD clinical hyaline membrane disease

CHN carbon, hydrogen, and nitrogen • central hemorrhagic necrosis • Certified Hemodialysis Nurse • child neurology • Chinese (hamster) • community health network

CHO carbohydrate *also* C • Chinese hamster ovary • cholesterol *also* C, CH, Ch, CHOL, chol • chorea • cyclophosphamide, hydroxydaunorubicin, and Oncovin (vincristine)

C_{H2O} water clearance

Cho choline

choc chocolate

CHOI considered characteristic of osteogenesis imperfecta

CHOL, chol cholesterol *also* C, CH, Ch, CHO

c̄hold withhold

Chole cholecystectomy

chol est cholesterol esters

CHOP cyclophosphamide,

hydroxydaunomycin, Oncovin (vincristine), and prednisone

CHOR cyclophosphamide, hydroxydaunorubicin, Oncovin (vincristine), and radiation

CHP capillary hydrostatic pressure • charcoal hemoperfusion • child psychiatry • comprehensive health planning • coordinating hospital physician • cutaneous hepatic porphyria

ChP chest physician

CHPX, chpx chickenpox *also* CHIX, Cp

CHQ chlorquinol (topical anti–infective)

CHR Cercarien–Hüllen–Reaktion (test)

chr chromosome • chronic *also* chron

c hr candle hour

c–hr curie–hour *also* ci–hr

ChRBC chicken red blood cell *also* CRBC

ChrBrSyn chronic brain syndrome

CHRIS Cancer Hazards Ranking and Information System

chron chronic *also* chr • chronological

CHRS cerebrohepatorenal syndrome • congenital hereditary retinoschisis

CHS central hypoventilation syndrome • Chediak–Higashi syndrome •

cholinesterase • chondroitin sulfate compression hip screw • contact hypersensitivity

CHSD Children's Health Services Division

CHSS cooperative health statistics system

CHT closed head trauma • contralateral head turning

ChTg chymotrypsinogen

ChTK chicken thymidine kinase

CHU closed head unit

CHV canine herpesvirus

CI cardiac index • cardiac insufficiency • cell immunity • cell inhibition • cephalic index • cerebral infarction • cesium implant • chain initiating • chemical ionization • chemotactic index • chemotherapeutic index • chronically infected • clinical impression • clinical investigator/ investigation • clomipramine • clonus index • closure index • cochlear implant • coefficient of intelligence • colloidal iron • colony inhibition • color index • complete iridectomy • confidence interval • contamination index • *Colour Index* • continuous infusion • coronary insufficiency • corrected count increment • crystalline insulin • cytotoxic index

Ci curie *also* C, c, CU, cu

CIA canine inherited ataxia • chronic idiopathic anhidrosis • chymotrypsin inhibitor activity • colony-inhibiting activity

CIAA competitive insulin autoantibodies

CIAED collagen–induced autoimmune ear disease

CIB cytomegalic inclusion bodies

CIB, cib crying–induced bronchospasm • [L. *cibus*] food

CIBD chronic inflammatory bowel disease

CIBHA congenital inclusion–body hemolytic anemia

CIBP chronic intractable benign pain

CIC cardioinhibitor center • Certified Infection Control • circulating immune complex • constant initial concentration • coronary intensive care

CICA cervical internal carotid artery

CICE combined intracapsular cataract extraction

CICU cardiac intensive care unit • cardiovascular inpatient care unit • coronary intensive care unit

CID Central Institute for the Deaf • central integrative deficit • cervical immobilization device • chick infective dose • combined immunodeficiency disease • cytomegalic inclusion disease

CIDEP chemically–induced dynamic electron polarization

CIDP chronic inflammatory demyelinating polyradioneuropathy

CIDS cellular immunodeficiency syndrome • continuous insulin delivery system

CIE countercurrent immunoelectrophoresis • counterimmunoelectrophoresis *also* CIEP • crossed immunoelectrophoresis *also* CIEP

CIEA continuous infusion epidural analgesia

CIE–C counter-immunoelectrophoresis-colorimetric

CIE–D counter-immunoelectrophoresis-densitometric

CIEP counterimmuno-electrophoresis *also* CIE • crossed immuno-electrophoresis *also* CIE

CIF cartilage induction factor • claims inquiry form • cloning inhibitory factor

CIG, cigs cigarettes • cold–insoluble globulin

CIg intracytoplasmic immunoglobulin

cIgM cytoplasmic immunoglobulin M

CIH carbohydrate–induced hyperglyceridemia • Certificate in Industrial Health • children in hospital

CIHD chronic ischemic heart disease

ci–hr curie–hour *also* c–hr

CII Carnegie Interest Inventory

CIIA common internal iliac artery

CIIPS chronic idiopathic intestinal pseudo–obstruction syndrome

CIIS Cattell Infant Intelligence Scale

CIL Center for Independent Living

CIM cimetidine • cortical induction of movement • cortically induced movement • Cumulated Index Medicus

Ci/mL curies per milliliter

CIMS chemical ionization mass spectrometry • clinical information scale • Conflict in Marriage Scale

CIN cerebriform intradermal nevus • cervical intraepithelial neoplasia • chronic interstitial nephritis • cinoxacin

C$_{IN}$, C$_{in}$ inulin clearance

CIN 1, CIN I cervical intraepithelial neoplasia, grade 1

CIN 2, CIN II cervical intraepithelial neoplasia, grade 2

CIN 3, CIN III cervical intraepithelial neoplasia, grade 3

CINE chemotherapy–induced nausea and emesis • cineangiogram

CIOP chromosomally incompetent ovarian failure

CIP Carcinogen Information Program • Cardiac Injury Panel • cellular immunocompetence profile • chronic idiopathic polyradiculoneuropathy • chronic inflammatory polyneuropathy *also* CIPN

CIPD chronic inflammatory polyradiculoneuropathy, demyelinating • chronic intermittent peritoneal dialysis

CIPF clinical illness promotion factor

CIPN chronic inflammatory polyneuropathy *also* CIP

cir circuit • circular • circumference *also* Circ, circ

Circ, circ circulation • circumcision *also* circum • circumference *also* cir

circ & sen circulation and sensation

circum circumcision *also* Circ, circ

CIRR cirrhosis

CIS carcinoma in situ • catheter–induced spasm • central inhibitory state • Chemical Information Service • clinical information system

CI–S calculus index, simplified

CIS cingulate sulcus

CISCA cisplatin,

cyclophosphamide, and Adriamycin (doxorubicin)

cis–DDP *cis*–diamminedichloroplatinum (cisplatin)

CIT citrate *also* cit • combined intermittent therapy • conjugated–immunoglobulin technique • conventional immunosuppresive therapy • conventional insulin therapy

cit citrate *also* CIT

cit disp [L. *cito dispensetur*] dispense quickly

CIU chronic idiopathic urticaria

CIV Chilo iridescent virus • common iliac vein • continuous intravenous (infusion)

CIVII continuous intravenous insulin infusion

CIXU constant infusion excretory urogram

CJD Creutzfeldt–Jakob disease

CJR centric jaw relationship

CJS Creutzfeldt–Jakob syndrome

CK calf kidney • chicken kidney • cholecystokinin • choline kinase • contralateral knee *also* ck • creatine kinase • cyanogen chloride

CK$_1$, CK$_2$, CK$_3$ isoenzymes of creatine kinase

ck check(ed) • contralateral knee *also* CK

CK–BB creatine kinase BB band • isoenzyme of

creatine kinase with brain subunits

CKC cold–knife conization

CKG cardiokymograph/cardiokymography

CK–ISO creatine kinase isoenzyme

CK–MB isoenzyme of creatine kinase with muscle and brain subunits

CK–MM isoenzyme of creatine kinase with muscle subunits

CK–PZ cholecystokinin–pancreozymin

CKW clockwise

CL capacity of the lung • capillary lumen • cardinal ligament • cardiolipin • cell line • center line • centralis lateralis • chemiluminescence • chest and left arm (lead in electrocardiography) • cholelithiasis • cholesterol–lecithin • chronic leukemia • cirrhosis of liver • clamp lamp • clear liquid • cleft lip • clinical laboratory • cloudy *also* cl, cldy • complex loading • compliance of the lungs *also* C_L • composite lymphoma • confidence level • contact lenses • continence line • corpus luteum *also* cl • cricoid lamina • criterion level • critical list • current liabilities • cutis laxa • cycle length • cytotoxic lymphocyte

CL1–CL5 Papanicolaou class 1 through 5

C–L consultation–liaison (psychiatry)

C$_L$ compliance of the lungs *also* CL • constant domain of L chain

Cl chloride *also* chlor • chlorine • clavicle • clear • clinic *also* cl • clonus • closure *also* cl • colistin

cL centiliter *also* cl

cl centiliter *also* cL • clavicle • cleft • clinic *also* Cl • closure *also* Cl • cloudy *also* CL, cldy • corpus luteum *also* CL

CLA Certified Laboratory Assistant • cervico-linguoaxial • community living arrangements • contralateral local anesthesia • cyclic lysine anhydride

CLAH congenital lipoid adrenal hyperplasia

C lam cervical laminectomy

CLAS congenital localized absence of skin

class. classification

CLAV, clav clavicle

CLB chlorambucil • curvilinear body

CLBBB complete left bundle–branch block

CLC Charcot–Leyden crystal • cork, leather, and celastic (orthotic)

CL/CP cleft lip and cleft palate

CLD central language disorder • chronic liver disease • chronic lung disease • congenital limb deficiency • crystal ligand field

cld cleared • colored

CLDH choline dehydrogenase

CLDM clindamycin

cldy cloudy *also* CL, cl

CLE centrilobular emphysema • continuous lumbar epidural (anesthesia)

CLED cystine–lactose electrolyte–deficient (agar)

cler clear

CLF cardiolipin fluorescence (antibody) • cholesterol–lecithin flocculation

CLH chronic lobular hepatitis • cutaneous lymphoid hyperplasia

CLI corpus luteum insufficiency

CLIA Clinical Laboratories Improvement Act

CLIF cloning inhibitory factor • *Crithidia luciliae* immunofluorescence

Clin, clin clinic

Clin Path clinical pathology

Clin Proc clinical procedure(s)

CLINPROT Clinical Cancer Protocols

CLIP cerebral lipidosis (without visceral involvement and with onset of disease past infancy) • corticotropin–like intermediate lobe peptide

CLL cholesterol–lowering lipid • chronic lymphatic leukemia • chronic lymphocytic leukemia • cow lung lavage

CLLE columnar–lined lower esophagus

cl liq clear liquid

CLML Current List of Medical Literature

CLMN complete lower motor neuron (lesion)

clmp clumped

CLMV cauliflower mosaic virus

CLN computer liaison nurse

CLO cod liver oil

CLOF clofibrate

C–loop anatomical position (shape) of duodenum

CLOT R clot retraction

CLP chymotrypsin–like protein • cleft lip with cleft palate *also* CL&P • cycle length, paced

CL&P cleft lip and palate *also* CLP

CIP clinical pathology

Clpal cleft palate *also* CP

CLRO community leave for reorientation

CLS Clinical Laboratory Scientist

CLSH corpus luteum stimulating hormone

CLSL chronic lymphosarcoma (cell) leukemia

CLSP clinical laboratory specialist

CLT Certified Laboratory Technician • chronic lymphocytic thyroiditis • clinical laboratory technician/technologist • clot lysis time • clotting time

CLV constant linear velocity

CL VOID clean voided specimen (urine)

ClVPP chlorambucil, vinblastine, procarbazine, and prednisone

CLX cloxacillin

clysis hypodermoclysis

CM California mastitis (test) • calmodulin • capreomycin • carboxymethyl cellulose *also* CMC • cardiac monitor • cardiac muscle • cardiomyopathy *also* CMP • Caucasian male • cell membrane • center of mass • centrum medianum • cerebral mantle • cervicle mucus • chemotactic migration • Chick–Martin (coefficient) • chloroquine–mepacrine • chondromalacia • chopped meat (medium) • chylomicron • circular muscle • circulating monocyte • clinical medicine • coccidioidal meningitis • cochlear microphonic(s) • common migraine • community meeting • competing message • complete medium • complications *also* cm • conditioned medium • congenital malformation • congestive myocardiopathy • continuous murmur • contrast medium • copulatory mechanism • costal margin • cow's milk • culture medium • cystic mesothelioma • cytometry • cytoplasmic membrane • [Fr. *crête manche*] narrow–diameter endosseous screw implant • [L. *cras mane*] tomorrow morning *also* cm

C/M counts per minute *also* CPM, cpm

C&M cocaine and morphine

Cm curium • maximal clearance *also* C_m

C_m maximal clearance

cM centimorgan

cm centimeter *also* CENT, cent. • complications *also* CM • costal margin • [L. *cras mane*] tomorrow morning *also* CM

cm² square centimeter

cm³ cubic centimeter *also* CC, cc

CMA *Candida* metabolic antigen • Certified Medical Assistant • chronic metabolic acidosis • compound myopic astigmatism • cow's milk allergy • cultured macrophages

CMAF centrifuged microaggregate filter

c magnum [L. *cochleare magnum*] tablespoon/ tablespoonful

CMAmg corticomedial amygdaloid (nucleus)

CMAP compound muscle/ motor action potential

CMB carbolic methylene blue • Central Midwives' Board • chloromercuribenzoate

CMBBT cervical mucous basal body temperature

CMC carboxymethylcellulose *also* CM • care management continuity • carpometacarpal • cell–mediated cytolysis/ cytotoxicity • chloramphenicol *also* C, chloro, CP • Chloromycetin • chronic mucocutaneous candidiasis *also* CMCC • critical micellar concentration • cyclophosphamide, methotrexate, and CCNU (lomustine)

CMCC chronic mucocutaneous candidiasis *also* CMC

CMCt care management continuity (across settings)

CMD childhood/congenital muscular dystrophy • count median diameter (of particles) • cytomegalic disease

CME cervical mediastinal exploration • cervical mucous extract • continuing medical education • crude marijuana extract • cystic/ cystoid macular edema

CMER current medical evidence of record

CMF calcium–magnesium free • catabolite modular factor • chondromyxoid fibroma • cortical magnification factor • craniomandibulofacial • cyclophosphamide, methotrexate, and fluorouracil

CMFE calcium and magnesium free plus ethylenediaminetetraacetic acid

CMFH cyclophosphamide, methotrexate, fluorouracil, and hydroxyurea

CMFP cyclophosphamide, methotrexate, fluorouracil, and prednisone

CMF–TAM cyclophosphamide, methotrexate, fluorouracil, and tamoxifen

CMFV cyclophosphamide, methotrexate, fluorouracil, and vincristine

CMFVP cyclophosphamide, methotrexate, fluorouracil, vincristine, and prednisone

CMG canine myasthenia gravis • chopped meat glucose (medium) • congenital myasthenia gravis • cyanmethemo-globin • cystometrogram/cystometrography

CMGN chronic membranous glomerulonephritis

CMGS chopped meat–glucose–starch (medium)

CMGT chromosome–mediated gene transfer

CMH congenital malformation of heart

CMHC community mental health center

CMHN Community Mental Health Nurse

cm H_2O centimeters of water (cuff pressure)

CMI carbohydrate metabolism index • care management integration • cell–mediated immunity • cell multiplication inhibition • chronically mentally ill • chronic mesenteric ischemia • circulating microemboli index • computer–managed instruction • Cornell Medical Index

CMID cytomegalic inclusion disease

c/min cycles per minute *also* cpm

CMIR cell–mediated immune response

CMIT Current Medical Information and Terminology

CMJ carpometacarpal joint

CMK chloromethyl ketone • congenital multicystic kidney

CML cell–mediated lymphocytotoxicity/lympholysis • cell–mediated lysis • chronic myelocytic/myelogenous/myeloid leukemia • cross midline • count median length

CMM cell–mediated mutagenesis • cutaneous malignant melanoma

cmm cubic millimeter *also* cu mm, mm^3

cm/m² centimeters per square meter

CMME chloromethyl methyl ether (carcinogen at technical grade)

CMML chronic myelomonocytic leukemia

CMN caudal mediastinal node • cystic medial necrosis

CMN–AA cystic medial necrosis of ascending aorta

CMO calculated mean organism • cardiac minute output • card made out • Chief Medical Officer • comfort measures only • corticosterone methyl oxidase

cMO centimorgan

CMoL chronic monoblastic/ monocytic leukemia

CMOMC cell meeting our morphologic criteria

C–MOPP cyclophosphamide, mechlorethamine, Oncovin (vincristine), procarbazine, and prednisone

CMOR craniomandibular orthopedic repositioning device

CMOS complementary metal– oxide semiconductor (logic)

CMP cardiomyopathy *also* CM • cervical mucus penetration • chondromalacia patellae • competitive medical plans • comprehensive medical plan • cytidine monophosphate

CMP–FX complement fixation

CMPGN chronic membranoproliferative glomerulonephritis

CMPT cervical musus penetration test

CMR cerebral metabolic rate • common mode rejection • crude mortality ratio

CMRG cerebral metabolic rate of glucose

CMRL cerebral metabolic rate of lactate

CMRNG chromosomally mediated resistant *Neisseria gonorrhoeae*

CMRO, CMRO$_2$ cerebral metabolic rate of oxygen

CMRR common mode rejection ratio (of amplifiers)

CMS cardiomediastinal silhouette • central material section/supply • cervical mucous solution • Christian Medical Society • chromosome modification site • chronic myelodysplastic syndrome • circulation motion sensation • clean, midstream (urine) • click murmur syndrome • clofibrate–induced muscular syndrome • Clyde Mood Scale • council of medical staffs

CMS, cms [L. *cras mane sumendus*] to be taken tomorrow morning

cm/s centimeters per second

CMSS circulation, motor (ability), sensation, and swelling

CMSUA clean, midstream urinalysis

CMT California mastitis test • cancer multistep therapy • catechol methyltransferase • Certified Medical Transcriptionist • Charcot–Marie–Tooth (disease/syndrome) • chronic motor tic • circus movement tachycardia • continuous memory test • Current Medical Terminology

CMTD Charcot–Marie–Tooth disease

CMU cardiac monitoring unit • chlorophenyldimethylurea • complex motor unit

CMUA continuous motor unit activity

CMV cisplatin, methotrexate, and vinblastine • controlled/conventional mechanical ventilation • cool mist vaporizer • cucumber mosaic virus • cytomegalic (inclusion) virus • cytomegalovirus

CMVS culture midvoid specimen

CMVIG cytomegalovirus immune globulin

CN caudate nucleus • cellulose nitrate • charge nurse • child nutrition • clinical nursing • cochlear nucleus • congenital nephrosis • congenital nystagmus • cranial nerve • Crigler–Najjar (syndrome) • cyanogen • cyanosis neonatorum • [L. *cras nocte*] tomorrow night *also* cn

C/N carbon to nitrogen (ratio) • carrier to noise (ratio) • contrast to noise ratio

Cn color naming • cyanide

cn [L. *cras nocte*] tomorrow night *also* CN

CNA calcium nutrient agar • chart not available

CNAG chronic narrow angle glaucoma

CNAP cochlear nucleus action potential

CNB cutting needle biopsy

CNBr cyanogen bromide (poisonous vapor)

CNC clear, no creamy (layer)

CNCbl cyanocobalamin

CND canned • cannot determine

CNDC chronic nonspecific diarrhea of childhood

CNE chronic nervous exhaustion • concentric needle electrode • could not establish

CNEMG concentric needle electromyography

CNF chronic nodular fibrositis • congenital nephrotic (syndrome), Finnish • cyclophosphamide, Novantrone (mitoxantrone), and fluorouracil

CNH central neurogenic hyperpnea/hyperventilation • community nursing home

CNHD congenital nonspherocytic hemolytic disease

CNK cortical necrosis of kidneys

CNL cardiolipin natural lecithin

CNM Certified Nurse–Midwife • computerized nuclear morphometry

CNMT Certified Nuclear Medicine Technologist

CNN congenital nevocytic nevus

CNOR Certified Nurse, Operating Room

CNP community nurse practitioner • continuous negative pressure • cranial nerve palsy • cyclic nucleotide phosphodiesterase

CNPase cyclic nucleotide phosphohydrolase

CNPV continuous negative pressure ventilation

CNRN Certified Neuroscience Registered Nurse

CNRS citrated normal rabbit serum

CNS central nervous system • clinical nurse specialist • computerized notation system • cyanide sulfonate (sulfocyanate)

cns [l. *cras nocte sumendus*] to be taken tomorrow night

CNSD chronic nonspecific diarrhea

CNSHA congenital nonspherocytic hemolytic anemia

CNS–L central nervous system leukemia

CNSN Certified Nutrition Support Nurse

CNT could not test • current night terrors

CNV choroidal neovascularization • contingent negative variation • cutaneous necrotizing vasculitis

CO candidal onychomycosis • carbon monoxide • cardiac output • castor oil • casualty officer • centric occlusion • cervical orthosis • choline oxidase • coenzyme *also* Co • community organization • compound • control • corneal opacity • crossover

C/O, c/o check out • complains of • complaints • in care of

CO₂ carbon dioxide

Co cobalt • coenzyme *also* CO

Co I coenzyme I

Co II coenzyme II

57Co, Co 57 cobalt isotope

60Co, Co 60 cobalt isotope

co [L. *compositus*] compounded/compound • cutoff

COA calculated opening area • cervico–oculoacusticus (syndrome)

CoA coarctation of the aorta *also* CA, C of A • coenzyme A

COAD chronic obstructive airway/arterial disease

COAG, coag chronic open angle glaucoma • coagulation/coagulated

COAG PD coagulation profile–diagnosis

COAG PP coagulation profile–presurgery

COAGSC coagulation screen

COAP cyclophosphamide, Oncovin (vincristine), arabinosylcytosine, and prednisone

coarc coarctation (of aorta)

CoASH uncombined coenzyme A

CoA–SPC coenzyme A–synthesizing protein complex

COB chronic obstructive bronchitis • cisplatin, Oncovin (vincristine), and bleomycin • coordination of benefits

COBOL common business–oriented language

COBRA Consolidated Omnibus Budget Reconciliation Act

COBS cesarean (section)–obtained barrier–sustained (animals) • chronic organic brain syndrome

COBT chronic obstruction of biliary tract

COC cathodal opening clonus *also* COCL, COCl • cathodal opening contraction • coccygeal *also* Coc, coc • combination oral contraceptive

Coc, coc coccygeal *also* COC

Cocci coccidioidomycosis

coch, cochl [L. *cochleare*] spoonful

cochl amp [L. *cochleare amplum*] heaping spoonful

cochl mag [L. *cochleare magnum*] dessert spoonful

cochl parv [L. *cochleare parvum*] teaspoonful *also* c parvum

COCI Consortium on Chemical Information

COCL, COCl cathodal opening clonus *also* COC

coct [L. *coctio*] boiling

COD cause of death • chemical oxygen demand • codeine *also* cod. • condition on discharge

cod. codeine *also* COD

CODATA Committee on Data for Science and Technology

COD–MD cerebro–oculardysplasia–muscular dystrophy

COE court–ordered examination

coeff coefficient

COEPS cortical originating extrapyramidal system

COF cut–off frequency

CoF cobra (venom) factor • cofactor

C of A coarctation of aorta *also* CA, CoA

COFS cerebro–oculofacial–skeletal (syndrome)

COG Central Oncology Group • clinical obstetrics and gynecology • cognitive (function tests)

COGN cognition

COGTT cortisone–primed oral glucose tolerance test

COH carbohydrate

COHB, CoHb carboxyhemoglobin

COHSE Confederation of Health Service Employees

COI Central Obesity Index

COL, col colicin • colony • color/colored • column • cost of living • [L. *cola*] strain

COLAT, colat [L. *colatus*] strained

COLD chronic obstructive lung disease

COLD A, cold agg cold agglutinin (titer)

colet [L. *coletur*] let it be strained

COLL, coll collect/collection/collective • colloidal • [L. *collyrium*] eyewash *also* COLLYR, collyr

collun [L. *collunarium*] nose wash

COLLUT, collut [L. *collutorium*] mouthwash

coll vol collective volume

COLLYR, collyr [L. *collyrium*] eyewash *also* COLL, coll

col/mL colonies per milliliter

color colorimetry, including

spectrophotometry and photometry • [L. *coloretur*] let it be colored

colp, colpo colporrhaphy • colposcopy

COM chronic otitis media • computer output on microfilm • cyclophosphamide, Oncovin (vincristine), and methotrexate • cyclophoshamide, Oncovin (vincristine), and methyl–CCNU (semustine)

com commitment

COMA cyclophosphamide, Oncovin (vincristine), methotrexate, and arabinosylcytosine

COMB cyclophosphamide, Oncovin (vincristine), methyl–CCNU (semustine), and bleomycin

comb. combination/combine

COMF, comf comfortable

com fix complement fixation *also* CF

COMLA cyclophosphamide, Oncovin (vincristine), methotrexate, leucovorin, and arabinosylcytosine

comm commission/commissioner • committee • communicable *also* commun

commun communicable *also* comm

commun dis communicable disease

COMP complication •

cyclophosphamide, Oncovin (vincristine), methotrexate, and prednisone

comp compare/comparable/ comparative · compensation/ compensated · complaint · composition *also* compn · compound/compounded *also* C, compd, CP, cpd · compress/compression · computer

compd compound/ compounded *also* C, comp, CP, cpd

compet competition

compl completion/completed *also* cpl · complication/ complicated *also* complic

complic complication/ complicated *also* compl

compn composition *also* comp

COMS chronic organic mental syndrome

COMT catechol methyltransferase

COMTRAC computer–based (case) tracing

CON certificate of need

Con concanavalin

con [L. *contra*] against *also* cont

Con A concanavalin A

Con A–HRP concanavalin A– horseradish peroxidase

conc, concentr concentrated/ concentrations

concis [L. *concisus*] cut

cond condensation/

condensed · condition/ conditional/conditioned · conductivity

cond ref conditioned reflex *also* CR

cond resp conditioned response *also* CR

cone conization (of cervix) *also* coniz

conf [L. *confectio*] a confection · conference

cong congenital *also* congen · congress · [L. *congius*] gallon

congen congenital *also* cong

congr congruent

coniz conization (of cervix) *also* cone

conj conjunctiva/conjunctival

conjug conjugated/ conjugation

CONPADRI I cyclophosphamide, Oncovin (vincristine), L–phenyl- alanine mustard, and Adriamycin (doxorubicin)

CONPADRI II CONPADRI I plus high dose methotrexate

CONPADRI III CONPADRI I plus intensified doxorubicin

CONS consultation *also* cons

cons conserve/conservation/ conservative · consultant/ consultation *also* CONS · [L. *conserva*] keep

consperg [L. *consperge*] dust, sprinkle

const constant

constit constituent

cont [L. *contra*] against *also*
con • [L. *contusus*]
bruised • containing/
contains • contents •
continue/continuation •
contusions

contag contagion/contagious

conter [L. *contere*] rub
together

contin [L. *continuetur*] let it
be continued

contr contraction

contra contraindicated

contralat contralateral

cont rem [L. *continuetur
remedium*] let the medicine
be continued

contrib contributory

contrit [L. *contritus*] broken
down

contrx contraction

contus [L. *contusus*] bruised

conv convalescence/
convalescent/
convalescing •
conventional (rat) •
convergence/convergent

CONV HOSP convalescent
hospital

conv strab convergent
strabismus

COOD chronic obstructive
outflow disease

coord coordination/
coordinated

COP capillary osmotic
pressure • change of
plaster • cicatricial ocular
pemphigoid • cicumoval

precipitin • coefficient of
performance • colloid
oncotic/osmotic pressure •
cyclophosphamide, Oncovin
(vincristine), and
prednisone

COPA cyclophosphamide,
Oncovin (vincristine),
prednisone, and Adriamycin
(doxorubicin)

COP–BLAM
cyclophosphamide, Oncovin
(vincristine), prednisone,
bleomycin, Adriamycin
(doxorubicin), and
Matulane (procarbazine)

COPC community–oriented
primary care

COPD chronic obstructive
pulmonary disease

COPE chronic obstructive
pulmonary emphysema

COPI California Occupational
Preference Inventory

COP$_i$ colloid osmotic pressure
in interstitial fluid

COPP cyclophosphamide,
Oncovin (vincristine),
procarbazine, and
prednisone

COP$_p$ colloid osmotic pressure
in plasma

COPRO coproporphyria/
coproporphyrin

CoQ coenzyme Q

coq [L. *coque*] boil

coq in s a [L. *coque in
sufficiente aqua*] boil in
sufficient water

coq s a [L. *coque secundum
artem*] boil properly

coq simul [L. *coque simul*] boil together

COR [L. *corpus*] body · cardiac output recorder · comprehensive outpatient rehabilitation (facility) · conditioned orientation reflex (audiometry) · coroner · corrosion/corrosive · cortisone

Cor Congo red *also* CR

cor coronary · correction/corrected *also* corr

CORA conditioned orientation reflex audiometry

CORD chronic obstructive respiratory disease · Commissioned Officer Residency Deferment

corr corrected *also* cor · correspondence

CORT Certified Operating Room Technician

cort cortex *also* C · cortical

CORTIS cortisol

COS Chief of Staff · clinically observed seizure ·

cos change of shift

COSMIS Computer System for Medical Information Systems

COSTAR Computer–stored Ambulatory Record

COSTEP Commissioned Officer Student Training and Extern Program

COT colony overlay test · content of thought · continuous oxygen therapy · contralateral

optic tectum · critical off-time

CO₂T total carbon dioxide content

COTA Certified Occupational Therapy Assistant

COTD cardiac output by thermodilution

COTe cathodal opening tetanus

COTH Council of Teaching Hospitals

COTRANS Coordinated Transfer Application System

COTX cast off, to x–ray *also* CRTX

COU cardiac observation unit

coul coulomb

COV crossover value

CoVF cobra venom factor

COWAT Controlled Oral Word Association Test

COWS cold to opposite and warm to same side (Hallpike caloric stimulation response)

COX coxsackie virus

CP candle–power *also* cp · capillary pressure · carbamoyl phosphate · cardiac pacing · cardiac performance · cardiac pool · cardiopulmonary *also* C/P · cardiopulmonary performance · cell passaged · central pit · centric position · cerebellopontine · cerebral palsy · certified prosthetist • ceruloplasmin • cervical probe • chemically pure *also* cp • chest pain • child psychiatry • child psychology • chloramphenicol *also* C, chloro, CMC • chloropurine • chloroquine–primaquine • chondrodysplasia punctata • chondromalacia patellae • chronic pain • chronic pancreatitis • chronic pyelonephritis • cicatricial pemphoid • circular polarization • cisplatin • cleft palate *also* Clpal • clinical pathology • closing pressure • clottable protein • cochlear potential • code of practice • cold pressor • color perception • combination product • combining power • complete physical • compound *also* C, comp, compd, cpd • compressed • constant pressure • coproporphyrin/coproporphyria • coracoid process • cor pulmonale • cortical plate • costal plaque • C peptide • creatine phosphate • creatine phosphokinase • cross–linked protein • crude protein • current practice • cyclophosphamide *also* CY, Cy, CYC, CYCLO • cyclophosphamide and prednisone • cystosarcoma phyllodes • cytosol protein

C/P cardiopulmonary *also* CP • cholesterol–phospholipid (ratio)

C&P compensation and pension • complete and

pain–free (range of motion) • cystoscopy and pyelography

Cp ceruloplasmin • chickenpox *also* Chix, CHPX, chpx • peak concentration • phosphate clearance *also* C_p

C_p constant pressure • phosphate clearance *also* Cp

cP centipoise *also* cp

cp candle–power *also* CP • centipoise *also* cP • chemically pure *also* CP • compare *also* CF, cf

CPA carboxypeptidase A • cardiophrenic angle • cardiopulmonary arrest • carotid phonoangiography • cerebellopontine angle • chlorophenylalanine • chronic pyrophosphate arthropathy • circulating platelet aggregate • costophrenic angle • cyclophosphamide • cyproterone acetate

C3PA complement 3 proactivator (convertase)

CPAF chlorpropamide–alcohol flushing

Cpah, C_{pah} p–aminohippuric acid clearance

CPAI central principal axis of inertia

CPAN Certified Post–Anesthesia Nurse

CPA/OPG carotid phonoangiography/oculoplethysmography

CPAP continuous positive airway pressure

c parvum [L. *cochleare*

parvum] teaspoonful *also* cochl parv

CPB cardiopulmonary bypass • competitive protein binding

CPBA competitive protein-binding analysis/assay

CPBS cardiopulmonary bypass surgery

CPBV cardiopulmonary blood volume

CPC cerebellar Purkinje cell • cerebral palsy clinic • cetylpyridinium chloride • chronic passive congestion • circumferential pneumatic compression • clinico-pathologic conference • committed progenitor cell

CPCL congenital pulmonary cystic lymphangiectasia

CPCN capitated primary care network

CPCP chronic progressive coccidioidal pneumonitis

CPCR cardiopulmonary–cerebral resuscitation

CPCS circumferential pneumatic compression suit • clinical pharmaco-kinetics consulting service

CPD calcium pyrophosphate deposition • calcium pyrophosphate dihydrate • cephalopelvic disproportion • childhood polycystic disease • chorioretinopathy and pituitary dysfunction • chronic peritoneal dialysis • citrate–phosphate–dextrose • contact potential difference • contagious

pustular dermatitis • critical point drying • cyclopentadiene

cpd compound *also* C, comp, compd, CP

CPDA, CPD–A citrate–phosphate–dextrose–adenine

CPDD calcium pyrophosphate deposition disease • *cis*–platinum diamminedichloride

CPDL cumulative population doubling level

CPE cardiac/cardiogenic pulmonary edema • chronic pulmonary emphysema • compensation, pension, and education • complete physical examination *also* CPX • complex partial epilepsy • corona–penetrating enzyme • cytopathic/cytopathogenic effect

CPEHS Consumer Protection and Environmental Health Service

CPEO chronic progressive external ophthalmoplegia

CPF clot–promoting factor • contraction peak force

CP&FD cephalopelvic disproportion and fetal distress

CPG capillary blood gases • carotid phonoangiogram

CPGN chronic proliferative/progressive glomerulonephritis

CPH Certificate in Public

Health • chronic paroxysmal hemicrania • chronic persistent hepatitis

CPHA Commission on Professional and Hospital Activities

CPI California Personality Inventory • Cancer Potential Index • congenital palatopharyngeal incompetence • constitutional psychopathic inferiority • coronary prognostic index • cysteine proteinase inhibitor

CPIB chlorophenoxyisobutyrate

CPID chronic pelvic inflammatory disease

CPIP chronic pulmonary insufficiency of prematurity • common peak developed isovolumetric pressure

CPK creatine phosphokinase

CPKD childhood polycystic kidney disease

CPKI, CPKISO creatinine phosphokinase isoenzyme(s)

CPL caprine placental lactogen • conditioned pitch level • congenital pulmonary lymphangiectasia

C/PL cholesterol to phospholipid ratio

cpl complete/completed *also* compl

CPLM cysteine–peptone–liver (infusion) medium

CPM central pontine myelinosis • chlorpheniramine maleate • Clinical Practice Model • cognitive–perceptual–motor • Colored Progressive Matrices • continue present management • continuous passive motion (device) • counts per minute *also* C/M, cpm • cyclophosphamide • chloroethyl cyclohexylnitrosourea (lomustine), procarbazine, and methotrexate

cpm counts per minute *also* C/M, CPM • cycles per minute *also* c/min

CPmax peak (maximum) serum concentration

CPMDI computerized pharmacokinetic model–driven (drug) infusion

CPMG Carr–Purcell–Meiboom–Gill (spin–echo technique)

CPMI central principal moments of inertia

CP min trough (minimum) serum concentration

CPMM constant passive motion machine

CPMP computer–patient management problems

CPMS chronic progressive multiple sclerosis

CPMV cowpox mosaic virus

CPN carboxypeptidase N • chronic polyneuropathy • chronic pyelonephritis

CPNM corrected perinatal mortality

CPNP/A Certified Pediatric Nurse Practitioner/ Associate

CPP cancer proneness phenotype • canine pancreatic polypeptide • cerebral perfusion pressure • cryoprecipitrate

CPPB continuous positive–pressure breathing

CPPD calcium pyrophosphate dihydrate • chest percussion and postural drainage *also* CP&PD

CP&PD chest percussion and postural drainage *also* CPPD

CPPT coronary primary prevention trial

CPPV continuous positive–pressure ventilation

CPR cardiac and pulmonary rehabilitation • cardiac pulmonary reserve • cardiopulmonary resuscitation • centripetal rub • cerebral cortex perfusion rate • chlorophenyl red • cochleopalpebral reflex • cortisol production rate • cumulative potency rate • customary, prevailing, and reasonable

CPRAM controlled partial rebreathing anesthesia method

CPRS Children's Psychiatric Rating Scale • Comprehensive Psychiatric Rating Scale • Comprehensive Psychopathological Rating Scale

CPS carbamyl phosphate synthetase • cardioplegic perfusion solution • cardiopulmonary support • characters per second • Child Personality Scale • Child Protective Services • chloroquine, pyrimethamine, and sulfisoxazole • clinical performance score • clinical pharmacokinetic service • coagulase-positive staphylococci • complex partial seizure • constitutional psychopathic state • contagious pustular stomatitis • C–polysaccharide • cumulative probability of success • current population survey

cps counts per second • cycles per second *also* c/s

CPSC Consumer Product Safety Commission

CPT carnitine palmityltransferase • carotid pulse tracing • chest physiotherapy • child protection team • choline phosphotransferase • ciliary particle transport • clinical pharmacokinetics team • cold pressor test • combining power test • continuous performance task/test • Current Procedural Terminology

CPTH chronic posttraumatic headache • C–terminal parathyroid hormone

CPU caudate putamen • central processing unit

CPUE chest pain of unknown etiology

CPV canine parvovirus · cytoplasmic polyhidrosis virus

CPVD congenital polyvalvular disease

CPX complete physical examination *also* CPE

CPZ cefoperazone *also* (antibacterial) · chlorpromazine · Compazine (prochlorperazine dimaleate)

CQ chloroquine · chloroquine–quinine · circadian quotient · conceptual quotient

CQA concurrent quality assurance

CQM chloroquine mustard

CR calcification rate · calculus removal/removed · calorie restricted · cardiac rehabilitation · cardiorespiratory · caries resistant · cartilage residue · case report · cathode ray · central ray · centric relation · chest and right arm (lead in electrocardiography) · chest roentgenogram/ roentgenography · chief resident · child–resistant (bottle top) · choice reaction · chromium *also* Cr · chronic rejection · clinical record · clinical research · closed reduction · clot retraction · coefficient (of fat) retention · colon resection · colony–reared (animal) · colorectal · complement receptor · complete remission · complete response/ responders · conditioned reflex/response *also* cond ref, cond resp · congenital rubella · Congo red *also* Cor · contact record · continuous reinforcement · controlled release/ respiration/response · conversion rate · cooling rate · correct response · corticoresistant · cranial *also* Cr, cran · creamed · creatinine *also* Cr, Cre, creat · cresyl red · critical ratio · crown–rump (length) *also* CRL, CRM

C&R cardiac and respiratory · convalescence and rehabilitation · cystocopy and retrograde

Cr chromium *also* CR · cranium/cranial *also* CR, cran · creatinine *also* CR, Cre, creat · crown

^{51}Cr, Cr 51 chromium isotope

cr [L. *cras*] tomorrow

CRA central retinal artery · chronic rheumatoid arthritis · colorectal anastomosis

CRABP cellular retinoic acid– binding protein

CRAG cerebral radionuclide angiography

CRAMS circulation, respiration, abdomen, motor, and speech

cran cranium/cranial *also* CR, Cr

CRAO central retinal artery occlusion

crast [L. *crastinus*] for tomorrow

CRBBB complete right bundle–branch block

CRBC chicken red blood cell *also* ChRBC

CRBP cellular retinol–binding protein

CRC cardiovascular reflex conditioning • child–resistant container • clinical research center • colorectal carcinoma • concentrated red (blood) cell • Crisis Resolution Center • cross–reacting cannabinoids

CR&C closed reduction and cast

CrC1 creatinine clearance

CRCS cardiovascular reflex conditioning system

CRD childhood rheumatic disease • child–restraint device • chorioretinal degeneration • chronic renal disease • chronic respiratory disease • completely randomized design • complete reaction of degeneration • cone–rod dystrophy • congenital rubella deafness • crown–rump distance (fetal measurement)

CRE cumulative radiation effect

Cre, creat creatinine *also* CR, Cr

CREA–S creatinine urin spot (test)

CRENA crenated (red blood cells)

crep [L. *crepitus*] crepitation

CREST calcinosis cutis, Raynaud's phenomenon, esophageal motility disorder, sclerodactyly, and telangiectasia (syndrome)

CRF case report form • chronic renal failure • chronic respiratory failure • citrovorum rescue factor • coagulase–reacting factor • continuous reinforcement • corticotropin–releasing factor

CRFK Crandell feline kidney cells

CRG cardiorespirogram

CRH corticotropin–releasing hormone

CRHL Collaborative Radiological Health Laboratory

CRHV cottontail rabbit herpesvirus

CRI Cardiac Risk Index • catheter–related infection • chronic renal insufficiency • Composite Risk Index • concentrated rust inhibitor • congenital rubella infection • cross–reactive idiotype

CRIE crossed radioimmuno-electrophoresis

CRIS controlled release infusion syndrome

Crit, crit critical • hematocrit *also* H'crit, HCT, Hct, hemat, HMT

CRL cell repository line • Certified Record Librarian • complement

receptor location/
lymphocyte • crown–rump
length *also* CR, CRM

CRM certified raw milk •
Certified Reference
Materials • contralateral
remote masking • cross–
reacting material • crown–
rump measurement *also* CR,
CRL

CRNA Certified Registered
Nurse Anesthetist

cRNA chromosomal
ribonucleic acid

CRNF chronic rheumatoid
nodular fibrositis

cr nn cranial nerves *also* cr ns

CRNP Certified Registered
Nurse Practitioner

cr ns, crns cranial nerves

CRO cathode ray oscillograph/
oscilloscope • centric
relation occlusion

CROP cyclophosphamide,
rubidazone, Oncovin
(vincristine), and
prednisone

CROS contralateral routing of
signal

CRP chronic relapsing
pancreatitis • confluent,
reticulate papillomatosis •
corneal–retinal potential •
coronary rehabilitation
program • C–reactive
protein • cyclic adenosine
monophosphate receptor
protein

CrP creatine phosphate •
phosphocreatine

CRPA C–reactive protein
antiserum

CRPD chronic restrictive
pulmonary disease

CRPF chloroquine–resistant
Plasmodium falciparum •
contralateral renal plasma
flow

CRS catheter–related sepsis •
caudal regression
syndrome • central supply
room • Chinese restaurant
syndrome • colorectal
surgery • compliance of
the respiratory system •
congenital rubella syndrome

CRSP comprehensive renal
scintillation procedure

CrSp craniospinal

CRST calcinosis cutis,
Raynaud's phenomenon,
sclerodactyly, and
telangiectasia (syndrome) •
corrected sinus recovery
time

CRT cadaver renal transplant •
cardiac resuscitation team •
cathode ray tube • central
reaction time • certified
also C • Certified Record
Technique • choice
reaction time • chromium
release test • complex
reaction time • computed
renal tomography • copper
reduction test • corrected
retention time • cortisone
resistant thymocyte •
cranial radiation therapy

CRTP Consciousness Research
and Training Project

CrTr crutch training *also* CT

CRTT Certified Respiratory
Therapy Technician

CRTX cast removed, take x–
ray *also* COTX

CRU cardiac rehabilitation unit • clinical research unit

CRV central retinal vein

CRVF congestive right ventricular failure

CRVO central retinal vein occlusion

CRY–AB cryptococcal antibody

CRY–AG cryptococcal antigen

cryo cryoglobulin, cryoprecipitate, cryosurgery, cryotherapy

crys, cryst crystal, crystalline/crystallinized

CRYST crystal examination screen

CS calf serum • carcinoid syndrome • cardiogenic shock • caries susceptible • carotid sheath • carotid sinus • cat scratch (disease) *also* CSD • celiac sprue • central service • central supply • cerebrospinal • cervical spine *also* C–S, C–spine • cervical stimulation • cesarean section *also* C/S, C–section, C sect • chemical sympathectomy • chest strap • cholesterol stone • chondroitin sulfate • chorionic somato-mammotropin • chronic schizophrenia • cigarette smoke (solution) • cigarette smoker • citrate synthase • clinical (laboratory) scientist • clinical stage • clinical state • close supervision • Cockayne syndrome •

colistin • Collet–Sicard (syndrome) • completed stroke • completed suicide • concentrated strength (of solution) • conditioned stimulus • congenital syphilis • conjunctival secretion • conjunctiva–sclera • conscious/consciousness *also* Cs, cs • constant spring • consultation service • contact sensitivity • continue same (treatment) • continuing smoker • continuous stripping • control serum • convalescence/convalescent • convalescent status • coronary sclerosis • coronary sinus • corpus striatum • cortical spoking • corticoid sensitive • corticosteroid • crush syndrome • current smoker • current strength • Cushing syndrome • cycloserine • cyclosporin *also* CSP • [L. *colla sinistra*] with the left hand

C–S cervical spine *also* CS, C–spine

C/S cesarean section *also* CS, C–section, C sect • Cost–Stirling (antibody) • culture and sensitivity *also* C&S

C&S conjunctiva and sclera • cough and sneeze • culture and sensitivity *also* C/S • culture and susceptibility

C4S chondroitin 4–sulfate

C$_s$ standard clearance *also* Cs • static (lung) compliance *also* CST, Cst, C$_{st}$, C$_{stat}$

Cs case *also* cs • cell surface antigen • cesium • consciousness *also* CS, cs • standard clearance *also* C$_S$

cS centistoke *also* cSt

cs case *also* Cs • conscious/ consciousness *also* CS, Cs

c/s cycles per second *also* cps

CSA canavaninosuccinic acid • chondroitin sulfate A • colon–specific antigen • colony– stimulating activity • compressed spectral assay • controlled substance analog • cross–sectional area • cyclosporin A *also* CsA, CyA

CsA cyclosporin A *also* CSA, CyA

CSAD cysteine sulfinic acid decarboxylase

CSAP colon–specific antigen protein

CSB caffeine sodium benzoate • Cheyne–Stokes breathing • contaminated small bowel

CSB I&II Chemistry Screening Batteries I and II

CSBF coronary sinus blood flow

CSBO complete small bowel obstruction

CSC [Fr. *coup sur coup*] blow on blow (administration of small doses of drugs at short intervals) • central serous choroidopathy • cigarette smoke condensate • collagen sponge contraceptive • cornea,

sclera, and conjunctiva • cryogenic storage container

C/S & CC culture and sensitivity and colony count

CSCD Center for Sickle Cell Disease

CSCI continuous subcutaneous infusion

CSCT comprehensive support care team

CSD carotid sinus denervation • cat scratch disease *also* CS • combined system disease • conditionally streptomycin dependent • conduction system disease • cortically spreading depression • craniospinal defect • critical stimulus duration

CS&D cleaned, sutured, and dressed

CSE clinical–symptom/self– evaluation (questionnaire) • cross–sectional echocardiography

C–section, C sect cesarean section *also* CS, C/S

CSER cortical somatosensory evoked response

CSF cancer family syndrome • cerebrospinal fluid • circumferential shortening fraction • colony– stimulating factor • coronary sinus flow

CSFH cerebrospinal fluid hypotension

CSFP cerebrospinal fluid pressure

CSFV cerebrospinal fluid volume

CSF–WR cerebrospinal fluid–Wassermann reaction

CSGBM collagenase soluble glomerular basement membrane

CSH carotid sinus hypersensitivity • chronic subdural hematoma • cortical stromal hyperplasia

C–Sh chair shower

CSI calculus surface index • cancer serum index • cavernous sinus infiltration • cholesterol saturation index

CSICU cardiac surgery intensive care unit

CSII continuous subcutaneous insulin infusion

CSIIP continuous subcutaneous insulin infusion pump

CSIN Chemical Substances Information Network

CSIS clinical supplies and inventory system

CSL cardiolipin synthetic lecithin

CSLU chronic stasis leg ulcer

CSM carotid sinus massage • cerebrospinal meningitis • circulation, sensation, mobility • Committee on Safety of Medicines • Consolidated Standards Manual • cornmeal, soybean, milk

CSMA chronic spinal muscular atrophy

CSMB Center for Study of Multiple Births

CSME cotton–spot macular edema

CSMMG Chartered Society of Massage and Medical Gymnastics

CSN carotid sinus nerve

CS(NCA) Clinical (Laboratory) Scientist Certified by the National Certification Agency (for Medical Laboratory Personnel)

CSNRT, cSNRT corrected sinus node recovery time *also* CSRT

CSNS carotid sinus nerve stimulation

CSO common source outbreak • copied standing orders

CSOM chronic serous/suppurative otitis media

CSP carotid sinus pressure • cavum septi pellucidi • cell surface protein • cellulose sodium phosphate • chemistry screening profile • Cooperative Statistical Program • criminal sexual psychopath • cyclosporin *also* CS

C–spine cervical spine *also* CS, C–S

CSR central supply room • Cheyne–Stokes respiration • continued stay review • corrected sedimentation rate • corrected survival rate • corrective septorhinoplasty • cortisol secretion rate • cumulative survival rate

CSRT corrected sinus (node) recovery time *also* CSNRT, cSNRT

CSS Cancer Surveillance System · carotid sinus stimulation · carotid sinus syndrome · chewing, sucking, swallowing · chronic subclinical scurvy · Churg–Strauss syndrome · coronary sinus stimulation · cranial sector scan

CSSD central sterile supply department

CST cardiac stress test · cavernous sinus thrombosis · Certified Surgical Technician · Compton scatter tomography · contraction stress test · convulsive shock therapy · cosyntropin stimulation test · static (lung) compliance *also* C$_S$, Cst, C$_{st}$, C$_{stat}$

Cst, C$_{st}$, C$_{stat}$ static (lung) compliance

cSt centistoke *also* cS

CSTI Clearinghouse for Scientific and Technical Information

CSU cardiac surgery unit · cardiac surveillance unit · cardiovascular surgery unit · casualty staging unit · catheter specimen of urine · Central Statistical Unit (of Venereal Disease Research Laboratory) · clinical specialty unit

CSUF continuous slow ultrafiltration

CSV chick syncytial virus

CSW Certified Social Worker · current sleepwalker

CT calcitonin · calf testis · cardiac tamponade · cardiothoracic (ratio) · Cardiovascular Technologist · carotid tracing · carpal tunnel · cationic trypsinogen · cell therapy · center thickness · cerebral thrombosis · cerebral tumor · cervical traction *also* CXTX · chemotaxis *also* CTX · chemotherapy · chest tube · chloramine T · chlorothiazide · cholera toxin · chordae tendineae · chronic thyroiditis · chymotrypsin · circulation time · classic technique · clotting time · coagulation time · coated tablet · cobra toxin · cognitive therapy · coil test · collecting tubule · combined tumor · compressed tablet · computed tomography · connective tissue · continue treatment · continuous–flow tub · contraction time · controlled temperature · Coombs test · corneal thickness · corneal transplant · coronary thrombosis · corrected transposition · corrective therapy · cortical thickness · cough threshold · crest time · crutch training *also* CrTr · cystine–tellurite (medium) · cytotechnologist · cytotoxic therapy

C/T compression to traction

ratio • cross–match to transfusion ratio

Ct carboxyl terminal *also* C–terminal

C$_{T-1824}$ T–1824 (Evans blue) clearance

CTA [L. *catamenia*] menses *also* Cta • chemotactic activity *also* CA • chromotropic acid • clear to auscultation • computed tomoangiography • congenital trigeminal anesthesia • cyproterone acetate • cystine trypticase agar • cytoplasmic tubular aggregate • cytotoxic assay

Cta [L. *catamenia*] menses *also* CTA

CTAB cetyltrimethylammonium bromide *also* CTBM

C–TAB cyanide tablet

CTAC Cancer Treatment Advisory Committee • Carrow Test for Auditory Comprehension • cetyltrimethylammonium chloride

CTAL cortical thick ascending limb

ctant [L. *cum tanto*] with the same amount

CTAP computed tomography during arterial portography • connective tissue activating peptide

CT(ASCP) Cytotechnologist (American Society of Clinical Pathologists)

CTAT computed transaxial tomography

CTB ceased to breathe

CTBA cetrimonium bromide

CTBM cetyltrimethyl-ammonium bromide *also* CTAB

CTC chlortetracycline • computer–assisted tomographic cisternography • cultured T cell

CTCL cutaneous T–cell (leukemia/lymphoma)

ctCO$_2$ concentration of total carbon dioxide

CTD carpal tunnel decompression • chest tube drainage • congenital thymic dysplasia • connective tissue disease • Corrective Therapy Department

CT&DB cough, turn, and deep breathe

CTDW continues to do well

CTE calf thymus extract • cultured thymic epithelium

CTEM conventional transmission electron microscopy

C–terminal carboxyl terminal *also* Ct

CTF cancer therapy facility • certificate *also* Cert, cert • Colorado tick fever • cytotoxic factor

CTG cardiotocography • chymotrypsinogen

C/TG cholesterol–triglyceride (ratio)

CTGA complete transposition of great arteries

CTH ceramide trihexoside · clot to hold

CTI certification of terminal illness

CTIU cardiac–thoracic intensive care unit *also* CTU

CTL cervical, thoracic, and lumbar · cytotoxic T lymphocyte

ctl contact lens

CTLD chlorthalidone (diuretic and antihypertensive agent)

CTLL cytotoxic T–lymphocyte line

CTLSO cervicothora-columbosacral orthosis

CTM cardiotachometer · *Chlamydia* transport media · Chlor–Trimeton (antihistaminic) · continuous tone masking · cricothyroid muscle

CTMM computed tomographic metrizamide myelography

CT/MPR computed tomography with multiplanar reconstructions

CTN calcitonin · computed tomography number

C&TN BLE color and temperature normal, both lower extremities

cTNM (clinical) staging of tumors (tumors, nodes, and metastases) as determined by noninvasive examination

CTP comprehensive treatment plan · cytidine triphosphate · cytosine triphosphate

C–TPN cyclic total parenteral nutrition

CTPP cerebral tissue perfusion pressure

CTPV coal tar pitch volatiles

CTPVO chronic thrombotic pulmonary vascular obstruction

CTR cardiothoracic ratio · carpal tunnel release

ctr center

CTS carpal tunnel syndrome · composite treatment score · computed tomographic scanner · computed topographic scanner · contralateral threshold shift · corticosteroid

CTSP called to see patient

CTT cefotetan · central tegmental tract · compressed tablet triturate · computed transaxial tomography

CTU cardiac–thoracic unit *also* CTIU · centigrade thermal unit · constitutive transcription unit

CTUWSD chest tube under water–seal drainage

CTV cervical and thoracic vertebrae

CTW central terminal of Wilson · combined testicular weight

CTX cefotaxime · cerebrotendinous xanthomatosis · chemotaxis *also* CT · chemotoxins · contraction *also* CTXN · Cytoxan (cyclophosphamide)

CTx cardiac transplantation

CTXN contraction *also* CTX

CTZ chemoreceptor trigger zone • chlorothiazide

CU cardiac unit • casein unit • cause unknown • chymotrypsin unit • clinical unit • color unit • contact urticaria • control unit • convalescent unit • curie *also* C, c, Ci, cu

Cu [L. *cuprum*] copper

Cu–7 Copper–7 (intrauterine contraceptive device)

C$_u$ urea clearance

cu cubic *also* C, c • curie *also* C, c, Ci, CU

CuB copper band

CUC chronic ulcerative colitis

cu cm cubic centimeter *also* CC, cc, cm^3

CUD cause undetermined • congenital urinary (tract) deformities

CUE cumulative urinary excretion

cu ft cubic foot

CUG cystidine, uridine, and guanidine • cystourethrogram/ cystourethrography

CuHVL copper half–value layer

cu in cubic inch

cuj [L. *cujus*] of which

cuj lib [L. *cujus libet*] of whatever you please

cult culture

CUM cumulative report

cum cubic micrometer *also* μm^3

cu m cubic meter *also* m^3

CUMITECH Cumulative Techniques and Procedures in Clinical Microbiology

cu mm cubic millimeter *also* cmm, mm^3

CUP carcinoma unknown primary

CUPS carcinnma of unknown primary site

CUR curettage

cur cure/curative • current

curat [L. *curatio*] dressing

CURN Conduct and Utilization of Research in Nursing

CUS chronic undifferentiated schizophrenia • contact urticaria syndrome

CUSA Cavitron ultrasonic surgical aspirator

cusp. cuspid

CUT chronic undifferentiated type (schizophrenia)

CuTS cubital tunnel syndrome

cu yd cubic yard

CV cardiovascular • carotenoid vesicle • cell volume • central venous • cerebrovascular • cervical vertebra • chikungunya virus • cisplatin and Vepeside (etoposide) • closed vitrectomy • closing volume • coefficient of variation • color vision • concentrated volume •

conducting vein • conduction velocity • consonant vowel (syllable) • contrast ventriculography • conventional ventilation • conversational voice • corpuscular volume • Coxsackie virus *also* Cvirus • cresyl violet • critical value • crystal violet • curriculum vitae • cutaneous vasculitis • [L. *cras vespere*] tomorrow evening *also* cv • [L. *conjugata vera*] true conjugate (diameter of pelvic inlet)

C/V coulomb per volt

Cv specific heat at constant volume

C$_v$ constant volume (specific heat capacity)

cv [L. *cras vespere*] tomorrow evening *also* CV

CVA cardiovascular accident • cerebrovascular accident • cervicovaginal antibody • chronic villous arthritis • costovertebral angle • cresyl violet acetate • cyclophosphamide, vincristine, and Adriamycin (doxorubicin)

CVA–BMP cyclophosphamide, Oncovin (vincristine), Adriamycin (doxorubicin), BCNU (carmustine), methotrexate, and procarbazine

CVAH congenital virilizing adrenal hyperplasia

C–Vasc cerebral vascular (profile study)

CVAT costovertebral angle tenderness

CVB CCNU (lomustine), vinblastine, and bleomycin • chorionic villi biopsy

CVC central venous catheter • consonant vowel consonant (syllable)

CVCT cardiovascular computed tomography

CVD cardiovascular disease *also* CD • cerebrovascular disease • cerebrovascular disorder • collagen vascular disease • color vision deviant

cvd curved

CVE cerebrovascular evaluation

CVEB cisplatin, vinblastine, etoposide, and bleomycin

CVF cardiovascular failure • central visual field • cervicovaginal fluid • cobra venom factor

CVG contrast ventriculography

CVH cervicovaginal hood • combined ventricular hypertrophy • common variable hypogamma-globulinemia

CVHD chronic valvular heart disease

CVI cardiovascular insufficiency • cerebrovascular insufficiency • common variable immunodeficiency *also* CVID • continuous venous infusion • Cox Uphoff International (tissue expander)

CVID common variable immunodeficiency *also* CVI

Cvirus Coxsackie virus *also* CV

CVL clinical vascular laboratory

CVM cardiovascular monitor • cyclophosphamide, vincristine, and methotrexate

CVN central venous nutrient

CVO central vein occlusion • central venous oxygen • Chief Veterinary Officer • circumventricular organs • [L. *conjugata vera obstetrica*] obstetric conjugate (of pelvic inlet)

C$_v$O$_2$ mixed venous oxygen content

CVOD cerebrovascular obstructive disease

CVOR cardiovascular operating room

CVP cardiac valve procedure • cardioventricular pacing • cell volume profile • central venous pressure • cerebrovascular profile • cyclophosphamide, vincristine, and prednisone

CVP lab cardiovascular–pulmonary laboratory

CVPP cyclophosphamide, vincristine, prednisone, and procarbazine

CVR cardiovascular–renal (disease) *also* CVRD • cardiovascular resistance • cardiovascular–respiratory • cardiovascular review • cephalic vasomotor response • cerebrovascular resistance

CVRD cardiovascular–renal disease *also* CVR

CVRI cardiovascular resistance index

CVRR cardiovascular recovery room

CVS cardiovascular surgery • cardiovascular system • challenge virus strain • chorionic villi sampling • clean voided specimen

CVSF conduction velocity of slower fibers

CVSU cardiovascular specialty unit

CVT central venous temperature • congenital vertical talus

CVT–ICU cardiovascular–thoracic intensive care unit

CVTP–ICU cardiovascular–thoracic intensive care unit

CVTR charcoal viral transport medium

CVTS cardiovascular–thoracic surgery

CVUG cysto–void urethrogram

CW cardiac work • careful watch • case work/worker • cell wall • chemical warfare • chemical weapon • chest wall • children's ward • clockwise *also* cw • compare with • continuous wave *also* cw • cotton wool (spots) *also* C–W, CWS • crutch walking *also* c/w

C–W cotton wool (spots) *also* CW

C/W compatible/consistent with *also* c/w

cw clockwise *also* CW • continuous wave *also* CW

c/w compatible/consistent with *also* CW • crutch walking *also* CW

CWBTS capillary whole blood true sugar

CWD cell wall defective • continuous–wave Doppler

CWDF cell wall–deficient form (bacteria)

CWE cotton–wool exudates

CWF Cornell Word Form

CWI cardiac work index

CWL cutaneous water loss

CWMS color, warmth, movement sensation

CWOP childbirth without pain *also* CWP

CWP childbirth without pain *also* CWOP • coal worker's pneumoconiosis

CWS cell wall skeleton • chest wall stimulation • Child Welfare Service • cold water soluble • comfortable walking speed • cotton–wool spots *also* CW, C–W

CWT cold water treatment

Cwt, cwt hundredweight

CX cancel • cerebral cortex • cervix *also* Cx • chest x–ray (film) *also* Cx, CXR • cloxacillin • critical experiment • culture • cylinder axis

Cx cancel • cervix *also* CX •

circumflex • chest x–ray (film) *also* CX, CXR • clearance • complex • complication • contraction *also* C • convex

CXM cefuroxime • cyclohexamide

CxMT cervical motion tenderness

CXR chest x–ray (film) *also* CX, Cx

CXTX cervical traction *also* CT

CY calendar year • cyanogen *also* Cy • cyclophosphamide *also* CP, Cy, CYC, CYCLO

Cy cyanogen *also* CY • cyclophosphamide *also* CP, CY, CYC, CYCLO • cyst • cytarabine

cy copy

CyA cyclosporin A *also* CSA, CsA

CyADIC cyclophosphamide, Adriamycin (doxorubicin), and DIC (dacarbazine)

cyath [L. *cyathus*] a glassful

CYC cyclophosphamide *also* CP, CY, Cy, CYCLO

cyc cyclazocine • cycle • cyclotron

CYCLO, CyClo cyclophosphamide *also* CP, CY, Cy, CYC • cyclopropane

Cyclo C cyclocytidine hydrochloride

Cyd cytidine

CYE charcoal yeast extract (meduim)

CYL casein yeast lactate (medium)

cyl cylinder • cylindrical lens

CYN cyanide

CYNAP cytotoxicity negative, absorption positive

CYP cyproheptadine

CYS cystoscopy

Cys cyclosporin • cysteine *also* C

CYSTO, cysto cystogram • cystoscopy

CYT cyclophosphamide • cytochrome

Cyt cytosine

cyt cytology/cytologic *also* cytol • cytoplasm/ cytoplasmic

cytol cytology/cytologic *also* cyt

CYTOMG cytomegalovirus

Cyt Ox cytochrome oxidase

cyt sys cytochrome system

CY–VA–DIC cyclophosphamide, Oncovin (vincristine), Adriamycin (doxorubicin), and DTIC (dacarbazine)

CZ cefazolin

Cz central midline placement of electrodes in electroencephalography

CZD cefazedone

CZI crystalline zinc insulin

CZP clonazepam

D cholecalciferol • coefficient of diffusion • dacryon *also* dac • date *also* d • daughter *also* da • day *also* d, da • dead *also* d • dead air space • debye • deceased *also* d, DEC, dec, dec'd, decd • deciduous *also* DEC, dec • decimal reduction time • decrease *also* d, DC, D/C, DEC, dec, DECR, decr • degree *also* d, DEG, Deg, deg • density *also* d • dental • dermatology/dermatologist/dermatologic • detail response • deuterium *also* d • deuteron *also* d • development(al) *also* dev, devel • deviation *also* DEV, dev • dextro– *also* d • dextrose • dextrorotatory *also* d • diagnosis *also* Diag, diag • diagonal *also* Diag, diag • diameter *also* d, Dia, dia, diam • diarrhea *also* d • diastole *also* dias • diathermy • didymium (praseodymium) • died *also* d • difference *also* DIFF, Diff, diff • diffusion/diffusing *also* DIFF, diff • dihydrouridine • diopter *also* d • diplomate *also* Dip • disease *also* dis • (electric) displacement • distal *also* d, dist • diuresis • diurnal *also* d • diverticulum • divorced *also* d, div • dominant *also* DOM, dom • donor • dorsal • [L. *dosis*] dose *also* d, dos • drive • drug • dual • duodenum/duodenal • duration *also* d • dwarf • [L. *da*] give *also* d • [L. *detur*] let it be given *also* d, det • [L. *dexter*] right *also* d, dex • unit of vitamin D potency

$\overline{\text{D}}$ mean dose

$\frac{1}{\text{D}}$ diffusion resistance

D1—D12 first through twelfth dorsal vertebra *also* D_1—D_{12}

D_1—D_{12} first through twelfth dorsal nerve • first through twelfth dorsal vertebra *also* D1—D12

1–D one–dimensional

2–D two–dimensional

D/3 distal third

3–D delayed double diffusion (test) • three–dimensional

2,4–D 2,4–dichlorophenoxyacetic acid

D dead space gas (subscript)

D– stereochemical structure

d atomic orbital with angular momentum quantum number 2 • date *also* D • [L. *dies*] day *also* D, da • dead *also* D • deceased *also* D, DEC, dec, dec'd, decd • deci– • decrease/decreased *also* D, DC, D/C, DEC, dec, DECR, decr • degree *also* D • density *also* D • deoxyribose • deuterium *also* D • deuteron *also* D • dextro– (right, clockwise) *also* D • diameter *also* D, Dia, dia, diam • diarrhea *also* D • died *also* D • diopter *also* D • distal *also* D, dist • diurnal *also* D • divorced *also* D, div • dorsal • dose *also* D, dos • doubtful • duration *also* D • dyne •

[L. *da*] give *also* D • [L. *detur*] let it be given *also* D, det • relative to rotation of a beam of polarized light • [L. *dexter*] right *also* D, dex

1/d daily, one per day

2/d twice a day

d– dextrorotary

DA dark agouti (rat) • daunomycin and cytosine • decubitus angina • degenerative arthritis • delayed action • delivery awareness • Dental Assistant • developmental age • diabetic acidosis • diagnostic arthroscopy • differentiation antigen • diphenylchlorarsine • direct admission • direct agglutination • disability assistance • disaggregated • dispense as directed *also* DAD • dopamine • drug addict/addiction • drug aerosol • ductus arteriosus • [L. *da*] give *also* D, d

D–A donor–acceptor

D/A date of admission • digital–to–analog (converter) • discharge and advise

dA deoxyadenosine *also* dAdo

da daughter *also* D, dau • day *also* D, d • deca–

DAA dehydroacetic acid

DA/A drug/alcohol addiction

DAB days after birth • diaminobutyric acid • dimethylaminoazobenzene • dysrhythmic aggressive behavior

DAC diazacholesterol • digital–to–analog converter • disabled adult child • disaster assistance center • Division of Ambulatory Care

dac dacryon *also* D

DACA dissecting aneurysm of the coronary artery

DACL Depression Adjective Check List

DACT dactinomycin (actinomycin D)

DAD diffuse alveolar damage • dispense as directed *also* DA • drug administration device

DADA dichloroacetic acid diisopropylammonium salt

DADDS diacetyldiaminodiphenyl sulfone

dAdo deoxyadenosine *also* dA

DADPS diphenylaulfone

DAE diphenylanthracene endoperoxide • diving air embolism

DAF delayed auditory feedback

DAFT Draw–A–Family test

DAG diacylglycerol

DAGT direct antiglobulin test

DAH disordered action of the heart

DAHEA Department of Allied Health Education and Accreditation

DAHM Division of Allied Health Manpower

DAI diffuse axonal injury

DAL drug analysis laboratory

daL, dal decaliter

DALA δ–aminolevulinic acid

DALE Drug Abuse Law Enforcement

DAM degraded amyloid • diacetylmonoxime • diacetylmorphine • discriminant analytic model

dam decameter

DAMA discharge against medical advice

dAMP deoxyadenylic acid

DANA drug–induced antinuclear antibodies

dand [L. *dandus*] to be given

D and C dilation and curettage *also* DC, D&C

DAO diamine oxidase • duly authorized officer

DAP data acquisition processor • delayed after polarization • depolarizing afterpotential • diabetes–associated peptide • diahydrogalactital, Adriamycin (doxorubicin), and Platino (cisplatin) • dihydroxyacetone phosphate • dipeptidyl amino peptidase *also* DAT • direct (latex) agglutination pregnancy (test) *also* DAPT • Draw–A–Person (test) • dynamic aortic patch

DAPRU Drug Abuse Prevention Resource Unit

DAPST Denver Auditory Phoneme Sequencing Test

DAPT diaminophenyl-thiazole • direct (latex) agglutination pregnancy test *also* DAP

DAR daily affective rhythm • dual asthmatic reaction

DARF direct antiglobulin rosette–forming

DARP drug abuse rehabilitation program

DARTS Drug and Alcohol Rehabilitation Testing System

DAS death anxiety scale • delayed anovulatory syndrome • developmental apraxia of speech • dextroamphetamine sulfate • died at scene

DASE Denver Articulation Screening Examination

DASH Distress Alarm for the Severely Handicapped

DASI Developmental Activities Screening Inventory

DASP double antibody solid phase

DAT daunorubicin, arabinosylcytosine, and thioguanine • delayed–action tablet • dementia of the Alzheimer type • dental aptitude test • diet as tolerated • differential agglutination test/titer • Differential Aptitude Test • dipeptidyl amino peptidase *also* DAP • diphtheria antitoxin • direct agglutination test • direct antiglobulin (Coombs) test • Disaster Action Team (of Red Cross)

DATE dental auxiliary teacher education

DAU Dental Auxiliary Utilization

dau daughter *also* D, da

DAUNO daunorubicin *also* DRB

DAV duck adenovirus

DAW dispense as written

DB Baudelocque diameter • database • date of birth *also* D/B, DOB • deep breath • dense body • dextran blue • diabetic • diagonal band • diet beverage • direct bilirubin • disability • distobuccal • double–blind (study) • dry bulb • duodenal bulb • Dutch belted (rabbit)

D/B date of birth *also* DB, DOB

dB decibel

db diabetes

DBA dibenzanthracene • *Dolichos biflorus* agglutinin

DBAE dihydroxyboryl-aminoethyl

DBC dibencozide • dye–binding capacity

DB&C deep breathing and coughing

DBCL dilute blood clot lysis (method)

DBCP dibromochloropropane

DBD definite brain damage • dibromodulcitol

DBDG distobuccal developmental groove

DBE deep breathing exercise • dibromoethane

DBED dibenzylethylenediamine dipenicillin (penicillin G benzathine)

DBF disturbed bowel function

DBH dacarbazine, carmustine, and hydroxyurea • dopamine β–hydroxylase

DBI development at birth index

DBIL, D bili direct bilirubin

DBIOC database input/output control

DBIP Discrimination by Identification of Pictures

dBk decibels above 1 kilowatt

dbl double

DBM database management • decarboxylase base Moeller • diabetic management • dibromo-mannitol • dobutamine

dBm decibels above 1 milliwatt

DBMC dystrophica bullosa Mendes da Costa

DBMG mandelonitrile β–glucuronide

DBMS database management systems

DBO distobucco–occlusal

db/ob diabetic obese (mouse)

DBP demineralized bone powder • diastolic blood pressure • dibutyl phthalate • distobuc-copulpal • Döhle body panmyelopathy • di-*tert*-butyl peroxide *also* DTBP

DBQ debrisoquin(e)

DBR direct bilirubin · disordered breathing rate

DBS deep brain stimulation · Denis Browne splint · despeciated bovine serum · dibromsalicil · diminished breath sounds · direct bonding system · Division of Biological Standards

DBT disordered breathing time · dry bulb temperature

DBW desirable body weight

dBW decibels above 1 watt

DBZ dibenzamine

DC daily census · data communication · daunorubicin and cytarabine · decarboxylase · decrease *also* D, d, D/C, DEC, dec, DECR, decr · deep compartment · degenerating cell · Dental Corps · deoxycholate · descending colon · dextran charcoal · diagonal conjugate (diameter) · diagnostic center · diagnostic code · differentiated cell · diffuse cortical · digit copying · dilation and curettage *also* D and C, D&C · dilation catheter · diphenylcyanarsine · direct and consensual *also* D&C · direct Coombs (test) · direct current *also* dc · Direction Circular · discharge *also* D/C · discontinue *also* D/C, d/c, dc · distal colon · distocervical · Doctor of Chiropractic · donor cells ·

dorsal column · duodenal cap · dyskeratosis congenita

DC65 Darvon compound 65

D/C decrease *also* D, d, DC, DEC, dec, DECR, decr · diarrhea/constipation · discharge *also* DC · discontinue *also* DC, d/c, dc

D&C dilation and curettage *also* D and C, DC · direct and consensual *also* DC · drugs and cosmetics

dC deoxycytidine

dc direct current *also* DC · discontinue *also* DC, D/C, d/c

d/c discontinue *also* DC, D/C, dc · discharge (vaginal)

DCA deoxycholate–citrate agar · deoxycholic acid · desoxycorticosterone acetate · dicarboxylic acid · dichloroacetate

DCAG double coronary artery graft

DCB dichlorobenzidine · dilutional cardiopulmonary bypass

DC&B dilation, curettage, and biopsy

DCBE double contrast barium enema

DCBF dynamic cardiac blood flow

DCC day care center · dextran–coated charcoal · dicyclohexylcarbodiimide *also* DCCD · Disaster Control Center · dorsal cell column · double concave *also* DCc, DDc

DCc double concave *also* DCC, DDc

DCCD dicyclohexylcarbo-diimide *also* DCC

DCCF dural carotid–cavernous fistula

DCCMP daunomycin, cyclocytidine, 6–mercaptopurine, and prednisolone

DC$_{CO2}$ diffusing capacity for carbon dioxide

DCD Dennis Test of Child Development

D/c'd discontinued

DCDA deuterium with cesium dihydrogen arsenate

DCE delayed contrast enhancement • designated compensable event • demosterol–to–cholesterol enzyme

DCF direct contrifugal flotation • dopachrome conversion factor

DCFM Doppler color flow mapping

DCG desoxycorticosterone glucoside • disodium cromoglycate • dynamic electrocardiogram

DCH delayed cutaneous hypersensitivity

DCHA dicyclohexylamine

DCHFB dichlorohexa-fluorobutane

DCHN dicylohexylamine nitrate/nitrite

DCI dichloroisoprenaline • dichloroisoproterenol

DCIS ductal carcinoma in situ

DCL dicloxacillin • diffuse/disseminated cutaneous leishmaniasis • digital counter/locator

DCLS deoxycholate citrate lactose saccharose (agar)

DCM dichloromethane • dichloromethotrexate • dilated cardiomyopathy • Doctor of Comparative Medicine • dyssynergia cerebellaris myoclonica

DCMO dihydrocarboxa-nilidomethyloxathin

DCMP daunorubicin, cytarabine, 6–mercapto-purine, and prednisone

dCMP deoxycytidylic acid • deoxycytidine monophosphate

DCMX dichloro–*m*–xylenol

DCMXT dichloromethotrexate

DCN Data Collection Network (medical records) • delayed conditioned necrosis • dorsal column nucleus • dorsal cutaneous nerve

DCNU chloroethyl-nitrosoglucosyl urea (chlorozotocin)

D$_{CO}$ diffusing capacity for carbon monoxide

DCP calcium phosphate, dibasic • dicalcium phosphate • dichlorophene • discharge planner • District Community Physician • dynamic compression plate

DCPC dichlorodiphenylmethyl carbinol

DCPM daunorubicin, cytarabine, prednisolone, and mercaptopurine

DCPN direction–changing positional nystagmus

DCPU dorsal caudate putamen

DCR dacryocystorhinostomy • delayed cutaneous reaction • direct cortical response

DCS decompression sickness • dense canalicular system • diffuse cortical sclerosis • disease control serum • dorsal column stimulation/stimulator

DCSA double–contrast shoulder arthrography

DCT daunorubicin, cytarabine, and thioguanine • deep chest therapy • direct Coombs test • distal convoluted tubule • diurnal cortisol test • dynamic computed tomography

DCTM delay computer tomographic myelography

DCTMA desoxycorticosterone trimethylacetate

dCTP deoxycytidine triphosphate

DCTPA desoxycorticosterone triphenylacetate

DCU dichloral urea

DCV dacarbazine, CCNU (lomustine), and vincristine

DCX double–charge exchange

DCx double convex

DD dangerous drug • day of delivery • degenerative disease • delusional disorder • dependent drainage • detrusor dyssynergia • developmental disability • developmental disability • dialysis dementia • diaper dermatitis • died of the disease • differential diagnosis *also* D/D, DDX, DDx, DIAGNO, diff diag • digestive disease • Di Guglielmo disease • disk diameter • discharged dead • discharge diagnosis • Distortion of Dots • double diffusion • double dose • down drain • drug dependence • dry dressing • Duchenne dystrophy • Dupuytren disease

DD, dd [L. *de die*] daily • [L. *detur ad*] let it be given to

D/D differential diagnosis *also* DD, DDX, DDx, DIAGNO, diff diag

D→D discharge to duty

D&D diarrhea and dehydration

Dd unusual detail response

dD confabulated detail response

DDA Dangerous Drugs Act • dideoxyadenosine • digital differential analyzer • digital display alarm

DDAVP, dDAVP deamino–8–D–arginine vasopressin (desmopressin acetate)

DDC dangerous drug cabinet • dideoxycytidine (zalcitabine) • diethyldithiocarbamate (diethyldithiocarbamic

acid) • dihydrocollidine •
dihydroxyphenylalanine
decarboxylase • direct
display console •
diverticular disease of colon

DDc double concave *also*
DCC, DCc

DDD defined daily dose •
degenerative disk disease •
dense deposit disease •
dichlorodiphenyldichloro-
ethane • dihydroxy-
dinaphthyl disulfide

DDE dichlorodiphenyl-
dichloroethylene • direct
data entry

DDFS distant–disease–free
survival

DDG deoxy–D–glucose

DDGB double–dose
gallbladder
(cholecystogram)

DDHT double dissociated
hypertropia

DDI dideoxyinosine
(didanosine) • dressing dry
and intact

DDIB Disease Detection
Information Bureau

dd in d [L. *de die in diem*]
from day to day

DDM Doctor of Dental
Medicine

DDMS degenerative dense
microsphere

dDNA denatured DNA

DDP diamminedi-
chloroplatinum (cisplatin) •
density–dependent
phosphoprotein • difficult–

denture patient •
distributed data processing

DDR diastolic descent rate •
discharged during referral

DDS damaged disk syndrome •
Demon Dropout Scale •
dendrodendritic
synaptosome • dental
distress syndrome •
depressed DNA synthesis •
dialysis disequilibrium
syndrome • diaminodi-
phenylsulfone (dapsone) *also*
DDSO • directional Doppler
sonography • Director of
Dental Services • disease
disability scale • Doctor of
Dental Surgery • dodecyl
sulfate • double decidual
sac • dystrophy–dystocia
syndrome • dystrophy–
dystonia syndrome

Dds detail response to small
white space

DDSc Doctor of Dental
Science

DDSO diaminodiphenyl-
sulfone (dapsone) *also* DDS

DDST Denver Developmental
Screening Test

DDT dichlorodiphenyl-
trichloroethane
(chlorophenothane) •
ductus deferens tumor

DDTP drug dependence
treatment program

ddTTP dideoxythymidine
triphosphate

DDVP dimethyldichlorovinyl
phosphate (dichlorvos)

DDW double distilled water

DdW detail response
elaborating the whole

DDX, DDx differential diagnosis *also* DD D/D, DIAGNO, diff diag

DE dendritic expansion • deprived eye • diagnostic error • digestive energy • dose equivalent • dream elements • drug evaluation • duodenal exclusion • duration of ejection

D$_5$E$_{48}$ 5% dextrose and electrolyte 48% (solution)

2DE two–dimensional echocardiography

D&E diet and elimination • dilation and evacuation

de edge detail

DEA dehydroepiandrosterone • diethylamine • diethanolamine • Drug Enforcement Agency

DEA # Drug Enforcement Agency number (physicians' federal narcotic number)

DEA–D, DEAE–D diethyl-aminoethyl dextran

DEAE diethylaminoethanol • diethylaminoethyl (cellulose)

DEB diepoxybutane • diethylbutanediol • dystrophic epidermolysis bullosa

deb debridement

DEBA diethylbarbituric acid

debil debility

DEBS dominant epidermolysis bullosa simplex

deb spis [L. *debita*

spissutudine] of proper consistency

DEC deceased *also* D, d, dec, dec'd, decd • deciduous *also* D, dec • decimal • decimeter • decrease *also* D, d, DC, D/C, dec, DECR, decr • deoxycholate citrate • diethylcarbamazine • dynamic environmental conditioning (cycle) • [L. *decanta*] pour off

Dec decant *also* dec

dec decant *also* Dec • deciduous *also* D, DEC • decompose/ decomposition • deceased *also* D, d, DEC, dec'd, decd • decrease/decreased *also* D, d, DC, D/C, DEC, DECR, decr

decd, dec'd deceased *also* D, d, DEC, dec

DECEL, decel deceleration

DECO decreasing consumption of oxygen

decoct decoction

decomp decomposition/ decompose

decon decontamination

dec(R) decrease, relative

DECR, decr decrease/ decreased *also* D, d, DC, D/ C, dec

DECUB, decub [L. *decubitus*] lying down

DED date of expected delivery • defined exposure dose • delayed erythema dose

de d in d [L. *de die in diem*] from day to day

DEEG depth electroencephalogram/ electroencephalography • depth electography

DEET diethyltoluamide

DEF decayed, extracted, or filled • defecation *also* def • deficiency • duck embryo fibroblast

def defecation *also* DEF • deficiency/deficient *also* defic • definite, definition

defib defibrillate/defibrillation

defic deficiency/deficient *also* def

deform deformed/deformity

DEG, Deg, deg degeneration/ degenerative *also* degen • degree *also* D, d

degen degeneration/ degenerative *also* DEG, Deg, deg

deglut [L. *deglutiatur*] let it be swallowed

DEH dysplasia epiphysealis hemimelica

DEHFT developmental hand function test

DEHS Division of Emergency Health Services

dehyd dehydration/dehydrated

DEJ, dej dentoenamel junction

del deletion • delivery • delusion

deliq deliquescence/ deliquescent

delta (Δ, δ) fourth letter of the Greek alphabet

Δ absence of heat in a reaction • delta gap • difference (mathematics) • double bond

δ fourth in a series or group • heavy chain of immunoglobulin D

DEM, Dem Demerol (meperidine)

DEN dengue • diethylnitrosamine

denat denatured

denom denominator

DENT Dental Exposure Normalization Technique

Dent, dent dentistry/dentist/ dental/dentition • [L. *dentur*] let it be given

dent tal dos [L. *dentur tales doses*] give of such doses

DEP diethylpropanediol • diethyl pyrocarbonate • dilution end point

dep dependent • deposit • [L. *depuratus*] purified

DEPA diethylenephosphoramide

DEPC diethylpyrocarbonate

depr depression/depressed

DEPS distal effective potassium secretion

DEP ST SEG depressed ST segment

Dept, dept department

DER disulfiram–ethanol reaction

DeR degeneration reaction

der derivative of chromosome • derive

deriv derivative/derived

DERM, Derm, derm
dermatology/dermatologist/
dermatologic

DES dermal–epidermal
separation • dialysis
encephalopathy syndrome •
diethylstilbestrol • diffuse
esophageal spasm •
disequilibrium syndrome •
doctor's emergency service

DESAT, desat desaturated

desc descent/descending/
descendant

DESI drug efficacy study
implementation

DEST dichotic environmental
sounds test

destil, dest [L. *destilla,
destillatus*] distill/distilled

DET diethyltryptamine

det determine • [L. *detur*] let
it be given *also* D, d

Det–6 detroid–6 (human
sternum marrow cells)

determ, determin
determination/determined

det in dup, det in 2 plo [L.
detur in duplo] let twice as
much be given

detn detention

detox detoxification

d et s [L. *detur et signetur*] let
it be given and labeled

DEUC direct electronic
urethrocystometry

DEV deviant/deviation *also*
D • duck embryo
vaccine • duck embryo
virus

dev develop/development(al)
also D • deviate/deviation
also D

devel development *also* D, dev

DevPd developmental
pediatrics

DEVR dominant exudative
vitreoretinopathy

DEX dexamethasone

dex [L. *dexter*] right

DF decapacitation factor
(sperm) • decayed and
filled (permanent teeth) •
decontamination factor •
deferoxamine • deficiency
factor • defined flora
(animal) • degree of
freedom • dengue fever •
desferrioxamine • diabetic
father • diaphragmatic
function • diastolic
filling • dietary fiber •
digital fluoroscopy •
discriminant function •
disseminated foci •
distribution factor • dome
fragment • dorsiflexion •
drug free • dry (gas)
fractional (concentration) •
dye free

df decayed and filled
(deciduous teeth) • degrees
of freedom

DFA diet for age • difficulty
falling asleep • direct
fluorescence antibody
(test) • dorsiflexion assist

DFB dinitrofluorobenzene •
dysfunctional (uterine)
bleeding

DFC deletion of final
consonants • dry–filled
capsule

DFD defined formula diets • degenerative facet disease • diisopropylphosphoro-fluoridate

DFDD difluorodiphenyl-dichloroethane

DFDT difluorodiphenyl-trichloroethane

DFE diffuse fasciitis with eosinophilia • distal femoral epiphysis

DFECT dense fibroelastic connective tissue

DFG direct forward gaze

DFI disease–free interval(s)

DFM decreased fetal movement

DFMC daily fetal movement count

DFMO difluoromethylor-nithine

DFMR daily fetal movement record

DFO, DFOM deferoxamine

DFP diastolic filling period • diisopropylfluorophos-phonate

DF³²P radiolabeled diisopropylfluorophos-phonate

DFR diabetic floor routine • dialysate filtration rate

DFRC deglycerolized frozen red cells

DFS disease–free survival • dynamic flow study

DFSP dermatofibrosarcoma protuberans

DFT defibrillation threshold • discrete Fourier transforms

DFT₄ dialyzable free thyroxine

DFU dead fetus in utero • dideoxyfluorouridine

DFV diarrhea with fever and vomiting

DFX desferrioxamine

DG dark ground • dentate gyrus • deoxyglucose *also* 2DG • diagnosis *also* Dg • diastolic gallop • diglyceride • distogingival • Duchenne–Griesinger (disease)

Dg diagnosis *also* DG

dg decigram *also* dgm

2DG 2–deoxy–D–glucose *also* DG

DGCI delayed gamma camera image

DGE delayed gastric emptying • density gradient electrophoresis

DGF digoxin–like factor

DGI disseminated gonococcal infection

DGL deglycyrrhizined liquorice

DGM ductal glandular mastectomy

dgm decigram *also* dg

dGMP deoxyguanosine monophosphate • deoxyguanylic acid

DGMS Division of General Medical Services

DGN diffuse glomerulonephritis

DGP deoxyglucose phosphate

DGR Degranol (mannomustine)

DGS diabetic glomerulosclerosis

dGTP deoxyguanosine triphosphate

DGV dextrose, gelatin, Veronal (solution)

DGVB dextrose–gelatin–Veronal buffer

DH daily habits • day hospital • dehydrocholic acid • dehydrogenase • delayed hypersensitivity • dental habits • dental hygienist • dermatitis herpetiformis • developmental history • diaphragmatic hernia • diffuse histiocytic (lymphoma) • disseminated histoplasmosis • dominant hand • dorsal horn • ductal hyperplasia • Dunkin–Hartley (guinea pig)

D/H deuterium/hydrogen (ratio)

DHA dehydroascorbic acid • dehydroepiandrosterone *also* DHEA • dihydroacetic acid • dihydroxyacetone • district health authority

DHAD dihydroxybis(hydroxy-ethylaminoethyl)amino-anthraquinone dihydro-chloride (mitoxantrone hydrochloride)

DHAP dihydroxyacetone phosphate

DHAS dehydroepiandros-terone sulfate

DHB dihydroxybenzoic acid

DHBS dihydrobiopterin synthetase

DHBV duck hepatic B virus

DHC dehydrocholate • dehydrocholesterol

DHCA deep hypothermia and circulatory arrest

DHCC dihydroxychole-calciferol

DHD district health department

DHE dihydroergocryptine *also* DHEC, DHK • dihydroergotamine

DHEA dehydroepiandrosterone *also* DHA

DHEAS dehydroepiandros-terone sulfate

DHEC dihydroergocryptine *also* DHE, DHK

DHES Division of Health Examination Statistics

DHEW Department of Health, Education, and Welfare (now Department of Health and Human Services)

DHF dengue hemorrhagic fever • dorsihyperflexion

DHFR dihydrofolate reductase

DHFS dengue hemorrhagic fever shock (syndrome)

DHg Doctor of Hygiene

DHHS Department of Health and Human Services

DHI Dental Health International • dihydroisocodeine • dihydroxyindole

DHIA dehydroisoandrosterol

DHK dihydroergocryptine *also* DHE, DHEC

DHL diffuse histiocytic lymphoma

DHM dihydromorphine

DHMA dihydroxymandelic acid

DHO deuterium hydrogen oxide · dihydroergocornine *also* DHO 180

DHO 180 dihydroergocornine *also* DHO

DHODH dihydroorotate dehydrogenase

DHP dehydrogenated polymer · dihydroprogesterone · dihydroxyacetone phosphate

DHPc dorsal hippocampus

DHPG dihydroxyphenyl-ethylene glycol · dihydroxyphenylglycol · dihydroxyproproxymethylguanine (ganciclovir)

DHPR dihydropteridine reductase

dhPRL decidual prolactin

DHR delayed hypersensitivity reaction

DHS delayed hypersensitivity · dihydrostreptomycin *also* DHSM · duration of hospital stay · dynamic hip screw

D–5–HS dextrose 5% in Harman solution

DHSM dihydrostreptomycin *also* DHS

DHSS dihydrostreptomycin sulfate

DHST delayed hypersensitivity test

DHT dehydrotestosterone · dihydroergotoxine · dihydrotachysterol · dihydrotestosterone · dihydrothymine · dihydroxypropyltheophylline · dissociated hypertropia

DHTP dihydrotestosterone propionate

DHy, DHyg Doctor of Hygiene

DHZ dihydralazine

DI date of injury · Debrix Index · defective interfering · degradation index · dentinogenesis imperfecta · deoxyribonucleic acid index · (Beck) Depression Inventory · desorption ionization · deterioration index · detrusor instability · diabetes insipidus · diagnostic imaging · diaphragmatic · disability insurance · dispensing information · distal intestine · distoincisal · double indemnity · dorsal interosseous · dorsoiliacus · drug information · drug interactions · dyskaryosis index · dyspnea index

D&I debridement and irrigation · dry and intact

D$_I$ insulin dialysance

DI didymium · Diego blood group

dl inside detail

DIA depolarization–induced automaticity · diabetes *also* Dia, diab

DIA Diego antigen

Dia, dia diathermy *also* diath • diameter *also* D, d, diam

Dia, diab diabetes/diabetic *also* DIA

DIAC diiodothyroacetic acid

Diag, diag diagnosis *also* D • diagram • diagonal *also* D

DIAGNO diagnosis *also* DD, D/D, DDX, DDx, diff diag

diam diameter *also* D, d, Dia, dia

diaph diaphragm/diaphragmatic *also* DI, DPH

DIAR dextran–induced anaphylactoid reaction

dias diastole/diastolic *also* D

DIAS BP diastolic blood pressure

diath diathermy *also* Dia, dia

DIATH SW diathermy short wave

DIAZ diazepam

DIB Diagnostic Interview for Borderlines • disability insurance benefits • dot immunobinding

DIC differential interference contrast (microscopy) • diffuse intravascular clotting/coagulation • dimethyltriazenoimidazole carboxamide (dacarbazine) • disseminated intravascular coagulopathy/coagulation • drug information center

dic dicentric

DICD dispersion–induced circular dichroism

diclox dicloxacillin

DID dead of intercurrent disease • delayed ischemia deficit • double immunodiffusion (technique) • dystonia–improvement–dystonia

DIDD dense intramembranous deposit disease

DIDMOAD diabetes insipidus, diabetes mellitus, optic atrophy, and deafness (syndrome) *also* DIMOAD

DIE died in emergency (room)

dieb alt [L. *diebus alternis*] on alternate days

dieb secund [L. *diebus secundis*] every second day

dieb tert [L. *diebus tertiis*] every third day

DIEDA diethyliminodiacetic acid

Diet. Tech. Dietetic Telchnician

DIF diffuse interstitial fibrosis • diflunisal • direct immuno-fluorescence • dose increase factor

dif differential (blood count) *also* DIFF, Diff, diff

DIFF, diff difference *also* D, Diff • differential (blood count) *also* dif, Diff • diffusion *also* D

Diff difference/different *also* D, DIFF, diff • differential (blood count) *also* dif, DIFF, diff

diff diag differential diagnosis *also* DD, D/D, DDX, DDx, DIAGNO

DIFP diffuse interstitial fibrosing pneumonitis · diisopropyl fluorophosphonate

DIG digitalis *also* dig. · digitoxin · digoxin

dig. [L. *digeretur*] let it be digested · digitalis *also* DIG

dig. tox digitalis toxicity

DIH died in hospital

DIHPPA diiodohydroxy-phenylpyruvic acid

DIJOA dominantly inherited juvenile optic atrophy

DIL, dil dilute/dilution/diluted *also* dilut · drug–induced lupus · drug information log

Dil Dilantin · dilation *also* dil

dilat dilatation

DILD diffuse interstitial lung disease

DILE drug–induced lupus erythematosus

diln dilution

Diluc, diluc [L. *diluculo*] at daybreak

dilut dilute/dilution/diluted *also* DIL, dil

DIM diminish *also* dim. · divalent ion metabolism

dim. diminish *also* DIM · [L. *dimidus*] one–half

DIMOAD diabetes insipidus, diabetes mellitus, optic atrophy, and deafness (syndrome) *also* DIDMOAD

dIMP deoxyinosine monophosphate (deoxyinosinate)

DIMS disorders of initiating and maintaining sleep

DIMSA disseminated intravascular multiple systems activation

d in dup [L. *detur in duplo*] give twice as much

d in p aeq [L. *dividetur in partes aequales*] divide into equal parts

diopt diopter

DIP desquamative interstitial pneumonia/pneumonitis · dichlorophenolindophenol · diisopropyl phosphate · distal interphalangeal (joint) *also* DIPJ · drip–infusion pyelogram · drug–induced parkinsonism · dual–in-line package (integrated circuits)

Dip diplomate *also* D

dip diploid

DIPA diisopropylamine

DIPC diffuse interstitial pulmonary calcification

DIPF diisopropylphospho-fluoridate

diph diphtheria

diph–tox diphtheria toxoid

diph–tox AP alum–precipitated diphtheria toxoid

DIPJ distal interphalangeal joint *also* DIP

DIR director · double isomorphous replacement

Dir, dir direct · [L. *directione*] direction · director

DIRD drug–induced renal disease

dir prop [L. *directione propria*] with proper direction

DIS Diagnostic Interview Schedule · dislocation *also* dis, disloc

DI–S Debris Index–Simplified

dis disability/disabled *also* DSBL · disease *also* D · dislocation *also* DIS, disloc · distance · distribution *also* dist

disc discontinue

disch discharge(d)

DISH diffuse/disseminated idiopathic skeletal hyperostosis

DISIDA diisopropylimino-diacetic acid

disinfect. disinfection

disloc dislocation/dislocated *also* DIS, dis

disod disodium

D₅ISOM dextrose 5% in Isolyte M

disp dispensary/dispense

dispo disposition

diss dissolve(d)

dissem disseminated/dissemination

dist distal *also* D, d · distill(ed)/distillation · distribute/distribution *also* dis · district

dist fr distinguished from

distill. distillation

DIT diet–induced thermogenesis · diiodotyrosine · drug–induced thrombocytopenia

dITP deoxyinosine triphosphate

DIV double–inlet ventricle

div divergence/divergent · divide(d)/division · divorced *also* D, d · [L. *dividetur*] devide

DIVA digital intravenous angiography

DIVBC disseminated intravascular blood coagulation

DIVC disseminated intravascular coagulation

div in par aeq [L. *dividetur in partes aequales*] divide into equal parts

DJD degenerative joint disease

DJS Dubin–Johnson syndrome

DK dark *also* dk · decay · degeneration of keratinocytes · Déjérine–Klumpke (syndrome) · diabetic ketoacidosis *also* DKA · diet kitchen · diseased kidney · dog kidney (cells)

dk dark *also* DK

DKA diabetic ketoacidosis *also* DK · did not keep appointment

DKB deep knee bends · dideoxykanamycin B

DKDP deuterium with

potassium dihydrogen phosphate

dkg decagram

dkL, dkl decaliter

dkm decameter

DKP dibasic potassium phosphate • dikalium phosphate • diketopiperazine

DKTC dog kidney tissue culture

DKV deer kidney virus

DL danger list • dansyl lysine • deep lobe • developmental level • diagnostic laparoscopy • difference limen (threshold) • diffuse lymphoma • diffusing capacity of lung *also* D_L • direct laryngoscopy • directed listening • disabled list • distolingual • Donath–Landsteiner (antibody) *also* D–L • drug level • [L. *dosis letalis*] lethal dose

D–L Donath–Landsteiner (antibody) *also* DL

DL– equal quantities of D and L enantiomorphs (formerly *dl–*)

D_L diffusing capacity of lung *also* DL

dL, dl deciliter

DLA, DLa distolabial

D–L Ab Donath–Landsteiner antibody

DLAI, DLaI distolabioincisal

DLAP, DLaP distolabiopulpal

DLB diffuse and lymphoblastic • direct laryngoscopy and bronchoscopy

DLC differential leukocyte count • double–lumen catheter

DLCO, DL_{CO}, D_{LCO} carbon monoxide diffusing capacity of the lungs

$DLCO_2$, D_{LCO2} carbon dioxide diffusing capacity of the lungs

$D_{LCO}{}^{SB}$ single–breath carbon monoxide diffusing capacity of lungs

$D_{LCO}{}^{SS}$ steady–state carbon monoxide diffusing capacity of lungs

DLE delayed light emission • dialyzable leukocyte extract • discoid lupus erythematosus • disseminated lupus erythematosus

D_1LE diagonal 1 lower extremity

D_2LE diagonal 2 lower extremity

DLF digitalis–like factor • digoxin–like factor • dorsolateral funiculus

DLG distolingual groove

DLI distolinguoincisal • double label index

DLIF digoxin–like immunoreactive factors

DLIS digoxin–like immunoreactive substance

DLLI dulcitol lysine lactose iron (agar)

DLMP date of last menstrual period

DLNMP date of last normal menstrual period

DLO distolinguo–occlusal

D₁O₂, D_LO2 diffusing capacity of lungs for oxygen

DLP delipidized serum protein • developmental learning problems • direct linear plotting • dislocation of patella • distolinguopulpal • dysharmonic luteal phase

D₅LR dextrose 5% in lactated Ringer (solution)

DLS daily living skills

DLT dihydroepiandrosterone loading test

DLV defective leukemia virus

DLWD diffuse lymphocytic, well differentiated

DM dermatologist/ dermatology • dermatomyositis • Descemet membrane • dextromaltose • dextromethorphan • diabetes mellitus • diabetic mother • diastolic murmur • diffuse mixed • diphenylaminechlorarsine • distant metastases • dopamine • dorsomedial • dose modification • double membrane • double minute (chromosome) • dry matter • duodenal mucosa • membrane diffusing capacity

D_M membrane component of diffusion

dM decimorgan

dm decimeter

dm² square decimeter

dm³ cubic decimeter

DMA dimethyladenosine • dimethylamine • di- methylaniline • dimethyl- arginine • direct memory access/address (computers)

DMAARD delayed– mechanism–of–action antirheumatic drug

DMAB dimethylamino- benzaldehyde (Ehrlich reagent) *also* DMABA • dimethylaminoazobenzene

DMABA dimethylamino- benzaldehyde (Ehrlich reagent) *also* DMAB

DMAC dimethylacetamide

DMAD disease–modifying antirheumatic drug *also* DMARD

DMAE dimethylaminoethanol

DMARD disease–modifying antirheumatic drug *also* DMAD

DMAS dimethylamine sulfate

DMC dactinomycin, methotrexate, and cyclophosphamide • demeclocycline • dichlorodiphenyl- methylcarbinol • dimethylcysteine • direct microscopic count

DMCC direct microscopic clump count

DMCM dimethoxyethyl- carboline carboxylate

DMCT, DMCTC dimethyl-chlortetracycline

DMD desmethyldiazepam *also* DMDZ • disease–modifying drug • Doctor of Dental Medicine • Duchenne muscular dystrophy

DMDS dimethyl disulfide

DMDT dimethoxydiphenyl-trichloroethane

DMDZ desmethyldiazepam *also* DMD

DME degenerative myoclonus epilepsy • dimethyl diester • dimethyl ether • diphasic meningo-encephalitis • director of medical education • dropping mercury electrode • drug–metabolizing enzyme • Dulbecco modified Eagle (medium) *also* DMEM • durable medical equipment

DMEM Dulbecco modified Eagle medium *also* DME

DMF decayed, missing, and filled (teeth) • dimethyl-formamide *also* DMFA • diphasic milk fever

DMFA dimethylformamide *also* DMF

DMFS decayed, missing, or filled surfaces (permanent teeth)

dmfs decayed, missing, or filled surfaces (deciduous teeth)

DMG dimethylglycine

DMGBL dimethyl–γ–butyrolactone

DMGG dimethylguanyl-guanidine

DMH Department of Mental Health/Hygiene • diffuse mesangial hypercellularity • dimethylhydrazine

DMI defense mechanism inventory • desipramine • desmethylimipramine • Diagnostic Mathematics Inventory (psychologic testing) • diaphragmatic myocardial infarct • direct migration inhibition

DMKA diabetes mellitus ketoacidosis

DML diffuse mixed lymphoma • distal motor latency

DMM dimethylmyleran • disproportionate micromelia

DMN dimethylnitrosamine *also* DMNA • dorsal motor nucleus (of vagus)

DMNA dimethylnitrosamine *also* DMN

DMO dimethyloxazolin-dinedione

DMOOC diabetes mellitus out of control

DMP diffuse mesangial proliferation • dimethylphosphate • dimethylphthalate • dura mater prosthesis

DMPA depomedroxy-progesterone acetate

DMPE dimethoxyphenyl-ethylamine

DMPP dimethylphenyl-piperazinium

DMPS dysmyelopoietic syndrome

DMRF dorsal medullary reticular formation

DMS delayed microembolism syndrome • delayed muscle soreness • demarcation membrane system • dense microsphere • Department of Medicine and Surgery • dermatomyositis • diagnostic medical sonography • diffuse mesangial sclerosis • dimethyl sulfate • dimethyl sulfoxide *also* DMSO • Doctor of Medical Science • dysmyelopoietic syndrome

dms double minute sphere

DMSA dimercaptosuccinic acid • disodium monomethanearsonate

DMSO dimethylsulfoxide *also* DMS

DMT dermatophytosis • dimethyltryptamine • Doctor of Medical Technology

DMTU dimethylthiourea

DMU dimethanolurea

D,M,V,P disk, macula, vessels, periphery

DMX diathermy, massage, and exercise

DN Deiters nucleus • dextrose–nitrogen (ratio) • diabetic neuropathy • dibucaine number • dicrotic notch • Diploma in Nursing • District Nurse • down • dysplastic nevus

D/N dextrose/nitrogen ratio

D&N distance and near (vision)

Dn dekanem

dn decinem

DNA deoxyribonucleic acid • did not answer • did not attend • does not apply

DNAP deoxyribonucleic acid polymerase

DNA–P deoxyribonucleic acid phosphorus

DNAse, DNase deoxyribonuclease

DNB dinitrobenzene • dorsal noradrenergic bundle

DNBP dinitrobutylphenol

DNBT dinitroblue

DNC did not come • dinitrocarbanilide

DNCB dinitrochlorobenzene

DND died a natural death

DNE Director of Nursing Education • Doctor of Nursing Education

DNFB dinitrofluorobenzene (Sanger reagent)

DNI do not intubate

DNKA did not keep appointment

DNL diffuse nodular lymphoma • disseminated necrotizing leukoencephalopathy

DNLL dorsal nucleus of lateral lemniscus

DNO District Nursing Officer

DNOC dinitro–orthocresol

DNOCHP dinitro–*o*–cyclohexyphenol

DNP deoxyribonucleoprotein • dinitrophenol

DNPH dinitrophenylhydrazine

DNPM dinitrophenol–morphine

DNPT diethylnitrophenyl thiophosphate (parathion) *also* DNTP

DNR daunorubicin • did not respond • do not report • do not resuscitate • dorsal nerve root

DNS dansyl • de novo synthesis • deviated nasal septum • diaphragmatic nerve stimulation • (doctor) did not see (patient) • did not show • Doctor of Nursing Services • do not show • do not substitute • dysplastic nevus syndrome

D₅NS, D₅NSS dextrose 5% in normal saline solution

DNT did not test

DNTP diethylnitrophenyl thiophosphate (parathion) *also* DNPT

DNUA distillable nonurea adductable

DNV dorsal nucleus of vagus

DO diamine oxidase (histaminase) • diet order • digoxin • dissolved oxygen • disto–occlusal • Doctor of Osteopathy • doctor's orders • doxycycline • drugs only

D–O directive–organic

D/O disorder

D₀ oxygen diffusion

do [L. *dicto*] the same, as before

DOA date of admission • date of arrival • dead on arrival • duration of action

DOAC Dubois oleic albumin complex

DOA–DRA dead on arrival despite resuscitative attempts

DOAP daunorubicin, Oncovin (vincristine), araC (cytarabine), and prednisone

DOB date of birth *also* DB, D/B • dobutamine • doctor's order book

DOC date of conception • deoxycholate • deoxycorticosterone • diabetes out of control *also* doc, DOOC • died of other causes • diet of choice • drug of choice

doc diabetes out of control *also* DOC, DOOC • doctor *also* DR, Dr • document/documentation

DOCA deoxycorticosterone acetate

DOCG deoxycorticosterone glucoside

DOCLINE Documents On–Line

DOCS, DOCs deoxycorticoids

DOcSc Doctor of Ocular Science

DOC–SR deoxycorticosterone secretion rate

DOD date of death • date of discharge • died of disease • dissolved oxygen deficit

DOE date of examination • desoxyephedrine • direct observation evaluation • dyspnea on exertion

DOES disorders of excessive sleepiness

DOET dimethoxy-ethylamphetamine

DOFOS disturbance of function occlusion syndrome

DOH Department of Health

DOHb Dohle bodies

DOI date of injury • died of injuries

DOL day of life (followed by number)

dol dolorimetric unit (of pain intensity)

DOLV double–outlet left ventricle

DOM deaminated *O*–methyl metabolite • Department of Medicine • dimethoxy-methylamphetamine • dissolved organic matter • dominance/dominant *also* D, dom

dom dominant/dominance *also* D, DOM • domestic

DOMA dihydroxymandelic acid

DON diazo–oxonorleucine • Director of Nursing

don. [L. *donec*] until

donec alv sol fuerit [L.

donec alvus soluta fuerit] until bowels are opened (until a bowel movement takes place)

DOOC diabetes out of control *also* DOC, doc

DOOR deafness, onycho–osteodystrophy, and mental retardation (syndrome)

DOPA, dopa dihydroxy-phenylalanine (methyldopa)

DOPAC dihydrophenylacetic acid

dopase dihydroxy-phenylalanine oxidase

DOPC determined osteogenic precursor cell

DOPE disease–oriented physician education

DOPP dihydroxyphenyl-pyruvate

DOPS diffuse obstructive pulmonary syndrome • dihydroxyphenylserine

Dors dorsal

DORV double–outlet right ventricle

DoRx date of treatment

DOS day of surgery • deoxystreptamine • disk operating system • Doctor of Ocular Science • Doctor of Optical Science

dos dosage/dose *also* D, d

DOSC Dubois oleic serum complex

DOSS Department of Social Services • dioctyl sodium

sulfosuccinate (docusate sodium) • distal over–shoulder strap

DOT date of transcription • date of transfer • died on (operating) table • Doppler ophthalmic test

DOTC Dameshek oval target cell

DOU direct observation unit

DOV discharged on visit

DOX, Dox doxorubicin

DP data processing • deep pulse • definitive procedure • degradation product • degree of polymerization • deltopectoral • dementia praecox • dense plate • dental prosthesis • dental prosthodontics • developed pressure • dexamethasone pretreatment • diaphragmatic plaque • diastolic pressure • diffuse precipitation • diffusion pressure • digestible protein • diphosgene • diphosphate • dipropionate • directional preponderance • disability pension • discharge planning • discriminating power • disopyramide phosphate • displaced person • distal phalanx • distal pit • distopulpal • Doctor of Podiatry • donor's plasma • dorsalis pedis • driving pressure • dyspnea • D–penicillamine *also* DPA, d–pen • [L. *directione propria*] with proper direction *also* dp

dp [L. *directione propria*] with proper direction *also* DP

DPA Department of Public Assistance • Designed Plan Agencies (medical records) • dextroposition of aorta • diphenolic acid • diphenylamine • diphenylalanine • dipicolinic acid • dipropylacetate • D–penicillamine *also* DP, d–pen • dual photon absorptiometer • dynamic physical activity

DPB days postburn

DPC delayed primary closure • desaturated phosphatidylcholine • direct patient care • discharge planning coordinator • distal palmar crease

DPD depression pure disease • desoxypyridoxine hydrochloride • diffuse pulmonary disease • diphenamid

DPDA phosphorodiamidic anhydride

DPDL diffuse poorly differentiated lymphoma

DPDT, dpdt double–pole double–throw (switch)

DPE Death Personification Exercise (psychology) • dipiperidinoethane

d–pen D–penicillamine *also* DP, DPA

DPF Dental Practitioners' Formulary

DPFR diastolic pressure–flow relationship

DPG diphosphoglycerate · displacement placentogram

DPGN diffuse proliferative glomerulonephritis

DPGP diphosphoglycerate phosphatase

DPH Department of Public Health · diaphragm *also* DI, diaph · diphenhydramine · diphenylhexatriene · diphenylhydantoin · Doctor of Public Health/ Hygiene *also* DrPH

DPharm Doctor of Pharmacy

DPhC Doctor of Pharmaceutical Chemistry

DPhc Doctor of Pharmacology

DPHN Doctor of Public Health Nursing

DPI daily permissible intake · days postinoculation · dietary protein intake · drug prescribing index

DPIF Drug Product Information File

DPJ dementia paralytica juvenilis

DPL diagnostic peritoneal lavage · dipalmitoyl lecithin · distopulpolingual

DPLa distopulpolabial

DPM dipyridamole · disabling pansclerotic morphea · discontinue previous medication · disintegrations per minute *also* dpm · Doctor of Physical Medicine · Doctor of Podiatric Medicine · dopamine · drops per minute

dpm disintegrations per minute *also* DPM

DPN dermatosis papalosa nigra · diabetic polyneuropathy · diphosphopyridine nucleotide

DPNase diphosphopyridine nucleotide

DPNH diphosphopyridine nucleotide (nicotinamide adenine dinucleotide, reduced)

DPP differential pulse polarography · dimethoxyphenylpenicillin

DPPC dipalmitoylphos- phatidylcholine

DPR doctor/population ratio

DPS dimethylpolysiloxane (simethicone—antiflatulent)

dps disintegrations per second

DPSS Department of Public Social Service

DPST, dpst double–pole single–throw (switch)

DPT Demerol, Phenergan, and Thorazine · department · dichotic pitch (discrimination) test · diphosphothiamine · diphtheria–pertussis–tetanus (vaccine) · diphtheric pseudotabes · dipropyltryptamine

DPTA diethylenetriamine penta–acetic acid

DPTI diastolic pressure–time index

DPTP diphtheria, pertussis, tetanus, poliomyelitis (vaccines)

DPTPM diphtheria, pertussis, tetanus, poliomyelitis, measles (vaccines)

DPU delayed pressure urticaria

DPUD duodenal peptic ulcer disease

DPW distal phalangeal width

DPX dextropropoxyphene

DQ development quotient

DR degeneration reaction • Déjérine–Roussey (syndrome) • delivery room • deoxyribose • diabetic retinopathy *also* dr • diagnostic radiology • distribution ratio • diurnal rhythm • doctor *also* doc, Dr • donor–related • dorsal raphe • dorsal root *also* dr • dose ratio • drug receptor • reaction of degeneration (muscle fibers)

Dr doctor *also* doc, DR • rare detail response

dr diabetic retinopathy *also* DR • dorsal root *also* DR • drachm • drain • dram • dressing *also* DRSG, drsg, dsg • unusual rare detail response

DRA despite resuscitation attempts • dextran–reactive antibody • disease–resistant antigen • drug–related admissions

DRAM dynamic random access memory

dr ap dram, apothecaries' (weight)

DRAT differential rheumatoid agglutination test

DRB daunorubicin *also* DAUNO

DRBC denatured red blood cell • dog red blood cell *also* DRC • donkey red blood cell

DRC damage risk criteria • dendritic reticulum cell • dog red (blood) cell *also* DRBC

DRC, DRC dorsal root, cervical

dRCA distal right coronary artery

DRE digital rectal examination

DREF dose reduction effectiveness factor

D reg. diseased region

DRESS depth–resolved surface (coil) spectroscopy

DREZ dorsal root entry zone

DRF daily replacement factor (of lymphocytes) • dose–reduction factor

DRG Diagnosis–Related Groups • dorsal respiratory group • dorsal root ganglion

drg, DRGE drainage/draining *also* drng

DrHyg Doctor of Hygiene

DRI Discharge Readiness Inventory

dRib deoxyribose

DRID double radial immunodiffusion • double radioisotope derivative

DRL differential reinforcement of low (response rates)

DRL, DRI dorsal root, lumbar

DRME Division of Research in Medical Education

DRMS drug reaction–monitoring system

DrMT Doctor of Mechanotherapy

DRN dorsal raphe nucleus

drng drainage *also* drg, DRGE

DRnt diagnostic roentgenology

DRO differential reinforcement of other (behavior)

DRP digoxin reduction product • dorsal root potential

DrPH Doctor of Public Health/Hygiene *also* DPH

DRQ discomfort relief quotient

DRR dorsal root reflex

DRS descending rectal septum • drowsiness • Duane retraction syndrome • dynamic renal scintigraphy • Dyskinesia Rating Scale

DRS, DRs dorsal root, sacral

DRSG, drsg dressing *also* dr, dsg

DRT, DRT dorsal root, thoracic

DRUB drug (screen)–blood

DS dead (air) space • Debré–Semelaigne (syndrome) • deep sedative • deep sleep • defined substrate • dehydroepiandrosterone sulfate • Déjérine–Sottas (syndrome) • delayed sensitivity • dendritic spine • density (optical)

standard • dental surgery • deprivation syndrome • dermatan sulfate • dermatology and syphilology *also* D&S • desynchronized sleep • dextran sulfate • dextrose–saline • dextrose stick • diaphragm stimulation • diastolic murmur • difference spectroscopy • diffuse scleroderma • digit span • dihydrostrepto-mycin • dilute strength • dioptric strength • Disaster Services (of Red Cross) • discharge summary • discrimination score • discriminative stimulus • disoriented • disseminated sclerosis • dissolved solids • donor's serum • Doppler sonography • double strength • double subordinance • Down syndrome • driving signal • drug store • dry swallow • duration of systole

D–S Doerfler–Stewart (test)

D/S dextrose and sodium chloride • dextrose/saline

D&S dermatology and syphilology *also* DS • diagnostic and surgical • dilation and suction

D–5–S dextrose 5% in saline (solution)

Ds associative detail response to white space

ds double–stranded (DNA, RNA)

DSA digital subtraction angiography/

arteriography • disease–susceptible antigen

DSACT,D–SACT direct sinoatrial conduction time

DSAP disseminated superficial actinic porokeratosis

DSAS discrete subaortic stenosis

Dsb single–breath diffusing (capacity)

DSBB double sheath bronchial brushing

DSBL disabled *also* dis

DSBT donor–specific blood transfusion

DSC decussation (of) superior cerebellar (peduncles) • differential scanning colorimeter • disodium chromoglycate *also* DSCG • Doctor of Surgical Chiropody • Down syndrome child

DSc Doctor of Science

DSCF Doppler–shifted constant frequency

DSCG disodium cromoglycate *also* DSC

DSCT dorsal spinocerebellar tract

DSD depressed spectrum disease • depression sine depression • discharge summary dictated • dry sterile dressing

DSDB direct self–destructive behavior

DSDDT double–sampling dye dilution technique

dsDNA double–stranded deoxyribonucleic acid

DSDS daughter sites of dimer strands

DSE digital subtraction echocardiogram • Doctor of Sanitary Engineering

d seq [L. *die sequente*] on the following day

DSF disulfiram • dry sterile fluff

DSG dry sterile gauze

dsg dressing *also* dr, DRSG, drsg

DSH deliberate self–harm • dexamethasone–suppressible hyperaldosteronism

DSHR delayed skin hypersensitivity reaction

DSI deep shock insulin • Depression Status Inventory • drug–seeking index

DSIM Doctor of Science in Industrial Medicine

DSIP delta sleep–inducing peptide

dslv dissolve

DSM dextrose solution mixture • *Diagnostic and Statistical Manual (of Mental Disorders)* • dihydrostreptomycin • dried skim milk

DSO distal subungual onychomycosis

DSP decreased sensory perception • delayed sleep phase • dibasic sodium phosphate • digital signal processor • digital subtraction phlebography

DSp digit span

DSPC disaturated phosphatidylcholine

DSR distal splenorenal • double simultaneous recording • dynamic spacial reconstructor

DSRF drainage subretinal fluid

dsRNA double–stranded ribonucleic acid

DSRS distal splenorenal shunt

DSS dengue shock syndrome • Developmental Sentence Scoring • dioctyl sodium sulfosuccinate • disability status scale • docusate sodium

DSSEP dermatomal somatosensory evoked potential

DST desensitization test • desensitization time • dexamethasone suppression test • dihydrostreptomycin • disproportionate septal thickening • donor–specific transfusion

D–S test Doerfler–Stewart test

D–stix Dextrostix

DSU day surgery unit • double setup

DSUH directed suggestion under hypnosis

DSV digital subtraction ventriculography

DSVP downstream venous pressure

DSWI deep surgical wound infection

DSy digit symbol

DT Déjérine–Thomas (syndrome) • delirium tremens *also* DT's • dental technician • depression of transmission • dietetic technician • differently tested • digitoxin • diphtheria–tetanus (immunization) • diphtheria toxoid • discharge tomorrow • dispensing tablet • distance test (hearing) • dorsalis tibialis • double tachycardia • doubling time (of tumor size) • duration of tetany *also* Dt • dye test

D/T date of treatment • deaths/ total (ratio)

D&T diagnosis and treatment • dictated and typed

Dt duration of tetany *also* DT

dT deoxythymidine

DTA differential thermoanalysis

DTB dedicated time block

DTBC D–tubocurarine *also* DTC, dTc

DTBN di–*tert*–butyl nitroxide

DTBP di–*tert*–butyl peroxide *also* DBP

DTC, dTc day treatment center • differentiated thyroid carcinoma • D–tubocurarine *also* DTBC

DTD, dtd [L. *detur talis dosis*] give such a dose • [L. *dosis therapeutica die*] daily therapeutic dose

dTDP deoxythymidine diphosphate

DTE dessicated thyroid extract

2–D TEE two–dimensional transesophageal echocardiography

DTF detector transfer function

D–TGA, d–TGA dextro-transposition of great arteries

DTH delayed–type hypersensitivity (reaction)

dThd thymidine

DTIC (dimethyl-triazeno)imidazole carboxamide (dacarbazine)

DTICH delayed traumatic intracerebral hemorrhage

D time dream time

DTLA Detroit Tests of Learning Aptitude

DTM dermatophyte test medium

DTMA deoxycorticosterone trimethylacetate

DTMC ditrichloro-methylcarbinol

DTMP, dTMP deoxythmidine monophosphate • de novo thymidylate (synthesis)

DTMV$_{max}$ diastolic transmembrane voltage, maximum

DTN diphtheria toxin, normal

DTO deodorized tincture of opium

DTP diphtheria–tetanus–pertussis (vaccine) • distal tingling on percussion (Tinel sign)

DTPA diethylenetriamine pentaacetic acid

DTPT dithiopropylthiamine

DTR deep tendon reflex

DTRTT digital temperature recovery time test

DTS dense tubular system • diphtheria toxin sensitivity • discrete time sample • donor transfusion, specific

DTs, DT's delirium tremens *also* DT

DTT device for transverse traction • diagnostic and therapeutic team • diphtheria–tetanus toxoid • direct transverse reaction • dithiothreitol

dTTP deoxythymidine triphosphate

DTUS diathermy, traction, and ultrasound

DTV due to void

DT–VAC diphtheria–tetanus vaccine

DTVMI Developmental Test of Visual Motor Integration

DTVP Developmental Test of Visual Perception

DTX detoxification

DTZ diatrizoate

DU decubitus ulcer • density (optical) unknown • deoxyuridine • dermal ulcer • diabetic urine • diagnosis undetermined • diazouracil • diffuse and undifferentiated • dog unit • dose unit • duodenal ulcer • duroxide uptake • Dutch (rabbit)

D$_U$ urea dialysance

dU deoxyuridine

du dial unit

DUA dorsal uterine artery

DUB Dubowitz (score) • dysfunctional uterine bleeding

dUDP deoxyuridine diphosphate

D₁UE diagonal 1 upper extremity

D₂UE diagonal 2 upper extremity

DUF Doppler ultrasonic flowmeter

DUI driving under the influence

DUID driving under the influence of drugs

DUL diffuse undifferentiated lymphoma

dulc [L. *dulcis*] sweet

DUM dorsal unpaired median (axon, neuron)

dUMP deoxyuridine monophosphate

DUNHL diffuse undifferentiated non–Hodgkins lymphoma

duod duodenum/duodenal

dup duplicate/duplication

DUR Drug Usage Review • duration *also* dur

dur duration *also* DUR • [L. *duris*] hard

dur dol, dur dolor [L. *durante dolore*] while pain lasts

DUS Doppler ultrasound stethoscope

DUSN diffuse unilateral subacute neuroretinitis ("wipe–out" syndrome)

DUV damaging ultraviolet

DV dependent variable • dilute volume (of solution) • distance vision • distemper virus • domiciliary visit • dorsoventral • double vibrations (unit of frequency of sound waves) *also* dv • double vision *also* dv

D&V diarrhea and vomiting • disks and vessels (re: ophthalmology)

dv double vibrations (unit of frequency of sound waves) *also* DV • double vision *also* DV

DVA desacetylvinblastine amide (vindesine) • distance visual acuity • duration of voluntary apnea (test)

D/V_A diffusion per unit of alveolar volume

D value decimal reduction time

DVB *cis*–diamminedi-chloroplatinum, vindesine, and bleomycin • divinylbenzene

DVC direct visualization of vocal cords • divanillalcy-clohexanone

DVCC Disease Vector Control Center

DVD dissociated vertical deviation • double–vessel disease

DVDALV double–vessel disease with abnormal left ventricle

DVE duck virus enteritis

DVH Division for the Visually Handicapped

DVI atrioventricular sequential pacing • digital vascular imaging (system) *also* DVIS • Doppler (systolic) velocity index

DVIS digital vascular imaging system *also* DVI

DVIU direct vision internal urethrotomy

DVL deep vastus lateralis

DVLP daunomycin, vincristine, L–asparaginase, and prednisone

DVM digital voltmeter • Doctor of Veterinary Medicine

DVMS Doctor of Veterinary Medicine and Surgery

DVN dorsal vagal nucleus

DVPA daunorubicin, vincristine, prednisone, and L–asparaginase *also* DVPL– ASP

DVPL–ASP daunorubicin, vincristine, prednisone, and L–asparaginase *also* DVPA

DVR derotational varus osteotomy • digital vascular reactivity • Doctor of Veterinary Radiology • double valve replacement

DVS Doctor of Veterinary Science *also* DVSc • Doctor of Veterinary Surgery

DVSA digital venous subtraction angiography

DVSc Doctor of Veterinary Science *also* DVS

DVT deep vein/deep venous thrombosis

DVTS deep venous thromboscintigram

DVXI direct vision times one

DW daily weight • deionized water • dextrose in water *also* D/W • distilled water • doing well *also* D/W • dry weight • whole response to detail

D/W dextrose in water *also* DW • doing well *also* DW • dry to wet

D₅W, D5/W dextrose 5% in water (solution)

dw dwarf (mouse)

DWA died from wounds

DWD died with disease

DWDL diffuse well– differentiated lymphocytic (lymphoma)

DWI driving while impaired • driving while intoxicated

DWMI deep white–matter infarct

DWRT delayed work recall test

DWS Disaster Warning System

DWT Dichotic Word Test

dwt pennyweight

DX Dextran • dicloxacillin

Dx diagnosis

DXD, Dxd discontinued

DXM dexamethasone (suppression test)

DXR deep x–ray • doxorubicin

DXRT, DXT deep x–ray therapy *also* DXT

DXT deep x–ray therapy *also* DXRT, DXT • dextrose

dXTP deoxyxanthine triphosphate

D–XYL *d*–xylose (in urine)

DY dense parenchyma • Dyke–Young (syndrome)

Dy dysprosium

dy dystrophia muscularis

dyn dynamics • dyne • dynamometer

dysp dyspnea

DZ diazepam *also* DZP • disease *also* Dz • dizygotic/dizygous • dizziness

Dz, dz disease *also* DZ

DZAPO daunorubicin, azacytidine, araC (cytarabine), prednisone, and Oncovin (vincristine)

DZP diazepam *also* DZ

DZT dizygotic twins

E air dose • cortisone (compound E) • edema *also* ed • einstein (unit of energy) • elastance • electric affinity *also* E_O, EA • electric charge *also* e • electric field vector • electrode potential • electromagnetic force • electron *also* e • embryo *also* Emb • emmetropia • encephalitis • endangered (animal) • endogenous • endoplasm • enema *also* En, en, enem • energy • engorged • enterococcus • enzyme • eosinophil • epicondyle • epinephrine *also* EPI, epineph • error • erythrocyte *also* Er, er, ERY, Ery, eryth • erythroid • erythromycin *also* EM, ETM • esophagus *also* ES, ESO, esoph • esophoria (for distance) • ester *also* est • estradiol *also* E–diol • ethanol *also* ET, ETH, ETOH • ethmoid (sinus) • ethyl *also* ET, Et • etiocholanolone • etiology • exa– • examiner • exercise *also* Ex, ex, exer • expectancy (wave) • expected frequency in a cell of a contingency table • experiment(al) *also* exp, exper , exptl • expired (died) *also* exp • expired (gas) *also* exp • expired (air) • extension *also* EXT • extinction (coefficient) • extraction fraction • extraction ratio • extralymphatic • eye • glutamic acid • internal energy • kinetic energy of a particle • mathematical expectation • redox potential • [Ger. *entgegen*]

E

opposite (stereodescriptor to indicate configuration at a double bond) • vectorcardiography electrode (midsternal) • vitamin E

E* lesion on erythrocyte cell membrane at site of complement fixation

E′ esophoria (for near)

E˙ standard electrode potential

E⁻, e⁻ negative electron

E⁺, e⁺ positron (positive electron)

E_O electric affinity *also* E, EA

E_1 estrone

E_2 17–β–estradiol

E_3 estriol *also* Es

E_4 estetrol

4E four plus edema

e base of natural logarithms • early • egg transfer • electric charge *also* E • electron *also* E • elementary charge • erg • [L. *ex*] from

EA early antigen • educational age • egg albumin • elbow aspiration • electric affinity *also* E, E_O • electro-acupuncture *also* EAC • electroanesthesia • electrophysiologic abnormality • embryonic antigen/antibody • emergency area • endocardiographic amplifier • enteral alimentation •

enteroanastomosis • enzymatic active • epiandrosterone • erthrocyte antibody • erythrocyte antisera • esophageal atresia • esterase activity • estivoautumnal (malaria) • ethacrynic acid

E→A "E to A" (in pulmonary consolidation, all vowels including "e" heard as "a" through stethoscope)

E&A evaluate and advise

ea each

EAA electroacupuncture analgesia • electrothermal atomic absorption • essential amino acid • extrinsic allergic alveolitis

EAB elective abortion • Ethics Advisory Board • extra–anatomic bypass

EABV effective arterial blood volume

EAC Ehrlich ascites carcinoma • electroacupuncture *also* EA • erythema action (spectrum) • erythema annulare centrifugum • erthrocyte, antibody, complement • external auditory canal

EACA ε–aminocaproic acid

EACD eczematous allergic contact dermatitis

EAD extracranial arterial disease

ead [L. *eadem*] the same

E–ADD epileptic attentional deficit disorder

EAE experimental allergic

encephalitis/encephalomyelitis • experimental autoimmune encephalitis/encephalomyelitis

EAF emergency assistance to families

EAG electroantennogram • electroatriogram

EAHF eczema, asthma, and hay fever (complex)

EAHLG equine antihuman lymphoblast globulin

EAHLS equine antihuman lymphoblast serum

EAI Employment and Adaptation Index • erythrocyte antibody inhibition

EAL electronic artificial larynx

EAM external acoustic/auditory meatus

EAMG experimental autoimmune myasthenia gravis

EAN experimental allergic neuritis

EANG epidemic acute nonbacterial gastroenteritis

EAO experimental allergic orchitis

EAP electroacupuncture • epiallopregnanolone • erythrocyte acid phosphatase • evoked action potential

EAQ eudismic affinity quotient

e–aq aqueous electron

EAR electroencephalographic audiometry • expired air resuscitation

Ea R [Ger. *Entartungs–Reaktion*] reaction of degeneration

ear ox ear oximetry

EAST external rotation, abduction, stress test

EAT ectopic atrial tachycardia • Edinburgh Articulation Test • Education Apperception Test • Ehrlich ascites tumor • electroaerosol therapy • experimental autoimmune thymitis/thyroiditis

EATC Ehrlich ascites tumor cell

EAU experimental autoimmune uveitis

EAV equine abortion virus • extra–alveolar vessel

EAVC enhanced atrioventricular conduction

EAVM extramedullary arteriovenous malformation

EB elbow bearing • elementary body • endometrial biopsy • epidermolysis bullosa • Epstein–Barr (virus) *also* E–B • esophageal body • estradiol benzoate *also* E$_2$B • ethidium bromide • Evans blue (dye)

E–B Epstein–Barr (virus) *also* EB

E $_2$B estradiol benzoate *also* EB

EBA epidermolysis bullosa acquisita/atrophicans • extrahepatic biliary atresia

EBAB equal breath sounds bilaterally

EBC esophageal balloon catheter

EBCDIC extended binary–coded decimal interchange code

EBD epidermolysis bullosa dystrophica

EBDD epidermolysis bullosa dystrophica dominant

EBDR epidermolysis bullosa dystrophica recessive

EBEA Epstein–Barr (virus) early antigen *also* EBVEA

EBF erythroblastosis fetalis *also* EF

EBG electroblepharogram/electroblepharography

EBI emetine and bismuth iodide • erythroblastic islands • estradiol–binding index

EBK embryonic bovine kidney

EBL erythroblastic leukemia • estimated blood loss

EBL/S estimated blood loss/surgery

EBM electrophysiologic behavior modification • expressed breast milk

EBNA Epstein–Barr (virus) nuclear antigen *also* EBVNA

E/BOD electrolyte biochemical oxygen demand

EBP epidural blood patch • estradiol–binding protein

EBS elastic back strap • electrical brain stimulation/stimulator • epidermolysis bullosa simplex

EBSS Earle balanced salt solution

EBT early bedtime • ethylsulfonylbenzaldehyde thiosemicarbazone (subathizone) • external beam (photon) therapy

EBV effective blood volume • Epstein–Barr virus

EB–VCA Epstein–Barr viral capsid antigen

EBVDNA Epstein–Barr virus—determinated nuclear antigen

EBVEA Epstein–Barr virus, early antigen *also* EBEA

EBVNA Epstein–Barr virus, nuclear antigen *also* EBNA

EBZ epidermal basement zone

EC econazole • effect of closing (of eyes in electroencephalography) • effective concentration • ejection click • electrochemical • electron capture • Ellis–van Creveld (syndrome) • embryonal carcinoma • emetic center • endothelial cell • enteric–coated (tablet) • entering/entrance complaint • enterochromaffin • entorhinal cortex • environmental complexity • enzyme–treated cell • epidermal cell • epithelial cell • equalization–cancellation • Erb–Charcot (syndrome) • esophageal carcinoma • ether–chloroform (mixture) *also* E–C • excitation–contraction *also* E–C • excitatory center • experimental control • external carotid •

external conjugate • extracellular • extracellular compartment • extracellular concentration • extra-cranial • extruded cell • eye care • eyes closed

E.C. Enzyme Commission (of International Union of Biochemistry)

E–C ether–chloroform (mixture) *also* EC • excitation–contraction *also* EC

E/C endoscopy/cystoscopy • estriol/creatinine (ratio) • estrogen/creatinine (ratio)

EC$_{50}$ median effective concentration

ECA electric control activity • electrocardioanalyzer • enterobacterial common antigen • epidemiologic catchment area • ethacrynic acid (diuretic) • ethylcarboxylate adenosine • external carotid artery

E–CABG endarterectomy and coronary artery bypass grafting

ECAO enterocytopathogenic avian orphan (virus)

ECAT emmission computed axial tomography

ECB electric cabinet bath

ECBD exploration of common bile duct

ECBO enterocytopathogenic bovine orphan (virus)

ECBV effective circulating blood volume

ECC edema, clubbing, and cyanosis • electro-

corticogram • embryonal
cell carcinoma •
emergency cardiac care •
endocervical cone •
endocervical curettage •
estimated creatinine
clearance • external
cardiac compression •
extracorporeal circulation •
extrusion of cell cytoplasm

ECCE extracapsular cataract
extraction

ECCO enterocytopathogenic
cat orphan (virus)

ECCO₂R extracorporeal
carbon dioxide removal

ECD electrochemical
detection/detector •
electron capture detector •
endocardial cushion
defect • enzymatic cell
dispersion

ECDB encourage to cough and
deep breathe

ECDEU early clinical drug
evaluation unit

ECDO enterocytopathogenic
dog orphan (virus)

ECE early childhood
education • endocervical
ecchymosis • equine
conjugated estrogen

ECEMG evoked compound
electromyography

ECEO enterocytopathogenic
equine orphan (virus)

ECF East Coast fever •
effective capillary flow •
eosinophilic chemotactic
factor • erythroid colony
formation • *Escherichia
coli* filtrate • extended care
facility • extracellular fluid

ECF–A, ECFA eosinophilic
chemotactic factor of
anaphylaxis

ECF–C eosinophilic
chemotactic factor—
complement

ECFMG Educational
Commission on Foreign
Medical Graduates

ECFMS Educational Council
for Foreign Medical
Students

ECFV extracellular fluid
volume *also* EFV

ECG electrocardiogram/
electrocardiography *also*
EKG

ECGF endothelial cell growth
factor

ECGS endothelial cell growth
supplement

ECH epichlorohydrin •
extended care hospital

ECHINO echinocyte

ECHO echocardiogram/
echocardiography *also*
Echo •
enterocytopathogenic
human orphan (virus) *also*
EcHO • etoposide,
cyclophosphamide,
hydroxydaunomycin
(Adriamycin), and Oncovin
(vincristine) • ultrasound

EcHO enterocytopathogenic
human orphan (virus) *also*
ECHO

Echo echocardiogram/
echocardiography *also*
ECHO • echoencephalo-
gram/echoencephalography
also Echo EG

Echo EG echoencephalogram/ echoencephalography *also* Echo

ECI electrocerebral inactivity • eosinophilic cytoplasmic inclusion • extracorporeal irradiation (of blood) *also* ECIB

ECIB extracorporeal irradiation of blood *also* ECI

EC–IC extracranial– intracranial

ECIL extracorporeal irradiation of lymph

ECK extracellular kalium (potassium)

ECL electrogenerated chemiluminescence • emitter–coupled logic • enterochromaffin–like (type) • euglobulin clot lysis • extent of cerebral lesion • extracapillary lesions

eclec eclectic

ECLT euglobulin clot lysis time

ECM embryonic chick muscle • erythema chronicum migrans • external cardiac massage • external chemical messenger • extracellular material • extracellular matrix

ECMO enterocytopathogenic monkey orphan (virus) • extracorporeal membrane oxygenator/oxygenation

ECMP enterocoated micro-spheres of pancrelipase

ECN extended care nursery

E.C.No. Enzyme Commission Number

ECochG electrocochleography

ECoG electrocorticogram/ electrocorticography

E. coli *Escherichia coli*

ECP effector cell precursor • electronic claims processing • endocardial potential • eosinophil cationic protein • erythrocyte coproporphyrin • erythroid committed precursor • *Escherichia coli* polypeptide • estradiol cyclopentanepropionate • external cardiac pressure • external counterpulsation • free cytoporphyrin in erythrocytes

ECPD external counterpressure device

ECPO enterocytopathogenic porcine orphan (virus)

ECPOG electrochemical potential gradient

ECPR external cardiopulmonary resuscitation

ECR electrocardiographic response • emergency chemical restraint

ECRB extensor carpi radialis brevis

ECRL extensor carpi radialis longus

ECRO enterocytopathogenic rodent orphan (virus)

ECS elective cosmetic surgery • electrocerebral silence • electroconvulsive shock • electronic claims submission • electroshock • extracellular space

ECSO enterocytopathogenic swine orphan (virus)

ECSP epidermal cell surface protein

ECT electroconvulsive therapy • emission computed tomography • enhanced computed tomography • enteric–coated tablet • euglobulin clot test • European compression technique (bone screw and internal fixation) • extracellular tissue

ECTA Everyman's Contingency Table Analysis

ECTEOLA epichlorohydrin and triethanolamine

ECU environmental control unit • extended care unit • extensor carpi ulnaris

ECV extracellular volume • extracorporeal volume

ECVD extracellular volume of distribution

ECVE extracellular volume expansion

ECW extracellular water

ED early differentiation • ectodermal dysplasia • ectopic depolarization • effective dose • Ehlers–Danlos (syndrome) • elbow disarticulation • electrodiagnosis *also* EDX, EDx, El Dx • electro-dialysis • electron diffraction • elemental diet • embryonic death •

emergency department • emotional disorder/disturbance • emotionally disturbed • end diastole • entering diagnosis • Entner–Doudoroff (metabolic pathway) • enzyme deficiency • epidural • epileptiform discharge • equilibrium dialysis • equine dermis (cells) • erythema dose • ethylenediamine • ethynodiol • evidence of disease • exertional dyspnea • extensive disease • extensor digitorum • external diameter • external dyspnea • extra–low dispersion

E–D ego–defense

ED$_{50}$ median effective dose

E$_d$ depth dose

ed edema *also* E

EDA electrodermal activity • electrodermal audiometry • electrolyte–deficient agar • electron donor–acceptor (interaction) • end–diastolic area

EDAM electron–dense amorphous material

EDAP Emergency Department Approval for Pediatrics

EDAX energy dispersive x–ray analysis

EDB early dry breakfast • ethylene dibromide • extensor digitorum brevis

EDBP erect diastolic blood pressure

EDC effective dynamic

compliance • electrodesiccation and curettage *also* ED&C • emergency decontamination center • end–diastolic count • estimated date of conception • estimated/ expected date of confinement • expected delivery, cesarean • extensor digitorum communis

ED&C electrodessication and curettage *also* EDC

EDCI energetic dynamic cardiac insufficiency

EDCS end–diastolic chamber stiffness • end–diastolic circumferential stress

EDCT early distal proximal tubule

EDD effective drug duration • end–diastolic dimension • enzyme–digested delta (endotoxin) • estimated discharge date • estimated due date • expected date of delivery

EDDA expanded duty dental auxiliary

edent edentulous

EDF end–diastolic flow • extradural fluid

EDG electrodermography

EDH epidural hematoma • extradural hematoma

EDICP electron–dense iron–containing particle

EDIM epidemic diesease of infant mice • epizootic diarrhea of infant mice

E–diol estradiol *also* E

EDL end–diastolic (segment) length • end–diastolic load • estimated date of labor • extensor digitorum longus

ED/LD emotionally disturbed and learning disabled

EDM early diastolic murmur • extramucosal duodenal myotomy

EDMA ethylene glycol dimethacrylate

EDN electrodesiccation • eosinophil–derived neurotoxin

EDOC estimated date of confinement

EDP electron–dense particle • electronic data processing • emergency department physician • end–diastolic pressure

EDPA ethyldiphenyl-propenylamine

EDQ extensor digiti quinti

EDR early diastolic relaxation • edrophonium • effective direct radiation • electrodermal response • electrodialysis (with) reversed (polarity)

EDRF endothelium–derived relaxing factor

EDS edema disease of swine • egg drop syndrome • Ego Development Scale • Ehlers–Danlos syndrome • energy–dispersive spectrometer • excessive daytime sleepiness • extended data stream • extradimensional shift

EDT end–diastolic (cardiac wall) thickness

EDTA ethylenediamine-tetraacetic acid (edathamil, edetic acid)

EdU eating disorder unit

EDV end–diastolic volume

EDVI end–diastolic volume index

EDW estimated dry weight

EDWGT emergency drinking water germicidal tablet

EDWTH end–diastolic wall thickness

EDX, EDx electrodiagnosis *also* ED, El Dx

EDXA energy–dispersive x–ray analysis

EE embryo extract • end–expiration • end–to–end (anastomosis) *also* E–E • end–to–end (bite, occlusion) • energy expenditure • *Enterobacteriaceae* enrichment (broth) • equine encephalitis • ethynyl estradiol • expressed emotion • external ear • eyes and ears *also* E&E

E–E end–to–end (anastomosis) *also* EE • erythema–edema (reaction)

E&E eyes and ears *also* EE

EEA electroencephalic audiometry • elemental enteral alimentation • end–to–end anastomosis

EEC ectrodactyly–ectodermal dysplasia–clefting

(syndrome) • enteropathogenic *Escherichia coli*

EECD endothelial–epithelial corneal dystrophy

EECG electroencephalogram/ electroencephalography *also* EEG

EEDQ ethoxycarbonyl-ethoxydihydroquinoline

EEE eastern equine encephalomyelitis • edema, erythema, and exudate • experimental enterococcal endocarditis • external eye examination

EEEP end–expiratory esophageal pressure

EEEV eastern equine encephalomyelitis virus

EEG electroencephalogram/ electroencephalography *also* EECG

EEGA electroen-cephalographic audiometry

EEG T Electroencephalo-graphic Technologist

EELS electron energy loss spectroscopy

EEM ectodermal dysplasia–ectrodactyly–macular dystrophy (syndrome) • erythema exudativum multiforme

EEME ethynylestradiol methyl ether

EEMG evoked electromyogram

EENT eye, ear, nose, and throat

EEP end–expiratory pressure • equivalent effective photon

EEPI extraretinal eye position information

EER electroencephalographic response

EERP extended endocardial resection procedure

EES erythromycin ethylsuccinate • ethyl ethanesulfate

EESG evoked electrospinogram

EEV encircling endocardial ventriculotomy

EF ectopic focus • edema factor • ejection factor • ejection fraction • elastic fibril/fiber • electric field • elongation factor • embryo–fetal • embryo fibroblast • emergency facility • emotional factor • encephalitogenic factor • endothoracic fascia • endurance factor • eosinophilic fasciitis • epithelial focus • equivalent focus • erythroblastosis fetalis *also* EBF • erythrocytic fragmentation • essential findings • exophthalmic factor • exposure factor • extended field (radiation therapy) • extrafine • extra food • extrinsic factor

EFA essential fatty acid • extrafamily adoptee

EFAD essential fatty acid deficiency

EFBW estimated fetal body weight

EFC elastin fragment concentration • endogenous fecal calcium

EFDA expanded function dental assistant

EFE endocardial fibroelastosis

eff effect • efferent *also* effer • efficient • effusion

effect. effective

effer efferent *also* eff

EFFU epithelial focus–forming unit

EF–G elongation factor G

EFHBM eosinophilic fibrohistiocytic (lesion of) bone marrow

EFL effective focal length • external fluid loss

EFM electronic fetal monitoring • external fetal monitoring

EFP effective filtration pressure • endoneural fluid pressure

EFPS epicardial fat pad sign

EFR effective filtration rate

E FRAG erythrocyte (red blood cell) fragility (test)

EFS electric field stimulation

EFT Embedded Figures Test

EFV extracellular fluid volume *also* ECFV

EFVC expiratory flow–volume curve

EFW estimated fetal weight

EF/WM ejection fraction/wall motion

EG enteroglucagon • Erb–Goldflam (syndrome) • esophagogastric • esophagogastrectomy • external genitalia

EGA estimated gestational age

EGAT Educational Goal Attainment Tests

EGBPS equilibrium–gated blood pool study

EGBUS external genitalia and Bartholin, urethral, and Skene (glands)

EGC early gastric cancer • epithelioid–globoid cell

EGD esophagogastro-duodenoscopy

EGDF embryonic growth and development factor

EGF epidermal growth factor

EGFR epidermal growth factor receptor

EGG electrogastrogram/ electrogastrography

EGH equine growth hormone

EGJ esophagogastric junction

EGL eosinophilic granuloma of lung

EGLT euglobulin lysis time

EGM electrogram • extracellular granular material

EGN experimental glomerulonephritis

EGOT erythrocytic glutamic oxaloacetic transaminase

EGR erythrocyte glutathione reductase

EGRA equilibrium–gated radionuclide angiography

EGS electric galvanic stimulation • ethylene glycol succinate

EGT ethanol gelation test

EGTA esophageal gastric tube airway • ethyleneglycoltetraacetic acid

EH early healed • educationally/emotionally handicapped • enlarged heart • enteral hyperalimentation • environment and heredity *also* E&H • epidermolytic hyperkeratosis • epoxide hydratase • essential hypertension • extramedullary hematopoiesis

E&H environment and heredity *also* EH

E$_h$, eH oxidation–reduction potential *also* E$_O$+ and E^O)

EHA Environmental Health Agency

EHAA epidemic hepatitis–associated antigen

EHB elevate head of bed

EHBA extrahepatic biliary atresia

EHBD extrahepatic bile duct

EHBF estimated hepatic blood flow • exercise hyperemia blood flow • extrahepatic blood flow (clearance)

EHC enterohepatic circulation • enterohepatic clearance • essential hypercholesterolemia • extended health care • extrahepatic cholestasis

EH–CF *Entamoeba histolytica*–complement fixation

EHD electrohemodynamics • epizootic hemorrhagic disease

EHDA, EHDP ethanehydroxy-diphosphonic acid (etidronate sodium)

EHDV epizootic hemorrhagic disease virus

EHE epithelioid hemangioendothelioma

EHEC enterohemorrhagic *Escherichia coli*

EHF electrohydraulic fragmentation • epidemic hemorrhagic fever • exophthalmos–hyperthyroid factor • extremely high factor • extremely high frequency

EHH esophageal hiatal hernia

EHL effective half–life (of radioactive substance) • electrohydraulic lithotripsy • endogenous hyperlipidemia • Environmental Health Laboratory • essential hyperlipidemia • extensor hallucis longus

EHME Employee Health Maintenance Examination

EHMS electrohydrodynamic ionization mass spectrometry

EHO extrahepatic obstruction

EHP Environmental Health Perspectives • excessive heat production • extra high potency

EHPAC Emergency Health Preparedness Advisory Committee

EHPH extrahepatic portal hypertension

EHPT Eddy hot plate test

EHSDS Experimental Health Services Delivery System

EHT essential hypertension

EHV equine herpesvirus

EI electrolyte imbalance • electron impact • electron ionization • emotionally impaired • enzyme inhibitor • eosinophilic index • excretory index • external intervention

E/I expiration/inspiration (ratio)

E&I endocrine and infertility

EIA electroimmunoassay • enzyme immunoassay • equine infectious anemia • exercise–induced asthma

EIAB extracranial–intracranial arterial bypass

EIB exercise–induced bronchoconstriction/bronchospasm

EIC elastase inhibition capacity • enzyme inhibition complex

EICDT Ego–Ideal and Conscience Development Test

EICT external isovolumic contraction time

EID egg–infectious dose • electroimmunodiffusion • electronic induction desorption • electronic infusion device

EIEC enteroinvasive *Escherichia coli*

EIEE early infantile epileptic encephalopathy

EIF, eIF erythrocyte initiation factor • eukaryotic initiation factor

EIM excitability–inducing material

EIMS electron ionization mass spectrometry

EIP elective interruption of pregnancy • end–inspiratory pause • end–inspiratory pressure • extensor indicis proprius

EIPS endogenous inhibitor of prostaglandin synthase

EIRnv extra–incidence rate in nonvaccinated (groups)

EIRP effective isotropic radiated power

EIRv extra–incidence rate in vaccinated (groups)

EIS endoscopic injection scleropathy • Epidemic Intelligence Service • Environmental Impact Statement

EISA electroencephalogram interval spectrum analysis

EIT erythroid iron turnover

EIV external iliac vein

EJ ejection (fraction) • elbow jerk • external jugular

EJB ectopic junctional beat

EJP excitation junction potential

ejusd [L. *ejusdem*] of the same

EK enterokinase • erythrokinase

EKC epidemic keratoconjunctivitis

EKG electrocardiogram/ electrocardiography *also* ECG

EKV erythrokeratodermia variabilis

EKY electrokymogram/ electrokymography

EL early latent • Eaton–Lambert (syndrome) *also* E–L • egg lecithin • electroluminescence • elixir *also* el, Elix, Elx • erythroleukemia • exercise limit • external lamina

E–L Eaton–Lambert (syndrome) *also* EL • external lids

El elastase

el elbow *also* ELB, elb • elixir *also* EL, Elix, Elx

ELA endotoxin–like activity

ELAS extended lymphadenopathy syndrome

ELAT enzyme–linked antiglobulin test

ELB early light breakfast • elbow *also* el, elb

elb elbow *also* ELB, el

ELBW extremely low birth weight

ELD egg lethal dose

El Dx electrodiagnosis *also* ED, EDX, EDx

elec, elect. electricity/ electric • electuary (confection)

elem elementary

elev elevation/elevated/ elevator

ELF elective low forceps (delivery)

ELG eligible

ELH egg–laying hormone • endolymphatic hydrops

ELI endomyocardial lymphocytic infiltrates • Environmental Language Inventory • exercise lability index

ELIA enzyme–labeled immunoassay

ELICT enzyme–linked immunocytochemical technique

ELIEDA enzyme–linked immunoelectrodiffusion assay

ELISA enzyme–linked immunoadsorbent assay

Elix, elix elixir *also* EL, el, Elx

ELLIP, ELLP ellipotocyte

ELM Early Language Milestone (Scale) • external limiting membrane • extravascular lung mass

ELMT elements (on urinalysis)

ELOP estimated length of program

ELOS estimated length of stay • extralymphatic organ site

ELP early labeled peak • elastase–like protein • electrophoresis • endogenous limbic potential • Estimated Learning Potential

ELPS excessive lateral pressure syndrome

ELR Equal Listener Response (scale)

ELS Eaton–Lambert syndrome • electron loss spectroscopy • extralobar sequestration

ELSS emergency life support system

ELT euglobulin lysis test/time

ELU extended length of utterance

ELV erythroid leukemia virus

Elx elixir *also* EL, el, Elix

elytes electrolytes

EM early memory • effective masking • ejection murmur • electromagnetic *also* em • electro-mechanical • electron micrograph • electron microscopy/microscope *also* E/M, EMC, E–MICR • electrophoretic mobility • Embden–Meyerhof (glycolytic pathway) *also* E–M • emergency medicine • emmetropia (normal vision) *also* Em • emotional (disorder) • emotionally (disturbed) • emphysema *also* emph • ergonovine maleate • erythema migrans • erythema multiforme • erythrocyte mass • erythromycin *also* E, ETM • esophageal manometry • esophageal motility • excreted mass • extensive metabolizers • external monitor

E–M Embden–Meyerhof
(glycolytic pathway) *also*
EM

E/M electron microscope/
microscopy *also* EM, EMC,
E–MICR

E&M endocrine and metabolic

Em emmetropia *also* EM

em electromagnetic *also* EM

e/m ratio of (electron) charge
to mass

EMA electronic microanalyzer •
emergency assistance/
assistant • emergency
medical attendant •
endomysial antibody •
epithelial membrane antigen

EMA–CO etoposide,
methotrexate, actinomycin
D (dactinomycin), and
citrovorum factor
(leucovorin)

EMAD equivalent mean age at
death

EMAP evoked muscle action
potential

EMB embryology •
endometrial biopsy •
endomyocardial biopsy •
engineering in medicine and
biology • eosin–methylene
blue (agar) • ethambutol •
explosive mental behavior •
explosive motor behavior

Emb, emb embolus • embryo
also E • embryology *also*
embryol

EMBASE *Excerpta Medica
Database*

embryol embryology *also*
Emb, emb

EMC electron microscopy *also*
EM, E/M, E–MICR •
emergency medical care •
encephalomyocarditis •
endometrial curettage •
essential mixed
cryoglobulinemia

EMC&R emergency medical
care and rescue

EMCRO Experimental
Medical Care Review
Organization

EMCV encephalomyocarditis
virus

EMD electromechanical
dissociation • esophageal
mobility disorder

EMEM Eagle minimal essential
medium

EMER electromagnetic
molecular electronic
resonance

emer, emerg emergency

EMF electromagnetic
flowmeter • electromotive
force *also* emf •
endomyocardial fibrosis •
erythrocyte maturation
factor • evaporated milk
formula

emf electromotive force *also*
EMF

EMG electromyelogram/
electromyelography •
electromyogram/
electromyography •
emergency *also* emer,
emerg • essential
monoclonal gammopathy •
exomphalos, macroglossia,
and gigantism (syndrome) •
eye movement gauge

EMGN extramembranous glomerulonephritis

EMGORS electromyogram sensors

EMI electromagnetic interference • emergency medical information

EMIC emergency maternal and infant care

E–MICR electron microscopy *also* EM, E/M, EMC

EMIT enzyme multiplication immunoassay technique • enzyme–multiplied immunoassay test

EMJH Ellinghausen–McCullough–Johnson–Harris (medium)

EML effective mandibular length

EMLB erythromycin lactobionate

EMLD external muscle layer damaged

EMM erythema multiforme major

EMMA eye movement measuring apparatus

EMMV extended mandatory minute ventilation

EMO Epstein–Macintosh–Oxford (inhaler) • exophthalmos, myxedema circumscriptum praetibiale, and osteoarthropathia hypertrophicans (syndrome)

emot emotion/emotional

EMP electrical membrane property • electromagnetic pulse • Embden–Meyerhof pathway • epimacular

proliferation • external membrane protein • extramedullary plasmacytoma

emp [L. *ex modo praescripto*] as directed • [L. *emplastrum*] plaster

EMPEP erythrocyte membrane protein • electrophoretic pattern

emph emphysema *also* EM

EMPP ethylmethylpiperidino-propiophenone

emp vesic [L. *emplastrum vesicatorium*] blistering plaster

EMR educable mentally retarded • electromagnetic radiation • emergency mechanical restraint • empty, measure, and record • essential metabolism ratio • ethanol metabolic rate • eye movement recording

EMS early morning specimen • early morning stiffness • electrical muscle stimulation • emergency medical service(s) • emergency medical system • endometriosis • eosinophilia myalgia syndrome • ethyl methanesulfonate • extramedullary site

EMT emergency medical tag • emergency medical team • Emergency Medical Technician • emergency medical treatment

EMT–A Emergency Medical Technician–Ambulance

EMT–I Emergency Medical Technician–Intermediate

EMT–P Emergency Medical Technician–Paramedic

EMU early morning urine • electromagnetic unit *also* emu

emu electromagnetic unit *also* EMU

emul emulsion

EMV eye, motor, voice (Glasgow coma scale)

EMVC early mitral valve closure

EMW electromagnetic waves

EN electronarcosis • endocardial *also* ENDO • enrolled nurse • enteral nutrition • erythema nodosum

En, en enema *also* E, enem

E 50% N extension 50% of normal

ENA extractable nuclear antibodies/antigen

END early neonatal death • elective node dissection • endocrinology • endorphin • enhancement Newcastle disease

end. endoreduplication

ENDO endocardial *also* EN • endodontics *also* Endo • endoscopy • endotracheal *also* Endo, ET

Endo endodontics *also* ENDO • endotracheal *also* ENDO, ET

endocr endocrine/ endocrinology

ENDOR electron nuclear double resonance

endos endosteal

ENE ethylnorepinephrine

ENeG electroneurography

enem enema *also* E, En, en

ENF Enfamil

ENG electroneurography • electronystagmogram/ electronystagmography • engorged

ENI elective neck irradiation

ENK enkephalin

ENL erythema nodosum leprosum

enl enlarged/enlargement

ENNS Early Neonatal Neurobehavior Scale

Eno enolase

ENP extractable nucleoprotein

ENR eosinophilic nonallergic rhinitis • extrathyroidal neck radioactivity

ENS enteral nutritional support • enteric nervous system • ethylnorsuprarenin

ENT ear, nose, and throat • extranodular tissue

ENTOM entomology

ENV ethylmitrosourea

env envelope (of cell)

environ environment/ environmental

enz enzymatic/enzyme

EO effect of opening (eyes) • elbow orthosis • eosinophil *also* EOS, eos, eosin • eosinophilia • ethylene oxide *also* ETOX • eyes open

E_O electric affinity • skin (epidermis) dose (radiation)

E_O^+, E^O oxidation–reduction potential

EOA effective orifice area • erosive osteoarthritis • esophageal obturator airway • examination, opinion, and advice

EOB emergency observation bed

EOC enema of choice

EO CT eosinophil count

EOD electrical organ discharge • entry on duty • every other day *also* eod

eod every other day *also* EOD

EOE ethiodized oil emulsion

EOF end of field • end of file

E of M error of measurement

EOG electro–oculogram/ electro–oculography • electro–olfactogram/ electro–olfactography

EOJ extrahepatic obstructive jaundice

EOL end of life

EOM equal ocular movement • error of measurement • external otitis media • extraocular movement • extraocular muscle

EOMA emergency oxygen mask assembly

EOM F & Conj extraocular movements full and conjugate

EOMI extraocular muscles intact

EOMS extraocular movements/ muscles

EOP emergency outpatient • endogenous opioid peptides

EOR emergency operating room • exclusive OR (binary logic)

EORA elderly onset rheumatoid arthritis

EOS eligibility on–site • eosinophil *also* EO, eos, eosin

eos, eosin eosinophil *also* EO, EOS

EOT effective oxygen transport

EOU epidemic observation unit

EOWPVT Expressive One–Word Picture Vocabulary Test

EP ectopic pregnancy • edible portion • electrophoresis • electrophysiologic/ electrophysiology • electroprecipitin • elopement precaution • emergency physician • emergency procedure • endogenous pyrogen • endoperoxide • endorphin • end point • enteropep-tidase • environmental protection • enzyme product • eosinophilic pneumonia • ependymal (cell) • epicardial • epithelium/epithelial *also* EPI, EPITH • erythrocyte protoporphyrin •

erythrophagocytosis • erythropoietic porphyria • erythropoietin *also* Ep, EPO • esophageal pressure • esophoria • evoked potential • extreme pressure

Ep erythropoietin *also* EP, EPO

E&P estrogen and progesterone

EPA eicosapentaenoic acid • Environmental Protection Agency • erect posterior–anterior (projection) • ethylphenacemide • exophthalmos–producing activity • extrinsic plasminogen activator

EPAP expiratory positive airway pressure

EPAQ Extended Personal Attributes Questionnnaire

EPA/RCRA Environmental Protection Agency Resource Conservation and Recovery Act

EPB Environmental Pre–Language Battery • extensor pollicis brevis

EPC electronic pain control • end–plate current • epilepsia partialis continua • external pneumatic compression

EPCA external pressure circulatory assistance

EPCG endoscopic pan-creatocholangiography

EPD effective pressor dose

EPDML epidemiology/epidemiologic

EPE erythropoietin–producing enzyme

EPEA expense per equivalent admission

EPEC enteropathogenic *Escherichia coli*

EPEG etoposide

EPF early pregnancy factor • endocarditis parietalis fibroplastica • endothelial proliferating factor • Enfamil premature formula • exophthalmos–producing factor

EPG eggs per gram • electropneumography/electropneumogram • ethanolamine phosphoglyceride

EPH edema–proteinuria–hypertension • extensor proprius hallucis

EPI Emotions Profile Index • epileptic *also* epil • epinephrine *also* E, epineph • epithelium/epithelial *also* EP, EPITH • epitheloid cells • epitympanic • evoked potential index • exocrine pancreatic insufficiency • extrapyramidal involvement • Eysenck Personality Inventory

Epi epicardium • epiglottis

epid epidemic

epig epigastric

epil epilepsy/epileptic *also* EPI

epineph epinephrine *also* E, EPI

EPIS, epis episiotomy • episode • epistaxis

epistom [L. *epistomium*] stopper (on mouth of bottle)

EPITH, epith epithelium/epithelial *also* EP, EPI

EPK early prenatal karyotype

EPL effective patient life · essential phospholipids · extensor pollicis longus · external plexiform layer

EPM electron probe microanalysis · electronic pacemaker · electrophoretic mobility · energy–protein malnutrition

EPO erythropoietin *also* EP, Ep · exclusive provider organization · expiratory port occlusion

EPP end–plate potential · equal pressure point · erythropoietic protoporphyria

EPPS Edwards Personal Preference Schedule

EPQ Eysenck Personality Questionnaire

EPR electron paramagnetic resonance · electrophrenic respiration · emergency physical restraint · estradiol production rate · extraparenchymal resistance

EPROM erasable programmable read–only memory

EPS elastosis perforans serpiginosa · electrophysiologic study · enzymatic pancreatic secretion · exophthalmos–producing substance · expressed prostatic secretion · extrapyramidal side effect · extrapyramidal symptom · extrapyramidal syndrome

ep's epithelial cells

EPSD E–point to septal distance

EPSDT Early and Periodic Screening, Diagnosis, and Treatment

EPSE extrapyramidal side effects

EPSEM equal probability of selection method

epsilon (E, ε) fifth letter of Greek alphabet

ε chain of hemoglobin · dielectric constant · fifth in a series or group · heavy chain of immunoglobulin E · molar absorption coefficient · molar absorptivity · molar extinction coefficient · permittivity · specific absorptivity

EPSP excitatory postsynaptic potential

EPSS E–point septal separation

EPT early pregnancy test · Eidetic Parents Test · endoscopic papillotomy

EPTE existed prior to enlistment

EPTFE expanded polytetrafluoroethylene

EPTS existed prior to service

EPXMA electron probe x–ray microanalyzer

EQ educational quotient ·

encephalization quotient •
energy quotient • equal
to • equilibrium *also* eq

Eq, eq equation *also* eqn •
equivalent *also* equiv

eq equal • equilibrium *also*
EQ

EQA external quality
assessment

eqn equation *also* Eq, eq

equip equipment

equiv equivalency/equivalent
also Eq, eq • equivocal

ER early reticulocyte •
efficacy ratio • ejection
rate • electroresection •
emergency room •
endoplasmic reticulum *also*
er • enhanced
reactivation • enhancement
ratio • environmental
resistance • epigastric
region • equine
rhinopneumonia •
equivalent roentgen (unit) •
erythrocyte receptor •
esophageal rupture •
estradiol receptor •
estrogen receptor • evoked
response • expiratory
reserve • extended release
(tablet) • extended
resistance • external
reduction • external
resistance • external
rotation • extraction ratio •
eye research

ER⁻ decreased estrogen
receptor

ER⁺ increased estrogen
receptor

ER+ estrogen receptor–positive

E&R equal and reactive •
examination and report

Er erbium • erythrocyte *also*
E, er, ERY, Ery, eryth

er endoplasmic reticulum *also*
ER • erythrocyte *also* E,
Er, ERY, Ery, eryth

ERA electrical response
audiometry • electrical
response activity •
electroencephalic response
audiometry • estradiol
receptor assay • estrogen
receptor assay • evoked
response audiometry

ERB ethnic relational behavior

ERBF effective renal blood
flow

ERC endoscopic retrograde
cholangiography •
enterocytopathogenic
human orphan–rhino–
coryza (virus) • (pupils)
equal, reactive, and
contracting • erythro-
poietin–responsive cell

ERCP endoscopic retrograde
cannulation of pancreatic
(duct) • endoscopic
retrograde cholangiopan-
creatography • endoscopic
retrograde choledocho-
pancreatography

ERD early retirement with
disability • evoked
response detector

ERDA Energy Research and
Development
Administration

ERE external rotation in
extension

ERF external rotation in
flexion

erf error function

ERFC, E–RFC erythrocyte rosette–forming cell

ERG electrolyte replacement with glucose • electron radiography • electroretinography/ electroretinogram

erg energy unit *also* e

ERH egg–laying release hormone

ERHD exposure–related hypothermia death

ERI Environmental Response Inventory • erythrocyte rosette inhibitor

ERIA electroradioimmuno- assay

ERL effective refractory length

ERM electrochemical relaxation method • extended radical mastectomy

ERP early receptor potential • effective refractory period • emergency room physician • endocardial resection procedure • endoscopic retrograde pancreatography • equine rhinopneumonitis • estrogen receptor protein • event–related (brain) potential

ERPF effective renal plasma flow

ERPLV effective refractory period of the left ventricle

ERR, err. error

ERS endoscopic retrograde sphincterotomy

ERSP event–related slow– brain potential

ERT esophageal radionuclide transit • estrogen replacement therapy • external radiation therapy

ERV equine rhinopneumonitis virus • expiratory reserve volume

ERY erysipelas • erythrocyte *also* E, Er, er, Ery, eryth

Ery erythrocyte *also* E, Er, er, ERY, eryth

eryth erythema • erythrocyte *also* E, Er, er, ERY, Ery

ES Ego Strength (test) • ejection sound • elastic suspensor • electrical stimulus/electrical stimulation *also* Es • electroshock • elopement status (psychology) • emergency service • emission spectrometry • endometritis–salpingitis • endoscopic sclerosis • endoscopic sphincterotomy • end stage • end systole • end–to–side (anastomosis) *also* E–S, ETS • environmental stimulation • enzyme substrate • epileptic syndrome • esophageal scintigraphy • esophagus *also* E, ESO, esoph • esophoria • esterase *also* EST • exfoliation syndrome • Expectation Score • experimental study • exsmoker • exterior surface • extrasystole • [L. *enema saponis*] soap enema *also* es

E–S end–to–side (anastomosis) *also* ES, ETS

Es einsteinium • electrical stimulation *also* ES • estriol *also* E$_3$

es [L. *enema saponis*] soap enema *also* ES

ESA end–to–side anastomosis

ESAP evoked sensory (nerve) action potention

ESB electrical stimulation of brain

ESC electromechanical slope computer • end–systolic count • erythropoietin–sensitive stem cell

ESCA electron spectroscopy for chemical analysis

ESCC electrolyte steroid cardiopathy by calcification • epidural spinal cord compression

ESCH electrolyte steroid–produced cardiopathy (characterized by) hyalinization

ESCN electrolyte and steroid cardiopathy with necrosis

ESCS Early Social Communication Scale

ESD electronic summation device • electron–stimulated desorption • emission spectrometric detector • end–systolic dimension • environmental sex determination • esophagus, stomach, and duodenum • esterase D • exoskeletal device

ESE [Ger. *electrostatische Einheit*] electrostatic unit

ESEP elbow sensory potential

ESF electrosurgical filter • erythropoiesis–stimulating factor • external skeletal fixation

ESFL end–systolic force–length (relationship)

ESG electrospinogram • estrogen

ESI Ego State Inventory • enzyme substrate inhibitor • epidural steroid injection • extent of skin involvement

ES–IMV expiration–synchronized intermittent mandatory ventilation

ESL end–systolic (segment) length • English as a second language

ESLD end–stage liver disease

ESM ejection systolic murmur • endothelial specular microscope • ethosuximide

ESMIS Emergency Medical Services Management Information System

ESN educationally subnormal • estrogen–stimulated neurophysin

ESN(M) educationally subnormal–moderate

ESN(S) educationally subnormal–severe

ESO electrospinal orthosis

ESO, eso, esoph esophagoscopy • esophagus *also* E, ES

esoph steth esophageal stethoscope

ESP early systolic paradox • effective sensory projection • effective systolic pressure • electrosensitive point • endometritis–salpingitis–peritonitis • end–systolic pressure • eosinophil stimulation promoter • epidermal soluble protein • especially *also* esp • evoked synaptic potential • extrasensory perception

esp especially *also* ESP

ESPA electrical stimulation–produced analgesia

ESPQ Early School Personality Questionnaire

ESR electric skin resistance • electron spin resonance *also* esr • erythrocyte sedimentation rate

esr electron spin resonance *also* ESR

ESRD end–stage renal disease

ESRF end–stage renal failure

ESRS extrapyramidal symptom rating scale

ESS empty sella (turcica) syndrome • endostreptosin • erythrocyte–sensitizing substance • euthyroid sick syndrome • excited skin syndrome

ess essence • essential

ess neg essentially negative

EST electric shock threshold • electroshock therapy • electroshock threshold • endodermal sinus tumor • esterase *also* ES • exercise stress test

est ester *also* E • estimation/estimated

esth esthetics/esthetic

ESU, esu electrostatic unit • electrosurgical unit

E–sub excitor substance

ESV end–systolic (ventricular) volume • esophageal valve

ESVI end–systolic volume index

ESVS epiurethral suprapubic vaginal suspension

ESWL extracorporeal shock–wave lithotripsy

ESWS end–systolic wall stress

ET Ebbinghaus Test • edge thickness • educational therapy • effective temperature • ejection time • electroneurodiagnostic technologist • embryo transfer • endotoxin • endotracheal *also* ENDO, Endo • endotracheal tube *also* ETT • endurance time • enterostomal therapy/therapist • epithelial tumor • esotropia/esotropic • essential thrombocythemia • essential tremor • ethanol *also* E, ETH, ETOH • ethyl *also* E, Et • etiocholanolone test • etiology *also* et, etio, etiol • eustachian tube • exchange transfusion • exercise test • exercise treadmill • expiration time • extracellular tachyzoite

ET′ esotropia for near

E(T) intermittent esotropia

E/T effector to target ratio

ET$_1$ esotropia at near

ET$_3$ erythrocyte triiodothyronine

ET$_4$ effective thyroxine (test)

Et ethyl *also* E, ET

et etiology *also* ET, etio, etiol

ETA eicosatetraenoic acid • electron–transfer agent • endotracheal airway • endotracheal aspirates • estimated time of arrival • ethionamide

eta (H, η) seventh letter of Greek alphabet

η absolute viscosity

ETAB extrathoracic–assisted breathing

et al [L. *et alibi*] and elsewhere • [L. *et alii*] and others

E$_2$TBG estradiol–testosterone–binding globulin

ETC estimated time of conception

ET$_c$ corrected ejection time

etc [L. *et cetera*] and so forth

E$_T$CO$_2$ end–tidal carbon dioxide concentration

ETD eustachian tube dysfunction

ETE end–to–end (anastomosis)

ETEC enterotoxigenic *Escherichia coli* • enterotoxin of *Escherichia coli*

ETF electron–transferring flavoprotein • eustachian tube function

ETH elixir terpin hydrate • ethanol *also* E, ET, ETOH • ethionamide Ethrane (enflurane) • ethmoid

eth ether *also* Et$_2$O

ETHC, ETH/C elixir terpin hydrate with codeine

ETI ejective time index

ETIO etiocholanolone

etio, etiol etiology *also* ET, et

ETK erythrocyte transketolase

ETL expiratory threshold load

ETM erythromycin *also* E, EM

Et$_3$N triethylamine

ETO estimated time of ovulation • ethylene oxide • eustachian tube obstruction

EtO ethylene oxide

Et$_2$O ether *also* eth

ETOH, EtOH ethanol *also* E, ET, ETH • ethyl alcohol (consumption, dependency)

ETOP elective termination of pregnancy *also* ETP

ETOX ethylene oxide *also* EO

ETP elective termination of pregnancy *also* ETOP • electron transfer/transport particle • entire treatment period • ephedrine, theophylline, and phenobarbital • eustachian tube pressure

ETR effective thyroxine ratio • epitympanic recess • estimated thyroid ratio

ETS Educational Testing Service • electrical transcranial stimulation • end–to–side (anastomosis) *also* ES, E–S

ETT endotracheal tube *also* ET • epinephrine tolerance test • esophageal transit time • exercise tolerance test • exercise treadmill test • extrapyramidal thyroxine • extrathyroidal thyroxine

ETTN ethyltrimethylol-trimethane trinitrate

ETU emergency and trauma unit • emergency treatment unit

ETV educational television • extravascular thermal volume

ETX ethosuximide

ETYA eicosatetroenoic acid

EU Ehrlich unit • emergency unit • endotoxin unit • entropy unit • enzyme unit • esophageal ulcer • esterase unit • etiology unknown • excretory urography • expected utility

Eu europium • euryon

EUA examination under anesthesia/anesthetic

EUCD emotionally unstable character disorder

EUG extrauterine gestation

EUL expected upper limit

EUM external urethral meatus

EUP extrauterine pregnancy

EURONET European On–Line Network

EUROTOX European Committee on Chronic Toxicity Hazards

EUS external urethral sphincter

eust eustachian

EUV extreme ultraviolet (laser)

EV emergency vehicle • enterovirus • epidermodysplasia verruciformis • esophageal varices • estradiol valerate • eversion *also* ev, ever. • evoked (response) • excessive ventilation • expected value • extravascular

eV, ev electron volt

ev eversion *also* EV, ever.

EVA ethylene vinyl acetate • ethyl violet azide (broth)

EVAC, evac evacuation/evacuated/evacuate

eval evaluation/evaluate/evaluated

evap evaporation/evaporated

EVCI expected value of clinical information

EVD external ventricular drainage

eve evening

ever. eversion/everted *also* EV, ev

EVF ethanol volume fraction

EVG electroventriculogram

EVI endocardial, vascular, interstitial

EVLW extravascular lung water

EVM electronic voltmeter · extravascular mass

evol evolution

EVP evoked visual potential

EVR endocardial viability ratio · evoked visual response

EVS endoscopic variceal sclerosis

EVSD Eisenmenger ventricular septal defect

EVTV extravascular thermal volume

EW emergency ward

ew elsewhere

EWB estrogen withdrawal bleeding

EWHO elbow–wrist–hand orthosis

EWI Experiential World Inventory

EWL egg–white lysozyme · evaporation water loss

EWSCLs extended–wear soft contact lenses

EWT erupted wisdom teeth

E(X) expected value of the random variable X

Ex, ex exacerbation · exaggerated *also* exag · examination/examined *also* exam. · example · excision *also* exc · exercise *also* E, exer · exophthalmos · exposure · extraction *also* EXT

ex aff [L. *ex affinis*] of affinity

EXAFS extended x–ray absorption fine structure (spectroscopy)

exag exaggerated *also* Ex, ex

exam. examination/examined/ examine *also* Ex, ex

ex aq [L. *ex aqua*] in water

EXBF exercise hyperemia blood flow

exc except · excision *also* Ex, ex

EXD ethylxanthic disulfide

exec executive

ExEF ejection fraction during exercise

EXELFS extended electron–loss line fine structure

exer exercise *also* E, Ex, ex

EXGBUS external genitalia, Bartholin (gland), urethral (gland), and Skene (gland)

ex gr [L. *ex grupa*] of the group of

exhib [L. *exhibeatur*] let it be displayed

exist. existing

EXO exonuclease · exophoria

EXP experienced · exploration · expose

Exp expiration/expiratory/ expire *also* espir · expectorant *also* exp, expec, expect

exp expected · expectorant *also* Exp, expec, expect · experiment(al) *also* E, exper, exptl · expired *also* E · exploration/ exploratory · exponent ·

exponential function • exposed/exposure

expec, expect. expectorant *also* Exp, exp

exper experiment(al) *also* E, exp, exptl

ExPGN extracapillary proliferative glomerulonephritis

expir expiration/expiratory/ expired *also* Exp

exp lap exploratory laparotomy

expn expression

exptl experimental *also* E, exp, exper

EXREM external radiation– emission–man (radiation dose)

EXS externally supported • extrinsically supported

exsicc [L. *exsiccatus*] dried out

EXT extension *also* E •

external *also* ext • extract/ extraction *also* Ex • extremity *also* ext, extr

ext extension • extensor • exterior • external *also* EXT • extract • extremity *also* EXT, extr

ext aud external auditory

extd extended • extracted

Ext FHR external fetal heart rate (monitoring)

ext fd fluid extract

extr extremity *also* EXT, ext

extrap extrapolate/ extrapolation

extrav extravasation

ext rot external rotation

EXTUB extubation

EXU excretory urogram

EY egg yolk • epidemiology year

EYA egg yolk agar

Ez eczema

F bioavailability • [L. *frater*] brother • conjugative plasmid in F+ bacterial cells • degree of fineness of abrasive particles • facial • facies • factor *also* Fac • Fahrenheit *also* Fahr • failure • fair • false • family *also* fam • farad *also* f, far. • Faraday constant • fascia • fasting (test) • fat (dietary) • father *also* FR • fecal • feces • Fellow • female *also* Fe, fe, FEM, fem • fermentative • fermi • fertility (factor) • fetal • fibroblast • fibrous (protein) • Ficol • field of vision • filament *also* fil • fine • finger • firm • flexed • flexion *also* f • flow (of blood) • fluid • fluoride • fluorine • flutter wave • focal length • focus • foil • fontanel • foot *also* f, ft • foramen • force • form/forma *also* f • formula • formulary • fossa • fractional (composition of gas in gasphase) • fracture *also* Fr, frac, fract, Frx, Fx, fx, FXR • fragment of antibody • free • French (gauge, scale) *also* FR, Fr • frequency *also* f, freq • frontal • frontal electrode placement in electroencephalography • full (diet) • function *also* fn, FXN • fundus • fusion beat • gilbert (unit of magnetomotive force) • Helmholz free energy • hydrocortisone (compound F) • inbreeding coefficient • [L. *fiat*] let it be made • (luminous) flux • [L. *fac*] make *also* f • phenylalanine • [L. *filius*] son •

variance ratio • vectorcardiography electode (left foot)

F′ hybrid F plasmid • secondary focal point (of lens)

˙F degree Fahrenheit

F+ bacterial cell with an F plasmid • good form response

F− bacterial cell lacking an F plasmid • fluoride • poor form response

F/ full upper denture

/F full lower denture

(F) final

F₁, F₂, etc. first, second, etc. filial generation

F₃ TFT—trifluorothymidine

FI—FXIII factor I through XIII (blood)

F344 Fischer 344 (rat)

f atomic orbital with angular momentum quantum number 3 • farad *also* F, far. • femto– • fingerbreadth *also* FB, fb • fission • flexion *also* F • fluid • focal • following *also* ff • foot *also* F, ft • form/forma *also* F • fostered (experimental animal) • frequency *also* F, freq • frequently • [L. *fiant, fiat*] let them be made • [L. *fac*] make *also* f

FA false aneurysm • Families Anonymous • Fanconi anemia • far advanced •

fatty acid • febrile antigen • femoral artery • fertilization antigen • fetal age • fibrinolytic activity • fibroadenoma • fibrosing alveolitis • field ambulance • filterable agent • filterable/filtered air • first aid • fluorescein angiography • fluorescent antibody • fluorescent assay • fluoroalanine • folic acid • follicular area • foramen • forearm • fortified aqueous (solution) • free acid • Freund adjuvant • Friedreich ataxia • functional activities • fusaric acid • fusidic acid

F/A fetus active

fa fatty (rat)

FAA folic acid antagonist • formaldehyde, acetic acid, and alcohol (solution)

FAAD fetal activity acceleration determination

FAAP family assessment adjustment pass

FAA sol formalin, acetic acid, and alcohol solution

FAB fast atom bombardment • formalin ammonium bromide • fragment (of immunoglobulin G involved in) antigen binding *also* Fab • French–American–British (leukemia classification system) • functional arm brace

Fab fragment (of immunoglobulin G involved in) antigen binding *also* FAB

F(ab′)₂ fragment (of immunoglobulin G) after digestion with the enzyme pepsin

FABER flexion, abduction, and external rotation

Fabere flexion, abduction, external rotation, and extension

FABF femoral artery blood flow • folic acid binding protein

FAB/MS fast atom bombardment mass spectrometry

FABP fatty acid–binding protein • folic acid–binding protein

FAC femoral arterial cannulation • ferric ammonium citrate • fetal abdominal circumference • fluorouracil, Adriamycin (doxorubicin), and cyclophosphamide • fractional area concentration • free available chlorine

Fac factor *also* F

Facb fragment, antigen, and complement binding

FACES (unique) facies, anorexia, cachexia, and eye and skin (syndrome)

FACH forceps to after–coming head

FAC–LEV fluorouracil, Adriamycin (doxorubicin), cyclophosphamide, and levamisole

FACMTA Federal Advisory Council on Medical Training Aids

FACNHA Foundation of American College of Nursing Home Administrators

FACOSH Federal Advisory Committee on Occupational Safety and Health

FACP ftorafur, Adriamycin (doxorubicin), cyclophosphamide, and platinol (cisplatin)

FACS fluorescence–activated cell sorter • fluorouracil, Adriamycin (doxorubicin), cyclophosphamide, and streptozocin

FACT Flanagan Aptitude Classification Test

FAD familial Alzheimer dementia • familial autonomic dysfunction • Family Assessment Device • fetal abdominal diameter • fetal activity–acceleration determination • flavin adenine dinucleotide *also* FADN

FADF fluorescent antibody dark–field

FADH₂ flavin adenine dinucleotide (reduced form)

FADIR flexion (in) adduction and internal rotation

Fadire flexion, adduction, internal rotation, and extension

FADN flavin adenine dinucleotide *also* FAD

FADU fluorometric analysis of DNA unwinding

FAE fetal alcohol effect

FAF fatty acid free • fibroblast–activating factor

FAGA full–term appropriate for gestational age

FAH Federation of American Hospitals

Fahr Fahrenheit *also* F

FAI first aid instruction • functional aerobic impairment • functional assessment inventory

FAJ fused apophyseal joints

FALG fowl anti–mouse lymphocyte globulin

FALL fallopian

FALP fluoro–assisted lumbar puncture

FAM fluorouracil, Adriamycin (doxorubicin), and mitomycin C

Fam, fam family/familial *also* F

FAMA fluorescent antibody to membrane antigen (test)

fam doc family doctor *also* FD, FMD

FAME fatty acid methyl ester • fluorouracil, Adriamycin (doxorubicin), and methyl CCNU (semustine)

fam hist family history

FAMMM familial atypical mole malignant melanoma • familial atypical multiple mole melanoma (syndrome)

fam per par familial periodic paralysis

fam phys family physician *also* FP

FAM–S fluorouracil, Adriamycin (doxorubicin), mitomycin C, and streptozotocin

FAN fuchsin, amido black, and naphthol yellow

FANA fluorescent antinuclear antibody

FANCAP fluids, aeration, nutrition, communication, activity, and pain (re: nursing)

FANCAS fluids, aeration, nutrition, communication, activity, and stimulation

F and R force and rhythm (of pulse)

FANPT Freeman Anxiety Neurosis and Psychosomatic Test

FANSS & M fundus anterior, normal size and shape, and mobile

FAP familial adenomatous polyposis • familial amyloid polyneuropathy • fatty acid poor • fatty acids polyunsaturated • femoral artery pressure • fibrillating action potential • fixed action pattern • frozen animal procedure

FAQ Family Attitudes Questionnaire

FAR flight aptitude rating • fractional albuminuria rate

FAR immediate good function followed by accelerated rejection

far. farad/faradic *also* F, f

FARS Fatal Accident Reporting System

FAS fatty acid synthetase • fetal alcohol syndrome

FASC free–standing ambulatory surgical center

fasc fasciculation • fasicle • fasciculus

FASF Factor Analyzed Short Form

FAST Filtered Audiometer Speech Test • flow–assisted short term (balloon catheter) • fluorescent allegosorbent test • fluorescent antibody staining technique

FAT family attitudes test • fast axoplasmic transport • fluorescent antibody technique/test • food awareness training

FATG fat globules

F₁ATPase F_1 adenosine triphosphatase

FATSA Flowers Auditory Test of Selective Attention

FAV feline ataxia virus • floppy aortic valve • fowl adenovirus

FAZ Fanconi–Albertini–Zellweger (syndrome) • foveal avascular zone

FB factor B • fasting blood (sugar) *also* FBS • feedback • fiberoptic bronchoscopy *also* Fib. bronc, FOB • fingerbreadth *also* f, fb • foreign body

F/B forward bending

fb fingerbreadth *also* f, FB

f–b face–bow

FBA fecal bile acid

FBC full blood count • functional bactericidal concentration

FBCOD foreign body of the cornea, oculus dexter (right eye)

FBCOS foreign body of the cornea, oculus sinister (left eye)

FBCP familial benign chronic pemphigus

FBD fibrocystic breast disease • functional bowel disease/disorder

FBE full blood examination

FBEC fetal bovine endothelial cell

FBF forearm blood flow

FBG fasting blood glucose • fibrinogen *also* fbg, FG, FGN • foreign body–type granuloma

fbg fibrinogen *also* FBG, FG, FGN

FBH familial benign hypercalcemia

FBHH familial benign hypocalciuric hypercalcemia

FBI flossing, brushing, and irrigation

FBL fecal blood loss • follicular basal lamina

FBM fetal breathing movement

FBP femoral blood pressure • fibrin/fibrinogen breakdown product

FBR [Ger. *Frischblut*] fresh–blood reaction

FBRCM fingerbreadth below right costal margin

FBS fasting blood sugar *also* FB • feedback signal • feedback system • fetal bovine serum

FBSS failed back surgery syndrome

FBU fingers below umbilicus (measurement)

FBW fasting blood work

FC family conference • fasciculus cuneatus • fast component (of neuron) • febrile convulsion • fecal coli (broth) • feline conjunctivitis • ferric citrate • fever, chills • fibrocystic • fibrocyte • financial class • finger clubbing • finger counting • flexion contracture • flucytosine *also* 5–FC • Foley catheter *also* F cath • form (response determined by) color • foster care • free cholesterol • frontal cortex • functional capacity • functional class

F/C fever and chills • flare and cell *also* F+C

F&C foam and condom

F+C flare and cell *also* F/C

5–FC 5–fluorocytosine *also* FC

Fc centroid frequency • foot–candle *also* fc, ftc • fragment, crystallizable (of immunoglobulin) • shade response to black areas

Fc' fragment crystallized in

minute quantities
(immunoglobulin) • shade
response to light gray area

fc foot–candle *also* Fc, ftc

FCA ferritin–conjugated
antibodies • fracture,
complete, angulated •
Freund complete adjuvant

F cath Foley catheter *also* FC

FCC familial colonic cancer •
femoral cerebral catheter •
follicular center cells •
fracture complete and
compound • fracture
compound and comminuted

fcc face–centered–cubic

FCCC fracture complete,
compound, and comminuted

FCCL follicular center cell
lymphoma

FCD feces collection device •
fibrocystic disease •
fibrocystic dysplasia •
focal cytoplasmic
degradation • fracture
complete and deviated

FCDB fibrocystic disease of
breast

FCE fluorouracil, cisplatin, and
etoposide

FCF fetal cardiac frequency •
fibroblast chemotactic
factor

FCFC fibroblast colony–
forming cells

FCG French catheter gauge

FCH, FCHL familial combined
hyperlipidemia

FCI fixed cell
immunofluorescence •
food–chemical intolerance

F–CL fluorouracil and calcium
leucovorin

fcly face lying (position)

FCM fetal cardiac motion •
flow cytometric/cytometry

FCMC family–centered
maternity care

FCMD Fukuyama–type
congenital muscular
dystrophy

FCMN family–centered
maternity nursing

FCMW Foundation for Child
Mental Welfare

FCP fasting chemistry
profile • final common
pathway • fluorouracil,
cyclophosphamide, and
prednisone • Functional
Communication Profile (of
aphasic adults)

FCR flexor carpi radialis •
fractional catabolic rate

FcR Fc receptor

FCRA fecal collection
receptacle assembly

FCRB flexor carpi radialis
brevis

FCRC Frederick Cancer
Research Center

FCS fecal containment
system • feedback control
system • fetal calf serum

FCSNVD fever, chills,
sweating, nausea, vomiting,
and diarrhea

FCT food composition table

FCU flexor carpi ulnaris

FCV forced vital capacity

FCVD fracture complete and varus deformity

FCVDS Framingham Cardiovascular Disease Survey

FCx frontal cortex

FD failure to descend • familial dysautonomia • family doctor *also* fam doc, FMD • fan douche • fatal dose • fetal danger • fetal demise • fetal distress • fibrinogen derivative • field desorption • Filatov–Dukes (disease) • fixed and dilated *also* F&D • fluorescence depolarization • fluphenazine decanoate • focal disease • focal distance • Folin–Denis (assay) • follicular diameter • foot drape • forceps delivery • freedom from distractability • freeze–dried • frequency deviation • full denture

F/D fracture/dislocation *also* Fx–dis

F&D fixed and dilated *also* FD

Fd animo–terminal portion of heavy chain of immunoglobulin • ferredoxin • fundus

FD$_{50}$ median fatal dose

FDA Food and Drug Administration • [L. *frontodextra anterior*] right frontal anterior (position of fetus)

FDBL fecal daily blood loss

FDC frequency dependence of compliance • perfluoro-decalin (blood substitute)

FD&C Food, Drug, and Cosmetic (Act) *also* FFDCA

FDCPA Food, Drug, and Consumer Product Agency

FDCT Franck Drawing Completion Test

FDD Food and Drugs Directorate

FDDC ferric dimethyldithiocarbonate

FDDQ Freedom from Distractibility Deviation Quotient

FDDS Family Drawing Depression Scale

FDE female day–equivalent • final drug evaluation

FDF fast death factor • further differentiated fibroblast

FDG fluorodeoxyglucose

FDG, fdg feeding

FDGF fibroblast–derived growth factor

FDH familial dysalbuminemic hyperthyroxinemia

FDI first dorsal interosseus

FDIU fetal death in utero

FDL flexor digitorum longus

FDLMP first day of last menstrual period

FDLV fer de lance virus

FDM fetus of diabetic mother

FDNB fluorodinitrobenzene (Sanger reagent)

FDP fibrin/fibrinogen degradation product *also* fdp • flexor digitorum profundus • [L. *frontodextra posterior*] right frontal posterior (position of fetus) • fructose diphosphate

fdp fibrin/bibrinogen degradation product *also* FDP

FDPALD fructose diphosphate aldolase

FDPase fructose diphosphatase

FDQB flexor digiti quinti brevis

FDR fractional disappearance rate • frequency dependence of resistance

FDS flexor digitorum sublimis • flexor digitorum superficialis • for duration of stay

FDT [L. *frontodextra transversa*] right frontal transverse (position of fetus)

F₃dTMP trifluorothymidylate

F_3dTMP trifluorothymidylate

FdUMP fluorodeoxyuridylate

FDV Friend disease virus

FDZ fetal danger zone

FE fatty ester • fecal emesis • fetal erythroblastosis • fetal erythroblastosin • fluid extract • fluorescing erythrocyte • forced expiratory • formalin and ethanol • freely eating

Fe female *also* F, fe, FEM, fem • [L. *ferrum*] iron *also* Fer

fe female *also* F, Fe, FEM, fem

feb febrile • [L. *febris*] fever

feb dur [L. *febre durante*] while the fever lasts

FEBP fetal estrogen–binding protein

FEC fluorouracil, etoposide, and cisplatin • forced expiratory capacity • free erythrocyte coproporphyrin *also* FECP • freestanding emergency center • Friend erythroleukemia cell

FECG fetal electrocardiogram

F_{ECO2} fractional concentration of carbon dioxide in expired gas

FECP free erythrocyte coproporphyrin *also* FEC

FECT factor VIII correctional time: fibroelastic connective tissue

FECV functional extracellular (fluid) volume

FeD, Fe def iron (ferrum) deficiency

FEE forced equilibrating expiration

FEEG fetal electroencephalogram

FEF Family Evaluation Form • forced expiratory flow

FEF₅₀ forced expiratory flow after 50% of vital capacity has been expelled

FEF₅₀/FIF₅₀ ratio of expiratory flow to inspiratory flow at 50% of forced vital capacity

FEFV forced expiratory flow volume

FEHBP Federal Employee Health Benefits Program

FEIBA factor VIII inhibitor bypassing activity

FEKG fetal electrocardiogram

FEL familial erythrophagocytic lymphohistiocytosis

FELC Friend erythroleukemia cell

FeLV feline leukemia virus *also* FLV

FEM femoral *also* fem • femur *also* fem • finite element method • fluid–electrolyte malnutrition

fem female *also* F, Fe, fe • feminine • femoral *also* FEM • femur *also* Fem

fem intern [L. *femoribus internus*] at inner side of thighs

Fem–pop femoral–popliteal (bypass)

FEN fluid, electrolytes, and nutrition

FENa, FE_Na fractional excretion of sodium

FENF fenfluramine

F_EO2 fractional concentration of oxygen in expired gas

FEP fluorinated ethylene–propylene (polymer) • free erythrocyte porphyrin • free erythrocyte protoporphyrin *also* FEPP

FEPB functional electronic peroneal brace

FEPP free erythrocyte protoporphyrin *also* FEP

FER flexion, extension, and rotation • fractional esterification rate

Fer [L. *ferrum*] iron *also* Fe

fert fertility • fertilized

ferv [L. *fervens*] boiling

FES Family Environment Scale • fat embolism syndrome • flame emission spectroscopy • forced expiratory spirogram • functional electrical stimulation

FESA finite element stress analysis

FeSV feline sarcoma virus

FET field–effect transistor • Fisher exact test • fixed erythrocyte turnover • forced expiratory time

fet fetus

FETE Far Eastern tick–borne encephalitis

FETI fluorescence energy transfer immunoassay

Fe/TIBC iron saturation of serum transferrin

FETs forced expiratory time in seconds

FEUO for external use only

FEV familial exudative vitreoretinopathy • forced expiratory volume

fev fever

FEV₁ forced expiratory volume in one second

FEVB frequency ectopic ventricular beat

FEV_t forced expiratory volume timed

FEV₁/VC ratio of one–second forced expiratory volume to vital capacity

FEXE formalin, ethanol, xylol, and ethanol

FeZ iron zone

FF degree of fineness of abrasive particles • fat–free (diet) • father factor • fear of failure • fecal frequency • fertility factor *also* F factor • fields of Forel • filtration factor • filtration fraction • fine fiber • fine fraction • finger flexion • finger–to–finger *also* f→f • fixation fluid • fixing fluid • flat feet • flip–flop (electronic logic circuitry) • fluorescent focus • force fluids *also* ff • forearm flow • forward flexion • foster father • Fox–Fordyce (disease) • free fraction • fresh frozen • fundus firm *also* ff • further flexion

F&F filiform (bongie) and follower • fixes and follows

fF ultrafine fiber • ultrafine fraction

ff following *also* f • force fluids *also* FF • fundus firm *also* FF

f→f finger–to–finger *also* FF

FFA female–female adaptor • free fatty acid

F factor fertility factor *also* FF

FFAP free fatty acid phase

FFB fast feedback • flexible fiberoptic bronchoscopy

FFC fixed flexion contracture • free from chlorine

FFCS forearm flexion control strap

FFD fat–free diet • focus–film distance

FFDCA Federal Food, Drug, and Cosmetic Act *also* FDCA

FFDW fat–free dry weight

FFE fecal fat excretion

FFEM freeze fracture electron microscopy

FFF degree of fineness of abrasive particles • field–flow fractionation • flicker fusion frequency (test)

FFG free fat graft

FFI fast food intake • free from infection • fundamental frequency indicator

FFIT fluorescent focus inhibition test

FFM fat–free mass • five–finger movement

FFP fresh frozen plasma

FFR frequency–following response

FFROM full, free range of motion

FFS failure of fixation suppression • fat–free solid • fat–free supper • fee for service • flexible fiberoptic sigmoidoscopy

FFT fast Fourier transform • flicker fusion test • flicker fusion threshold

FFTP first full–term pregnancy

FFU focus–forming unit

FFW fat–free weight

FFWC fractional free–water clearance

FFWW fat–free wet weight

FG fasciculus gracilis • fast–glycolytic (muscle fiber) • fast green • Feeley–Gorman (agar) *also* F–G • fibrin glue • fibrinogen *also* FBG, fbg, FGN • field gain • Flemish giant (rabbit) • French gauge

F–G Feeley–Gorman (agar) *also* FG

fg femtogram

FGAR formylglycinamide ribonucleotide

FGB fully granulated basophil

FGC fibrinogen gel chromatography

FGD fatal granulomatous disease

FGDS fibrogastro-duodenoscopy

FGF father's grandfather • fibroblast growth factor • fresh gas flow

FGG focal global glomerulosclerosis • fowl γ–globulin

FGL fasting gastrin level

FGLU fasting glucose

FGM father's grandmother

FGN fibrinogen *also* FBG, fbg, FG • focal glomerulonephritis

FGP fundic gland polyps

FGRN finely granular

FGS fibrogastroscopy • focal glomerular sclerosis

FGT female genital tract • fluorescent gonorrhea test

FGU French gauge, urodynamic

FH familial hypercholesterolemia *also* FHC • family history *also* FH$_X$ • Fanconi–Hegglin (syndrome) • fasting hyperbilirubinemia • favorable histology • femoral hypoplasia • fetal head • fetal heart *also* FHT • fibromuscular hyperplasia *also* FMH • Ficoll–Hypaque (technique) • floating hospital • follicular hyperplasia • Frankfort horizontal (plane of skull) • fundal height

fh fostered by hand (experimental animal) • [L. *fiat haustus*] let a draught be made

FH$_4$ folacin • tetrahydrofolic acid

FHA familial hypoplastic anemia • filamentous hemagglutinin • filterable hemolytic anemia • fimbrial hemagglutinin

FHC familial hypercholesterolemia *also* FH • family health center • Ficoll–Hypaque centrifugation • Fuchs heterochromic cyclitis

FHCH fortified hexachlorocyclohexane

FHD family history of diabetes

FHF fetal heart frequency • fulminant hepatic failure

FHH familial hypocalciuric hypercalcemia • family history of hirsutism • fetal heart heard

FHI Fuchs heterochromic iridocyclitis

FHIP family health insurance plan

FHL flexor hallucis longus • functional hearing loss

FHLDL familial hypercholesterolemia, low density lipoprotein

FHM fathead minnow (cells) • fetal heart motion

FH–M fumarate hydratase, mitochondrial

FHMI family history of mental illness

FHN family history negative

FHNH fetal heart not heard

FHP family history positive

FHR familial hypophos-phatemic rickets • fetal heart rate • fetal heart rhythm

FHRDC family history, research diagnostic criteria

FHR–NST fetal heart rate nonstress test

FHS fetal heart sound • fetal hydantoin syndrome

FH–S fumarate hydratase, soluble

FHT fetal heart *also* FH • fetal heart tone

FHTG familial hypertri-glyceridemia

FH–UFS femoral hypoplasia–unusual facies syndrome

FHVP free hepatic venous pressure

FH$_x$ family history *also* FH

FI fasciculus interfascicularis • fever caused by infection • fibrinogen *also* FIB, fib. • fiscal intermediary • fixed interval (schedule) • flame ionization • forced inspiration • fronto–iliacus • functional inquiry

FIA fluorescent immunoassay • Freund incomplete adjuvant

FIB fibrin • fibrinogen *also* FI, fib. • fibrositis • fibula

fib. fiber • fibrillation *also* fibrill • fibrinogen *also* FI, FIB

fibrill fibrillation *also* fib.

Fib. bronc fiberoptic bronchoscopy *also* FB, FOB

FIC functional inhibitory concentration

FICA Federal Insurance Contributions Act

FI$_{CO2}$, FICO$_2$ fractional concentration of carbon dioxide in inspired gas

FID father in delivery • flame ionization detector • free induction decay • fungal immunodiffusion

FIF feedback inhibition factor • (human) fibroblast interferon *also* FIFN • forced inspiratory flow • formaldehyde–induced fluorescence

FIFN (human) fibroflast interferon *also* FIF

FIFR fasting intestinal flow rate

fig. figure

FIGD familial idiopathic gonadotropin deficiency

FIGLU formiminoglutamic acid

FIGO International Federation of Gynecology and Obstetrics (classification of tumor staging)

FIH fat–induced hyperglycemia

FIL father–in–law

fil filament *also* F

FILAR filariasin

filt filter, filtration

FIM field ion microscopy • functional independence measure

FIME fluorouracil, ICRF–159 (razoxane), and methyl–CCNU (semustine)

FIN fine intestinal needle

F–insulin fibrous insulin

FI$_{02}$, FiO$_2$ forced inspiratory oxygen • fraction of inspired oxygen

FIP feline infectious peritonitis

FIPT periarteriolar transudate

FIQ full scale intelligence quotient

FIR far infrared • fold increase in resistance

FIRDA frontal irregular rhythmic delta activity (electroencephalography)

FIRO–B Fundamental Interpersonal Relations Orientation—Behavior

FIRO–F Fundamental Intepersonal Relations Orientation—Feelings

FIS forced inspiratory spirogram

FISP fast imaging with steady–state precision

FISS Flint Infant Security Scale

Fiss, fiss fissure

fist. fistula

FIT Flanagan Industrial Tests • fluorescein isothiocyanate *also* FITC • fusion–inferred threshold (test)

FITC fluorescein isothiocyanate *also* FIT • fluorescein isothiocyanate, conjugated

FITT frequency, intensity, time, and type (exercise)

FIUO for internal use only

FIV$_1$ forced inspiratory volume in one second

FIVC forced inspiratory vital capacity

F–J Fisher–John (melting point method)

FJN familial juvenile nephrophthisis

FJRM, FJROM full joint range of movement/motion

FJS finger joint size

FK Feil–Klippel (syndrome) • feline kidney • Foster Kennedy (syndrome) •

functioning kasai (Belgian Congo anemia)

FL factor level • fatty liver • feline leukemia • femur length • fetal length • fibers of Luschka • fibroblast–like • filtered load *also* Fl, fl • filtration leukapheresis • flavomycin • fluorescein • flutamide and leuprolide acetate • focal length • Friend leukemia (cell) *also* FLC • frontal lobe • full liquids (diet) • functional length • functioning kasai

Fl florentiam

Fl, fl filtered load *also* FL • fluid • fluorescence *also* fluores

fL femtoliter *also* fl

fl femtoliter *also* fL • flank • flexion/flexible • fluid *also* FLD, fld • flutter

FL–2 feline lung (cell)

FLA fluorescent–labeled antibody • [L. *frontolaeva anterior*] left frontal anterior (position of fetus)

Fla, fla [L. *fiat lege artis*] let it be done according to rule of the art

flac flaccidity/flaccid

Fl Ang fluorescein angiography

FLASH fast low–angle shot

flav [L. *flavus*] yellow

FLC fatty liver cell • fetal liver cell • Friend leukemia cell *also* FL

FLD fatty liver disease •

fibrotic lung disease • fluid *also* Fl, fl, fld • flutamide and leuprolide acetate depot

fld field • fluid *also* Fl, fl, FLD

fld ext fluid extract *also* fldxt

fl dr fluid dram

fld rest. fluid restriction

fl drs fluff dressing

fldxt fluid extract *also* fld ext

FLES Fairview Language Evaluation Scale

FLEX Federation Licensing Examination

flex. flexor/flexion

flex sig flexible sigmoidoscopy

FLGA full–term, large for gestational age

FLK funny–looking kid (syndrome)

FLKS fatty liver and kidney syndrome

FLM fasciculus longitudinalis medialis

floc, flocc flocculation

flor [L. *flores*] flowers (mineral substance in powdery state after sublimation)

fl oz fluid ounce

FLP [L. *frontolaeva posterior*] left frontal posterior (position of fetus)

FLPR flurbiprofen

FLS fatty liver syndrome • fibrous long–spacing (collagen) • flashing lights and/or scotoma • flow–

limiting segment • Functional Life Scale

FLSA follicular lymphosarcoma

FLSP fluorescein–labeled serum protein

FLT [L. *frontolaeva transversa*] left frontal transverse (position of fetus)

FLTA Fullerton Language Test for Adolescents

FLTAC Fisher–Logemann Test of Articulation Competence

FLU fluphenazine *also* FPZ

FLU A influenza A virus

fluores fluorescent/ fluorescence *also* Fl, fl

fluoro fluoroscopy

fl up flare–up • follow up

FLV feline leukemia virus *also* FeLV • Friend leukemia virus

FLW fasting laboratory work

FLZ flurazepam

FM face mask • facilities management • fathom • feedback mechanism • fetal movement • fibromuscular • filtered mass • flavin mononucleotide • flowmeter • fluid movement • fluorescent microscopy • foramen magnum • forensic medicine • formerly married • foster mother • frequence modulation • Friend–Moloney (antigen) • functional movement •

fusobacteria micro– organisms • [L. *fiat mistura*] make a mixture *also* fm

F&M firm and midline (uterus)

Fm fermium

fm femtometer • from *also* fr • [L. *fiat mistura*] make a mixture *also* FM

FMA Frankfort–mandibular plane angle

FMAC fetal movement acceleration test

FMB full maternal behavior

FMC family medicine center • fetal movement count • flight medicine clinic • focal macular choroidopathy

FMD family medical doctor *also* fam doc, FD • fibromuscular dysplasia • foot–and–mouth disease

FMDV foot–and–mouth disease virus

FME full–mouth extraction

FMEL Friend murine erythroleukemia

FMEN familial multiple endocrine neoplasia

FMET, F–met, fMet formylmethionine

FMF familial Mediterranean fever • fetal movement felt • flow microfluorometry • forced midexpiratory flow

FMFD1 familial multiple factor deficiency 1

FMG fine mesh gauze • foreign medical graduate

FMGEMS Foreign Medical Graduate Examination in Medical Sciences

FMH family medical history · fat–mobilizing hormone · fetomaternal hemorrhage · fibromuscular hyperplasia *also* FH

FML flail mitral leaflet · fluorometholone (anti–inflammatory)

FMN first malignant neoplasm · flavin mononucleotide · frontomaxillo–nasal (suture)

FMNH, FMNH$_2$ reduced form of flavin mononucleotide

fmol femtomole

FMP fasting metabolic panel · first menstrual period

FMR fetal movement record · Friend–Moloney–Rauscher (antigen)

FMS fat–mobilizing substance · fluorouracil, mitomycin, and streptozocin · full–mouth series (dental x–ray films)

FMSTB Frostig Movement Skills Test Battery

FMU first morning urine

FMULC free monoclonal urinary light chain

FMV fluorouracil, methyl–CCNU (semustine), and vincristine

FMX full–mouth x–ray

FN facial nerve · false negative *also* Fneg · fastigial nucleus ·

fibronectin · final nitrogen · finger–to–nose (coordination test) *also* F–N, F→N, FTN · fluoride number

F–N, F→N finger–to–nose (coordination test) *also* FN, FTN

fn function *also* F, FXN

FNA fine–needle aspiration

FNa filtered sodium

FNAB fine–needle aspiration biopsy

FNAC fine–needle aspiratory cytology

FNC fatty nutritional cirrhosis

FNCJ fine–needle catheter jejunostomy

FND febrile neutrophilic dermatosis · frontonasal dysplasia

Fneg false negative *also* FN

FNF false–negative fraction · femoral neck fracture · finger–nose–finger (coordination test)

FNH focal nodular hyperplasia

FNP Family Nurse Practitioner

fn p fusion point

FNR false–negative rate

FNS food and nutrition services · functional neuromuscular stimulation

FNT false neurochemical transmitter · finger to nose test

FO fast oxidative · fiberoptic · focus out · foot orthosis · foramen ovale • forced oscillation • foreign object • fronto–occipital (fetal position)

Fo fomentation/fomenting

FOAVF failure of all vital forces

FOB father of baby • fecal occult blood • feet out of bed • fiberoptic bronchoscope/bronchoscopy *also* FB, Fib. bronc • foot of bed • foreign object/body

FOBT fecal occult blood test

FOC father of child • fluid of choice • frequency of contact scale • fronto–occipital circumference

FOCAL formula calculation (computer language)

FOCMA feline oncornavirus–associated cell membrane antigen

FOD free of disease

FOEB feet over edge of bed

FOG fast–oxidative–glycolytic (fiber) • Fluothane, oxygen, and gas (nitrous oxide) • full–on gain

FOI flight of ideas

fol following

FOM figure of merit (measure of diagnostic value per radionuclide radiation dose) • floor of mouth

FOMI fluorouracil, Oncovin (vincristine), and mitomycin C

FOOB fell out of bed

FOOSH fell on outstretched hand

FOP fibrodysplasia ossificans progressiva • forensic pathology

FOPR full outpatient rate

FOR, For forensic

for. foreign • formula *also* form.

form. formula *also* for.

fort. [L. *fortis*] strong

FORTRAN formula translation (computer language)

FOS fiberoptic sigmoidoscope/sigmoidoscopy • fissura orbitalis superior • fractional osteoid surface • full of stool

found. foundation

FOV field of view

FOVI field of vision intact

FOW fenestration open window

FP false positive • family physician *also* fam phys • family planning • family practice • family practitioner • Fanconi–Petrassi (syndrome) • fibrinolytic potential • fibrinopeptide • filling pressure • filter paper • final pressure • first pass • fixation protein • flat plate • flavin phosphate • flavoprotein • flexor profundus • fluid pressure • fluorescence polarization • food poisoning • forearm pronated *also* fp • freezing point *also* fp • fronto-parietal • frozen plasma • full period • fundal pressure • fusion point

F–P femoral popliteal

F/P fluorescein to protein (ratio) • fluid–plasma (ratio)

F–6–P fructose–6–phosphate

Fp filtered phosphate • frontal polar electrode placement in electroencephalography

fp flexor pollicis • foot–pound • forearm pronated *also* FP • freezing point • [L. *fiat potio*] let a potion be made • [L. *fiat pulvis*] let a powder be made

FPA fibrinopeptide A *also* fpA • filter paper activity • fluorophenylalanine

fpA fibrinopeptide A *also* FPA

FPAL full–term (deliveries), premature (deliveries), abortion(s), living (children)

FPB femoral popliteal bypass • fibrinopeptide B • flexor pollicis brevis

FPC familial polyposis coli • family planning clinic • family practice center • fish protein concentrate • forced pair copulation • frozen packed cells

FPCL fibroblast–populated collagen lattice

FPD fetopelvic disproportion • fixed partial denture • flame photometric detector

FPDD familial pure depressive disease

FPE first–pass effect

FPF false–positive fraction • fibroblast pneumocyte factor

FPG fasting plasma glucose • fluorescence plus Giemsa (stain) • focal proliferative glomerulonephritis *also* FPGN

FPGN focal proliferative glomerulonephritis *also* FPG

FPH$_2$ of flavin phosphate, reduced

FPHA family planning health assistant

FPHE formaldehyde/formalin–treated pyruvaldehyde–stabilized human erythrocytes

FPHx family psychiatric history

FPI femoral pulsatility index • formula protein intolerance • Freiburger Personality Inventory

FPIA fluorescence–polarization immunoassay

f pil [L. *fiant pilulae*] let pills be made

FPK fructose–6–phosphokinase

FPL fasting plasma lipid • flexor pollicis longus

FPLA fibrin plate lysis area

FPM filter paper microscopic (test) • full passive movements

fpm feet per minute

FPN ferric chloride, perchloric acid, and nitric acid (solution)

FPNA first–pass nuclear angiocardiography

FPO freezing point osmometer

FPP free portal pressure

FPPH familial primary pulmonary hypertension

FPR fluorescence photobleaching recovery • fractional proximal resorption

FPRA first–pass radionuclide angiogram

FPS fetal PCB (polychlorinated biphenyl) syndrome • footpad swelling • foot–pound–second (system) *also* fps

fps feet per second • foot–pound–second (system) *also* FPS • frames per second

FPT fixed parenchymal turnover

FPU Family Participation Unit

FPV fowl plague virus

FPVB femoral–popliteal vein bypass

FPZ fluphenazine *also* FLU

FPZ–D fluphenazine decanoate

FR failure rate (contraception) • father *also* F • Favre–Racouchot (disease) • feedback regulation • fibrinogen related • Fischer–Race (notation) • fixed ratio • flocculation reaction • flow rate • fluid restriction • fluid retention • free radical • French (guage, scale) *also* F, Fr • frequency of respiration • frequent relapses • Friend (virus) • full range • functional residual

(capacity) • [L. *formatio reticularis*] reticular formation

F&R force and rhythm (of pulse)

Fr fracture *also* F, frac, fract, Frx, Fx, fx, FXR • francium • franklin (unit charge) • French (guage, scale) *also* F, FR

fr fried • from *also* fm

FRA fibrinogen–related antigen • fluorescent rabies antibody

fra fragile site (chromosome in cytogenetics)

frac, fract fracture *also* F, Fr, Frx, Fx, fx, FXR

FRACON framycetin, colistin, and nystatin

fract fraction *also* FX

fract dos [L. *fracta dosi*] in divided doses

FRACTS fractional urines

frag fragile/fragility • fragment

FRAP fluorescence recovery after photobleaching

FRAT free radical assay technique

fra(X) fragile X (chromosome) • fragile X (syndrome)

FRBB, Fr BB fracture of both bones *also* Fx BB

FRBS fast red B salt

FRC frozen red cells • functional reserve/residual capacity (of lungs)

FRCD fixed ratio combination drugs

FRD flexion–rotation–drawer

FRE Fischer rat embryo • flow–related enhancement

FREIR Federal Research on Biological and Health Effects of Ionizing Radiation

frem [L. *fremitus vocalis*] vocal fremitus

freq frequency *also* F, f

FRF fasciculus retroflexus • filtration replacement fluid • follicle–stimulating hormone–releasing factor

FRH follicle–stimulating hormone–releasing hormone *also* FSH–RF

FRHS fast–repeating high sequence

frict friction (rub)

Fried Friedman (test for pregnancy)

frig [L. *frigidus*] cold

FRJM full range joint motion/ movement

FRM full range of motion *also* FROM

FRN fully resonant nucleus

FRNS frequently relapsing nephrotic syndrome

FROM full range of motion *also* FRM

FROS front routing of signal

FRP functional refractory period

FRPS functional resting position splint

FR r, fr r friction rub

FRS ferredoxin–reducing substance • first rank symptom • furosemide *also* FSM, FUR

FRT Family Relations Test • full recovery time

Fru, fru fructose

frust [L. *frustillatim*] in small pieces

FRV functional residual volume

Frx fracture *also* F, Fr, frac, fract, Fx, fx

FS factor of safety • Fanconi syndrome • Felty syndrome • fetoscope • field stimulation • fine structure • fingerstick • fire setter (psychology) • Fisher syndrome • flexible sigmoidoscopy • food service • forearm supination • for skin • Fourier series • fracture, simple • fracture site • fragile site • Freeman–Sheldon (syndrome) • Friesinger score • frozen section *also* FZ • full–scale (IQ) • full and soft (diet) *also* F&S • full strength • function study • functional shortening • (human) foreskin (cells)

F/S female, spayed (animal)

F&S full and soft (diet) *also* FS

FSA fetal sulfoglycoprotein antigen

fsa [L. *fiat secundum artem*] let it be made skillfully *also* fsar

fsar [L. *fiat secundum artem*

reglas] let it be made according to the rules of the art *also* fsa

FSB fetal scalp blood • Fokes sentence builder • full spine board

FSBG finger–stick blood gas

FSBM full–strength breast milk

FSBT Fowler single breath test

FSC Forer Sentence Completion (Test) • fracture simple and comminuted • fracture simple and complete • free secretory component • free–standing clinic

FSCC fracture simple, complete, and comminuted

FSD focus–skin distance • fracture simple and depressed • full–scale deflection

FSDQ Frost Self–Description Questionnaire

FSE fetal scalp electrode • filtered smoke exposure

FSF fibrin stabilizing factor (factor XIII)

FSG fasting serum glucose • focal sclerosing glomerulonephritis *also* FSGN • focal segmental glomerulosclerosis

FSGA full–term, small for gestational age

FSGHS focal segmental glomerular hyalinosis and sclerosis

FSGN focal sclerosing glo-merulonephritis *also* FSG

FSGO floating spherical gaussian orbital

FSGS focal segmental glomerulosclerosis

FSH fascioscapulohumeral • focal and segmental hyalinosis • follicle–stimulating hormone

FSH/LR–RH follicle–stimulating hormone and luteinizing hormone–releasing hormone

FSHMD facioscapulohumeral muscular dystrophy

FSH–RF follicle–stimulating hormone–releasing factor *also* FRH

FSH–RH follicle–stimulating hormone–releasing hormone

FSI foam stability index • Food Sanitation Institute • Function Status Index

FSIA foot shock–induced analgesia

FSIQ Full–Scale Intelligence Quotient

FSL fasting serum level • fixed slit light

FSM furosemide *also* FRS, FUR

F–SM/C fungus, smear and culture

FSP familial spastic paraplegia • fibrin/ fibrinogen split products • fibrinolytic split products • fine suspended particulate • free secretory piece

F–SP [L. *forma specialis*] special form (taxonomy)

FSR film screen radiography · fragmented sarcoplasmic reticulum · fusiform skin revision

FSS Familiar Sensory Stimulation · Fear Survey Schedule · focal segmental sclerosis · Freeman–Sheldon syndrome · French steel sound · front support strap · full–scale score · functional systems scale

FSST Full–Scale Score Total

FST foam stability test

FSU family service unit

FSV feline fibrosarcoma virus

FSW field service worker

FT false transmitter · family therapy · fast twitch · feeding tube · ferritin *also* F_t · ferromagnetic tamponade · fetal tonsil · fibrous tissue · filling time · finger tapping · fingertip · follow through (after barium meal) · formol toxoid · Fourier transform · free thyroxine · full term · function test

FT$_3$ free triiodothyronine

FT$_4$ free (unbound) thyroxine

F$_t$ ferritin *also* FT

ft foot/feet *also* F, f · [L. *fiat or fiant*] let there be made

FTA fluorescein treponema antibody (test) · fluorescent titer antibody · fluorescent treponemal antibody

FTA–ABS, FTA–Abs fluorescent treponemal antibody absorption (test)

F–TAG fast–binding target–attaching globulin

FTAT fluorescent treponemal antibody test

FTB fingertip blood

FTBD fit to be detained · full–term, born dead

FTBE focal tick–borne encephalitis

FTBS Family Therapist Behavioral Scale

FTC frames to come (optometry) · frequency threshold curve

ftc foot candle *also* Fc, fc

ft catapl [L. *fiat cataplasma*] let a poultice be made

ft cerat [L. *fiat ceratum*] let a poultice be made

ft collyr [L. *fiat collyrium*] let an eyewash be made

FTD failure to descend · femoral total density

FTE full–time equivalent (resident)

ft emuls [L. *fiat emulsio*] let an emulsion be made

ft enem [L. *fiat enema*] let an enema be made

FTF finger to finger (test)

FTFTN finger to finger to nose (test)

FTG full–thickness graft

ft garg [L. *fiat gargarisma*] let a gargle be made

FTI free thyroxine index

FT₃I free triiodothyronine index

ft infus [L. *fiat infusum*] let an infusion be made

ft injec [L. *fiat injectio*] let an injection be made

FTIR functional terminal innervation ratio

FTKA failed to keep appointment

FTLB full–term live birth

ft lb foot pound

FTLFC full–term living female child

ft linim [L. *fiat linimentum*] let a liniment be made

FTLMC full–term living male child

FTM fluid thioglycolate medium • fractional test meal

ft mas [L. *fiat massa*] let a mass be made

ft mas div in pil [L. *fiat massa dividenda in pilulae*] let a mass be made and divided into pills

ft mist. [L. *fiat mistura*] let a mixture be made

FTN finger–to–nose (coordination test) *also* FN, F–N, F→N • full–term nursery

FTNB full–term newborn

FTND full–term normal delivery

FTNS functional transcutaneous nerve stimulation

FTNSD full–term, normal, spontaneous delivery

FTO fructose–terminated oligosaccharide

FTP failure to progress (in labor)

FTPA perfluorotripropylamine (blood substitute)

ft pil [L. *fiant pilulae*] let pills be made

ft pulv [L. *fiat pulvis*] let a powder be made

FTR for the record • fractional turnover rate

FTS Family Tracking System • feminizing testis syndrome • fingertips • [Fr. *facteur thymique sérique*] serum thymic factor

FTSG full–thickness skin graft

ft solut [L. *fiat solutio*] let a solution be made

ft suppos [L. *fiat suppositorium*] let a suppository be made

FTT failure to thrive • fat tolerance test • fraternal twins raised together • fructose tolerance test

ft troch [L. *fiat trochisci*] let lozenges be made

FTU fluorescence thiourea

ft ung [L. *fiat unguentum*] let an ointment be made

FTX field training exercise

FU fecal urobilinogen • Finsen unit *also* Fu • fluorouracil • follow–up *also* F/U • fractional urinalysis • fundus (at umbilicus) *also* F/U

F/U follow–up *also* FU • fundus at umbilicus *also* FU

F&U flanks and upper quadrants

F↑U fingers above umbilicus (measurement)

F↓U fingers below umbilicus (measurement)

5–FU 5–fluorouracil

FU–I, FU–II first, second set of follow–up data

Fu Finsen unit *also* FU

FUB found under bridge • functional uterine bleeding

FUC fucosidase

Fuc fucose

FU$_{CO}$ functional uptake of carbon monoxide

FUDR floxuridine • fluorodeoxyuridine

FUE fever of unknown etiology *also* FUO

FUFA free volatile fatty acid

fulg fulguration

FUM 5–fluorouracil and methotrexate • fumarase • fumarate • fumigation

FUMP fluorouridine monophosphate

FUN follow–up note

func, funct function/ functional

FUNG–C fungus culture

FUNG–S fungus smear

FUO fever of unknown origin *also* FUE

FUOV follow–up office visit

fu p fusion point

FUR fluorouracil riboside • fluorouridine • furosemide *also* FRS, FSM

FURAM ftorafur, Adriamycin (doxorubicin), and mitomycin C

FUS feline urologic syndrome • fusion

FUT fibrinogen uptake test

FUTP fluorouridine triphosphate

FV Fahr–Volhard (disease) • femoral vein • flow volume • fluid volume • formaldehyde vapors • Friend virus

FVA Friend virus anemia

FVC false vocal cord • filled voiding flow rate *also* FVFR • forced vital capacity

FVD fibrovascular tissue on disk

FVE fibrovascular tissue elsewhere • forced volume, expiratory

FVFR filled voiding flow rate *also* FVC

FVH focal vascular headache

FVIC forced inspiratory vital capacity

FVL femoral vein ligation • flow volume loop • force, velocity, length

FVM familial visceral myopathy

FVP Friend virus polycythemia

FVR feline viral rhinotracheitis • forearm vascular resistance

fvs [L. *fiat venae sectio*] let there be a cutting of a vein

FW Falconer–Weddell (syndrome) • Felix–Weil (reaction) • Folin–Wu (reaction) • forced whisper • fracturing wall • fragment wound

Fw F wave (fibrillatory wave, flutter wave)

fw fresh water

FWB full weight bearing

FWHM full width (of photopeak measured at) half maximal (count) (tomography) • full width (of line–spread function) half–maximal height

FWPCA Federal Water Pollution Control Administration

FWR Felix–Weil reaction • Folin–Wu reaction

FWW front wheel walker

FX factor X • fluoroscopy • fornix • fractional *also* F, fract, fx • frozen section *also* fx

Fx fracture *also* F, Fr, frac, fract, fx, FXR • fractional urine • friction

fx fractional *also* F, fract, FX • fracture *also* F, Fr, frac, fract, FXR • frozen section *also* FX

Fx BB fracture of both bones *also* FRBB, FrBB

Fx–dis fracture–dislocation *also* F/D

FXN function *also* F, fn

FXR fracture *also* F, Fr, frac, fract, Frx, Fx, fx

FY fiber year • fiscal year • framycetin • full year

FYI for your information

F–Y test fibrinogen qualitative test

FZ focal zone • frozen section *also* FS • furazolidone

FZRC frozen section red (blood) cell

Fz frontal midline placement of electrodes in electroencephalography

G acceleration (force) • conductance • force (pull of gravity) *also* g • gallop (heart sound) • ganglion • gap (in cell cycle) • gas *also* g • gastrin • gauge (of needle) *also* g, ga • gauss • gender *also* g, GEN • geometric efficiency • giga- • gingiva/gingival • glabella • globular (protein) • globulin • glucose *also* Glc, GLU, gluc • glycine *also* GLY • glycogen • gold inlay • gonidial (bacterial colony) • good • goose • grade *also* gr • Grafenberg spot • gram (stain) • gravida (pregnant) • gravitational constant • gravity (unit) • Greek • green *also* GRN, Grn • Gross (leukemia antigen) • guanidine • guanine • guanosine • gynecology • immunoglobulin G • unit of force of acceleration

G Gibbs free energy

G− gram–negative *also* GM−, GN, gr−, GrN

G+ gram–positive *also* GM+, GP, gr+, GrP

G° standard free energy

G₀ quiescent phase of cells leaving the mitotic cycle

G₁ presynthetic gap (phase of cells prior to DNA synthesis)

G₂ postsynthetic gap (phase of cells following DNA synthesis)

G$_{II}$, G−II hexachlorophene

G₄ dichlorophen

GI, GII, GIII, etc primigravida, secundigravida, tertigravida, etc *also* grav I, grav 2, grav 3, etc

G1 grid 1 (in electroencephalography)

G 1—G4 grade 1—4 (heart murmur)

G2 grid 2 (in electroencephalography)

G–6–PD glucose 6–phosphate dehydrogenase

g gas *also* G • gauge (of needle) *also* G, ga • gender *also* G, GEN • grain *also* GR, gr • gram *also* gm • gravity *also* gr, grav • group *also* GP, gp, grp • ratio of magnetic moment of a particle to Bohr magneton • standard acceleration due to gravity, 9.80665 m/s^2

g relative centrifugal force

g% gram percent (per deciliter) *also* g/dL, g/dl • gm

GA airway conductance *also* GAW, Gaw • Gamblers Anonymous • gastric analysis • gastric antrum • general anesthesia *also* gen–an • general appearance • gentisic acid • gestational age • Getting Along (psychologic test) • ginger ale *also* G'ale • gingivoaxial • glucoamylase • glucose/acetone • glucuronic acid • Golgi apparatus •

gramicidin A • granulocyte adherence • granuloma annulare • guessed average • gut–associated

Ga gallium • granulocyte agglutination

ga gauge (of needle) *also* G, g

GAA gossypol acetic acid

GABA γ–aminobutyric acid

GABA–T γ–aminobutyric acid transaminase

GABHS group A beta–hemolytic streptococcus *also* GABS

GABOA γ–amino–β–hydroxybutyric acid

GABOB γ–amino–β–hydroxybutyric

GABS group A beta–hemolytic streptococcus *also* GABHS

GAD generalized anxiety disorder • glutamic acid decarboxylase

GADH gastric alcohol dehydrogenase

GADS gonococcal arthritis/dermatitis syndrome

GAF giant axon formation

GAG glycosaminoglycan

GAHS galactorrhea–amenorrhea hyperprolactinemia syndrome

GAI guided affective imagery

GAIPAS General Audit Inpatient Psychiatric Assessment Scale

GAL galactosemia •

galactosyl • gallus adenolike (virus) • glucuronic acid lactone

Gal, gal. galactose • gallon

G–ALB globulin–albumin

G'ale ginger ale *also* GA

GALK galactokinase

gal/min gallons per minute

GalN galactosamine

GalNAc N–acetyl–D–galactosamine

gal–1–P galactose–1–phosphate

GALT galactose–1–phosphate uridyltransferase • gut–associated lymphoid tissue

GAL TT galactose tolerance test

GALV gibbon ape leukemia virus

GaLV gibbon ape lymphosarcoma virus

Galv, galv galvanic/galvanism/galvanized

gamma (Γ, γ) third letter of Greek alphabet

γ carbon separated from the carboxyl group by two other carbon atoms • chain of fetal hemoglobin • constituent of gamma protein plasma fraction • 10^{-4} gauss • heavy chain of immunoglobulin G • monomer in fetal hemoglobin • photon (gamma ray) • plasma protein (globulin) • third in a series or group

γ–BHC γ–benzene hexachloride (lindane) *also* GBH

γG immunoglobulin G

γ–HCD γ–heavy chain disease

GAMG goat anti-mouse immunoglobulin G

GAN giant axonal neuropathy

G and D growth and development

gang, gangl ganglion/ ganglionic

GAP Gardner Analysis of Personality (Survey) • glyceraldehyde phosphate

GAPD, GAPDH glycer- aldehyde–3–phosphate dehydrogenase

GAPO growth retardation, alopecia, pseudoanodontia, and optic atrophy (syndrome)

GAR genitoanorectal (syndrome) • goat anti– rabbit (gamma globulin)

Garg, garg gargle

GARGG goat anti-rabbit gamma globulin

GAS gastric acid secretion • gastroenterology • general adaptation syndrome • generalized arteriosclerosis • Glasgow Assessment Schedule • Global Assessment Scale • group A streptococcus

GASA growth–adjusted sonographic age

Gas Anal F&T gastric analysis, free and total

GAST, gastroc gastro- cnemius (muscle)

Gastro, gastro gastro- enterology • gastrointestinal

GAT gas antitoxin • gelatin agglutination test • Gerontological Apperception Test • group adjustment therapy

GATase 6-alkyl guanine alkyl transferase

GATB General Aptitude Test Battery

GAU geriatric assessment unit

gav gavage

GAW, Gaw airway conductance *also* GA

GAZT glucuronide derivative of azidothymidine

GB gallbladder • Gilbert– Beh(et (syndrome) • glass bead • glial bundle • goofball (barbiturate pill) • Gougerot–Blum (syndrome) • Guillain– Barré (syndrome)

G&B good and bad (days)

GBA ganglionic blocking agent • gingivobuccoaxial

G banding Giemsa banding (stain)

GBBS group B beta–hemolytic streptococcus *also* GBS

GBCE Grassi Basic Cognitive Evaluation

GBD gallbladder disease • gender behavior disorder • glassblower's disease • granulomatous bowel disease

GBE *Ginkgo biloba* extract

GBG glycine–rich β–glycoprotein • gonadal steroid–binding globulin

GBH γ–benzene hexachloride (lindane) *also* γ–BHC • graphite, benzalkonium, heparin

GBI globulin–bound insulin

GBIA Guthrie bacterial inhibition assay

GBL γ–butyrolactone • glomerular basal lamina

GBM glomerular basement membrane

GBMI guilty but mentally ill

GBP galactose–binding protein • gastric bypass • gated blood pool

GBPS gallbladder pigment stones

GBq gigabequerel

GBS gallbladder series • gastric bypass surgery • glycerine–buffered saline • group B (β–hemolytic) streptococcus *also* GBBS • Guillain–Barré syndrome

GBSS Grey's balanced saline solution • Guillain–Barré–Strohl syndrome

GC ganglion cell • gas chromatography • gel chromatography • general circulation • general condition • geriatric care • geriatric chair • glucocorticoid • glycocholate • goblet cell • Golgi complex • gonococcal (infection) • gonococcus *also* GN • gonorrhea culture • good condition • Gougerot–

Carteaud (syndrome) • graham crackers • granular casts • granular cysts • granule cell • granulocyte cytotoxic • granulomatous colitis • granulosa cell • guanine cytosine • guanylcyclase

G–C gram–negative cocci

G+C gram–positive cocci

Gc gigacycle • group–specific component

GCA gastric cancerous area • giant cell arteritis

g–cal gram calorie (small calorie) *also* gm cal

GCB gonococcal base

GCDFP gross cystic disease fluid protein

GCDP gross cystic disease protein

GCF greatest common factor

GCFT gonococcal/gonorrhea complement–fixation test

GCI General Cognitive Index

GCII glucose–controlled insulin infusion

GCIIS glucose–controlled insulin infusion system

GCM good control maintained

g–cm gram–centimeter

GC–MS gas chromatography–mass spectrometry

GCN giant cerebral neuron

GCR glucocorticoid receptor • Group Conformity Rating

GCRC General Clinical Research Centers

GCS general clinical service • Generalized Contentment Scale • Glasgow Coma Scale • glucocorticosteroid • glutamylcysteine synthetase

Gc/s gigacycles per second

GCSA Gross cell surface antigen

GCSF granulocyte cell-stimulating factor

G–CSF granulocyte colony–stimulating factor

GCT general care and treatment • giant cell thyroiditis • giant cell tumor

GCU gonococcal urethritis

GCV great cardiac vein

GCVF great cardiac vein flow

GCW glomerular capillary wall

GCWM General Conference on Weights and Measures

GD gastroduodenal • general diagnostics • general dispensary • general duties • gestational day • Gianotti disease • gonadal dysgenesis • Graves disease • growth and development *also* G&D

G&D growth and development *also* GD

Gd gadolinium

gd good

GDA gastroduodenal artery • germine diacetate

GDB gas–density balance • guide dogs for the blind

GDC General Dental Council • giant dopamine–containing cell

GDF gel diffusion precipitin

GDH glucose dehydrogenase • glutamate dehydrogenase • glutamic acid dehydrogenase • glycerophosphate dehydrogenase • gonadotropic hormone • growth and differentiation hormone (in insects)

GDID genetically determined immunodeficiency disease

g/dL, g/dl grams per deciliter

GDM gestational diabetes mellitus

GDMO General Duties Medical Officer

gdn guardian

GDP gastroduodenal pylorus • gel diffusion precipitin • guanosine diphosphate

GDS Gesell Developmental Schedules • Global Deterioration Scale • gradual dosage schedule

GDT gel development time

GDW glass–distilled water

GE gainfully employed • Gänsslen–Erb (syndrome) • gastric emptying • gastroemotional • gastroenteritis • gastroenterology • gastroenterostomy • gastroesophageal • gastrointestinal endoscopy • gel electrophoresis • generalized epilepsy •

generator of excitation •
gentamicin *also* GENT,
GM • glandular
epithelium • Gsell–
Erdheim (syndrome)

G/E granulocyte/erythroid
(ratio)

Ge Gerbich red cell antigen •
germanium

GEC galactose elimination
capacity • glomerular
epithelial cell

GEE glycine ethyl ester

GEF glossoepiglottic fold •
gonadotropin–enhancing
factor

GEFT Group Embedded
Figures Test

GEH glycerol ester hydrolase

GEJ gastroesophageal junction

gel. gelatin

gel. quav [L. *gelatina quavis*]
in any kind of jelly

GEMS good emergency
mother substitute

GEN gender *also* G, g •
generation • genetics *also*
Gen, genet • genital *also*
gen, genit

Gen genetics *also* GEN,
genet • genus *also* gen

gen general *also* gen'l •
genital *also* GEN, genit •
genus *also* Gen

gen–an general anesthesia
also GA

GEN/ENDO general
anesthesia with
endotracheal intubation

genet genetic/genetics *also*
GEN, Gen

gen et sp nov [L. *genus et
species nova*] new genus
and species

genit genitalia/genital *also*
GEN, gen

gen'l general *also* gen

gen nov [L. *genus novum*]
new genus

gen proc general procedure

GENPS genital neoplasm–
papilloma syndrome

GENT, gent gentamicin *also*
GE, GM

GENTA/P gentamicin peak

GENTA/T gentamicin trough
(level)

GEP gastroenteropancreatic

GEPG gastroesophageal
pressure gradient

GER gastroesophageal reflux •
geriatrics *also* geriat •
granular endoplasmic
reticulum

Ger German

GERD gastroesophageal reflux
disease

geriat geriatrics/geriatric *also*
GER

GERL Golgi–associated
endoplasmic reticulum
lysosome

Geront gerontology/
gerontologist/gerontologic

GES glucose–electrolyte
solution • Group
Encounter Survey • Group
Environment Scale

GEST, gest gestation

GET gastric emptying time • graded (treadmill) exercise test

GET$\frac{1}{2}$ gastric emptying half–time

GETA general endotracheal anesthesia

GEU gestation, extrauterine

Gev, GeV giga electron volt

GEX gas exchange

GF gastric fistula • gastric fluid • germ–free • glass factor (tissue culture) • globule fibril • glomerular filtrate/filtration • gluten–free • grandfather *also* GR–FR • griseofulvin • growth factor • growth failure • growth fraction

G–F globular–fibrous (protein)

gf gram–force

GFA glial fibrillary acidic (protein) • global force applicator

G factor general factor (single variance common to different intelligence tests)

GFAP glial fibrillary acidic protein

GFD gluten–free diet • Goodenough Figure Drawing

GFFS glycogen– and fat–free solid

GFH glucose–free Hanks (solution)

GFI glucagon–free insulin • ground–fault interrupter

GFL giant follicular lymphoma

GFM good fetal movement

G forces acceleration forces

GFP γ–fetoprotein • gel–filtered platelet • glomerular filtered phosphate

GFR glomerular filtration rate • grunting, flaring, and retracting (neonate)

GFS global focal sclerosis

GFTA Goldman–Fristoe Test of Articulation

G–F–W Battery Goldman–Fristoe–Woodcock Auditory Skills Test Battery

GG gamma globulin • genioglossus • glyceryl guaiacolate • glycylglycine • guar gum

GGA general gonadotropic activity

GGCT ground glass clotting time

GGE generalized glandular enlargement • gradient gel electrophoresis

GGFC gamma globulin–free calf (serum)

GGG gambodium • [L. *gummi guttae gambiae*] gamboge • glycine–rich gamma–glycoprotein

GG or S glands, goiter, or stiffness (of neck) *also* GGS

GGM glucose–galactose malabsorption

GGPNA γ–glutamyl–p–nitroanilide

GGS glands, goiter, or stiffness (of neck) *also* GG or S

GGT γ–glutamyl transpeptidase *also* GGTP • γ–glutamyltransferase

GGTP γ–glutamyl transpeptidase *also* GGT

GGVB gelatin, glucose, and veronal buffer

GH Gee–Herter (disease) • general health • general hospital • genetically hypertensive (rat) • genetic hypertension • geniohyoid • Gilford–Hutchinson (syndrome) • glenohumeral • good health • growth hormone

GHAA Group Health Association of America

GHAG general high altitude questionnaire

GHB γ–hydroxybutyrate • γ–hydroxybutyric acid *also* GHBA

GHb glycosylated hemoglobin *also* GLYCOS Hb

GHBA γ–hydroxybutyric acid *also* GHB

GHD growth hormone deficiency

GHDT Goodenough–Harris Drawing Test

GHK Goldman–Hodgkin–Katz (equation)

GHPP Genetically Handicapped Persons Program

GHQ General Health Questionnaire

GHR granulomatous hypersensitivity reaction

GHRF growth hormone-releasing factor

GH–RH, GHRH growth hormone-releasing hormone

GH–RIF, GHRIF growth hormone release-inhibiting factor

GH–RIH, GHRIH growth hormone release-inhibiting hormone

GHV goose hepatitis virus

GHz gigahertz

GI gastrointestinal • gelatin infusion (medium) • gingival index • globin insulin • glomerular index • glucose intolerance • granuloma inguinale • growth inhibiting/inhibition

GI good impression (California Psychological Inventory)

gl gill ($\frac{1}{4}$ pint) *also* gl

GIA gastrointestinal anastomosis

GIB gastric ileal bypass • gastrointestinal bleeding

GIBF gastrointestinal bacterial flora

GIC gastric interdigestive contraction • general immunocompetence

GICA gastrointestinal cancer • gastrointestinal cancer antigen

GID gender identity disorder

GIDA Gastrointestinal Diagnostic Area

GIF gonadotropin–inhibitory factor (somatostatin) • growth hormone-inhibiting factor

GIFT gamete intrafallopian transfer • granulocyte immunofluorescence test

GIGO garbage in, garbage out (computers)

GIH gastric inhibitory hormone • gastrointestinal hemorrhage • gastrointestinal hormone • growth–inhibiting hormone

GII gastrointestinal infection

GIK glucose–insulin–potassium (solution)

GILCU gradual increase in length and complexity of utterance

GIM gonadotropin–inhibiting material

GIN glutamine

Ging, ging gingiva/gingival

g–ion gram–ion

GIP gstric inhibitory peptide/polypeptide • giant (cell) interstitial pneumonia/pneumonitis • glucose-dependent insulin–releasing peptide • glucose insulinotropic peptide • gonorrheal invasive peritonitis

GIR global improvement rating

GIS gas in stomach • gastrointestinal series • gastrointestinal symptom • gastrointestinal system • Gender Identity Service

GIT gastrointestinal tract •

glutathione–insulin transhydrogenase

GITS gastrointestinal therapeutic system

GITSG Gastrointestinal Tumor Study Group

GITT gastrointestinal transit time • glucose–insulin tolerance test

GIV gastrointestinal virus

GIV giga (electron) volts

giv give/given

GIWU gastrointestinal work–up

GJ gap junction • gastric juice • gastrojejunostomy

GK galactokinase • Gasser–Karrer (syndrome) • glomerulocystic kidney • glycerol kinase

GKA guinea pig keratocyte

GKN glucose–potassium–sodium

GL gastric lavage • Gilbert–Lereboullet (syndrome) • gland *also* gl • glomerular layer • glycolipid • glycosphingolipoid • granular layer • greatest length (fetus) • gustatory lacrimation

Gl [L. *glucinium*] beryllium • glabella

gl gill ($\frac{1}{4}$ pint) *also* gi • gland/glandular *also* GL

g/L, g/l grams per liter *also* gm/L, gm/l

GLA α–galactosidase • γ–linolenic acid • giant left atrium •

gingivolinguoaxial · D–glucaric acid

glac glacial

GLAD gold–labeled antigen detection (technique)

gland. glandular

GLAT glutamic acid, lysine, alanine, and tyrosine

glau glaucoma *also* glc

GLC gas–liquid chromatography

Glc glucose *also* G, GLU, gluc

glc glaucoma *also* glau

GlcA gluconic acid

GLC/MS gas–liquid chromatography/mass spectrometry

GlcN glucosamine

GlcNAc *N*–acetylglucosamine

GlcUA glucuronic acid

GLD globoid leukodystrophy · glutamate dehydrogenase *also* GLDH

GLDH glutamate dehydrogenase *also* GLD

GLH germinal layer hemorrhage · giant lymph node hyperplasia

GLI glicentin · glucagon–like immunoreactivity

GLIM generalized linear interactive model

glio glioma

GLL glabellolambda line (craniometric point)

GLM general linear model

Gln glucagon · glutamine

GLNH giant lymph node hyperplasia

GLO, Glo glyoxalase

GLO1 glyoxalase 1

Glob, glob globular · globulin

GLP Gambro Liendia Plate · glucose–L–phosphate · glycolipoprotein · good laboratory practice · group–living program

GLPP, GL–PP glucose, postprandial

GLR graphic level recorder

GLS generalized lymphadenopathy syndrome · guinea (pig) lung strip

GLTN glomerulotubulo-nephritis

GLTT glucose–lactate tolerance test

GLU, glu glucose *also* G, Glc, gluc · glucuronidase · glutamic acid · glutamine

GLU–5 five–hour glucose tolerance test

GluA glucuronic acid

GLUC glucosidase

Gluc, gluc glucose *also* G, Glc, GLU

GLUC–S urine glucose spot (test)

glucur glucuronide

glu ox. glucose oxidase

GLUT glucose transporter

GLV Gross leukemia virus

Glx glutamic acid ·

glutamine • glutaminyl and/or glutamyl (indicates uncertainty between Glu and Gln)

GLY, gly glycerite • glycerol *also* glyc • glycine *also* G • glycocoll • glycyl

glyc glyceride • glycerin • [L. *glyceritum*] glycerite • glycerol *also* GLY

GLYCOS Hb glycosylated hemoglobin *also* GHb

GM gastric mucosa • Geiger–MHller (counter) *also* G–M • general medical • general medicine • genetic manipulation • gentamicin *also* GE, GENT • geometric mean • giant melanosome • grand mal • grandmother *also* GR–MO • grand multiparity • granulocyte–macrophage • granulocyte–monocyte • growth medium • monosialoganglioside (genetic marker)

GM– gram–negative *also* G–, GN, gr–, GrN

GM+ gram–positive *also* G+, GP, gr+, GrP

G–M Geiger–MHller (counter) *also* GM

Gm gamma (allotype marker on heavy chains of immunoglobins)

gm gram *also* G, g

g/m gallons per minute

g–m gram–meter *also* gm–m

gm% grams percent (per deciliter) *also* g%, g/dL, g/dl

GMA glyceral methacrylate •

glycol methacrylate • gross motor activity

GMB gastric mucosal barrier • glioblastoma multiforme • granulomembranous body

GMBF gastric mucosal blood flow

GMC general medical clinic • grivet monkey cell

gm cal gram calorie (small calorie) *also* g–cal

GMCD grand mal convulsive disorder

GM–CFU granulocyte–macrophage colony–forming unit

GM–CSF granulocyte–macrophage colony–stimulating factor

GMCU gracilis myocutaneous unit

GMD geometric mean diameter • glycopeptide moiety (modified) derivative

GME graduate medical education

GMENAC Graduate Medical Education National Advisory Committee

GMEPP giant miniature end–plate potential

GMH germinal matrix hemorrhage

GMK green monkey kidney (cells)

GML glabellomeatal line • gut mucosal lymphocyte

g/mL, g/ml grams per milliliter

gm/L, gm/l grams per liter *also* g/L, gl

GMM Goldberg–Maxwell–Morris (syndrome)

gm–m gram–meter *also* g–m

GMO general medical officer

g–mol gram–molecule

GMP guanosine mono-phosphate • guanylic acid

G–MP G–myeloma proteins

3′,5′–GMP guanosine 3′,5′–cyclic phosphate

GMR gallops, murmurs, or rubs

GMS General Medical Service • glyceryl monostearate • Gomori methenamine silver (stain)

GM&S general medicine and surgery

GMT geometric mean (antibody) titer • gingival margin trimmer • Greenwich Mean Time

GMTs geometric mean (antibody) titers

GMV gram–molecular volume

GMW gram molecular weight

GN Gandy–Nanta (disease) • gaze nystagmus • glomerulonephritis • glucagon • glucose:nitrogen (ratio in urine) *also* G/N, G/Nr • gnotobiote • gonococcus *also* GC • graduate nurse • gram–negative *also* G–, GM–, gr , GrN

G/N glucose/nitrogen (ratio in urine) *also* GN, G/Nr

Gn gnathion • gonadotropin

GNA general nursing assistance

GNB gram–negative bacilli

GNBM gram–negative bacillary meningitis

GNC general nursing care • General Nursing Council • glandular neck cell

GNCA gastric noncancerous area

GND gram–negative diplococcus

gnd ground

GNID gram–negative intracellular diplococci

GNP Gerontologic Nurse Practitioner

GNR gram–negative rod *also* G–R

G/Nr glucose:nitrogen ratio (in urine) *also* GN, G/N

GnRF gonadotropin–releasing factor *also* GRF

GnRH gonadotropin–releasing hormone *also* GRH

GNS gerontologic nurse–specialist

G/NS glucose in normal saline

GNTP Graduate Nurse Transition Program

GO glucose oxidase *also* GOD • gonorrhea • Gordan–Overstreet (syndrome)

G&O gas and oxygen

Go Golgi • gonion

GOAT Galveston Orientation and Amnesia Test

GOBAB γ–hydroxy–β–aminobutyric acid

GOD generation of diversity • glucose oxidase *also* GO

GOD/POD glucose oxidase–perioxidase (method)

GOE gas, oxygen, and ether (anesthesia)

GOG Gynecologic Oncology Group (of National Cancer Institute)

GOH geroderma osteodysplastica hereditaria

GOL glabello–opisthion line

GΩ gigohm (one billion ohms)

GON gonococcal ophthalmia neonatorum

Gonio gonioscopy

GOO gastric outlet obstruction

GOQ glucose oxidation quotient

GOR gastroesophageal reflux • general operating room

GORT Gilmore Oral Reading Test • Gray Oral Reading Test

GOT glucose oxidase test • glutamic–oxaloacetic transaminase (aspartate aminotransferase) • goals of treatment

GOTM, GOT–M glutamic–oxaloacetic transaminase, mitochondrial

GOT–S glutamic–oxaloacetic transaminase, soluble

govt government

GP gastroplasty • general

paralysis • general paresis • general practice • general practitioner • general proprioception • general purpose • genetic prediabetes • geometric progression • globus pallidus • glucose phosphate • glucose production • glutathione peroxidase • glycero-phosphate • glycopeptide • glycoprotein • Goodpasture (syndrome) *also* GPS • gram–positive *also* G+, GM+, gr+ • group *also* g, gp, grp • guinea pig • gutta–percha

G/P gravida/para

G–1,6–P glucose–1,6–phosphate

G3P, G–3–P glyceraldehyde 3–phosphate

gp glycoprotein • group *also* g, GP, grp

GPA glutaraldehyde, picric acid, acetic acid • grade point average • gravida, para, abortus (subscript numbers after each category) *also* Gr PAB • guinea pig albumin

GPAIS guinea pig anti–insulin serum

G6PASE, G–6–Pase glucose–6–phosphatase

GPB glossopharyngeal breathing

GPBP guinea pig myelin basic protein

GPC gastric parietal cell • gel permeation chroma-tography • giant papillary conjunctivitis • glycerophosphorylcholine • gram–positive cocci • granular progenitor cell • guinea pig complement

GPC/TP glycerophosphorylcholine to total phosphate (ratio)

GPD glucose–6–phosphate dehydrogenase *also* G–6–PD • glycerophosphate dehydrogenase • guinea pig dander

G–6–PD glucose–6–phosphate dehydrogenase *also* GPD

G6PDA glucose–6–phosphate dehydrogenase, varient A

GPE glycerylphosphoryl-ethanolamine • guinea pig embryo

GPF glomerular plasma flow • granulocytosis–promoting factor

GPGG guinea pig gamma globulin

GPHN giant pigmented hairy nevus

GPHLV guinea pig herpes–like virus

GPHV guinea pig herpesvirus

GPI general paralysis/paresis of insane • Gingival–Periodontal Index • glucosephosphate isomerase • Gordon Personal Inventory • guinea pig ileum

GPIMH guinea pig intestinal mucosal homogenate

GPIPID guinea pig intraperitoneal infectious dose

GPK guinea pig kidney (antigen)

GPKA guinea pig kidney absorption (test)

G–PLT giant platelets

GPLV guinea pig leukemia virus

Gply gingivoplasty

GPM general preventive medicine • giant pigment melanosome

GPMAL gravida, para, multiple births, abortions, live births

GPN Graduate Practical Nurse

GPO group purchasing organization

GPP Gordon Personal Profile

GPPQ General Purpose Psychiatric Questionnaire

GPR good partial response • gram–positive rod *also* G+R

GPRBC guinea–pig red blood cell

GPS Goodpasture syndrome *also* GP • gray platelet syndrome • guinea pig serum • guinea pig spleen

GPT glutamic pyruvic transaminase • guinea pig trachea

GpTh group therapy *also* GT

GPTSM guinea pig tracheal smooth muscle

GPU guinea pig unit

GPUT galactose phosphate uridyl transferase

GPx glutathione peroxidase

GQAP general question–asking program

GR γ–ray • gamma roentgen *also* gr • gastric resection • generalized rash • general relief • general research • glucocorticoid receptor • glucose response • gluthathione reductase *also* GSR, GSSG–R • good recovery • grain *also* g, gr • granulocyte • gravid *also* gr, Grav

G–R gram–negative rod *also* GNR

G+R gram–positive rod *also* GPR

Gr Greek

gr gamma roentgen *also* GR • grade *also* G • graft • grain *also* g, GR • gravid *also* GR, Grav • gravity *also* g, grav • gray • great • gross *also* GRS

gr⁻ gram–negative *also* G⁻, GM–, GN, GrN

gr⁺ gram–positive *also* G⁺, GM+, GP, GrP

GRA gated radionuclide angiography • Gombarts reducing agent • gonadotropin–releasing agent

GRA⁺ Gombarts reducing agent–positive

Grad, grad. [L. *gradatim*] by degrees

grad. gradient • gradually • graduate

GRAE generally regarded as effective

GRAN Gombarts reducing agent–negative

gran granule/granulated

GRAS generally recognized as safe

Grav, grav gravid *also* GR

grav gravity *also* GR, gr

grav 1, grav 2, grav 3, etc first, second, third, etc. pregnancy *also* GI, II, III, etc. • pregnant once, twice, etc. • primigravida

GRD gastroesophageal reflux disease • gender role definition • β–glucuronidase *also* GRS, GUSB

grd ground

GRE gradient–echo • Graduate Record Examination

GREAT Graduate Record Examination Aptitude Test

GRF gonadotropin–releasing factor *also* GnRF • growth–hormone–releasing factor

GR–FeSV Gardner–Rasheed feline sarcoma virus

GR–FR grandfather *also* GF

GRG glycine–rich glycoprotein

GRH gonadotropin–releasing hormone *also* GnRH • growth hormone-releasing hormone

GRIF growth hormone release-inhibiting factor

GRL granular layer

GR–MO grandmother *also* GM

gr m p [L. *grosso modo pulverisatum*] ground in a coarse way

GRN granules · green *also* G, Grn

Grn glycerone · green *also* G, GRN

GrN gram–negative *also* G⁻, GM–, GN, gr⁻

gros [L. *grossus*] coarse

GRP gastrin–releasing peptide

GrP gram–positive *also* G⁺, GM+, GP, gr⁺

grp group *also* g, GP, gp

GrPAB pregnancy, birth, abortion (subscript numbers after each category) *also* GPA

GRPS glucose–Ringer–phosphate solution

GRS β–glucuronidase *also* GRD, GUSB · gross *also* gr

GRS&MIC gross and microscopic

GRT gastric residence time · Graduate Respiratory Therapist

GrTr graphite treatment

GRW giant ragweed (test)

gr wt gross weight

GS gallstone · Gardner syndrome · gastric shield · gastrocnemius soleus · generalized seizure · general surgery · Gilbert syndrome · Glanzmann–Saland (syndrome) · glomerular sclerosis · glucagon secretion · glutamine synthetase · goat serum · Goldenhar syndrome · graft survival · Gram stain · granulocyte substance · grip strength · group section · group specific *also* gs · Guérin–Stern (syndrome)

G/S glucose and saline

Gs gauss

gs group specific *also* GS

g/s gallons per second

GSA general somatic afferent (nerve) · Gross (sarcoma) virus antigen · group–specific antigen · guanidinosuccinic acid

GSB graduated spinal block

GSBG gonadal steroid–binding globulin

GSC gas–solid chromatography · gravity settling culture (plate)

G–SC guanosine–coupled spleen cell

GSCN giant serotonin–containing neuron

GSD genetically significant dose (of mutagenic radiation) · glutathione synthetase deficiency · glycogen storage disease

GSE general somatic efferent (nerve) · genital self–examination · gluten–sensitive enteropathy · grips strong and equal

GSF galactosemic fibroblast · genital skin fibroblast

GSH glomerulus–stimulating

hormone • golden Syrian hamster • growth–stimulating hormone • reduced glutathione

GSHP reduced glutathione peroxidase

GSI genuine stress incontinence

GSK glycogen synthetase kinase

GSN giant serotonin–containing neuron

GSP galvanic skin potential • general survey panel • glycogen synthetase phosphatase • glycosylated serum protein

GSPN greater superficial petrosal neurectomy

GSR galvanic skin resistance • galvanic skin response • generalized Shwartzman reaction • glutathione reductase *also* GR, GSSG–R

GSS gamete–shedding substance • Gerstmann–StraHssler syndrome

GSSG oxidized gluthathione

GSSG–R glutathione reductase *also* GR, GSR

GSSI Global Sexual Satisfaction Index

GSSR generalized Sanarelli–Schwartzman reaction

GST gluthathione–*S*–transferase • gold salt therapy • gold sodium thiomalate *also* GSTM • graphic stress telethermometry/thermography • group striction

GSTM gold sodium thiomalate *also* GST

GSW gunshot wound

GSWA gunshot wound to abdomen *also* GWA

GT gait • gait training • galactosyl transferase • Gamow–Teller • gastrostomy • gastrostomy tube *also* G–tube • Gee–Thaysen (disease) • generation time • genetic therapy • gingiva treatment • Glanzmann thrombasthenia • glucagon test • glucose tolerance • glucose transport • glucuronyl transferase • γ-glutamyltransferase • glutamyl transpeptidase • glycityrosine • grand total • granulation tissue *also* g/t • greater trochanter • great toe • group tensions • group therapy *also* GpTh

G&T gowns and towels

GT1—GT10 glycogen storage disease, types 1 to 10

gt [L. *gutta*] drop

g/t granulation time • granulation tissue *also* GT

GTB gastrointestinal tract bleeding

GTCS generalized tonic–clonic seizure

GTD gestational trophoblastic disease

GTF gastrostomy tube feedings • glucose tolerance factor • glucosyltransferase

GTG gold thioglucose

GTH gonadotropic hormone

GTM grade, location, (lymph node involvement), and metastases (Surgical Staging System for bone sarcomas)

GTN gestational trophoblastic neoplasia/neoplasm • glomerulotubulonephritis • glyceryl trinitrate (nitroglycerin)

GTO Golgi tendon organ

GTP glutamyl transpeptidase • guanosine triphosphate

GTR galvanic tetanus ratio • generalized time reflex • granulocyte turnover rate

GTS Gilles de la Tourette syndrome • glucose transport system

gts [L. *guttae*] drops *also* GTTS, gtts

GTSTD Grid Test of Schizophrenic Thought Disorder

GTT gelatin–tellurite–taurocholate (agar) • glucose tolerance test

GTTS, gtts [L. *guttae*] drops *also* gts

GTT3H glucose tolerance test 3 hours (oral)

G–tube gastrostomy tube *also* GT

GU gastric ulcer • genitourinary • glucose uptake • glycogenic unit • gonococcal urethritis • gravitational ulcer

[G]u concentration of glucose in urine

GUA group of units of analysis

Gua guanine

guid guidance

GUK guanylate kinase

GULHEMP general physique, upper extremity, lower extremity, hearing, eyesight, mentality, and personality

Guo guanosine

GUS genitourinary sphincter • genitourinary system

GUSB β–glucuronidase *also* GRD, GRS

gutt [L. *gutturi*] to the throat

guttat [L. *guttatim*] drop by drop

gutt quibusd [L. *guttis quibusdam*] with a few drops

GV gastric volume • gentian violet • germinal vesicle • granulosis virus • griseoviridin • Gross virus (nodule)

GVA general visceral afferent (nerve)

GVB gelatin–veronal buffer

GVBD germinal vesicle breakdown

GVE general visceral efferent (nerve)

GVF Goldman visual fields • good visual fields

GVH, GvH graft–versus–host (disease, reaction)

GVHD, GvHD graft–versus–host disease

GVHR, GvHR graft–versus–
host reaction

GVTY gingivectomy

GW germ warfare •
gigawatt • glycerin in
water • gradual
withdrawal • Gray–
Wheelwright • group work

G/W glucose in water

G&W glycerin and water

GWA gunshot wound of
abdomen *also* GSWA

GWBS global ward behavior
scale

GWE glycerin and water
enema

GWG generalized Wegener
granulomatosis

GWT gunshot wound of the
throat

GXD EKG graded exercise
electrocardiogram

GXP graded exercise program

GXT graded e xercise test

GY gynecologic disease

Gy gray (unit of absorbed dose
of ionizing radiation)

GYN, gyn gynecologic/
gynecologist/gynecology

GYS guaranteed yield strength

GZ Guilford–Zimmerman
(personality test)

GZAS Guilford–Zimmerman
Aptitude Survey

GZTS Guilford–Zimmerman
Temperament Survey

H [Ger. *Hauch* film] bacterial antigen in serologic classification of bacteria • deflection in His bundle in electrogram (spike) • [L. *haustus*] draft, drink *also* h, ht • electrically induced spinal reflex • enthalpy (physics) • fucosal transferase–producing gene • Hancock • Hartnup (disease) • head • heart *also* He, HT, ht • heavy • heelstick • height *also* h, Hgt, HT, ht • hemagglutination • hemisphere • hemolysis *also* HEM • henry • heparin *also* HEP, HP • hernia *also* her, hern • heroin • hetacillin • high • histidine *also* HI, Hi, HIS, His, Hist • history *also* Hist, hist, Hx, Hy • Hoffmann (reflex) • Holzknecht (unit) • homosexual *also* HOMO, homo • horizontal *also* h, hor, horiz • hormone • horse *also* Ho • hospital/hospitalization *also* Hosp, hosp, HX • hot • Hounsfield (unit) • hour *also* h, HR, hr • human • husband *also* husb • hydrogen • hydrolysis • hygiene *also* Hyg, hyg • hyoscine (scopolamine) • hypermetropia *also* (H), h, Hy • hyperopia *also* h, Hy • hyperphoria • hyperplasia • hypodermic *also* h • hypodermic (injection) • hypothalamus *also* HT, Hth, Hyp, hyp • magnetic field strength • magnetization • mustard gas • oersted • [Ger. *heller* lighter] region of sarcomere containing only myosin filaments •

H

vectorcardiography electrode (neck)

(H) hip • hypodermic *also* H

H+ hydrogen ion

[H+] hydrogen ion concentration

H$_0$ null hypothesis

H$_1$ alternative hypothesis • histamine receptor type 1

H^2 hiatal hernia

H1, ^{1}H, H^1 protium (light hydrogen)

H2, ^{2}H, H^2 deuterium (heavy hydrogen)

H3, ^{3}H, H^3 tritium

H$_3$ procaine hydrochloride

h [L. *hora decubitus*] at bedtime *also* hd, hor decub, hor som, HS, hs, h som • coefficient of heat transfer • [L. *haustas*] draft, drink *also* H, ht • hand–rearing (of experimental animals) • hecto • height *also* H, Hgt, HT, ht • henry • heteromorphic region • high • horizontal *also* H, hor, horiz • hour *also* H • human *also* H • human response • hundred • hypermetropia *also* H, Hy • hyperopia/hyperopic *also* H, Hy • hypodermic *also* H, (H) • negatively staining region of chromosome • Planck constant • specific enthalpy

HA halothane anesthesia • H

antigen • Hartley (guinea pig) • headache • hearing aid • heated • heated aerosol *also* ht aer • height age • hemadsorbent • hemadsorption (test) • hemagglutinating activity/ antibody/antigen • hemagglutination • hemolytic anemia • hemophiliac with adenopathy • hepatic adenoma • hepatic artery • hepatitis A • hepatitis–associated (virus) • herpangina • heterophil antibody • Heyden antibiotic • high anxiety • hippuric acid • histamine • histidine ammonia–lyase • histocompatibility antigen • Horton arteritis • hospital acquired • hospital administration *also* HAD, HAd • hospital admission • hospital apprentice • household activity • hyaluronic acid • hydroxyanisole • hydroxypatite • hyperalimentation • hyperandrogenism • hypermetropic astigmatism • hyperopia, absolute • hypersensitivity alveolitis • hypothalmic amenorrhea

H/A headache • head–to–abdomen (ratio)

HA1 hemadsorption (virus, type 1)

HA2 hemadsorption (virus, type 2)

Ha absolute hypermetropia • hahnium • hamster

H/a home with advice

HAA hearing aid amplifier • hemolytic anemia antigen • hepatitis A antibody *also* HAAb • hepatitis–associated antigen • hospital activity analysis

HAAb hepatitis A antibody *also* HAA

HAAg hepatitis A antigen

HABA hydroxybenzeneazo-benzoic acid

HABF hepatic artery blood flow

HAb/HAd horizontal abduction/adduction

habt [L.*habeatur*] let the patient have

HAC hexamethylmelamine, Adriamycin (doxorubicin), and cyclophosphamide

HAc acetic acid

HAChT high–affinity choline transport

HACR hereditary adenomatosis of colon and rectum

HACS hyperactive child syndrome

HAD hearing aid dispenser • hemadsorption *also* HAd • hexamethylmelamine, Adriamycin (doxorubicin), and *cis*–diammine-dichloroplatinum (cisplatin) • hospital administration/administrator *also* HA, HAd • human adjuvant disease • hypophysectomized alloxan diabetic

HAd hemadsorption *also* HAD • hospital

administration *also* HA, HAD

HADD hydroxyapatite deposition disease

HAd–I hemadsorption inhibition

HAE health appraisal examination • hearing aid evaluation • hepatic artery embolization • hereditary angioedema • hereditary angioneurotic edema

HAF hepatic arterial flow

HaF Hageman factor

HAFP human α–fetoprotein

HAG heat–aggregated globulin

HAGG hyperimmune antivariola gamma globulin

HAHTG horse antihuman thymus globulin

HAI hemagglutination inhibition (titer) *also* HI • hemagglutinin inhibition • hepatic arterial infusion

H&A Ins health and accident insurance

HAIR–AN hyperandrogenism, insulin resistance, and acanthosis nigricans (syndrome)

HaK hamster kidney

HAL haloperidol • halothane *also* hal, HALO • hepatic artery ligation • hyperalimentation

Hal halogen

hal halothane *also* HAL, HALO

halluc hallucination

HALO halothane *also* HAL, hal • hemorrhage, abruption, labor, placenta previa with mild bleeding

HALP hyperalphalipo-proteinemia

HALT Heroin Antagonist and Learning Therapy

HaLV hamster leukemia virus

HAM hearing aid microphone • helical axis of motion • hexamethylmelamine, Adriamycin (doxorubicin), and melphalan • human albumin microsphere • human alveolar macrophage • hypoparathyroidism, Addison disease, and mucocutaneous candidiasis (syndrome)

HAMA Hamilton Anxiety (Scale) • human antimouse antibody

HAMD Hamilton Depression (Scale)

HAMM human albumin minimicrosphere

Hams hamstrings *also* HS

HaMSV Harvey murine sarcoma virus

HAN heroin–associated nephropathy • hyperplastic alveolar nodule

HANA hemagglutinin neuraminidase

H and E hematoxylin and eosin (stain) *also* H&E

Handicp handicapped

HANE hereditary angioneurotic edema

HANES health and nutrition examination survey

H antigens [Ger. *Hauch*] flagella antigens of motile bacteria

HAP Handicapped Aid Program • held after positioning • heredopathia atactica polyneuritiformis • high–amplitude peristalsis • histamine acid phosphate • hospital–acquired pneumonia • humoral antibody production • hydrolyzed animal protein • hydroxyapatite (fractionation procedure)

HAPA hemagglutinating antipenicillin antibody

HAPC hospital–acquired penetration contact

HAPE high–altitude pulmonary edema

HAPO high–altitude pulmonary (o)edema

HAPS hepatic arterial perfusion scintigraphy

HAPTO haptoglobin *also* HP, Hp, Hpt

HAQ Headache Assessment Questionnaire

HAR high–altitude retinopathy

HAREM heparin assay rapid easy method

HARH high–altitude retinal hemorrhage

HARM heparin assay rapid method

harm. harmonic

HARPPS heat, absence of use, redness, pain, pus, swelling (symptoms of infection)

HARS Hamilton Anxiety Rating Scale

HAS Hamilton Anxiety Scale • health advisory service • highest asymptomatic (dose) • hospital administrative service • hospital advisory service • hyperalimentation solution • hypertensive arteriosclerotic

HASCHD hypertensive arteriosclerotic heart disease *also* HASHD

HASCVD hypertensive arteriosclerotic cardiovascular disease

HASHD hypertensive arteriosclerotic heart disease *also* HASCHD

HASP Hospital Admissions and Surveillance Program

HAsP health aspects of pesticides

HAT Halstead Aphasia Test • head, arms, and trunk • harmonic attenuation table/ test • heterophil antibody titer • hospital arrival time • hypoxanthine, aminopterin, and thymidine • hypoxanthine, azaserine, and thymidine

HATG horse anti-human thymocyte globulin

HATH Heterosexual Attitudes Toward Homosexuality (scale)

HATT hemagglutination treponemal test

HATTS hemagglutination treponemal test for syphilis

HAU hemagglutinating unit

haust [L. *haustus*] draft, drink

HAV hallux abducto valgus • hemadsorption virus • hepatitis A virus

HAVAB hepatitis A virus antibody

HAWIC Hamburg–Wechsler Intelligence Test for Children

HB head backward • health board • heart block *also* hb • heel to buttock • held backward • hemoglobin *also* Hb, Hbg, hemo, HG, Hg, hg, HGB, Hgb • hemolysis blocking • hepatitis B • His bundle • hold breakfast • hospital bed • housebound • Hutchinson–Boeck (disease) • hybridoma bank • hyoid body

HB1°, HB2°, HB3° first–, second–, third–degree heart block

Hb hemoglobin *also* HB, Hbg, hemo, HG, Hg, hg, HGB, Hgb

hb heart block *also* HB

HbA adult hemoglobin • hemoglobin A • hemoglobin α–chain

Hb A° hemoglobin determination

HbA$_1$ major component of adult hemoglobin

HbA$_2$ minor fraction of adult hemoglobin

HBAb, HBAB hepatitis B antibody

HBAC hyperdynamic β–adrenergic circulatory

HBAg, HbAg hepatitis B antigen

HbAS heterozygosity for hemoglobin A and hemoglobin S (sickle–cell trait)

HBB hemoglobin β (chain) • hospital blood bank • hydroxybenzylbenzimidazole

HbBC hemoglobin–binding capacity

HBBW hold breakfast for blood work

HB$_c$ hepatitis B core (antibody, antigen)

HB$_c$Ab, HBcAb, HBCAB hepatitis B core antibody

HbC hemoglobin C

HB$_c$Ag, HBcAg, HBCAG hepatitis B core antigen

HBCG heat–aggregated bacille Calmette–Guérin

HbCO carbon monoxide hemoglobin • carboxyhemoglobin

HB core hepatitis B core (antigen)

Hb CS hemoglobin Constant Spring

HBD has been drinking • hemoglobin δ chain • hydroxybutyric dehydrogenase *also* HBDH • hypophosphatemic bone disease

HbD hemoglobin D

HBDH hydroxybutyrate dehydrogenase

HBDT human basophil degranulation test

HBE hemoglobin ε chain • His bundle electrogram

HbE hemoglobin E

HBE$_1$ His bundle electrogram, distal

HBE$_2$ His bundle electrogram, proximal

HB$_e$Ab, HBeAb, HBEAB hepatitis B early antibody

HB$_e$Ag, HBeAg, HBEAG hepatitis B early antigen

HBF fetal hemoglobin *also* HbF • hand blood flow • hemispheric blood flow • hemoglobinuric bilious fever • hepatic blood flow • hypothalamic blood flow

HbF fetal hemoglobin *also* HBF • hemoglobin F

HBG1 hemoglobin γ chain A

HBG2 hemoglobin γ chain G

Hbg hemoglobin *also* HB, Hb, hemo, HG, Hg, hg, HGB, Hgb

HBGA had it before, got it again

HBGM home blood glucose monitoring

HbH hemoglobin H

HBHC home–based hospital care

Hb–Hp hemoglobin–haptoglobin (complex)

HBI hemibody irradiation • hepatobiliary imaging • high (serum)–bound iron

HBID hereditary benign intraepithelial dyskeratosis

HBIG, HBIg hepatitis B immunoglobulin

Hb$_{Kansas}$ mutant hemoglobin with low affinity for oxygen

HBL hepatoblastoma

HBLA human B–lymphocyte antigen

Hb$_{Lepore}$ hemoglobin Lepore

HBLLSB heard best at left lower sternal border

HBLUSB heard best at left upper sternal border

HBLV human B–lymphotropic virus

HBM Health Belief Model • hypertonic buffered medium

HbM hemoglobin M

HbMet methemoglobin *also* HiHb

HBO hyperbaric oxygen (therapy) *also* HBOT • hyperbaric oxygenation • oxygenated hemoglobin *also* HbO$_2$

HbO$_2$ oxygenated hemoglobin *also* HBO • hyperbaric oxygen • oxyhemoglobin

HBOT hyperbaric oxygen therapy *also* HBO

HBP hepatic binding protein • high blood pressure

HbP primitive (fetal) hemoglobin

HBPM home blood pressure monitoring

HBr hydrobromic acid

HbR methemoglobin reductase

HBS Health Behavior Scale • hepatitis B surface • hyperkinetic behavior syndrome

HbS sickle–cell hemoglobin • sulfhemoglobin

HB$_S$ hepatitis B surface (antibody, antigen)

HB$_S$A hepatitis B surface associated

HB$_S$Ab, HBsAb, HBSAB hepatitis B surface antibody

HB$_S$Ag, HBsAg, HBSAG hepatitis B surface antigen

HBsAg/adr hepatitis B surface antigen manifesting group–specific determinant *a* and subtype–specific determinants *d* and *r*

HBSC hemopoietic blood stem cell

HbSC sickle–cell hemoglobin C

HBSS Hanks balanced salt solution

HbSS homozygosity for hemoglobin S

HBSSG Hanks balanced salt solution plus glucose

HBT human brain thromboplastin • human breast tumor

HBV hepatitis B vaccine • hepatitis B virus • honey–bee venom

HBW high birth weight

H/BW heart–to–body weight (ratio) • height–to–body weight (ratio)

HbZ hemoglobin ζ chain • hemoglobin Z • hemoglobin ZHrich

HC hair cell • hairy cell • handicapped *also* HCAP, HCP • head check • head circumference • head compression • healthy control • heart cycle • heat conservation • heavy chain • heel cord • hemoglobin concentration • hemorrhage, cerebral • heparin cofactor • hepatic catalase • hepatocellular cancer • hereditary coproporphyria *also* HCP • Hickman catheter • high calorie *also* hg–cal • hippocampus • histamine challenge • histochemistry • home call • home care • homocystinuria • Hospital Corps • hospital course • hospitalized controls • house call • Huntington chorea • hyaline casts • hydranencephaly • hydraulic concussion • hydrocarbon • hydrocodone • hydrocortisone *also* HCT, Hyd • hydroxycorticoid *also* HOC • hyoid cornu • hypercholesterolemia • hypertropic cardiomyopathy

H&C hot and cold

Hc hydrocolloid

HCA health care aide • heart cell aggregate • hepatocellular adenoma • home care aide • Hospital Corporation of America • hydrocortisone acetate

HCAP handicapped *also* HC, HCP

H–CAP hexamethylmelamine, cyclophosphamide, Adriamycin (doxorubicin), and Platinol (cisplatin)

HCB hexachlorobenzene

HCC heat conservation center • hepatitis contagiosa canis (virus) • hepatocellular carcinoma • hepatoma carcinoma cell • hexachlorocyclohexane (lindane) *also* HCH, γ–HCH • history of chief complaint • hydroxycholecalciferol (vitamin D)

25–HCC 25–hydroxy-cholecalciferol

HCD health care delivery • heavy–chain disease (protein) • high caloric density • high carbohydrate diet *also* HICHO • homologous canine distemper (antiserum) • hydrocolloid dressing

HCF hereditary capillary fragility • high carbohydrate, high fiber (diet) • highest common factor • hypocaloric carbohydrate feeding

HCFA Health Care Financing Administration

HCFSH human chorionic follicle–stimulating hormone

HCFU hexylcarbamoyl-fluorouracil (carmofur–antineoplastic)

HCG, hCG human chorionic gonadotropin

HCGN hypocomplementemic glomerulonephritis

HCH hexachlorocyclohexane (lindane) *also* HCC, γ–HCH

Hch hemochromatosis

HCHO formaldehyde

HcImp hydrocolloid impression

HCIS Health Care Information System

HCL hairy–cell leukemia • hard contact lens *also* HCLs • hemacytology index • human cultured lymphoblasts

HCLF high carbohydrate, low fiber (diet)

HCLs hard contact lenses *also* HCL

HCM health care maintenance • health care management • hypertrophic cardiomyopathy

HCMM hereditary cutaneous malignant melanoma

HCMV human cytomegalovirus

HCN hereditary chronic nephritis • hydrocyanic acid • hydrogen cyanide

HCO carbohydrate

HCO₃– bicarbonate

HCP handicapped *also* HC, HCAP • hepatocatalase peroxidase • hereditary coproporphyria *also* HC • hexachlorophene • high cell passage

H&CP hospital and community psychiatry

HCQ hydroxychloroquine

HCR heme–controlled repressor • host–cell reactivation • human–controlled repressor • hydrochloric acid • hysterical conversion reaction

HCRE Homeopathic Council for Research and Education

H'crit hematocrit *also* Crit, crit, HCT, Hct, hemat, HMT

HCS Hajdu–Cheney syndrome • health care support • hourglass contraction of stomach • human chorionic somatomammotropin (human placental lactogen) *also* hCS, HCSM, hCSM • human chorionic somatotropin • human cord serum • hydroxy-corticosteroid

hCS human chorionic somatomammotropin (human placental lactogen) *also* HCS, HCSM, hCSM

HCSD Health Care Studies Division

HCSM, hCSM human chorionic somatomammotropin (human placental lactogen) *also* HCS, hcs

HCT Health Check Test • heart–circulation training • hematocrit *also* Crit, crit, H'crit, Hct, hemat, HMT • histamine challenge test • historic control trial • homocytotrophic • human calcitonin *also* hCT • human chorionic (placental)

thyrotropin *also* hCT • hydrochlorothiazide • hydrocortisone *also* HC, Hyd • hydroxycortisone

Hct hematocrit *also* Crit, crit, H'crit, HCT, hemat, HMT

hCT human calcitonin *also* HCT • human chorionic thyrotropin *also* HCT

hct hundred count

HCTC Health Care Technology Center

HCTD hepatic computed tomographic density • high cholesterol and tocopherol deficient

HCTS high cholesterol and tocopherol supplemented

HCTU home cervical traction unit

HCTZ hydrochlorothiazide

HCU homocystinuria • hyperplasia cystica uteri

HCV human coronary virus

HCVD hypertensive cardiovascular disease *also* HTCVD

HCVR hypercapnic ventilatory response

HCVS human corona virus sensitivity

HCWs health care workers

Hcy hemocyanin • homocysteine

HD Haab–Dimmer (syndrome) • Hajna–Damon (broth) • haloperidol decanoate *also* HLD • Hanganutziu–Deicher • Hansen disease • [L. *heloma*

durum] hard corn • hearing distance • heart disease • helium dilution • hemidiaphragm • hemodialysis • hemolytic disease • hemolysing dose • herniated disc • high density • high dose • hip disarticulation • Hirschsprung disease • histidine decarboxylase • Hodgkin disease • hormone dependent • hospital day also HOD • house dust • human diploid (cell) • Huntington disease • hydatid disease • hydroxydopamine also HDA • hypnotic dosage

HD# hospital day number

H&D Hunter and Driffield (curve)

HD$_{50}$ hemolyzing dose of complement that lyses 50% of sensitized erythrocytes

hd [L. *hora decubitus*] at bedtime *also* h, hor decub, hor som, HS, hs, h som • head *also* he

HDA hydroxydopamine *also* HD

HDAC, HDARAC high–dose cytarabine (araC)

HDBD hydroxybutyric dehydrogenase

HDBH hydroxybutyrate dehydrogenase

HDC histidine decarboxylase • human diploid cell • hypodermoclysis

HDCS human diploid cell strain • human diploid cell system

H and D curve Hurter and Driffield curve (re: radiology)

HDCV human diploid cell (rabies) vaccine

HDD half–dose depth • high dose depth

HDF high dry field • host defensive factor • human diploid fibroblast

HDFL human development and family life

HDFP Hypertension Detection and Follow–up Program

HDG high dose group

HDH heart disease history • Hostility and Direction of Hostility (questionnaire) *also* HDHQ

HDHQ Hostility and Direction of Hostility Questionnaire *also* HDH

HDI hemorrhagic disease of infants

HDL high density lipoprotein *also* HDLP

HDL–C high–density lipoprotein cholesterol

HDL–c high density lipoprotein–cell surface (receptor)

HDLP high density lipoprotein *also* HDL

HDLS hereditary diffuse leukoencephalopathy with spheroids

HDLW hearing distance, left, watch (distance from which watch ticking is heard by left ear)

HDM hexadimethrine

HDMP high–dose methylprednisolone

HDMTX high–dose methotrexate

HDMTX–CF high–dose methotrexate and citrovorum factor

HDMTX/LV high–dose methotrexate and leucovorin

HDN hemolytic disease of newborn • high–density nebulizer

hDNA deoxyribonucleic acid, histone

HDP hexose diphosphate • high–density polyethylene • hydroxydimethylpyrimidine

HDPAA heparin–dependent platelet–associated antibody

HDRF Heart Disease Research Foundation

HDRS Hamilton Depression Rating Scale

HDRV human diploid (cell strain) rabies vaccine

HDRW hearing distance, right, watch (distance from which watch ticking is heard by right ear)

HDS Hamilton Depression (Rating) Scale • Healthcare Data Systems • Health Data Services • health delivery system • herniated disc syndrome • Hospital Discharge Survey

HDU head–drop unit (curare standard) • hemodialysis unit

HDV hepatitis delta virus • hepatitis virus, type D

HDW hearing distance (with) watch

HDZ hydralazine

HE hard exudate • hektoen enteric (agar) • hemagglutinating encephalomyelitis • hemoglobin electrophoresis • hepatic encephalopathy • hereditary elliptocytosis • hollow enzyme • human enteric (virus) • hyperextension • hypogonadotropic eunuchoidism • hypophysectomy *also* hyp • hypoxemic episode

H–E heat exchanger

H&E hematoxylin and eosin (stain) *also* H and E • hemorrhage and exudate • heredity and environment

He heart *also* H, HT, ht • Hedstrom number • helium

he head *also* hd

HEA hexone–extracted acetone • human erythrocyte antigen

HEADSS home life, education level, activities, drug use, sexual activity, suicide ideation/attempts (adolescent medical history)

HEAL Health Education Assistance Loan

HEART Health Evaluation and Risk Tabulation

HEAT human erythrocyte agglutination test

HEB hematoencephalic barrier (blood–brain barrier)

hebdom [L. *hebdomada*] first week of life

HEC hamster embryo cell · Health Education Council · health evaluation center · human endothelial cell · hydroxyergocalciferol

HED hydrotropic electron donor · [Ger. *Haut–Erythem–Dosis*] skin erythema dose · [Ger. *Haut –Einheits–Dosis*] unit skin dose (of x–rays)

HeD helper determinant

HEDSPA ^{99m}Tc–etidronate (bone–imaging agent)

HEENT head, ears, eyes, nose, and throat

HEEP health effects of environmental pollutants

HEF hamster embryo fibroblast

HEG hemorrhagic erosive gastritis

HEHR highest equivalent heart rate

HEI high–energy intermediate · homogeneous enzyme immunoassay · human embryonic intestine (cell)

HE inj hyperextension injury

HEIR health effects of ionizing radiation · high–energy ionizing radiation

HEIS high–energy ion scattering

HEK human embryonic kidney (cell) · human embryo kidney

HEL hen egg–white lysozyme · human embryo lung (cell culture) · human embryonic lung (cell) · human erythroleukemia · human erythroleukemia line

HeLa cells continuously cultured carcinoma cell line used for tissue cultures (named for patient, Henrietta Lacks)

HELF human embryoic lung fibroblast

HELLP hemolysis, elevated liver enzymes, and low platelet (count)

HELM helmet cell

HELP Hawaii Early Learning Profile · Health Education Library Program · Health Emergency Loan Program · Health Evaluation and Learning Program · heat escape lessening posture · Heroin Emergency Life Project · Hospital Equipment Loan Project

HEM, Hem hematology *also* hemat · hemolysis/hemolytic *also* H · hemorrhage · hemorrhoid

hem hematuria

hemat hematocrit *also* Crit, crit, H'crit, HCT, Hct, HMT · hematology/hematologist *also* HEM, Hem

hematem hematemesis

hemi hemiparesis/hemiparalysis · hemiplegia · hemisphere

hemo hemoglobin *also* HB,

Hb, Hbg, HG, Hg, hg, HGB, Hgb • hemophilia

hemocyt hemocytometer

hemorr hemorrhage

HEMOSID hemosiderin

HEMPAS hereditary erythroblastic/erythrocytic multinuclearity with positive acidified serum

HEMRI hereditary multifocal relapsing inflammation

HEMS helicopter emergency medical services

HEN hemorrhages, exudates, and/or nicking

HEP hemolysis end point • heparin *also* H, HP • hepatic • hepatoerythropoietic porphyria • high egg passage (virus) • high–energy phosphate • histamine equivalent prick • human epithelial (cell) *also* HEp

HEp human epithelial (cell) *also* HEP

HEp–1 human cervical carcinoma cells

HEp–2 human laryngeal tumor cells

hEP human endorphin

hep hepatitis

HEPA hamster egg penetration assay • high–efficiency particulate air (filter)

HEP–AC hepatitis battery–acute

Hep/Clav hepatoclavicular

HEPM human embryonic palatal mesenchymal (cell)

HER hemorrhagic encephalopathy of rats

her. hernia *also* H, hern

herb. recent. [L. *herbarium recentium*] of fresh herbs

hered heredity/hereditary

hern hernia/herniated/herniation *also* H, her.

HERP human exposure (dose)/rodent potency

HERS Health Evaluation and Referral Service

HES health examination survey • hemotoxylin–eosin stain • human embryonic skin • human embryonic spleen • hydroxethyl starch • (acute) hypereosinophilic syndrome

HET Health Education Telecommunications • helium equilibration time

Het heterophil (antibody)

het heterozygous

HETE hydroxyeicosatetraenoic (acid)

HETP height equivalent to a theoretical plate (gas chromatography)

HEV health and environment • hemagglutination encephalomyelitis virus • hepatoencephalomyelitis virus • high endothelial venule • human enteric virus

HEW (Department of) Health, Education, and Welfare

HEX hexosaminidase

HEx hard exudate

Hex hexamethylmelamine *also* HM, HMM, HXM

HEX A hexosaminidase A (α–subunit)

Hexa–CAF hexamethyl-melamine, cyclophos-phamide, methotrexate, and fluorouracil

HEX B hexosaminidase B (β–subunit)

HF Hageman factor • half *also* hf • haplotype frequency • hard feces • hard filled (capsule) • harvest fluid • hay fever • head forward • head of fetus • heart failure • helper factor • hemofiltration • hemorrhagic factor • hemorrhagic fever • hepatocyte function • Hertz frequency • high–fat (diet) • high flow • high frequency *also* hf • hollow filter (dialyzer) • hot fomentation • house formula • human fibroblast • hydrogen fluoride (catalyst) • hyperflexion

H/F HeLa/fibroblast (hybrid)

Hf hafnium

hf half *also* HF • high frequency *also* HF

HFAK hollow–fiber artificial kidney

HFC hand–filled capsule • high–frequency current • histamine–forming capacity

HFCS high–fructose corn syrup

HFCWC high–frequency chest wall compression

HFD hemorrhagic fever of deer • high–fiber diet • high forceps delivery • hospital field director • Human Figure Drawing

HFDK human fetal diploid kidney (cell)

HFDL human fetal diploid lung (cell)

HFEC human foreskin epithelial cell

HFF human foreskin fibroblast

HFHL high–frequency hearing loss

HFI hereditary fructose intolerance • human fibroblast interferon *also* HFIF

HFIF human fibroblast interferon *also* HFI

HFJV high–frequency jet ventilation

HFL human fetal lung

HFM hemifacial microsomia *also* HM

HFO hard food orientation • high–frequency oscillation

HFOV high–frequency oscillatory ventilation

HFP hypofibrinogenic plasma

HFPPV high–frequency positive pressure ventilation

HFR heart frequency • high frequency (of) recombination

Hfr high frequency

Hfr mutant high–frequency recombination mutant

HFRS hemorrhagic fever with renal syndrome

HFS hemifacial spasm • Hospital Financial Support

hfs hyperfine structure

hFSH, HFSH human follicle–stimulating hormone

HFST hearing–for–speech test

HFT high–frequency transduction • high–frequency transfer

HFUPR hourly fetal urine production rate

HFV high–frequency ventilation

HG hand grip (exercise) • hemoglobin *also* HB, Hb, Hbg, hemo, Hg, hg, HGB, Hgb • herpes genitalis • herpes gestationis • Herter–Gee (syndrome) • Heschl gyrus • high glucose • human gonadotropin • human growth (factor) • Hutchinson–Gilford (syndrome) • hypoglycemia

Hg [L. *hydrargyrum* silver water] mercury *also* hydrarg

Hg, hg hectogram • hemoglobin *also* HB, Hb, Hbg, hemo, HG, HGB, Hgb

HGA homogentisate (homogentisic acid oxidase)

HGB, Hgb hemoglobin *also* HB, Hb, Hbg, hemo, HG, Hg, hg

hg–cal high calorie *also* HC

HGF human growth factor • hyperglycemic–glucogenolytic factor (glucagon)

Hg–F hemoglobin, fetal

HGG herpetic geniculate ganglionitis • human gamma globulin *also* hGG

hGG human gamma globulin *also* HGG

HGH, hGH high growth hormone • human (pituitary) growth hormone

HGM hog gastric mucin • human glucose monitoring

HGMCR human genetic mutant cell repository

HGO hepatic glucose output • hip guidance orthosis • human glucose output

HGP hepatic glucose production • hyperglobulinemia purpura

HGPRT, HG–PRTase hypo-xanthine–guanine phospho-ribosyltransferase

HGSHS Harvard Group Scale of Hypnotic Susceptibility

Hgt height *also* H, h, HT, ht

HH halothane hepatitis • hard of hearing *also* HOH • Head–Holms (syndrome) • healthy hemophiliac • Henderson and Haggard (inhaler) • hiatal hernia • holistic health • home health • home help • Hunter–Hurler (syndrome) • hydroxyhexamide •

hypergastrinemic
hyperchlorhydria •
hyperhidrosis •
hypogonadotropic
hypogonadism •
hyporeninemic
hypoaldosteronism

H/H, H&H hemoglobin and
hematocrit

Hh hemopoietic
histocompatibility

HHA Health Hazard
Appraisal • hereditary
hemolytic anemia • Home
Health Agency •
hypothalamic hypophyseal
adrenal (system)

HHAA hypothalamo–
hypophyseal–adrenal axis

HHB, HHb hypohemo-
globinemia • un–ionized
hemoglobin • reduced
hemoglobin

HHC home health care

HHCS high–altitude
hypertrophic
cardiomyopathy syndrome

HHD high heparin dose •
home hemodialysis •
hypertensive heart disease
also HTHD

HHE health hazard
evaluation •
hemiconvulsion–
hemiplegia–epilepsy
(syndrome)

HHFM high–humidity face
mask

HHG hypertrophic
hypersecretory gastropathy

HHH hyperornithinemia,
hyperammonemia, and

homocitrillinemia
(syndrome)

HHHO hypotonia, hypomentia,
hypogonadism, and obesity
(syndrome)

HHM hemohydrometry •
humoral hypercalcemia of
malignancy

H+Hm compound
hypermetropic astigmatism

HHN hand–held nebulizer

HHNC hyperosmolar
hyperglycemic nonketotic
coma

HHNK hyperglycemic
hyperosmolar nonketotic
(coma)

HHNKS hyperglycemic
hyperosmolar nonketotic
syndrome

HHPC hyperoxic–hypercapnic

HHRH hereditary
hypophosphatemic rickets
with hypercalciuria •
hypothalamic
hypophysiotropic–releasing
hormone

HHS (Department of) Health
and Human Services •
Hearing Handicap Scale •
hereditary hemolytic
syndrome • human
hypopituitary serum •
hyperkinetic heart syndrome

HHT head halter traction *also*
HHTx • hereditary
hemolytic telangiectasia •
hereditary hemorrhagic
telangiectasia • heterotopic
heart transplantation •
hydroxyheptadecatrienoic
(acid)

HHTA hypothalamohypo-
physeothyroidal axis

HHTx head halter traction *also*
HHT

HI head injury • health
insurance • hearing
impaired • heart infusion •
heat inactivated • heat
input • hemagglutination
inhibition (titer) *also* HAI •
hepatic insufficiency •
hepatobiliary imaging •
high impulsiveness •
histidine *also* H, Hi, HIS,
His, Hist • homoridal
ideation • hormone
dependent • hormone
insensitive • hospital
induced • hospital
insurance • humoral
immunity • hydriodic
acid • hydroxyindole •
hyperglycemic index •
hypomelanosis of Ito •
hypothermic ischemia

HI histamine • histidine *also*
H, HI, HIS, His, Hist

HIA heat infusion agar •
hemagglutination inhibition
antibody/assay

HIAA hydroxyindoleacetic acid

HIB *Haemophilus influenzae*
type b (vaccine) *also*
HITB • heart infusion
broth • hemolytic immune
body

HIBAC Health Insurance
Benefits Advisory Council

HIC Heart Information Center

H–ICD–A International
Classification of Diseases,
Adopted Code for Hospitals

HICHO high carbohydrate
(diet) *also* HCD

HICn cyanmethemoglobin

HID headache, insomnia, and
depression (syndrome) •
herniated intervertebral
disc • human infectious
dose • hyperkinetic
impulse disorder

HIDA hepatic 2,6–dimethyl-
iminodiacetic acid

HIE human intestinal
epithelium •
hyperimmunoglobulin E •
hypoxic–ischemic
encephalopathy

HIES hyperimunoglobulin E
syndrome

HIF higher integrative
function • higher
intellectual function •
histoplasma (tissue)
inhibitory factor •
Historical Information Form

HIFBS heat–inactivated fetal
bovine serum

HIFC hog intrinsic factor
concentrate

HIFCS heat–inactivated fetal
calf serum

HIg, HIG, hIG human
immunoglobulin

HIH hypertensive intracerebral
hemorrhage

HIHA high impulsiveness, high
anxiety

HIHb hemiglobin
(methemoglobin) *also*
HbMet

HII Health Industries Institute •
Health Insurance Institute •

hemagglutination inhibition immunoassay

HIL hypoxic–ischemic lesion

HILA high impulsiveness, low anxiety

HIM hemopoietic inductive microenvironment • hepatitis–infectious mononucleosis • hexosephosphate isomerase • Hill Interaction Matrix (psychologic test)

HIMC hepatic intramito-chondrial crystalloid

HIMP high–dose intravenous methylprednisolone

HIMT hemagglutination inhibition morphine test

Hind II, III restriction endonucleases from *Haemophilus influenzae*

H inf hypodermoclysis infusion

Hint. Hinton (flocculation test for syphilis)

HIO hypoiodism • hypoiodite (salt of hypoiodous acid)

HIOS high index of suspicion

HIP health illness profile • health insurance plan • hospital insurance program • humoral immunocompetence profile • hydrostatic indifference point

HiPIP high–potential iron protein

Hi Prot high protein *also* HiPro, HP

HIPO hemihypertrophy,

intestinal web, preauricular skin tag, and congenital corneal opacity (syndrome) • Hospital Indicator for Physicians Orders

HiPro, HiProt high protein (diet) *also* HP

HIR head injury routine • high irradiance response

HIRF histamine inhibitory releasing factor

HIS Hanover Intensive Score • Haptic Intelligence Scale • health information system • Health Intention Scale • Health Interview Survey • histidine *also* H, HI, Hi, His, Hist • hospital information system • hyperimmune serum • hyperimmunized suppressed

His histidine *also* H, HI, Hi, HIS, Hist

HISG human immune serum globulin

HISMS How I See Myself Scale (psychologic test)

HISSG Hospital Information Systems Sharing Group

HIST hospital in–service training

Hist, hist histidine *also* H, HI, Hi, HIS, His • histidinemia • history *also* H, Hx, Hy

HISTLINE History of Medicine On–Line

Histo histology • histoplasmin skin test

histol histologic/histologist/histology

HIT hemagglutination inhibition test • heparin–induced thrombocytopenia • histamine inhalation test • histamine ion transfer • Holtzman Inkblot Technique • hypertrophic infiltrative tendinitis • hypertrophied inferior turbinate

HITB, HITb *Haemophilus influenzae* type B (meningitis) *also* HIB

HITES hydrocortisone, insulin, transferrin, estradiol, and selenium

HITTS heparin–induced thrombosis–thrombocytopenia syndrome

HIU head injury unit • hyperplasia interstitialis uteri

HIV human immunodeficiency virus

HIVD herniated interverterbral disc

HIVIG HIV immunoglobulin

HIVIt high vitamin

HJ hepatojugular (reflux) *also* HJR • Howell–Jolly (bodies) *also* HJB

HJB Howell–Jolly bodies *also* HJ

HJR hepatojugular reflux *also* HJ

HK heat–killed • heel–to–knee • hexokinase • Hoffa–Kastert (syndrome) • human kidney (cell)

H–K hand–to–knee (test) • heel to knee (test) *also* HTK

H→K hand to knee (coordination)

HK1 hexokinase 1

HKAFO hip–knee–ankle–foot orthosis

HKAO hip–knee–ankle orthosis

HKC human kidney cell

HKH hyperkinetic heart syndrome

HKLM heat–killed *Listeria monocytogenes*

HKO hip–knee orthosis (splint)

HKS heel–knee–shin (test) • hyperkinesis syndrome

HL hairline • half–life (of radioactive element) • hallux limitus • haloperidol • harelip • hearing level • hearing loss • heart and lungs *also* H&L • heavy lifting • hectoliter • hemolysis • heparin lock *also* H/L • Hickman line • histiocytic lymphoma • histocompatibility locus • Hodgkin lymphoma • human leukocyte • human lymphocyte • hydrophil/lipophil (number) • hygienic laboratory • hyperlipidemia • hyperlipoproteinemia • hypertrichosis lanuginosa • latent hypermetropia • latent hyperopia • lateral habenular (nucleus)

H/L heparin lock *also* HL • hydrophil/lipophil (ratio) • hyperopia, latent *also* Hl • heart disease, low risk

H&L heart and lungs *also* HL

Hl hypermetropia, latent • hyperopia, latent *also* H/L

hL, hl hectoliter

HLA histocompatibility leukocyte antigen · histocompatibility locus antigen · homologous leukocyte antibody · human lymphocyte antibody · human lymphocyte antigen · hypoplastic left atrium

HLA human leukocyte antigen (system)

HLA–A, HLA–B, HLA–C, HLA–D, HLA–DR varieties of human leukocyte antigen

HLALD horse liver alcohol dehydrogenase

HLA–LD human lymphocyte antigen–lymphocyte defined

HLA negative heart, lungs, and abdomen negative

HLA–SD human lymphocyte antigen–serologically defined

HLB hydrophilic–lipophilic balance · hypotonic lysis buffer

HLBI human lymphoblastoid interferon

HLC heat loss center

HLCL human lymphoblastoid cell line

HLD haloperidol decanoate *also* HD · hepatolenticular degeneration · herniated lumbar disc · hypersensitivity lung disease · von Hippel–Lindau disease

HL–D haloperidol decamoate

HLDH heat–stable lactic dehydrogenase

HLE human leukocyte elastase

HLEG hydrolysate lactalbumin Earle glucose

HLF heat–labile factor · human lung field · human lung fluid

HLFCB horizontal laminar flow clean benches

HLH human luteinizing hormone *also* hLH · hypoplastic left heart (syndrome) *also* HLHS

hLH human luteinizing hormone *also* HLH

HLHS hypoplastic left heart syndrome *also* HLH

HLI hemolysis inhibition · human leukocyte interferon · human lymphocyte interferon

HLK, H–L–K heart, liver, and kidneys

HLN hilar lymph node · human Lesch–Nyhan (cell) · hyperplastic liver nodule

H&L OK heart and lungs normal

HLP hepatic lipoperoxidation · hind leg paralysis · hyperlipoproteinemia

HLR heart–lung resuscitation/ resuscitator

HLS Health Learning System · Hippel–Lindau syndrome

HLT heart–lung transplantation · human lipotropin · human lymphocyte transformation *also* hLT

hLT human lymphocyte transformation *also* HLT

hlth health

HLV herpes–like virus • hypoplastic left ventricle

HM hand motion • hand movement(s) • harmonic mean • health maintenance • heart murmur • heavily muscled • Heine–Medin (disease) • heloma molle (soft corn) • hemifacial microsomia *also* HFM • hepatic metabolism • hexamethylmelamine *also* Hex, HMM, HXM • Holter monitor/monitoring • hospital management • human milk • hydatidiform mole • hyperimmune mouse • hyperopia, manifest (hypermetropia) *also* Hm • hypoxic–metabolic

Hm hyperopia, manifest (hypermetropia) *also* HM

hm hectometer

HMA hemorrhages and microaneurysms

HMAC Health Manpower Advisory Council

HMAS hyperimmune mouse ascites (fluid)

HMB homatropine methylbromide

HMBA hexamethylene bisacetamide

HMC hand–mirror cell • health maintenance cooperative • heroin, morphine, and cocaine • hospital management

committee • hydroxymethyl cytosine • hyoscine–morphine–codeine

HMCCMP human mammary carcinoma cell membrane proteinase

HMD hyaline membrane disease

HMDP hydroxymethylene diphosphonate

HME Health Media Education • heat and moisture exchanger • heat, massage, and exercise *also* HMX

HMETSC heavy metal screen

HMF hydroxymethylfurfural

HMG high mobility group • human menopausal gonadotropin *also* hMG • hydroxymethylglutaric acid

hMG human menopausal gonadotropin *also* HMG

HMG CoA hepatic hydroxymethylglutaryl coenzyme A

HMI healed myocardial infarction

HMIS hospital medical information system

HMK high molecular weight kininogen *also* HMWK • homemaking

HML, hML human milk lysozyme

HM & LP hand motion and light perception

HMM heavy meromyosin (of muscle) • hexamethylmelamine *also* Hex, HM, HXM

HMMA 4–hydroxy–3–
methoxymandelic acid

HMO Health Maintenance
Organization • heart
minute output

HMP hexose monophosphate
pathway • hot moist
packs • human
menopausal • hydromotive
pressure

HMPA hexamethylphos-
phoramide

HMPG hydroxymethoxy-
phenylglycol

HMPS hexose monophosphate
shunt *also* HMS

HMPT hexamethylphosphoric
triamide

HMR histiocytic medullary
reticulosis

H–mRNA H–chain messenger
ribonucleic acid

HMRTE human milk reverse
transcriptase enzyme

HMS hexose monophosphate
shunt *also* HMPS • high
methacholine sensitivity •
hypermobility syndrome •
hypothetical mean strain

HMSAS hypertrophic
muscular subaortic stenosis

HMSN hereditary motor and
sensory neuropathy

HMSS Hospital Management
Systems Society

HMT hematocrit *also* Crit, crit,
H'crit, HCT, Hct, hemat •
hexamethylenetetramine
(methenamine) *also*
HMTA • histamine

methyltransferase •
hospital management team

hMT human molar thyrotropin

HMTA hexamethylene-
tetramine (methenamine)
also HMT

HMW high molecular weight

HMWC high molecular weight
component

HMWGP high molecular
weight glycoprotein

HMWK high molecular weight
kininogen *also* HMK

HMWM heavily muscled white
male

HMX heat, massage, and
exercise *also* HME

HN head and neck *also* H&N •
head nurse • Heller–
Nelson (syndrome) •
hemagglutinin
neuraminidase •
hematemesis neonatorum •
hemorrhage of newborn •
hereditary nephritis • high
nitrogen • hilar node •
histamine–containing
neuron • home nursing •
hospitalman • human
nutrition • hypertrophic
neuropathy

HN₂ mechlorethamine
(nitrogen mustard)

H&N head and neck *also* HN

hn [L. *hoc nocte*] tonight

HNA heparin–neutralizing
activity

HNB human neuroblastoma •
hydroxynitrobenzylbromide

HNC hypernephroma cell •

hyperosmolar nonketotic coma · hyperoxic normocapnic · hypothalamoneurohypophyseal complex

HNKDC hyperosmolar nonketotic diabetic coma

HNKDS hyperosmolar nonketotic diabetic state

HNLN hospitalization no longer necessary

H&N mot head and neck motion

HNP hereditary nephritic protein · herniated nucleus pulposus · human neurophysin

hnRNA heterogeneous nuclear ribonucleic acid

hnRNP heterogeneous nuclear ribonucleoprotein

HNS head and neck surgery · head, neck, and shaft (of bone) · home nursing supervisor

HNSHA hereditary nonspherocytic hemolytic leukemia

HNTD highest nontoxic dose

HNTLA Hiskey–Nebraska Test of Learning Aptitude

HNV has not voided

HO hand orthosis · Hematology–Oncology · heterotopic ossification · high oxygen · hip orthosis · Holt–Oram (syndrome) · house officer · hyperbaric oxygen · hypertrophic ossification

H/O, h/o history of

Ho holmium · horse *also* H

HOA hip osteoarthritis · hypertrophic osteoarthritis

Ho antigen low–frequency blood group antigen

HOAP–BLEO hydroxydaunomycin (doxorubicin), Oncovin (vincristine), araC (cytarabine), prednisone, and bleomycin

HoaRhLG horse anti-rhesus lymphocyte globulin

HoaTTG horse anti-tetanus toxoid globulin

HOB head of bed

HOB UPSOB head of bed up for shortness of breath

HOC Health Officer Certificate · human ovarian cancer · hydroxycorticoid *also* HC

HOCM high–osmolar contrast medium *also* HOM · hypertrophic obstructive cardiomyopathy

hoc vesp [L. *hoc vespere*] this evening

HOD hereditary opalescent dentin · Hoffer–Osmond Diagnostic · hospital day *also* HD · hyperbaric oxygen drenching

HOF hepatic outflow

HofF height of fundus

Hoff Hoffman (reflex)

HOG halothane, oxygen, and gas (nitrous oxide)

HOGA hyperornithinemia with gyrate atrophy

HOH hard of hearing *also* HH

HOI hospital onset of infection • hypoiodous acid

HoIg horse immunoglobulin

HOM hexamethylmelamine, Oncovin (vincristine), and methotrexate • high–osmolar (contrast) medium *also* HOCM

HOME Home Observation for Measurement of the Environment • Home Oriented Maternity Experience

Homeo, Homeop homeopathy

HOMO highest occupied molecular orbital • homosexual *also* H, homo

homo homosexual *also* H, HOMO

homolat homolateral

HOOD hereditary osteo–onychodysplasia

HOODS hereditary onycho–osteodysplasia syndrome

HOOI Hall Occupational Orientation Inventory

HOP high oxygen pressure • hydroxydaunomycin (doxorubicin), Oncovin (vincristine), and prednisone

HOPD hospital outpatient department

HOPE Healthcare Options Plan Entitlement • health–oriented physical education • holistic orthogonal parameter estimation

HOPI history of present illness *also* HPI

HOPP hepatic occluded portal pressure

hor, horiz horizontal *also* H, h

hor decub [L. *hora decubitus*] at bedtime *also* h, hd, hor som, HS, hs, h som

hor interm [L. *hora intermedia*] at the intermediate hour

hor som [L. *hora somni*] at bedtime *also* h, hd, hor decub, HS, hs, h som

hor un spat [L. *horae unius spatio*] at the end of one hour

HOS human osteosarcoma

HoS horse serum *also* HS

Hosp, hosp hospital/hospitalization *also* H, HX

HOST hypo–osmotic shock treatment

HOT human old tuberculin • hyperbaric oxygen therapy

HP *Haemophilus pleuropneumonia* • halogen phosphorus • handicapped person • haptoglobin *also* HAPTO, Hp, Hpt • hard palate • Harding–Passey (melanoma) • Harvard pump • hastening phenomenon • health professional • heater probe • heat production • heel–to–patella *also* H→P • hemiparesis • hemi-pelvectomy • hemiplegia *also* Hp • hemoperfusion • heparin *also* H, HEP • highly purified • high

potency • high power •
high pressure • high protein
(diet) *also* HiPro, Hi Prot •
Hodgen and Pearson
(suspension traction) *also*
H&P • horizontal plane •
horsepower • hospital
participation • hot pack •
hot pad • house physician •
human pituitary •
hybridoma product •
hydrocollator pack •
hydrogen peroxide •
hydrophilic petrolatum •
hydrophobic protein •
hydrostatic pressure •
hydroxyproline *also* HYP,
hyp, hypro • hydroxy-
pyruvate • hyperpara-
thyroidism *also* HPT,
HPTH • hyperphoria •
hypersensitivity
pneumonitis • hypertension
plus proteinuria •
hypoparathyroidism •
hypopharynx

H&P history and physical
(examination) *also* HPE •
Hodgen and Pearson
(suspension traction) *also*
HP

H→P heel–to–patella *also* HP

Hp haptoglobin *also* HAPTO,
HP, Hpt •
hematoporphyrin •
hemiplegia *also* HP

hp heaping • horsepower

HPA α–haptoglobin • *Helix
pomatia* agglutinin •
hemagglutinating penicillin
antibody • Hereford
Parental Attitude (Survey) •
human papilloma (virus) •
hypothalamic–pituitary–
adrenal (axis) *also* HPAA •

hypothalmo–pituitary–
adrenocortical (system)

HPAA hydroperoxy-
arachidonic acid •
hydroxyphenylacetic acid •
hypothalamo–pituitary–
adrenal axis *also* HPA

HPBC hyperpolarizing bipolar
cell

HPBF hepatotropic portal
blood factor

HPBL human peripheral blood
leukocyte

HPC hemangiopericytoma •
hippocampal pyramidal
cell • history (of) present
complaint • hydroxy-
phenylcinchoninic (acid) •
hydroxypropylcellulose

HPD hematoporphyrin
derivative • highly
probably drunk • high–
protein diet • home
peritoneal dialysis

HP–D Hough–Powell digitizer

HPE hepatic portoenter-
ostomy • high permeability
edema • history and
physical examination *also*
H&P • hydrostatic
pulmonary edema

HPETE hydroperoxy-
eicosatetraenoic acid

HPF heparin–precipitable
fraction • hepatic plasma
flow • high–pass filter •
high–power field
(microscope) *also* hpf •
hypocaloric protein feeding

hpf high power field
(microscope) *also* HPF

HPFH hereditary persistence of
fetal hemoglobin

hPFSH, HPFSH human pituitary follicle–stimulating hormone

HPG, hPG human pituitary gonadotropin

HPGe high–purity germanium

HPH halothane–percent–hour

HPI hepatic perfusion index · Heston Personality Inventory (Test) · history of present illness *also* HOPI

HPL human parotid lysozyme · human peripheral lymphocyte · human placental lactogen *also* hPL · hyperplexia

hPL human placental lactogen *also* HPL

HPLA hydroxyphenyllactic acid

HPLAC high–pressure liquid affinity chromatography

HPLC high–performance/high–power/high–pressure liquid chromatography

HPM Harding–Passey melanoma · hemiplegic migraine

HPMC human peripheral mononuclear cell

HPN home parenteral nutrition · hypertension *also* HT, HTN, hypn

hpn [L. *haustus purgans noster*] our own purgative draft

HPNS high–pressure neurologic syndrome

HPO high–pressure oxygen · hydroperoxide ·

hydrophilic ointment · hypertrophic pulmonary osteoarthritis · hypertrophic pulmonary osteoarthropathy

HPP, hPP hereditary pyropoikilocytosis · history (of) presenting problems · hydroxy-phenylpyruvate · hydroxy-pyrazolopyrimidine · human pancreatic polypeptide

2 HPP two hours postprandial (blood sugar)

HPPA hydroxyphenylpyruvic acid

HPPH hydroxyphenyl–phenylhydantoin

HPPO high partial pressure (of) oxygen · hydroxyphenyl pyruvate oxidase

HPR hospital peer review

HPr, hPr, HPRL human prolactin

HPRP human platelet–rich plasma

HPRT hot plate reaction time · hypoxanthine phospho-ribosyltransferase

HPS hematoxylin, phloxine, and saffron · Hermansky–Pudlak syndrome · high–protein supplement · His–Purkinje system · human platelet suspension · hypertrophic pyloric stenosis · hypothalamic pubertal syndrome

HPSL Health Professions Student Loan

HPT histamine provocation test • hot plate test • human placental thyrotropin *also* hPT • hyperparathyroidism *also* HPTH • hypothalmic–pituitary–thyroid

Hpt haptoglobin *also* HAPTO, HP, Hp

hPT human placental thyrotropin *also* HPT

HPTH hyperparathyroid hormone • hyperparathyroidism *also* HP, HPT

hPTH human parathyroid hormone I_{34} (teriparatide)

HPTIN human pancreatic trypsin inhibitor

HPTM home prothrombin time monitoring

HPV *Haemophilus pertussis* vaccine • hepatic portal vein • human papilloma virus • human parvovirus • hypoxic pulmonary vasoconstriction

HPVD hypertensive pulmonary vascular disease

HPV–DE high–passage virus–duck embryo (cell)

HPV–DK high–passage virus–dog kidney (cell)

HPVG hepatic portal venous gas

HPX high peroxide-containing (cell) • hypophysectomized *also* HX, hypox • partial hepatectomy

Hpx hemopexin (serum protein)

HPZ high–pressure zone

HQC hydroquinone cream

HR hallux rigidus • Halstead–Reitan (battery) *also* HRB • Hamman–Rich (syndrome) • Harrington rod • heart rate *also* HRT • hemirectococcygeus • hemorrhagic retinopathy • heterosexual relations (scale) • higher rate • high resolution • hormonal response • hospital record • hospital report • hour *also* H, hr • Howship–Romberg (syndrome) • human resources • hydroxyethylrutinosides (treatment of venous disorders) • hyperimmune reaction • hypoxic responder

2HR two–hour pregnancy test

H&R hysterectomy and radiation

hr hour *also* H, HR

HRA health risk appraisal • heart rate audiometry • high right atrial • high right atrium • histamine-releasing activity • Human Resources Administration

HRAE high right atrium electrocardiogram

HRANA histone–reactive antinuclear antibody

HRB Halstead–Reitan Battery *also* HR • histamine release (from) basophils

HRBC horse red blood cell

HRC help–rejecting complainer • high–resolution chromatography •

horse red cell • human rights committee

HRCT high–resolution computed tomography

HRE high–resolution electrocardiography • hormone–receptor enzyme

HREC hepatic reticuloendothelial cell

HREH high–renin essential hypertension

HREM high–resolution electron microscopy

HRF Harris return flow • histamine–releasing factor

HRH hypothalamic–releasing hormone

HRI Harrington rod instrumentation

HRIG, HRIg human rabies immunoglobulin

HRL head rotation (to) left

HRLA human reovirus–like agent

HRLM high–resolution light microscopy

hRNA heterogeneous ribonucleic acid

HRP high right parasternal (view) • high–risk pregnancy • histidine–rich protein • horseradish peroxidase

HRPD Hamburg Rating Scale for Psychiatric Disorders

HRR Hardy–Rand–Ritter (color vision test kit) • head rotation (to) right • heart rate range

HRRI heart rate retardation index

HRS Hamilton Rating Scale • hepatorenal syndrome • hormone receptor site • humeroradial synostosis

HRSA Health Resources and Services Administration

HRS–D Hamilton Rating Scale for Depression

HRT half relaxation time • heart rate *also* HR • hormone replacement therapy

HRTE human reverse transcriptase enzyme

HRTEM high–resolution transmission electron microscopy

HRV heart rate variability • human rotavirus

HRVL human reovirus–like

HS half strength • Hallervorden–Spatz (syndrome) • hamstrings *also* Hams • hand surgery • Hartmann solution • head sign • head sling • healthy subject • heart sound • heat stable • heavy smoker • heel spur • heel stick • Hegglin syndrome • heme synthetase • Henoch–Schönlein (syndrome) • heparin sulfate • hereditary spherocytosis • herpes simplex • hidradenitis suppurativa • high school • homologous serum • Hopelessness Scale • horizontally selective (visual cell) •

Horner syndrome • horse serum *also* HoS • hospital ship • hospital staff • hospital stay • hour of sleep • house surgeon • human serum • Hurler syndrome • hypereosinophilic syndrome • hypersensitivity • hypertonic saline

HS [L. *hora somni* hour of sleep] at bedtime *also* h, hor decub, hor som, h som

H/S helper–suppressor (ratio)

H→S heel–to–shin (test) *also* HTS

H&S hemorrhage and shock • hysterectomy and sterilization

H₂S Hering's law—EOM innervation, both eyes • Sherrington's law—EOM innervation, one eye

Hs hypochondriasis

hs [L. *hora somni* hour of sleep] at bedtime *also* h, HS, hor decub, hor som, h som

HSA Hazardous Substances Act • health service area • Health Services Administration • Health Systems Agency • horse serum albumin • human serum albumin *also* HuSA • hypersomnia–sleep apnea (syndrome)

HSAG HEPES (hydroxyethyl-piperazine ethanesulfonic acid)–saline–albumin–gelatin

HSAP heat–stable alkaline phosphatase

HSAS hypertrophic subaortic stenosis *also* HSS

HSBG heel–stick blood gas

HSC Hand–SchHller–Christian (disease) *also* HSCD • health sciences center • health screening center • hemopoietic stem cell • horizontal semicircular canal • human skin collagenase

HSCD Hand–SchHller–Christian disease *also* HSC

HSCL Hopkins Symptom Checklist

HS–CoA reduced coenzyme A

HSD honest significance difference • hydroxysteroid dehydrogenase

HSDA high single dose alternate day

HSDI Health Self–Determination Index

HSE health and safety executive • herpes simplex encephalitis • human serum esterase

Hse homoserine

HSF heated soybean flower • histamine–induced suppressor factor • histamine–sensitizing factor • hypothalamic secretory factor

HSG herpes simplex genitalis • hysterosalpingo-gram/hysterosalpinography

hSGF human skeletal growth factor

HSGP human sialoglycoprotein

HSHC hemisuccinate (of) hydrocortisone

HSI heat stress index • human seminal (plasma) inhibitor

HSK herpes simplex keratitis

HSL herpes simplex labialis

HSLC high–speed liquid chromatography

HSM hepatosplenomegaly • holosystolic murmur

HSMHA Health Services and Mental Health Administration

HSN Hanson–Street nail • hereditary sensory neuropathy • herpes simplex neonatorum

h som [L. *hora somni* hour of sleep] at bedtime *also* h, hd, hor decub, hor som, HS, hs

HSP Health Systems Plan • hemostatic screening profile • Henoch–Schönlein purpura • human serum prealbumin • human serum protein • hysterosalpingography

H spike His bundle electrogram deflection

HSPM hippocampal synaptic plasma membrane

HSPQ High School Personality Questionnaire

HSQB Health Standards and Quality Bureau

HSR Harleco synthetic resin • heated serum reagent • homogeneous staining region (of chromosome)

HSRC Health Services Research Center • Human Subjects Review Committee

HSRD hypertension secondary (to) renal disease

HSRI Health Systems Research Institute

HSRS Health–Sickness Rating Scale • Hess School Readiness Scale

HSS Hallervorden–Spatz syndrome • hepatic stimulator substance • high–speed supernatant • hypertrophic subaortic stenosis *also* HSAS

HSSE high soap suds enema

HST health screening test(s) • Hemoccult slide test • horseshoe tear

HSTF human serum thymus factor

HSTS human–specific thyroid stimulator

HSV herpes simplex virus • highly selective vagotomy

HSVE herpes simplex virus encephalitis

HSVtk herpes simplex virus thymidine kinase

HSyn heme synthase

HT hammertoe • Hand Test (psychologic test) • Hashimoto thyroiditis • hearing test • hearing threshold • heart *also* H, He, ht • heart test • heart tone *also* ht • heart transplantation/transplant • height *also* H, h, Hgt, ht • hemagglutination titer • high temperature • high tension *also* ht • Histologic Technologist • histo-technology • home treatment • hospital treatment • Hubbard tank • Huhner test • human thrombin • hydrocortisone test • hydrotherapy *also* hydro • hydroxytryptamine (serotonin) *also* 5–HT, HTA • hyperopia, total (hypermetropia) *also* Ht • hypertension *also* HPN, HTN, hypn • hyper-thyroidism • hypertrans-fusion • hypertropia • hypodermic tablet • hypothalamus *also* H, Ht, Hth, Hyp, hyp

3–HT 3–hydroxytyramine (dopamine)

5–HT 5–hydroxytryptamine (serotonin) *also* HTA

H&T hospitalization and treatment

H(T) intermittent hypertropia

Ht height of heart • hetero-zygote • hypermetropia, total • hyperopia, total *also* HT • hypothalamus *also* H, HT, Hth, Hyp, hyp

ht [L. *haustus*] draught, drink *also* H, h • heart *also* H, He, HT • heart tone *also* HT • heat • height *also* H, h, Hgt, HT • high tension *also* HT

HTA heterophil transplantation antigen • human thymocyte antigen • 5–hydroxytryptamine (serotonin) *also* HT, 5–HT • hypophysiotropic area (of hypothalamus)

HTACS human thyroid adenylcyclase stimulator

ht aer heated aerosol *also* HA

HT(ASCP) Histologic Technologist certified by Board of Registry of American Society of Clinical Pathologists

HTAT human tetanus antitoxin

HTB hot tub bath • house tube (feeding) *also* HTF • human tumor bank

HTC hepatoma cell • hepatoma tissue culture • homozygous typing cell • hypertensive crisis

HTCA human tumor colony assay

HTCVD hypertensive cardiovascular disease *also* HCVD

HTD human therapeutic dose

HTDW heterosexual development of women

HTF heterothyrotropic factor • house tube feeding *also* HTB

HTG hypertriglyceridemia

HTH homeostatic thymus hormone

Hth hypothalamus *also* H, HT, Ht, Hyp, hyp

HTHD hypertensive heart disease *also* HHD

HTI hemisphere thrombotic infarction • human tetanus immunoglobulin

HTIG homologous tetanus immune globulin

hTIg human tetanus immunoglobulin

HTK heel–to–knee (test) *also* H–K

HTL hamster tumor line • hearing threshold level • histologic technologist • histotechnologist • human T–cell leukemia • human T–cell lymphoma • human thymic leukemia

HTLA high titer, low acidity • human T–lymphocyte antigen

HTL(ASCP) Histotechnologist certified by the Board of Registry of the American Society of Clinical Pathologists

HTLV human T–cell leukemia/lymphoma/lymphotropic virus

HTLV–MA human T–cell leukemia virus–associated membrane antigen

HTN Hantaan(–to like virus) • hypertension also HPN, HT, hypn • hypertensive nephropathy

HTO heterotropic ossification • high tibial osteotomy • hospital transfer order

HTOH hydroxytryptophol

HTP House–Tree–Person (Projective Technique psychologic test) • hydroxytryptophan • hypothromboplastinemia

5–HTP 5–hydroxytryptophan

HTPN home total parenteral nutrition

HTR hypermetropia, right

HTS, hTS head traumatic syndrome • heel–to–shin (test) *also* H→S • hemangioma–thrombocytopenia syndrome • human thyroid–stimulating (hormone) *also* HTSH, hTSH • human thyroid stimulator

hTSAb human thyroid–stimulating antibody

HTSCA human tumor stem cell assay

HTSH, hTSH human thyroid–stimulating hormone *also* HTS

HTST high temperature–short time (pasteurization)

HTT hand thrust test

HTV herpes–type virus

HTVD hypertensive vascular disease *also* HVD

HTX hemothorax

HU head unit • heat unit • hemagglutinating unit • hemagglutinin unit • hemolytic unit • Hounsfield unit • human urinary • human urine • hydroxyurea *also* HUR, HYD • hyperemia unit

Hu human

HUC hypouricemia

HU–FSH human urinary follicle–stimulating hormone

HUI headache unit index

HUIFM human leukocyte interferon milieu

HUIS high–dose urea in invert sugar

HUK human urinary kallikrein

HUM heat (or hot packs), ultrasound, and massage • hematourimetry

hum. humerus

HUP Hospital Utilization Project

HUR hydroxyurea *also* HU, HYD

HURA health in underserved rural areas

HURT hospital utilization review team

HUS hemolytic–uremic syndrome • hyaluronidase unit for semen

HuSA human serum albumin *also* HSA

husb husband *also* H

HUTHAS human thymus antiserum

HUV human umbilical vein

HV hallux valgus • Hantaan virus • has voided • heart volume • Hemovac • hepatic vein • herpes virus • high voltage • high volume • home visit • hospital visit • hyperventilation

H&V hemigastrectomy and vagotomy

hv [L. *hoc vespere*] this evening

HVA homovanillic acid

HVc hyperstriatum ventrale, pars caudale

HVD hypertensive vascular disease *also* HTVD • hypoxic ventilatory drive

HVE hepatic venous effluence • high–voltage electrophoresis

HVEM high voltage electron microscope

HVF hepatocycle volume fraction

HVFP hepatic vein free pressure

HVG hematoxylin and van Gieson (stain) • host versus graft (disease, response)

HVGS high–voltage galvanic stimulation (physical therapy)

HVH *Herpesvirus hominis*

HVHMA *Herpesvirus hominis* membrane antigen

HVID horizontal visible iris diameter

HVJ hemagglutinating virus of Japan

HVL, hvl half–value layer

HVLP high volume, low pressure

HVLT high–velocity lead therapy

HVM hypothalamic ventromedial (nucleus)

HVPE high–voltage paper electrophoresis

HVPG hepatic venous pressure gradient

HVR hypoxic ventilatory response

HVS herpesvirus sensitivity • herpesvirus of Saimiri • hyperventilation

syndrome • hyperviscosity
syndrome

H vs A home versus (against)
advice

HVSD hydrogen–detected
ventricular septal defect

HVT half–value thickness •
herpesvirus (of) turkeys

HVTEM high–voltage
transmission electron
microscopy

HVUS hypocomplementemic
vasculitis urticaria
syndrome

HW Hayrem–Widal
(syndrome) • healing
well • heart weight •
hemisphere width •
heparin well • Hertwig–
Weyers (syndrome) •
housewife

HWB, hwb hot water bottle

HWE hot water extract

HWOK heel walking normal
(OK)

HWP hepatic wedge pressure •
hot wet pack • Hutchinson–
Weber–Pentz (syndrome)

HWRS Habits of Work and
Recreation Survey

HWS hot water soluble

HWY hundred woman years (of
exposure)

HX histiocytosis X •
hospitalization *also* H,
Hosp, hosp • hydrogen
exchange •
hypophysectomized *also*
HPX, hypox

Hx history *also* H, Hist, hist,

Hy • hypoxanthine *also*
Hyp, hyp

2–HxG di(hydroxy-
ethyl)glycine

HXIS hard x–ray imaging
spectrometer

HXM hexamethylmelamine
also Hex, HM, HMM

HXR hypoxanthine riboside

HY hypophysis *also* hyp

Hy history *also* H, Hist, hist,
Hx • hydraulics •
hydrostatics •
hypermetropia *also* H, h •
hyperopia *also* H, h •
hypothenar • hysteria *also*
hy, hys, hyst

hy hysteria *also* Hy, hys, hyst

HYD hydralazine • hydrated
to hydration • hydroxyurea
also HU, HUR

Hyd hydrocortisone *also* HC,
HCT • hydrostatics

hyd and tur hydration and
turgor

hydr hydraulic

hydrarg [L. *hydrargyrum* silver
water] mercury *also* Hg

hydro hydrotherapy *also* HT

hydrox hydroxyline

Hyg, hyg hygiene/hygienic/
hygienist *also* H

HYL, Hyl hydroxylysine

HYLO hyaline

HYP hydroxyproline *also* HP,
Hyp, hyp, hypro •
hypnosis *also* hypno

Hyp, hyp hydroxyproline *also*

HP, HYP, hypro ·
hyperresonance ·
hypertrophy · hypothalamus
also H, HT, Ht, Hth ·
hypoxanthine *also* Hx

hyp hypalgesia · hypophysis
also HY · hypo-
physectomy *also* HE

hyper A hyperactive

hyperal, hyper–al
hyperalimentation

hyper–IgE hyperimmuno-
globulinemia E

hyperpara hyperpara-
thyroidism

hypes hypesthesia

hyper T&A hypertrophy of
tonsils and adenoids

hypn hypertension *also* HPN,
HT, HTN

hypno hypnosis *also* HYP

hypo hypochromia ·
hypochromaria ·
hypodermic

hypo A hypoactive

hypox hypophysectomized
also HPX, HX

HYPP hypersegmented
neutrophil

HypRF hypothalamic releasing
factor

hypro hydroxyproline *also*
HP, HYP, Hyp, hyp

hys, hyst hysterectomy ·
hysteria *also* Hy, hy ·
hysterical

HZ herpes zoster

Hz hertz

HZFO hamster zona–free
ovum (test)

HZO herpes zoster ophthalmicus

HZV herpes zoster virus

I electric current • implantation • impression *also* IMP, imp • inactive *also* inac • incisor (permanent) • increased • independent *also* ind • index *also* ind • indicated • induction *also* Ind, ind • inhalation *also* INH, inhal • inhibition *also* inhib • inhibitor • initial • inosine • insoluble *also* insol • inspiration *also* Insp, inspir • inspired (gas) • insulin *also* IN, In, INS • intact (bag of waters) • intake • intensity • intensity of magnetism • intercalary (congenital limb absence) • intermediate *also* INT, int, Intmd • intestine • iodide • iodine • ionic strength • iris • isochromosome • isotope • isotropic (band, disk) • luminous intensity • moment of inertia • roman numeral one • vector cardiography electrode (right midaxillary line)

^{123}**I** iodine radioisotope

^{125}**I** iodine radioisotope

^{131}**I** iodine radioisotope

^{132}**I** iodine radioisotope

i incisor (deciduous) • insoluble • optically inactive (chemical)

IA ibotenic acid *also* ibo • image amplification • immune adherence • immunobiologic activity • impedance angle • inactive alcoholic • incidental appendectomy • incurred accidentally • Indian–American (Native

I

American) • indolaminergic–accumulating (cells) • indulin agar • infantile apnea • infantile autism • infected area • inferior angle • inhibitory antigen • internal auditory • intra–alveolar • intra–amniotic *also* i am • intra–aortic • intra–arterial • intra–articular • intra–atrial • intra–auricular • intrinsic activity • isonicotinic acid

I&A, I/A irrigation and aspiration

Ia immune (region)–associated antigen

IAA indoleacetic acid • infectious agent, arthritis • interruption (of) aortic arch • iodoacetic acid

I–3–AA indole–3–acetic acid

IAAR imidazoleacetic acid ribonucleotide

IAB Industrial Accident Board • intra–abdominal • intra–aortic balloon

IABA intra–aortic balloon assistance

IABC intra–aortic balloon catheter • intra–aortic balloon counterpulsation *also* IABCP

IABCP intra–aortic balloon counterpulsation *also* IABC

IABM idiopathic aplastic bone marrow

IABP intra–aortic balloon pump/pumping *also* IBP

IABPA intra–aortic balloon pumping assistance

IAC ineffective airway clearance • internal auditory canal • interposed abdominal compression • intra–arterial chemotherapy • Inventory of Anger Communications

IACB intra–aortic counterpulsation balloon

IAC–CPR interposed abdominal compressions—cardiopulmonary resuscitation

IACD implantable automatic cardioverter–defibrillator • intra–atrial conduction defect

IACP intra–aortic counterpulsation

IAD inactivating dose • inhibiting antibiotic dose • internal absorbed dose

IADH inappropriate antidiuretic hormone

IADHS inappropriate antidiuretic hormone syndrome

IAds immunoadsorption

IA DSA intra–arterial digital subtraction angiography

IAE intra–arterial electrocardiogram • intra–atrial electrocardiogram

IAFI infantile amaurotic familial idiocy

IAGT indirect antiglobulin test *also* IAT, IDAT

IAH idiopathic adrenal hyperplasia • implantable artificial heart

IAHA idiopathic autoimmune hemolytic anemia • immune adherence hemagglutination

IAHD idiopathic acquired hemolytic disease

IAI intra–abdominal infection

IAM Institute of Aviation Medicine • internal acoustic meatus • internal auditory meatus

I am intra–amniotic *also* IA

IAN idiopathic aseptic necrosis • intern admission note

I and O intake and output

IAO immediately after onset • intermittent aortic occlusion

IAP immunosuppressive acidic protein • innervated antral pouch • inosinic acid pyrophosphorylase • intermittent acute porphyria • islet–activating protein

IAR immediate asthmatic reaction • inhibitory anal reflex • iodine–azide reaction

IARF ischemic acute renal failure

IARSA idiopathic acquired refractory sideroblastic anemia

IAS idiopathic ankylosing spondylitis • immuno-suppressive acidic substance • infant apnea syndrome • interatrial septum • interatrial shunting • internal anal sphincter • intra–amniotic saline (infusion)

IASA interatrial septal aneurysm

IASD interatrial septal defect *also* ISD • interauricular septal defect

IASH isolated asymmetric septal hypertrophy

IASHS Institute for Advanced Study in Human Sexuality

IAT immunoaugmentative therapy • indirect antiglobulin test *also* IAGT, IDAT • instillation abortion time • invasive activity test • iodine azide test • Iowa Achievement Test

IAV interactive video • intermittent assisted ventilation • intra–arterial vasopressin

IAVM intramedullary arteriovenous malformation

IB Ibrahim–Beck (disease) • ileal bypass • immune balance • immune body • inclusion body *also* IncB • index (of body) build • infectious bronchitis • isolation bed

I–B interbody (vertebral)

Ib [L. *ibidem*] in the same place *also* ibid

IBA isobutyric acid

I band isotropic band (striated muscle fiber) *also* I disk

IBAT intravascular bronchoalveolar tumor

IBB intestinal brush border

IBBB intrablood–brain barrier

IBBBB incomplete bilateral bundle–branch block

IBC Institutional Biosafety Committee • iodine–binding capacity • iron–binding capacity • isobutyl cyanoacrylate *also* IBCA

IBCA isobutyl cyanoarcrylate *also* IBC

IBD infectious bowel disease • inflammatory bowel disease • irritable bowel disease • ischemic bowel disease

IBED Inter–African Bureau for Epizootic Diseases

IB–EP immunoreactive beta–endomorphin

IBF immature brown fat (cell) • immunoglobulin–binding factor

IBG insoluble bone gelatin

IBI intermittent bladder irrigation • ischemic brain infarction

ibid [L. *ibidem*] in the same place

IBILI indirect bilirubin

IBK infectious bovine keratoconjunctivitis

IBL immunoblastic lymphadenopathy

IBM inclusion body myositis • isotonic–isometric brief maximum

IBNR incurred but not reported

Ibo ibotenic acid *also* IA

IBOW intact bag of waters

IBP intra–aortic balloon pumping *also* IABP • iron–binding protein

IBPMS indirect blood pressure measuring system

IBQ Illness Behavior Questionnaire

IBR infectious bovine rhinotracheitis (virus)

IBRS Inpatient Behavior Rating Scale

IBRV infectious bovine rhinotracheitis virus

IBS imidazole–buffered saline • inside bathing solution • Interpersonal Behavior Survey • irritable bowel syndrome • isobaric solution

IBSA, IBSA immunoreactive bovine serum albumin • iodinated bovine serum albumin

IBT ink blot test (Rorschack test)

IBTR ipsilateral breast tumor recurrence

IBU ibuprofen • international benzoate unit

IBV infectious bronchitis vaccine • infectious bronchitis virus

IBW ideal body weight

IC [L. *inter cibos*] between meals *also* ic, int cib • icteric *also* ICT • ileocecal • iliococcygeal • iliorostal • immune complex • immune cytotoxicity •

immunocompromised • immunocytochemistry *also* ICC • impedence cardiogram • incomplete (diagnosis) • indirect calorimetry • indirect Coombs (test) • individual counseling • infection control • inferior colliculus • information content • inhibitory concentration • inner canthal (distance) • in- organic carbon • inspiratory capacity • inspiratory center • institutional care • integrated circuit • integrated concentration • intensive care • intercarpal • intercostal (space) *also* ICS, IS • intermediate care • intermittent catheterization *also* Ic • intermittent claudication • internal capsule • internal carotid • internal cerebral • internal cholecystectomy • internal conjugate (diameter) • International Classification • interstitial cell • interstitial change • intracameral • intracapsular • intracardiac • intracarotid • intracavitary • intracellular • intracellular concentration • intracerebral • intracisternal *also* ICI • intracoronary • intracranial • intracutaneous *also* i cut. • intrapleural catheter • irritable colon • islet cell (of pancreas) • isovolumic contraction

I/C invalid chair

IC$_{50}$ concentration that inhibits 50%

Ic intermittent catheterization *also* IC

Ic [L. *inter cibos*] between meals *also* IC, int cib

ICA Institute of Clinical Analysis • intercountry adoption • intermediate care area • internal carotid artery • intracranial anatomy • intracranial aneurysm • islet cell antibody

ICa ionized calcium

ICAb islet cell antibody

ICAF internal carotid artery flow

ICAO internal carotid artery occlusion

ICAP intracisternal A particle

ICAV intracavitary

ICB intracranial bleeding

ICBF inner cortical blood flow

ICBP intercellular binding protein • intracellular binding protein

ICBT intercostobronchial trunk

ICC immunocompetent cell • immunocytochemistry *also* IC • Indian childhood cirrhosis • intensive coronary care • interchromosomal crossing-over • intermediate cell column • intermittent clean catheterization • internal conversion coefficient • islet cell carcinoma

ICCE intracapsular cataract extraction

ICCE͞cPI intracapsular cataract extraction with peripheral iridectomy

ICCM idiopathic congestive cardiomyopathy

ICCU intensive coronary care unit

ICD immune complex disease • inclusion cell disease • induced circular dichroism • instantaneous cardiac death • Institute for Crippled and Disabled • intercanthal distance • internal cervical device • International Classification of Diseases (of World Health Organization) • intracervical device • intrauterine contraceptive device *also* IUCD, IUD • ischemic coronary disease • isocitrate dehydrogenase *also* ICDH • isolated conduction defect

ICDA International Classification of Diseases, Adapted (for use in United States)

ICDC implantable cardioverter/defibrillator catheter

ICDCD International Classification of Diseases and Causes of Death

ICD–CM International Classification of Diseases—Clinical Modification

ICDH isocitrate dehydrogenase *also* ICD • isocitric acid dehydrogenase *also* IDH

ICD–O International Classification of Diseases for Oncology

ICDS Integrated Child Development Scheme

ICE ice, compression, and

elevation · individual career exploration · iridocorneal endothelial (syndrome)

ICES ice, compression, elevation, and support

ICET (Forty–Eight) Item Counseling Evaluation Test

ICF indirect centrifugal flotation · intensive care facility · intercellular fluorescence · interciliary fluid · intermediate care facility · intracellular fluid · intravascular coagulation and fibrinolysis (syndrome)

ICFA incomplete Freund adjuvant *also* IFA · induced complement–fixing antigen

ICF–MR intermediate–care facility (for) mentally retarded

IC fx intracapsular fracture

ICG indocyanine green · isotope cisternography

ICGN immune complex-mediated glomerulonephritis

ICH idiopathic cortical hyperostosis · immunocompromised host · infectious canine hepatitis · intracerebral hematoma · intracerebral hemorrhage · intracerebral hypertension · intracranial hemorrhage · intracranial hypertension

ICHD ischemic coronary heart disease

ICHPPC International Classification of Health Problems in Primary Care

ICI Interpersonal Communication Inventory · intracardiac injection · intracisternal *also* IC

ICIDH International Classification of Impairments, Disabilities, and Handicaps

ICL intracorneal lens

ICM inner cell mass · intercostal margin · intracytoplasmic membrane · ion conductance modulator · ipsilateral competing message

ICN infection control nurse · intensive care neonatal · intensive care nursery · intermediate care nursery

ICNC intracerebellar nuclear cell

ICO impedance cardiac output

I coch intracochlear

ICP incubation period *also* IP · inductively coupled plasma · infection–control practitioner · infectious cell protein · intermittent catheterization protocol · intracranial pressure · intracytoplasmic

↑ICP increased intracranial pressure *also* IICP

ICPMM incisors, canines, premolars, and molars (permanent dentition formula)

ICPP intubated continuous positive–pressure

ICPS Interpersonal Cognitive Problem Solving

ICR (distance between) iliac crests • Institute for Cancer Research • intermittent catheter routine • international calibrated ratio • intracardiac catheter recording • intracranial reinforcement • ion cyclotron resonance

ICRD Index of Codes for Research Drugs

ICRETT International Cancer Research Technology Transfer

ICREW International Cancer Research Workshop

I–CRF immunoreactive corticotropin–releasing factor

ICRS Index Chemicus Registry System

ICRU International Commission on Radiological Units

ICS ileocecal sphincter • immotile cilia syndrome • impulse–conducting system • intensive care, surgical • intercellular space *also* IS • intercostal space *also* IC, IS • intracranial stimulation • irritable colon syndrome

ICSA islet cell surface antibody

ICSC idiopathic central serous chorioretinopathy

ICSH interstitial cell–stimulating hormone

ICSS intracranial self–stimulation

ICT icteric *also* IC • icterus *also* Ict, ict • immunoglobulin consumption test • indirect Coombs test/titer • inflammation (of) connective tissue • insulin coma therapy • insulin convulsive therapy • intensive conventional therapy • intermittent cervical traction *also* ICTX • interstitial cell tumor • intracardiac thrombus • intracranial tumor • intradermal cancer test • intraoral cariogenicity test • isovolumic contraction time *also* IVCT

Ict, ict icterus *also* ICT

ICT immunoreactive calcitonin

Ict Ind icteric index • icterus index *also* II

ICTS idiopathic carpal tunnel syndrome

ICTX intermittent cervical traction *also* ICT

ICU infant care unit • intensive care unit • intermediate care unit

I cut . intracutaneous *also* IC

ICV intracellular volume • intracerebroventricular *also* icv

Icv into cerebral ventricles • intracerebroventricular *also* ICV

ICVH ischemic cerebrovascular headache

ICW intact canal wall • intensive care ward • intercellular water • intracellular water

ICX immune complex

ID identification • identify • iditol dehydrogenase • ill–defined • immunodeficiency • immunodiffusion (test) • immunoglobulin deficiency • inappropriate disability • inclusion disease • index (of) discrimination • individual dose • induction delivery • infant death • infectious disease *also* inf dis • infective dose • inhibitory dose • inhomogeneous deposition • initial diagnosis • initial dose • initial dyskinesia • injected dose • inside diameter • insufficient data • interdigitating (cells) • internal diameter • interstitial disease • intradermal *also* i.d. • intraduodenal • isosorbide dinitrate *also* ISD, ISDN

I&D incision and drainage

ID$_{50}$ median infective dose

Id idiotypic • infradentale • interdentale

Id [L. *idem*] the same

i.d. [L. *in diem*] during the day • intradermal *also* ID

IDA image display and analysis • iminodiacetic acid • insulin–degrading activity • iron–deficiency anemia

Id ac [L. *idem ac*] the same as

IDAMIS Integrated Dose Abuse Management Informational Systems

IDARP Integrated Drug Abuse Reporting Process

IDAT indirect antiglobulin test *also* IAGT, IAT

IDAV immunodeficiency–associated virus

IDBR indirect bilirubin

IDBS infantile diffuse brain sclerosis

IDC idiopathic dilated cardiomyopathy • interdigitating cells

IDCF immunodiffusion complement fixation

IDCI intradiplochromatid interchange

I–D intensity–duration (curve)

IDD insulin–dependent diabetes *also* IDDM

IDDF investigational drug data form

IDDM insulin–dependent diabetes mellitus *also* IDD

IDDS implantable drug delivery system • investigational drug data sheet

IDDT immuno–double diffusion test

IDE inner dental epithelium • Investigational Device Exemption

ID/ED internaldiameter to external diameter (cardiac valve replacement ratio)

IDEM ischemic, drug, electrolyte, metabolic (effect)

IDFC immature dead female child

IDG interdisciplinary group •
intermediate–dose group

IDH isocitric acid
dehydrogenase *also* ICDH

IDH1 isocitrate dehydrogenase,
soluble *also* IDH–S

IDH2, IDH–M isocitrate
dehydrogenase,
mitochondrial

IDH–S isocitrate
dehydrogenase, soluble *also*
IDH1

IDI immunologically detectable
insulin • induction–
delivery interval •
interdentale inferius

IDIC Internal Dose Information
Center

I disk isotropic disk (striated
muscle fiber) *also* I band

IDK internal derangement (of)
knee (joint)

IDL intensity difference
limen • Index to Dental
Literature • intermediate–
density lipoprotein

IDM idiopathic disease of
myocardium • immune
defense mechanism •
indirect method • infant of
diabetic mother •
intermediate–dose
methotrexate

IDMC immature dead male
child • interdigestive
motility complex •
interdigestive motor
complex

IDMEC interdigestive
myoelectric complex *also*
IMC

ID–MS isotope dilution–mass
spectrometry

IDNA intercalary
deoxyribonucleic acid

Idon vehic [L. *idoneo
vehiculo*] in a suitable
vehicle

IDP imidoliphosphonate •
immunodiffusion
procedure • initial dose
period • inosine
diphosphate •
instantaneous diastolic
pressure

IDPase inosine diphosphatase

IDPH idiopathic pulmonary
hemosiderosis *also* IPH

IDPN β–iminodipropionitrile

IDR intradermal reaction

IDS immunity deficiency
state • infectious disease
service • inhibitor of DNA
synthesis • intraduodenal
stimulation •
investigational drug service

IDT immune diffusion test •
instillation delivery time •
interdivision time •
intradermal typhoid (and
paratyphoid vaccine)

IDU idoxuridine • iododeoxyuridine • Ivy dog unit

IdUA iduronic acid

IDUR, IdUrd idoxuridine

IDV intermittent demand
ventilation

IDVC indwelling venous
catheter

Idx cross–reactive idiotype

IE [Ger. *immunitäts Einheit*]

immunizing unit *also* IU,
ImmU • immunoelectro-
phoresis *also* IEP •
induced emesis • infectious
endocarditis • infective
endocarditis • inner ear •
intake energy (unit of
food) • internal ear •
internal elastica •
international unit (European
abbreviation) • intra-
epithelial • Introversion–
Extroversion (scale)

I/E, I:E inspiratory/expiratory
(ratio)

I&E internal and external

ie [L. *id est*] that is

IEA immediate early antigen •
immunoelectroadsorption •
immunoelectrophoretic
analysis • infectious equine
anemia • intravascular
erythrocyte aggregation

IEC injection electrode
catheter • inpatient
exercise center •
intraepithelial carcinoma •
ion–exchange
chromatography

IE Ca cx intraepithelial
carcinoma of cervix

IEE inner enamel epithelium

IEF isoelectric focusing

IEI isoelectric interval

IEL internal elastic lamina •
intimal elastic lamina •
intraepithelial lymphocyte

IEM immunoelectron
microscopy • inborn error
of metabolism

IEMG integrated
electromyogram

IEMT intermediate emergency
medical technician

IEOP immunoelectro–
osmophoresis

IEP immunoelectrophoresis
also IE • individualized
education program •
isoelectric point *also* IP

IER Institute of Educational
Research (intelligence test)

IES ingressive–egressive
sequence

I–E Scale internal versus
external (control of
reinforcement) scale

IF idiopathic fibroplasia •
ifosfamide *also* IFOS,
IFX • immersion foot •
immunofluorescence *also*
IFL • indirect
fluorescence • inferior
facet • infrared *also* IFR,
infra., IR • inhibiting
factor • initiation factor •
inspiratory force •
interferon *also* IFN, INF,
ITF • intermaxillary
fixation *also* IMF •
intermediate filament *also*
IMF • intermediate
frequency • internal
fixation • internal
friction • interstitial fluid
also ISF • intracellular
fluid • intrinsic factor •
involved field

IFA idiopathic fibrosing
alveolitis • immuno-
fluorescent antibody •
immunofluorescent assay •
incomplete Freund adjuvant
also ICFA • indirect
fluorescent antibody •
indirect fluorescent assay

IFAT indirect fluorescent antibody test

IFC inspiratory flow cartridge • intermittent flow centrifugation • intrinsic factor concentrate

IFCL intermittent flow centrifugation leukapheresis

IFCS inactivated fetal calf serum

IFDS isolated follicle– (stimulating hormone) deficiency syndrome

IFE immunofixation electrophoresis • interfollicular epidermis

IFF inner fracture face

IFGS interstitial fluids (and) ground substance

IFI Institutional Functioning Inventory (psychologic test)

IFIX immunofixation

IFL immunofluorescence *also* IF

IFLrA recombinant human leukocyte interferon A

IFM internal fetal monitoring • intrafusal muscle

IFN immunoreactive fibronectin • interferon *also* IF, INF, ITF

IFN–α (human leukocyte) interferon

IFN–β (human fibroblast) interferon

IFN–C partially pure human leukocyte interferon

If nec if necessary

IFOS ifosfamide *also* IF, IFX

IFP inflammatory fibroid polyp • insulin, Kendall compound F (hydrocortisone), and prolactin • intermediate filament protein • intrapatellar fat pad

IFR infrared *also* IF, infra., IR • inspiratory flow rate

IFRA indirect fluorescent rabies antibody (test)

IFRP International Fertility Research Program

IFS interstitial fluid space

IFT immunofluorescence technique • immuno-fluorescence test • International Frequency Tables

IFU interferon unit

IFV interstitial fluid volume *also* ISFV • intracellular fluid volume

IFX ifosfamide *also* IF, IFOS

IG immature granule • immune globulin • immunoglobulin *also* Ig • Inspector General • intragastric *also* ig

I–G insulin–glucagon

Ig immunoglobulin *also* IG

IG immunoreactive human gastrin

Ig intragastric *also* IG

IGA infantile genetic agranulocytosis

IgA immunoglobulin A

IgA1, IgA2 subclasses of immunoglobulin A

IGC intragastric cannula

IGD interglobal distance · isolated gonadotropin deficiency

IgD immunoglobulin D

IgD1, IgD2 subclasses of immunoglobulin D

IGDE idiopathic gait disorders of elderly

IGDM infant of mother with gestational diabetes mellitus

IGE impaired gas exchange

IgE immunoglobulin E

IgE1 subclass of immunoglobulin E

IGF insulin–like growth factor *also* ILGF

IGFET insulated gate field effect transistor

IgG immunoglobulin G

IgG1, IgG2, IgG3, IgG4 sub-classes of immunoglobulin G

IGH idiopathic growth hormone · immunoreactive growth hormone *also* IRGH

IGHD isolated growth hormone deficiency

IGI Institutional Goals Inventory

IGIM immune globulin, intramuscular

IGIV immune globulin, intravenous

IgM immunoglobulin M

IgM1 subclass of immunoglobulin M

IGP intestinal glycoprotein

IgQ immunoglobulin quantitation

IGR immediate generalized reaction · integrated gastrin response · intrauterine growth retardation

IGS inappropriate gonadotropin secretion

IgSC immunoglobulin–secreting cell

IGT impaired glucose tolerance · interpersonal group therapy · intragastric titration

IGTT intravenous glucose tolerance test

IGV intrathoracic gas volume *also* ITGV

IH idiopathic hirsutism · immediate hypersensitivity · incomplete healing · indirect hemagglutination · industrial hygiene · infectious hepatitis · inguinal hernia · inhibiting hormone · in hospital · inner half · inpatient hospital · intermittent heparinization · intracerebral hematoma · iron hematoxylin

IHA idiopathic hyperaldosteronism · immune hemolytic anemia · indirect hemagglutination antibody (test) · infusion hepatic arteriography

IHB incomplete heart block

IHBT incompatible hemolytic blood transfusion

IHBTD incompatible hemolytic blood transfusion disease

IHC idiopathic hemochromatosis • idiopathic hypercalciuria • immobilization hypercalcemia • inner hair cell (of cochlea) • intrahepatic cholestasis

IHCA isocapnic hyperventilation with cold air

IHCP Institute of Hospital and Community Psychiatry

IHD in–center hemodialysis • intraheptic duct(ule) • ischemic heart disease

IHG ichthyosis hystrix gravior

IHGD isolated human growth deficiency

IHH idiopathic hypogonadotropic hypogonadism • infectious human hepatitis

IHHS idiopathic hyperkinetic heart syndrome

IHMS (sodium) isonicotinylhydrazide methanesulfonate

IHO idiopathic hypertrophic osteoarthropathy

IHP idiopathic hypoparathyroidism • idiopathic hypopituitarism • interhospitalization period • inverted hand position

IHPC intrahepatic cholestasis

IHPH intrahepatic portal hypertension

IHPP Intergovernmental Health Project Policy

IHR intrahepatic resistance • intrinsic heart rate

IHRA isocapnic hyperventilation (with) room air

IHS Idiopathic Headache Score • inactivated horse serum • Indian Health Service • infrahyoid strap *also* IS

IHs iris hamartomas

IHSA iodinated human serum albumin

IHSC immunoreactive human skin collagenase

IHSS idiopathic hypertrophic subaortic stenosis

IHT insulin hypoglycemia test • intravenous histamine test • ipsilateral head turning

I5HT intraplatelet serotonin

IHW inner heel wedge

II icterus index *also* ict ind • image intensifier • insurance index • irradiated iodine • roman numeral two

IIA internal iliac artery

IIC integrated ion current

IICP increased intracranial pressure *also* ↑ICP

IICU infant intensive care unit

IID insulin–independent diabetes

IIDM insulin–independent diabetes mellitus

IIE idiopathic ineffective erythropoiesis

IIF immune interferon • indirect immunofluorescence

IIGR ipsilateral instinctive grasp reaction

IIIVC infrahepatic interruption of inferior vena cava

IIME Institute of International Medical Education

IIP idiopathic interstitial pneumonia • idiopathic intestinal pseudo–obstruction • indirect immunoperoxidase • Intra–and Interpersonal (Relations Scale)

IIS intensive immuno-suppression • intermittent infusion sets • International Institute of Stress

IIT ineffective iron turnover • integrated isometric tension

IJ ileojejunal *also* I–J • internal jugular (vein) • intrajejunal

I–J ileojejunal *also* IJ

IJC internal jugular catheter

IJD inflammatory joint disease

IJP inhibitory junction potential • internal jugular pressure

IJR idiojunctional rhythm

IJT idiojunctional tachycardia

IJV internal jugular vein

IK immobilized knee • [Ger. *Immunekörper*] immune body • immunoconglutinin • infusoria killing (unit) *also* IKU • interstitial keratitis

IKE ion kinetic energy

IKI iodine potassium iodide (Lugol solution)

IKU infusoria killing unit *also* IK

IL ileum • iliolumbar • immature lung • inciso-lingual • independent laboratory • insensible (weight) loss • inspiratory loading • intensity level • interleukin • intermediary letter • intestinal lympho-cyte • intralipid • intra-lumbar • intraocular lens

I–L intensity–latency

Il illinium (promethium)

Il intralesional

ILA insulin–like activity

ILa incisolabial

ILB infant, low birth (weight) *also* ILBW

ILBBB incomplete left bundle branch block

ILBW infant, low birth weight *also* ILB

ILC ichthyosis linearis circumflex • incipient lethal concentration

Ilc isoleucine *also* ILE, Ile, Ileu, ISL

ILD interstitial lung disease • ischemic leg disease • ischemic limb disease • isolated lactase deficiency

ILDCSI Individual Learning Disabilities Classroom Screening Instrument

ILE infantile lobar emphysema

ILE, Ile, Ileu isoleucine *also* Ilc, ISL

ILFC immature living female child

ILGF insulin–like growth factor *also* IGF

ILL intermediate lymphocytic lymphoma

Illic lag obturat [L. *illico lagena obturatur*] let the bottle be closed at once

ILM insulin–like material • internal limiting membrane

ILMC immature living male child

ILMI inferolateral myocardial infarct(ion)

ILo iodine lotion

ILP inadequate luteal phase • interstitial lymphocytic pneumonia

ILR irreversible loss rate

ILS idiopathic leucine sensitivity • idiopathic lymphadenopathy syndrome • increase in life span • infrared liver scanner • intralobular sequestration

ILSS integrated life support system • intraluminal somatostatin

ILVEN inflammatory linear verrucal epidermal nevus

IM idiopathic myelofibrosis *also* IMF • immuno-suppression method • *Index Medicus also* Ind Med • indomethacin *also* IMT, IND, INDO • industrial medicine *also* Ind–Med • infection medium • infectious mononucleosis *also*

INFM • inf mono • inner membrane • innocent murmur • inspiratory muscle • intermediate megaloblast • intermetatarsal • internal malleolus • internal mammary (artery) • internal medicine *also* Int Med • internal monitor • intestinal mesenchyme • intramedullary • intramuscular (injection site) • invasive mole

IMA inferior mesenteric artery • Interchurch Medical Assistance • internal mammary artery

IMAA iodinated macroaggregated albumin

IMAC ifosfamide, mesna uroprotection, Adriamycin (doxorubicin), and cisplatin

IMAG internal mammary artery graft

IMAI internal mammary artery implant

IMB intermenstrual bleeding

IMBC indirect maximal breathing capacity

IMC interdigestive migrating complex • interdigestive migrating contraction • interdigestive myoelectric complex *also* IDMEC • intestinal (mucosal) mast cell • intramedullary catheter

IMCU intermediate medical care unit

IMD immunologically mediated disease • inherited metabolic disorder

ImD$_{50}$ immunizing dose sufficient to protect 50% of subjects

IMDC intramedullary metatarsal decompression

IMDD idiopathic midline destructive disease

IME independent medical examination • independent medical examiner • indirect medical education

IMEM improved minimal essential medium

IMEM–HS improved minimal essential medium, hormone supplemented

IMET isometric endurance time

IMF idiopathic myelofibrosis *also* IM • ifosfamide, mesna uroprotection, methotrexate, and fluorouracil • inter-maxillary fixation *also* IF • intermediate filament *also* IF

IMG inferior mesenteric ganglion • internal medicine group (practice)

IMH idiopathic myocardial hypertrophy • indirect microhemagglutination (test)

IMHT indirect microhemagglutination test

IMI imipramine • immunologically measurable insulin • impending myocardial infarction • indirect membrane immuno-fluorescence • inferior myocardial infarction • intermeal interval • intramuscular injection

IMIC International Medical Information Center

IMIG intramuscular immunoglobulin

IML internal mammary lymphoscintigraphy

IMLA, IMLAD intramural left anterior descending (artery)

IMLC incomplete mitral leaflet closure

ImLy immune lysis

IMM inhibitor–containing minimal medium • internal medial malleolus

Immat immaturity/immature

IMMC interdigestive migrating motor complex

Immed immediately

Immobil immobilization/immobilize

ImmU immunizing unit *also* IE, IU

Immun immune/immunity/immunization

Immunol immunology

IMN internal mammary (lymph) node

IMP idiopathic myeloid proliferation • impacted *also* imp, Impx • important *also* imp • impression *also* I, imp • improved *also* imp • incomplete male pseudohermaphroditism • individual Medicaid practitioner • inosine monophosphate (inosinic acid) • Inpatient Multidimensional Psychiatric (scale) • intramembranous particle •

intramuscular (compartment) pressure

Imp impacted *also* IMP, Impx • important *also* IMP • impression *also* I, IMP • improved *also* IMP

IMPA incisal mandibular plane angle

IMPAC Immediate Psychiatric Aid and Referral Center

Imperf imperfect • imperforate

IMPEX immediate postexercise

IMPL impulse

IMPS Inpatient Multidimensional Psychiatric Scale

impvt improvement

Impx impacted *also* IMP, imp

IMR individual medical record • infant mortality rate • infectious mononucleosis receptor • Institute for Medical Research • institution for the metally retarded

IMRAD, IMRD introduction, materials and methods, results, and discussion (formal structure of scientific article)

IMS incurred (in) military service • Indian Medical Service • industrial methylated spirit • integrated medical services

IMSS in–flight medical support system

IMT indomethacin *also* IM, IND, INDO • induced muscular tension • inspiratory muscle training

ImU international milliunit

IMV inferior mesenteric vein • intermittent mandatory ventilation • intermittent mechanical ventilation • isophosphamide, methotrexate, and vincristine

IMVC, IMVIC, imvic indole, methyl red, Voges–Proskauer, and citrate (test)

IMVP idiopathic mitral valve prolapse

IN icterus neonatorum • impetigo neonatorum • incidence • incompatibility number • infantile nephrotic (syndrome) • infundibular nucleus • insulin *also* I, In, INS • intermediate nucleus • interneuron • internist *also* INT • interstitial nephritis • intranasal

In indium • inion • insulin *also* I, IN, INS • inulin

In. inch

In^2 square inch

In^3 cubic inch

INA infectious nucleic acid • inferior nasal artery

INAA instrumental neutron activation analysis

Inac inactive *also* I

INAD infantile neuroaxonal dystrophy • investigational new animal drug

INAH isonicotinic acid hydrazide

INB ischemic necrosis (of) bone

Inbr inbreeding

INC incisal • incision • incomplete *also* inc • inconclusive • incontinent *also* inc • increase *also* inc, incr • inside–the–needle catheter • interstitial nucleus of Cajal

Inc including *also* incl • incorporated

inc incisional • incompatibility • incomplete *also* INC • inconclusive • incontinent *also* INC • increase *also* INC, incr • increment *also* incr • incurred

Inc Ab incomplete abortion

IncB inclusion body *also* IB

INCD infantile nuclear cerebral degeneration

incid [L. *incide*] cut

incl including *also* Inc

Incomp, Incompl incomplete

incont incontinent

inc (R) increase (relative)

incr increase *also* INC, inc • increment *also* inc

INCS incomplete resolution, scan to follow

incur incurable

IND induced • indapamide • indomethacin *also* IM, IMT, INDO • industrial (medicine) *also* indust • investigational new drug

Ind induction (of labor) *also* ind

ind independent *also* I • index *also* I • indicate • indigent • indigo • indirect • induction *also* I, Ind

in d [L. *in dies*] daily • [L. *in die*] in a day

INDEP independent

indic indicated • indication

indig indigestion

INDIV individual

INDM infant (of) nondiabetic mother

Ind Med *Index Medicus also* IM

Ind–Med industrial medicine *also* IM

INDO indomethacin *also* IM, IMT, IND

indust industrial *also* IND

INE infantile necrotizing encephalomyelopathy

INEX inexperienced

in extrem [L. *in extremis*] in the last (hours of life)

INF infant *also* inf • infantile *also* inf • infarction • infected/infection *also* inf, infect., infx • infectious (disease) • infective • inferior *also* inf, infer. • infirmary *also* inf • information • infundibulum (of neurohypophysis) • infused • infusion *also* inf • interferon *also* IF, IFN, ITF • [L. *infunde*] pour in *also* inf

inf infancy • infant *also* INF • infantile *also* INF • infarct • infect • infected/infection *also* INF, infect., infx • inferior *also* INF, infer. • infirmary *also* INF • infusion *also* INF • [L. *infunde*] pour in *also* INF

in f [L. *in fine*] at the end •
finally

inf dis infectious disease *also*
ID

infect. infected/infective/
infection *also* INF, inf, infx

infer. inferior *also* INF, inf

infl inflamed • inflammation
also Inflamm • influence •
influx

Inflamm inflammation/
inflammatory *also* infl

infl proc inflammatory
process

INFM infectious
mononucleosis *also* IM, inf
mono

Inf MI inferior (wall)
myocardial infarction

inf mono infectious
mononucleosis *also* IM,
INFM

info information

infra. infrared *also* IF, IFR, IR

infx infection *also* INF, inf,
infect.

ING inguinal *also* ing •
isotope nephrogram

ing inguinal *also* ING

INH inhalation *also* I, inhal •
isonicotinic acid hydrazide
(isoniazid)

Inh inhaler

inhal inhalation *also* I, INH

INH–G isonicotinoylhydrazone
of D–glucuronic acid
lactone (glyconiazide)

inhib inhibition/inhibiting *also* I

INI intranasal insulin •
intranuclear inclusion
(agent)

inj injection *also* inject. •
injured • injurious •
injury

inject. injection *also* inj

inj enem [L. *injiciatur enema*]
let an enema be injected

INK injury not known

inl inlay

INN International
Nonproprietary Name

innerv innervated •
innervation

INO infantile nephrotic
(syndrome), other (types) •
internuclear
ophthalmoplegia

Ino inosine

INOC, inoc inoculate/
innoculation

inop inoperable

inorg inorganic

Inox inosine, oxidized

INP idiopathic neutropenia

INPAV intermittent negative
pressure–assisted
ventilation *also* INPV

INPEA isopropylnitro-
phenylethanolamine (β–
adrenergic blocker)

INPH iproniazid phosphate

INPRCNS, INPRONS
information processing in
central nervous system

IN–PT inpatient

in pulm [L. *in pulmento*] in
gruel

INPV intermittent negative pressure-(assisted) ventilation *also* INPAV

INQ inferior nasal quadrant

INR international normalized ratio

INREM internal roentgen equivalent man (radiation dose)

INS idiopathic nephrotic syndrome • insulin *also* I, IN, In • insurance *also* ins

ins insertion • insurance *also* INS • insured

INS Ab insulin antibody

insem insemination

insid insidious

insol insoluble *also* I

insp inspiration *also* I, inspir • inspect • inspection

inspir inspiration *also* I, Insp

INST instrumental (delivery)

Inst institute

Inst instrument

insuf, insuff insufficient • insufficiency • insufflation

INT intermediate *also* I, int, Intmd • intermittent *also* int, INTR • intermittent needle therapy • intern *also* int • internal *also* int, intern. • internist *also* IN, int • *p*–iodonitro-tetrazolium

int intact • integral • interest • intermediate *also* I, INT, Intmd • intermittent *also* INT, INTR • intern *also* INT • internal *also* INT, intern. • internist •

interval • intestinal *also* Intest • [L. *intime*] to the innermost

int cib [L. *inter cibos*] between meals *also* ic

INTEG integument

Intern . internal *also* INT, int

Internat international

Intertroch intertrochanteric

Intest intestine/intestinal *also* int

Int/Ext internal/external (rotation)

INTH intrathecal (anesthesia injection) *also* IT, ITh, i–thec

Int hist interval history

Intmd intermediate *also* I, INT, int

Int Med internal medicine *also* I, IM

Int noct [L. *inter noctem*] during the night

Int obst intestinal obstruction *also* IO

INTOX intoxication

INTR intermittent *also* INT, int

Intracal intracalvarium

Int–rot internal rotation *also* IR

Int trx intermittent traction *also* IT

INV inferior nasal vein

Inv invalid • inverse • inversion *also* inver • involuntary *also* invol

Inver inverted • inversion *also* inv

Invest. investigation

invet inveterate

Inv/Ev inversion/eversion

Inv ins inverted insertion

invol involuntary *also* inv

involv [L. *involve*] coat • involvement • involved

IO incisal opening • inferior oblique (eye muscle) • inferior olive • initial opening (pressure) • inside–out (vesicle) • intensive observation • internal os (cervix) • intestinal obstruction *also* int obst • intraocular (pressure)

I&O, I/O in and out • intake and output

Io ionium

IOA inner optic anlage

IOC in our culture • intern on call • intraoperative cholangiogram *also* IOCG

IOCG intraoperative cholangiogram *also* IOC

IOD injured on duty • integrated optical density • interorbital distance

IODM infant of diabetic mother

IOEBT intraoperative electron beam therapy

IOF intraocular fluid

IOFB intraocular foreign body

IOFNA intraoperative fine needle aspiration

IOH idiopathic orthostatic hypotension

IOI intraosseous infusion

IOL intraocular lens

IOLI intraocular lens implantation

IOM Institute of Medicine

IOML infraorbitomeatal line

ION ischemic optic neuropathy

IOP intraocular pressure

IOR index of response • information outflow rate

I or I illness or injuries

IORT intraoperative radiation therapy

IOS intraoperative sonography

IOT intraocular tension • intraocular transfer • ipsilateral optic tectum

IOTA information overload testing aid

iota (I, ι) ninth letter of Greek alphabet

IOU intensive (therapy) observation unit • international opacity unit

IOV initial office visit

IP icterus praecox • iliopsoas (muscle) • immune precipitate • immunoblastic plasma • immunoperoxidase • implantation (test) • inactivated pepsin • incisoproximal • incisopulpal • incontinentia pigmenti • incubation period *also* ICP • individualized plan • induced potential • induction period • industrial population • infection prevention • infundibular process • infundibulopelvic (ligament) • infusion pump • initial pressure •

inorganic phosphate • inosine phosphorylase • inpatient • in plaster • instantaneous pressure • Institut Pasteur • International Pharmacopoeia • interpeduncular (nucleus) • interphalangeal (joint, keratosis) *also* IPH • interpharyngeal • interpositus (nucleus) • interpupillary • intestinal pseudo–obstruction • intracellular proteolysis • intraperitoneal • ionization potential • isoelectric point *also* IEP • isoproterenol *also* IPT, IS, ISO, iso, ISP

IPA incontinentia pigmenti achromians • independent practice association • indole, pyruvic acid • intrapulmonary artery • isopropyl alcohol • invasive pulmonary aspergillosis

IPAO insulin–induced peak acid output

IPAR Institute of Personality Assessment and Research

I–para primipara *also* P, para I, primip

IPAT (Cattell's) Institute for Personality and Ability Testing (Anxiety Scale) • Iowa Pressure Articulation Test

IPB infrapopliteal bypass

IPC interpeduncular cistern • ion–pair chromatography • isopropyl chlorophenyl • isopropyl phenyl carbamate (propham)

IPCD infantile polycystic disease

IPCS intrauterine progesterone contraceptive system

IPD immediate pigment darkening • increase (in) pupillary diameter • incurable problem drinker • inflammatory pelvic disease • intermittent peritoneal dialysis • intermittent pigment darkening • interpupillary distance • Inventory of Psychosocial Development

IPE infectious porcine encephalomyelitis • initial psychiatric development • injury pulmonary edema • interstitial pulmonary emphysema

IPEH intravascular papillary endothelial hyperplasia

IPF idiopathic pulmonary fibrosis • infection–potentiating factor • International Primary Factors (Test Battery) • interstitial pulmonary fibrosis

IPFD intrapartum fetal distress

IPG impedance phlebograph • impedance plethysmography • inspiratory phase gas

IPGE immunoreactive prostaglandin E

IPH idiopathic portal hypertension • idiopathic pulmonary hemosiderosis *also* IDPH • infant passive hand • inflammatory papillary hyperplasia • interphalangeal (joint) *also* IP • intraparenchymal hemorrhage

IPHR inverted polypoid hamartoma (of) rectum

IPI Imagined Process Inventory • interphonemic interval • interpulse interval

IPIA immunoperoxidase infectivity assay

IPJ interphalangeal joint

IPK interphalangeal keratosis • intractable plantar keratosis

IPKD infantile polycystic kidney disease

IPL inner plexiform layer • interpupillary line • intrapleural

IPM impulses per minute • inches per minute • infant passive mitt

IPMI inferoposterior myocardial infarct(ion)

IPN infantile periarteritis nodosa • interim progress note • interpeduncular nucleus • interpenetrating polymer network

IPn interstitial pneumonitis

IPNA isopropylnoradrenaline (isoproterenol)

IPO improved pregnancy outcome • initial planning option

IPOF immediate postoperative fitting

IPOP immediate postoperative prosthesis

IPP independent practice plan • inferior point (of) pubic (bone) • inflatable penile prosthesis • inorganic pyrophosphate

also PPi, PP_i • inosine, pyruvate, and (inorganic) phosphate • intermittent positive pressure • intrahepatic portal pressure • intrapleural pressure

IPPA inspection, palpation, percussion, and auscultation

IPPB intermittent positive–pressure breathing

IPPB/I intermittent positive–pressure breathing/inspiratory

IPPB(R,V) intermittent positive–pressure breathing (respiration, ventilation)

IPPF immediate postoperative prosthetic fitting

IPPI interruption (of) pregnancy (for) psychiatric indication

IPPO intermittent positive–pressure (inflation with) oxygen

IPPR integrated pancreatic polypeptide response • intermittent positive–pressure respiration

IPPT Inter–Person Perception Test

IPPUAD immediate postprandial upper abdominal distress

IPPV intermittent positive–pressure ventilation

IPQ Intermediate Personality Questionnaire (for Indian Pupils) • intimacy potential quotient

IPR independent professional review • insulin production

rate • interval patency
rate • intraparenchymal
resistance • iproniazid

I–Pr isopropyl– (prefix
denoting 1–methylethyl
group)

IPRL isolated perfused rabbit
lung • isolated perfused rat
liver

IPRT interpersonal reaction
test

IPS idiopathic postprandial
syndrome • impulse per
second • infundibular
pulmonary stenosis • initial
prognostic score •
intermittent photic
stimulation (electroen-
cephalography) •
Interpersonal Perception
Scale • intraperitoneal
shock • ischiopubic
synchondrosis • *p*–
iodophenylsulfonyl (pipsyl)

Ips inches per second

IPSB intrapartum stillbirth

IPSC inhibitory postsynaptic
current

IPSF immediate postsurgical
fitting (of prosthesis)

IPSID immunoproliferative
small intestinal disease

IPSP inhibitory postsynaptic
potential

IPT immunoperoxidase
technique • immuno-
precipitation • intermittent
pelvic traction *also* IPTX •
interpersonal
psychotherapy •
ipratropium • isoproterenol
also IP, IS, ISO, iso, ISP

IPTG isopropylthiogalactoside

IPTH immunoreactive
parathyroid hormone

IPTX intermittent pelvic
traction *also* IPT

IPU inpatient unit

IPV inactivated poliomyelitis
(virus) vaccine •
inactivated polio vaccine •
inactived poliovirus
vaccine • incompetent
perforator vein • infectious
pustular vaginitis •
infectious pustular
vulvovaginitis (of cattle) •
intrapulmonary vein

IPVC interpolated premature
ventricular contraction

IPVD index of pulmonary
vascular disease

IPW interphalangeal width

IPZ insulin–protamine zinc

IQ intelligence quotient

Iq [L. *idem quod*] the same as

IQ&S iron, quinine, and
strychnine

IR ileal resection • immune
response *also* Ir •
immunization rate •
immunologic response •
immunoreactive *also* ir •
immunoreagent • index of
response • individual
reaction • inferior rectus
(muscle) • infrared *also* IR,
IFR, infra. • inside
radius • insoluble residue •
inspiratory reserve •
inspiratory resistance •
insulin receptor • insulin
requirement • insulin
resistance • insulin
response • integer ratio •
intelligence ratio • internal

reduction • internal resistance • internal rotation *also* int–rot • inversion recovery • inverted repeats • irritant reaction • isovolumetric relaxation

I–R Ito–Reenstierna (reaction, test)

I&R insertion and removal

Ir immune response (genes) *also* IR • iridium

Ir immunoreactive *also* IR • intrarectal • intrarenal

IRA immunoradioassay • immunoregulatory α–globulin • inactive renin activity

IR–ACTH immunoreactive adrenocorticotropic hormone

IRA–EEA ileorectal anastomosis with end–to–end anastomosis

IRB institutional review board

IRBBB incomplete right bundle–branch block

IRBC immature red blood cell *also* iRBC • infected red blood cell

IRBC immature red blood cell *also* IRBC

IRBP interphotoreceptor retinoid–binding protein

IRC indirect radionuclide cystography • infrared coagulator • inspiratory reserve capacity • instantaneous resonance curve • International Red Cross

IRCA intravascular red cell aggregation

IRCS International Research Communications System

IRCU intensive respiratory care unit

IRD isorhythmic dissociation

IRDS idiopathic respiratory distress syndrome • infant respiratory distress syndrome

IRE internal rotation in extension

IRF idiopathic retroperitoneal fibrosis • internal rotation (in) flexion

IRG immunoreactive gastrin • immunoreactive glucagon *also* IRGl • immunoreactive glucose

IRGH immunoreactive growth hormone *also* IGH

IRGl immunoreactive glucagon *also* IRG

IRH Institute for Research in Hypnosis • Institute of Religion and Health • intraretinal hemorrhage

IRHC immunoradioassayable human chorionic (somatomammotropin)

IRhCG immunoreactive human chorionic gonadotropin

IRHCS immunoradioassayable human chorionic somatomammotropin

IRhCS immunoreactive human chorionic somatomammotropin

IRhGH immunoreactive human growth hormone

IRhPL immunoreactive human placental lactogen

IRI immunoreactive insulin · insulin radioimmunoassay · insulin resistance index

IRIA indirect radioimmunoassay

Irid iridescent

IRI/G ratio of immunoreactive insulin to serum or plasma glucose

IRIg insulin–reactive immunoglobulin

IRIS interleukin regulation (of) immune system · International Research Information Service

IRM innate releasing mechanism

IRMA immunoradiometric assay · intraretinal microangiopathy · intraretinal microvascular abnormalities

IRNA immune ribonucleic acid · informational ribonucleic acid

IROS ipsilateral routing of signal

IRP immunoreactive plasma · immunoreactive proinsulin · incus replacement prosthesis · inhibitor (of) radical processes · insulin–releasing polypeptide · International Reference Preparation

IRR infrared refractometry · intrarenal reflux · irritation *also* Irr, irr

Irr, irr irradiation · irritation *also* IRR

Irreg irregularity · irregular

IRRIG, IRRG irrigate · irrigation

IRS immunoreactive secretin · infrared spectrophotometry · insulin receptor species

IRSA idiopathic refractory sideroblastic anemia · iodinated rat serum albumin

IRT immunoreactive trypsin · immunoreactive trypsinogen · instrument retrieval container · interresponse time · isometric relaxation time · item response theory (psychologic testing)

IRTO immunoreactive trypsin output

IRTU integrating regulatory transcription unit

IRU industrial rehabilitation unit · interferon reference unit

IRV inferior radicular vein · inspiratory reserve volume · inverse–ratio ventilation

IS ilial segment · immediate sensitivity · immune serum · immuno-suppression · incentive spirometer · index (of) saponification · index (of) sexuality · induced sputum · infant size · information system · infrahyoid strap *also* IHS · initial segment · [L. *in situ*] in original place · insertion sequence · insulin secretion · intercellular space *also* ICS · intercostal space *also* IC, ICS • interictal spike (in electroencephalography) • internal standard • interspace *also* i.s., ISP • interstitial space • interventricular septum *also* IVS • intracardial shunt • intraspinal • intrasplenic • intrastriatal • invalided (from) service • inventory (of) systems • Ionescu–Shiley (artificial cardiac valve) *also* I–S • ipecac syrup • Irvine syndrome • ischemic score • island *also* is. • isoproterenol *also* IP, IPT, ISO, iso, ISP

I–S Ionescu–Shiley (artificial cardiac valve) *also* IS

I–10–S invert sugar (10%) in saline

Is. island *also* IS • islet • isolation

I.s. in situ • interspace *also* IS, ISP

ISA intrinsic stimulating activity • intrinsic sympathomimetic activity • iodinated serum albumin • irregular spiking activity (in electroencephalography)

ISA₅ internal surface area of lung at volume of five liters

ISADH inappropriate secretion of antidiuretic hormone

IS and R information storage and retrieval *also* ISR

ISB incentive spirometry breathing

ISC immunoglobulin–secreting cell • insoluble collagen • intensive supportive care • International Statistical

Classification • intershift coordination • interstitial cell • intersystem crossing • irreversibly sickled cell • Isolette servo control

ISCCO intersterno-costoclavicular ossification

ISCF interstitial cell fluid

ISCN International System for (Human) Cytogenetic Nomenclature

ISCP infection surveillance and control program

ISCs irreversible sickle cells

ISD immunosuppressive drug • inhibited sexual desire • initial sleep disturbance • intensity (of service), severity (of illness), discharge (screens) • interatrial septal defect *also* IASD • interventricular septal defect *also* IVSD • isosorbide dinitrate *also* ISDN

ISDB indirect self–destructive behavior

ISDN isosorbide dinitrate *also* ID, ISD

ISE inhibited sexual excitement • integrated square error • ion–selective electrode

ISED Interview Schedule for Events and Difficulties

ISF interstitial fluid *also* IF

ISFET ion–specific field effect transducer

ISFV interstitial fluid volume *also* IFV

ISG immune serum globulin

ISH icteric serum hepatitis • isolated systolic hypertension

ISI infarct size index • initial slope index • injury severity index • International Sensitivity Index • International Slope index • interstimulus interval

ISIH interspike interval histogram

ISL interscapular line • inter-spinous ligament • iso-leucine *also* Ilc, ILE, Ile, Ileu

ISM intersegmental muscle

ISMA infantile spinal muscular atrophy

ISO International Standards Organization • isoproterenol *also* IP, IPT, IS, iso, ISP • isotropic *also* iso

Iso, iso isoproterenol *also* IP, IPT, IS, ISO, ISP • isotropic *also* ISO

Isol Isolette

Isol isolation/isolated

Is of Lang islands/islets of Langerhans

Isom isometric • isometrophic

IsoRAS isorenin–angiotensin system

Isox isoxsuprine

ISP distance between iliac spines • immunoreactive substance P • interspace *also* IS, i.s. • interspinal • intraspinal • isoproterenol *also* IP, IPT, IS, ISO, iso

ISPT interspecies (ovum) penetration test

ISPX Ionescu–Shiley pericardial xenograft

Isq [L. *in status quo*] unchanged

ISR information storage (and) retrieval *also* IS and R • Institute for Sex Research • Institute of Surgical Research • insulin secretion rate

ISS Injury Severity Scale • ion–scattering spectroscopy • ion surface scattering

IST insulin sensitivity test • insulin shock therapy • interstitiospinal tract • isometric systolic tension

ISTD insulin standard

I–sub inhibitor substance

ISW interstitial water

ISWI incisional surgical wound infection

ISY intrasynovial

IT iliotibial • immunity test • immunologic test • immunotherapy • implantation test • individual therapy • inferior temporal • inferior turbinate • information technology • inhalation test • inhalation therapist/ therapy • inspiratory time *also* I–time • insulin treatment • intact • intensive therapy • intentional tremor • intermittent traction *also* int trx • internal thoracic • interstitial tissue •

intertrochanteric • intertuberous (pelvic diameter) • intimal thickening • intolerance (and) toxicity • intracellular tachyzoite • intradermal test • intratesticular • intrathecal (anesthesia injection) *also* INTH, ITh, i–thec • intrathoracic • intratracheal *also* ITR • intratracheal tube • intratumoral *also* i–tumor • ischial tuberosity • isomeric transition (of radioactive isotopes)

I/T intensity/time (duration of contractions)

I–time inspiratory time *also* IT

ITA individual treatment assessment • inferior temporal artery • itaconic acid

ITAG internal thoracic artery graft

ITB iliotibial band

ITC imidazolyl–thioguanine chemotherapy • incontinence treatment center • Interagency Testing Committee

ITc International Table calorie

ITCP idiopathic thrombocytopenia purpura *also* ITP

ITCU intensive thoracic cardiovascular unit

ITCVD ischemic thrombotic cerebrovascular disease

ITD insulin–treated diabetic

ITE insufficient therapeutic effect • in the ear (hearing aid) • intrapulmonary interstitial emphysema

ITET isotonic endurance test

ITF interferon *also* IF, IFN, INF

ITFF intertrochanteric femoral fracture

ITFS iliotibial tract friction syndrome • incomplete testicular feminization syndrome

ITGV intrathoracic gas volume *also* IGV

ITh, i–thec intrathecal (anesthesia injection) *also* INTH, IT

ITI intertrial interval

ITLC instant thin–layer chromatography

ITLC–SG instant thin–layer chromatography—silica gel

ITM improved Thayer–Martin (medium) • intrathecal methotrexate

ITOU intensive therapy observation unit

ITP idiopathic thrombo-cytopenic purpura *also* ITCP • immunogenic thrombocytopenic purpura • inosine triphosphate • interim treatment plan • islet–cell tumor of the pancreas

ITPA Illinois Test of Psycholinguistic Abilities • inosine triphosphatase *also* ITPase

ITPase inosine triphosphatase *also* ITPA

ITQ Infant Temperament Questionnaire • inferior temporal quadrant

ITR intraocular tension recorder • intratracheal *also* IT

ITSC It Scale for Children (psychologic test)

ITSHD isolated thyroid stimulating hormone deficiency

ITT identical twins (raised) together • iliotibial tract • insulin tolerance test • internal tibial torsion • iron tolerance test

ITU intensive therapy unit

I–tumor intratumoral *also* IT

ITV inferior temporal vein

ITVAD indwelling transcutaneous vascular access device

ITX intertriginous xanthoma

ITyr monoiodotryrosine

IU immunizing unit *also* IE, ImmU • International Unit • intrauterine • in utero • indouracil

[I]U concentration of insulin in urine

Iu infectious unit

IUA intrauterine adhesion

IUC idiopathic ulcerative colitis • intrauterine catheter

IUCD intrauterine contraceptive device *also* ICD, IUD

IUD intrauterine death • intrauterine device *also* ICD, IUCD

IUDR idoxuridine • iododeoxyuridine

IUF isolated ultrafiltration

IUFB intrauterine foreign body

IUFD intrauterine fetal death • intrauterine fetal demise • intrauterine fetal distress

IUFGR intrauterine fetal growth retardation

IUG infusion urogram • intrauterine gestation • intrauterine growth

IUGR intrauterine growth rate • intrauterine growth retardation

IUI intrauterine insemination

IU/L International Unit per liter

IUM internal urethral meatus • intrauterine (fetally) malnourished • intrauterine malnourishment • intrauterine membrane

IU/min International Unit per minute

IUP intrauterine pregnancy • intrauterine pressure

IUPC intrauterine pressure catheter

IUPD intrauterine pregnancy, delivered

IUP,TBCS intrauterine pregnancy, term birth, cesarean section

IUP,TBLC intrauterine pregnancy, term birth, living child

IUP,TBLI intrauterine pregnancy, term birth, living infant

IUR intrauterine retardation

IUT intrauterine transfusion

IV ichthyosis vulgaris • interventricular • intervertebral • intravascular • intravenous • intraventricular *also* IVT • intravertebral • invasive • in vitro • in vivo • iodine value *also* iv • class 4 controlled substances

Iv iodine value *also* IV

IVAC intravenous accurate control (device)

IVAD implantable vascular access device

IVag intravaginal

IVAP in vivo adhesive platelet

IVAR insulin variable

IVB intraventricular block • intravitreal blood

IVBAT intravascular bronchioalveolar tumor

IVBC intravascular blood coagulation

IVC individually viable cell • inferior vena cava • inferior venacavagram/ venacavagraphy *also* IVCV • inspiratory vital capacity • inspired vital capacity • integrated vector control • intravascular coagulation • intravenous cholangiogram/ cholangiography *also* IVCh • intraventricular catheter • isovolumic contraction

IVCC intravascular consumption coagulopathy

IVCD intraventricular conduction defect • intraventricular conduction delay

IVCh intravenous cholangiogram/ cholangeography *also* IVC

IVCP inferior vena cava pressure

IVCT inferior vena cava thrombosis • intravenously (enhanced) computed tomography • isovolumic contraction time *also* ICT

IVCV inferior venacavagram/ venacavography *also* IVC

IVD intervertebral disk • intravenous drip

IVDA intravenous drug abuse(r)

IVDSA intravenous digital subtraction angiography

IVDU intravenous drug (use)

IVF interventricular foramen • intravascular fluid • intravenous fluid • in vitro fertilization • in vivo fertilization

IVFE intravenous fat emulsion

IVF–ET in vitro fertilization– embryo transfer

IVFT intravenous fetal transfusion

IVG isotopic ventriculogram

IVGTT intravenous glucose tolerance test

IVH intravenous hyperalimentation • intraventricular hemorrhage

IVIG intravenous immune globulin • intravenous immunoglobulin

IVJC intervertebral joint complex

IVL intravenous lock

IVLBW infant of very low birth weight

IVM immediate visual memory • intravascular mass

IVMP intravenous methylprednisolone

IVN intravenous nutrition

IVNF intravitreal neovascular frond

IVOX intravascular oxygenator

IVP intravenous push (dose) *also* IVp, IVPU • intravenous pyelogram/ pyelography • intraventricular pressure • intravesical pressure

IVp intravenous push (dose) *also* IVP, IVPU

IVPB intravenous piggyback (drug administration)

IVPD in vitro protein digestibility

IVPF isovolume pressure flow (curve)

IVPU intravenous push (dose) *also* IVP, IVp

IVR idioventricular rhythm • internal visual reference • intravaginal ring • isolated volume responder • isovolumic relaxation (time) *also* IVRT

IVRT isovolumic relaxation time *also* IVR

IVS inappropriate vasopressin secretion • intact ventricular septum • intervening sequence • interventricular septum *also* IS • intervillous space • irritable voiding syndrome

IVSD interventricular septal defect *also* ISD

IVSE interventricular septal excursion

IVT index (of) vertical transmission • intravenous transfusion • intraventricular *also* IV • isovolumic time

IVTTT intravenous tolbutamide tolerance test

IVU intravenous urogram/ urography

IVV influenza virus vaccine • intravenous vasopressin

IW inner wall

I–5–W invert sugar 5% in water

IWI inferior wall infarction • interwave interval

IWL insensible water loss

IWMI inferior wall myocardial infarct(ion)

IWML idiopathic white matter lesion

IWS Index of Work Satisfaction

IYS inverted Y–suspensor

IZ infarction zone

IZS insulin zinc suspension

J dynamic movement of inertia • electric current density • Jewish • joint *also* jnt, jt • joule • Joule's equivalent • journal *also* jour, jrl, jrnl • juice *also* j, jc • juvenile *also* juv • juxtapulmonary–capillary (receptor) • magnetic polarization • polypeptide chain in polymeric immuno-globulins • reference point following QRS complex, at beginning of ST segment • sound intensity

J flux (density)

J1, J2, J3, etc. Jaeger test type number 1, 2, 3, etc

j jaundice *also* jaund, JD • juice *also* J, jc

JA juvenile atrophy • juxta–articular

JAI juvenile amaurotic idiocy

JAMG juvenile autoimmune myasthenia gravis

JAS Jenkins Activity Survey (psychologic test) • Job Attitude Scale

jaund jaundice *also* j, JD

JBC Jesness Behavior Checklist

JBE Japanese B encephalitis

JC Jakob–Creutzfeldt (syndrome) • joint contracture • junior clinician

J/C joule per coulomb

jc juice *also* J, j

JCA juvenile chronic arthritis

JCAH Joint Commission on Accreditation of Hospitals

JCAHO Joint Commission on Accreditation of Healthcare Organizations

JCF juvenile calcaneal fracture

JCL job control language (computers)

JCML juvenile chronic myelocytic/myelogenous leukemia

JCP juvenile chronic polyarthritis

jct junction

JCV Jamestown Canyon virus

JD Janet disease • jaundice *also* j, jaund • jejunal diverticulitis • jugulodigastric (node) • juvenile delinquent • juvenile–onset diabetes *also* JDM, JOD, JODM

JDM juvenile–onset diabetes mellitus *also* JD, JOD, JODM

JDMS juvenile dermatomyositis

JE Japanese encephalitis • junctional escape

JEE Japanese equine encephalitis

JEJ, Jej, jej jejunum

JEMBEC agar plates for transporting cultures of gonococci

jentac [L. *jentaculum*] breakfast

JEPI Junior Eysenck Personality Inventory

JER Japanese erection ring · junctional escape rhythm

JEV Japanese encephalitis virus

JF joint fluid · jugular foramen · junctional fold

JFET junction field–effect transistor

JFS Jewish Family Service · jugular foramen syndrome

JG June grass (test) · juxtaglomerular *also* jg, j–g

jg, j–g juxtaglomerular *also* JG

JGA juxtaglomerular apparatus

JGC juxtaglomerular cell

JGCT juxtaglomerular cell tumor

JGI jejunogastric intussusception · juxtaglomerular granulation index · juxtaglomerular index

JGP juvenile general paralysis

JH juvenile hormone (of insects)

J_H heat transfer factor

JHA juvenile hormone analog

JHMO Junior Hospital Medical Officer

JHMV J Howard Mueller virus

JHR Jarisch–Herxheimer reaction

JI jejunoileal (bypass) · jejunoileitis · jejunoileostomy

JIB jejunoileal bypass

JIH joint interval histogram

JIS juvenile idiopathic scoliosis

JJ jaw jerk · jejunojejunostomy

JKD Junius–Kuhnt disease

J/kg joule per kilogram

JKST Johnson–Kenney Screening Test (psychologic test)

JL Jadassohn–Lewanowski (syndrome) · Jaffe–Lichtenstein (syndrome)

JLP juvenile laryngeal papilloma

JM josamycin · jugomaxillary

J_M mass transfer factor (in heat transfer)

JMD juvenile macular degeneration

JMH John Milton Hagen (antibody)

JMR Jones–Mote reactivity

JMS junior medical student

JND just noticeable difference

jnt joint *also* J

JOD juvenile–onset diabetes *also* JD, JDM, JODM

JODM juvenile–onset diabetes mellitus *also* JD, JDM, JOD

JOMAC judgment, orientation, memory, abstraction, and calculaltion

JOMACI judgment, orientation, memory, abstraction, and calculation intact

jour journal *also* J, jrl, jml

JP Jackson–Pratt (drain) • Jobst pump • joint protection *also* JTP • juvenile periodontitis

JPB junctional premature beat

JPC junctional premature contraction

JPD juvenile plantar dermatosis

JPI Jackson Personality Inventory

JPS joint position sense

JR Jolly reaction • junctional rhythm

JRA juvenile rheumatoid arthritis

jrl journal *also* J, jour, jml

JRAN junior resident admission note

Jr BF junior baby food

JRC joint replacement center

J receptor juxtapulmonary–capillary receptor

jrnl journal *also* J, jour, jrl

JS jejunal segment • Job syndrome • junctional slowing • Junkman–Schoeller (unit of thyrotropin)

J/s joule per second

JSI Jansky Screening Index (psychologic test)

JSU, JS unit Junkman–Schoeller unit (of thyrotropin)

JSV Jerry–Slough virus

JT jejunostomy tube

J/T joule per tesla

jt joint *also* J, jnt

jt asp joint aspiration

JTF jejunostomy tube feeding

JTP joint protection *also* JP

JTPS juvenile tropical pancreatitis syndrome

Ju jugale

jug. jugular

jug. comp jugular compression (test)

junct junction *also* Jx

juv juvenile *also* J

juxt [L. *juxta*] near

JV jugular vein • jugular venous (pressure, pulse)

JVC jugular venous catheter

JVD jugular venous distention

JVIS Jackson Vocational Interest Survey

JVP jugular vein pulse • jugular venous pressure • jugular venous pulse

JVPT jugular venous pulse tracing

JW Jehovah's Witness • jump walker

Jx junction *also* junct

JXG juvenile xanthogranuloma

K burst of diphasic slow waves in response to stimuli during sleep (in electroencephalography) • [Gr. *kalyx* cup] calix • [Ger. *Kapsel*, capsule] capsular antigen • carrying capacity (genetics) • cathode • coefficient of heat transfer • coefficient of scleral rigidity • cretaceous • dissociation constant • electron capture • electrostatic capacity • equilibrium constant • ionization constant • kalium (potassium) • kallikrein inhibiting unit • kanamycin *also* KM • Kell blood system • Kell factor • kelvin (SI fundamental unit of temperature) • keratometer • kerma • ketotifen • kidney • killer (cell) • kilo– *also* k • kilopermeability coefficient • kinetic energy *also* KE • knee *also* Kn, kn • lysine • modulus of compression • motor coordination (in General Aptitude Test Battery) • phylloquinone *also* K_1 • 1024 (number of bytes in kilobyte) • [L. *kalium*] potassium *also* Kal • ratio of curvature of flattest meridian of apical cornia (in fitting of contact lens) • one thousand *also* kilo • vitamin K

°K degree on the Kelvin scale (obsolete, now K)

K_1 phylloquinone *also* K

K–10 gastric tube

K

17K, 17–K 17–ketosteroid *also* 17–Keto, 17–KS

^{40}K radioactive potassium isotope

^{42}K radioactive potassium isotope

^{43}K radioactive potassium isotope

K_3 menadione

K_4 menadiol sodium diphosphate

k Boltzmann constant • constant • kilo– *also* K • rate of velocity constant • reaction rate constant

k magnetic susceptibility

KA alkaline phosphatase *also* AKP, ALK–P, alk phos, alk p'tase, ALP, AP • kainic acid • keratoacanthoma • keto acid • ketoacidosis • King–Armstrong (unit) *also* KA, KAU • kynurenic acid

K–A King–Armstrong (unit) *also* KA, KAU

K/A ketogenic/antiketogenic (ratio)

Ka cathode (kathode) • kallikrein

K_a acid ionization (dissociation) constant

kA kiloampere

KAAD kerosene, alcohol, acetic acid, and dioxane (mixture)

KAB knowledge, attitude, and behavior

KABC Kaufman Assessment Battery for Children

KABINS knowledge, attitude, behavior, and improvement in nutritional status

KAF conglutinogen–activating factor · killer–assisting factor · kinase–activating factor

KAFO knee–ankle–foot orthosis

Kal [L. *kalium*] potassium *also* K

KAO knee–ankle orthosis

KAP knowledge, aptitudes, (and) practices (fertility)

kappa (K, κ) tenth letter of Greek alphabet

κ magnetic susceptibility · one of two immunoglobulin light chains

KAS Katz Adjustment Scales (psychologic test)

KASH knowledge, abilities, skills, (and) habits

KAST Kindergarten Auditory Screening Test

KAT kanamycin acetyltransferase

kat katal (enzyme unit of measurement)

kat/L katal per liter

KAU King–Armstrong unit *also* KA, K–A

KB human oral epidermoid carcinoma cells · Kashin–Bek (disease) · ketone body · kilobyte · knee brace · knuckle–bender (splint)

K–B Kleihauer–Betke (test)

K/B knee–bearing (prosthesis)

K$_b$ base ionization constant · dissociation constant of a base

kb kilobase

kbp kilobase pair (nucleic acid molecules)

kBq kilobecquerel

KBr potassium bromide

KBS Klüver–Bucy syndrome

KC cathodal (kathodal) closing · keratoconus · keratoma climacterium · keratoconjunctivitis · knees to chest · knuckle cracking · Kupffer cell

kC kilocoulomb

kc kilocycle

K Cal, Kcal, kcal kilocalorie

KCC cathodal (kathodal) closing contraction *also* KSK · Kulchitzky cell carcinoma

KCCT kaolin–cephalin clotting time

K cell killer cell

KCG kinetocardiogram

kCi kilocurie

K complex slow waves related to sleep arousal (in electroencephalography)

kcps kilocycle per second *also* kc/sec, kc/s

KCS keratoconjunctivitis sicca

kc/sec, kc/s kilocycle per second *also* kcps

KCT, KCTe cathodal (kathodal) closing tetanus *also* KST

KD cathodal (kathodal) duration • Kawasaki disease • kidney donor • killed • knee disarticulation • knitted Dacron

K_d dissociation constant • distribution coefficient • partition coefficient

kd kilodalton *also* kdal

KDA known drug allergies

kdal kilodalton *also* kd

KDC cathodal (kathodal) duration contraction

KDO ketodeoxyoctonate • ketodeoxyoctonic acid

KDP potassium dihydrogen phosphate

KDS Kaufman Development Scale

KDSM keratinizing desquamative squamous metaplasia

KDT, KDTe cathodal (kathodal) duration tetanus

kdyn kilodyne

KE Kendall compound E (cortisone) • kinetic energy *also* K

K_e exchangeable body potassium

KED Kendrick extrication device

Kemo Tx chemical therapy (chemotherapy)

Kera keratitis

KERV Kentucky equine respiratory virus

keto 17–kerosteroid (test)

17–Keto 17–ketosteroids *also* 17–K, 17–KS

kev, keV kiloelectron volt

KF Kenner–fecal (medium) • kidney function • Klippel–Feil (syndrome)

kf flocculation rate in antigen–antibody reaction

KFAB kidney–fixing antibody

K factor γ–ray dose (roentgens per hour at 1 cm from 1–mCi point source of radiation)

KFAO knee–foot–ankle orthosis

KFD Kinetic Family Drawing • Kyasanur forest disease

KFR Kayser–Fleischer ring

KFS Klippel–Feil syndrome

kG kilogauss

kg kilogram *also* kilo

KG–1 Koeffler Golde–1 (cell line)

KGC Keflin (cephalothin), gentamicin, and carbenicillin

kg–cal kilogramcalorie

KGHT kidney Goldblatt hypertension

kg/cm² kilogram per square centimeter

KGDHC ketoglutarate dehydrogenase complex

kgf kilogram–force

kg/L kilogram per liter

kg–m kilogram–meter

kg–m/s² kilogram–meter per second squared

Kgn kininogen

kg/s, kgps kilogram per second

KGS ketogenic steroid

17–KGS 17–ketogenic steroid

KH Krebs–Henseleit (cycle)

K24H potassium in 24–hour urine

KHB Krebs–Henseleit bicarbonate

KHb potassium hemoglobinate *also* K hgb

KHC kinetic hemolysis curve

KHD kinky hair disease

KHF Korean hemorrhagic fever

K hgb potassium hemoglobinate *also* KHb

KHM keratoderma hereditaria mutilans

KHN Knoop hardness number (of solids)

KHS kinky hair syndrome · Krebs–Henseleit solution

kHz kilohertz

KI karyopyknotic index *also* KPI · knee immobilizer · Krönig isthmus

K$_i$ dissociation of enzyme–inhibitor complex · inhibition constant

KIA Kligler iron agar (medium)

KIC ketoisocaproate · ketoisocaproic acid

KICB killed intracellular bacteria

KID keratitis, ichthyosis, (and) deafness (syndrome)

KIDS Kent Infant Development Scale

kilo kilogram *also* kg · kilometer *also* km · one thousand *also* K

KIMSA Kirsten murine sarcoma (virus)

KIMSV, Ki–MSV Kirsten murine sarcoma virus

KIP key intermediary protein

KIS Krankenhaus Information System

KISS key integrative social system · kidney internal splint/stent · potassium iodide, saturated solution

KIT Kahn intelligence test

KIU kallikrein inactivation unit · kallikrein inhibiting unit

KJ, kj knee jerk

kJ kilojoule

KK knee kick

kkat kilokatal

KL kidney lobe · Klebs–Löffler (bacillus) · Kleine–Levin (syndrome)

kL kiloliter *also* kl

kl kiloliter *also* kL · [Ger. *Klang*] musical overtone (ringing, in acoustics)

KL–BET Kleihauer–Betke (test)

K level lowest level (of x–rays)

KLH keyhole limpet hemocyanin

KLS kidney(s), liver, (and) spleen • Kreuzbein lipomatous syndrome

KLST Kindergarten Language Screening Test

KM κ–immunoglobulin (light chain) • kanamycin *also* K • Kraepelin–Morel (disease)

Km, K$_m$ Michaelis constant (in enzyme assays) • Michaelis–Menten dissociation constant

km kilometer *also* kilo

km² square kilometer

kMc kilomegacycle

K–MCM potassium–containing minimal capacitation medium

kMc/s, kMcps kilomegacycle per second

KMDAT Key Math Diagnostic Arithmetic Test

KMEF keratin, myosin, epidermin, (and) fibrin (class of proteins)

kmps, km/s kilometer per second

KMV killed measles virus (vaccine)

Kn knee *also* K, kn • Knudsen number (low–pressure gas flow)

kN kilonewton

kn knee *also* K, Kn

K nail Küntscher nail

KNO keep needle open

knork knife and fork (physiatry)

KNRK Kirsten sarcoma virus in normal rat kidney (cell)

KO keep on (continue) *also* K/O • keep open *also* K/O • killed organism • knee orthosis • knocked out *also* KO'd

K/O keep on (continue) *also* KO • keep open *also* K/O

KOC cathodal (kathodal— obsolete) opening contraction

KO'd knocked out *also* KO

KOIS Kuder Occupational Interest Survey

kΩ kilohm

KOT Knowledge of Occupations Test

KP Kaufmann–Peterson (base) • keratic precipitate • keratitis punctata • keratoprecipitate • keratotic patch • kidney protein • kidney punch (trauma) • killed parenteral (vaccine)

K–P Kaiser–Permanente (diet)

kPa kilopascal

kPa·s/L kilopascal–second per liter

KPB ketophenylbutazone (kebuzone) • kalium (potassium) phosphate buffer

KPE Kelman phaco- emulsification

KPI karyopyknotic index *also* KI

KPM kilo/pound/meters

KPR key pulse rate • Kuder Preference Record

KPR–V Kuder Preference Record–Vocational

KPT kidney punch test (physical exam) • Kuder Performance Test

KPTI Kunitz pancreatic trypsin inhibitor

KPTT kaolin partial thromboplastin time

KPV killed parenteral vaccine • killed polio vaccine

KR knowledge (of) results • Kopper Reppart (medium)

Kr krypton

kR kiloroentgen

KRA Klinefelter–Reifenstein–Albright (syndrome)

KRB Krebs–Ringer bicarbonate (buffer) *also* KRBB

KRBB Krebs–Ringer bicarbonate buffer *also* KRB

KRBG Krebs–Ringer bicarbonate (buffer) (with) glucose

KRBS Krebs–Ringer bicarbonate solution

KRP Kolmer (test with) Reiter protein (antigen) • Krebs–Ringer phosphate

KRPS Krebs–Ringer phosphate (buffer) solution

KRRS kinetic resonance Raman spectroscopy

KS Kaposi sarcoma • Kartagener syndrome • Kawasaki syndrome • keratan sulfate • ketosteroid • Klinefelter syndrome • Kochleffel syndrome • Korsakoff syndrome • Kugel–Stoloff (syndrome) • Kveim–Siltzbach (test)

17–KS 17–ketosteroid *also* 17K, 17–K, 17–Keto

ks kilosecond

KSA knowledge, skills, and abilities

KSK [Ger. *Kathodenschließungs–Kontraktion*] cathodal closing contraction *also* KCC

KS/OI Kaposi sarcoma and opportunistic infections

KSP kidney–specific protein

K$_{sp}$ potassium solubility product

KST [Ger. *Kathodenschließungs–Tetanus*] cathodal closing tetanus *also* KCT, KCTe

KSU Kent State University (Speech Discrimination Test)

KT kidney transplant • kidney transplantation • kidney treatment • Klippel–Trenaunay (sydrome)

KTI kallikrein–trypsin inhibitor

KTS kethoxal thiosemicarbazone

KTSA Kahn Test of Symbol Arrangement

KTVS Keystone Telebinocular Visual Survey

KTWS Klippel–Trenaunay–Weber syndrome

KU kallikrein unit • Karmen unit • Kimbel unit • Kimbrel unit

Ku kurchatovium

KUB kidney and urinary bladder • (x–ray examination of) kidneys, ureter, and bladder

KUS kidney(s), ureter(s), and spleen

KV kanamycin–vancomycin • killed vaccine

kV, kv kilovolt

kVA kilovolt–ampere

KVBA kanamycin–vancomycin blood agar

kVcp, kvcp kilovolt constant potential

KVE Kaposi varicelliform eruption

KVLBA kanamycin–vancomycin laked blood agar

KVO keep vein open (IV lines)

KVO C D5W keep vein open with 5% dextrose in water

kVp, kvp kilovolt peak

KW Keith–Wagener (classification of eyeground findings) *also* KWB • Kimmelstiel–Wilson (syndrome) • Kugelberg–Welander (disease)

K$_w$ dissociation constant of water

kW, kw kilowatt

KWB Keith–Wagener–Barker (classification of eyeground findings) *also* KW

kWh, kW–hr, kw–hr kilowatt–hour

KWIC keyword in context (computers)

K wire Kirschner wire

KWOC keyword out (of) context (computers)

kyph kyphosis

KZ Kaplan–Zuelzer (syndrome)

L angular momentum • Avogadro constant/number • boundary *also* LIM • coefficient of induction • diffusion length • inductance • lambert (unit of luminance) *also* La • latent heat • latex *also* LX, Lx • Latin *also* Lat • left *also* (L), l, laev, lt, LT, lt • length *also* l • Lente insulin • lesser • lethal (Erlich's symbol for fatal) *also* l • leucine *also* LEU, Leu • lewisite • licensed (to practice) • lidocaine *also* LIDO • ligament, ligamentum *also* lgt, lig • light (chain of protein molecules) *also* LT, lt • light sense • lilac (indicator color) • lincomycin • lingual *also* ling • liquor • liter *also* l • liver *also* LIV • living *also* liv • longitudinal (section) • low/lower/lowest *also* LO • lumbar • lumen *also* lm • luminance • lung *also* LU, Lu • lymph • lymphocyte • lymphogranuloma • lysosome • [L. *libra*] pound *also* lb, lib • radiance • self–inductance • [L. *lues* pestilence] syphilis • [L. *limen*] threshold

(L) left *also* L, l, laev, lf, LT, lt • lunch

L$_0$ [L. *limes nul*] limes zero (neutralized toxin–antitoxin mixture)

L$_+$ limes tod (toxin–antitoxin mixture that contains one fatal dose in excess)

L–I, L–II, L–III first, second, or third stage of lues (syphilis)

L

L1—L5, L$_1$—L$_5$ first through fifth lumbar vertebra or lumbar nerve

L/3 lower third (of leg bone)

L– sterochemical structure

l left *also* L, (L), laev, lf, LT, lt • length *also* L • lethal *also* L • line • liter *also* L • long • longitudinal • radioactive constant • specific latent heat

l– levorotatory

LA lactic acid • language age • large amount • late abortion • late antigen • latex agglutination • Latin American • left angle • left angulation • left arm • left atrial (pressure) • left atrium (echocardiography image) • left auricle • leucine aminopeptidase *also* LAP • leukemia antigen • leukoagglutinating • levator ani (muscle) • lichen amyloidosis • Lightwood–Albright (syndrome) • linguoaxial • linoleic acid • lobuloalveolar • local anesthesia • long–acting (drug) • long–arm (cast) • low anxiety • Ludwig angina • lupus anticoagulant • lymphocyte antibody

L&A, L+A light and accomodation *also* l&a • living and active (family history) *also* l&a

LA50 total body surface area

of burn that will kill 50% of patients (lethal area)

La labial · lambert *also* L · lanthanum

la [L. *lege artis*] according to the art

l&a light and acomodation *also* L&A, L+A · living and active (family history) *also* L&A, L+A

LAA left atrial abnormality · left atrial appendage · left auricular appendage · leukemia–associated antigen · leukocyte ascorbic acid

LAAO L–amino acid oxidase

LAARD long–acting antirheumatic drug

LAB Leisure Activities Blank (psychology)

lab laboratory *also* LB · [Ger. *Lab* chymosin] rennet ferment coagulating milk

LABS Laboratory Admission Baseline Studies

LABVT left atrial ball–valve thrombus

LAC laceration *also* lac · La Crosse (arbovirus) · lactose · left atrial contraction · linguoaxio-cervical · long–arm cast · low amplitude contraction · lung adenocarcinoma cell

LaC labiocervical

lac laceration *also* LAC · lactate/lactation *also* lact

lac & cont lacerations and contusions

LACN local area communications network

lacr lacrimal

LACT Lindamood Auditory Conceptualization Test (psychology)

LAC T lactose tolerance

lact lactate/lactating/lactation *also* lac · lactic

LACT–ART lactate arterial

lact hyd lactalbumin hydrolysate

LAD lactic acid dehydrogenase *also* LADH · language acquisition device · left anterior descending (coronary artery) *also* LADCA · left axis deviation · linoleic acid depression · lipoamide dehydrogenase · lymphocyte–activating determinant

LADA laboratory animal dander allergy · left acromiodorsoanterior (position of fetus)

LADCA left anterior descending coronary artery *also* LAD

LADD lacrimoauriculo-dentodigital (syndrome) · left anterior descending diagonal (branch of coronary artery)

LADH lactic acid dehydrogenase *also* LAD · liver alcohol dehydrogenase

LADME liberation, absorption, distribution, metabolism, (and) excretion

LAD–MIN left axis deviation, minimal

LADP left acromiodorso-posterior (position of fetus)

LADu lobuloalveolar–ductal

LAE left atrial enlargement • long above–elbow (cast)

LAEDV left atrial end–diastolic volume

LAEI left atrial emptying index

LAESV left atrial end–systolic volume

laev [L. *laevus*] left *also* L, (L), l, lf, LT, lt

LAF laminar air flow • Latin American female • leukocyte–activating factor • low animal fat • lymphocyte–activating factor

LAFB left anterior fascicular block

LAFR laminar air flow room

LAFU laminar air flow unit

LAG labiogingival *also* LaG • linguoaxiogingival • lymphangiography/ lymphangiogram

LaG labiogingival *also* LAG

lag. [L. *lagena*] flask

LAH lactalbumin hydrolysate • left anterior hemiblock *also* LAHB • left atrial hypertrophy • lithium–aluminum hydride

LAHB left anterior hemiblock *also* LAH

LAHV leukocyte–associated herpesvirus

LAI labioincisal *also* LaI • latex (particle) agglutination inhibition • left atrial involvement • leukocyte adherence inhibition (assay)

LaI labioincisal *also* LAI

LAIF leukocyte adherence inhibition factor

LAIT latex agglutination inhibition test

LAK lymphokine–activated killer (cell)

LAL left axillary line • limulus amebocyte lysate • low air loss

LaL labiolingual

L–Ala L–alanine

LALI lymphocyte antibody lymphocytolytic interaction

LAM lactation amenorrhea method • laminar air flow • laminectomy *also* Lam, lam • L–asparaginase and methotrexate • late ambulatory monitoring • Latin American male • left anterior measurement • left atrial myxoma • lymph-angioleiomyomatosis

Lam, lam lamina • laminectomy *also* LAM • laminogram

LA–MAX maximal left atrial (dimension)

lambda (Λ, λ) eleventh letter of Greek alphabet

λ craniometric point • decay constant • junction of lambdoid and sagittal sutures (craniotomy) • one of two forms of immunoglobulin light chain • mean free path • thermal conductivity *also* TC • wavelength *also* WL

lam & fus laminectomy and fusion

lami laminotomy

LAMMA laser microprobe mass analyzer

LAN long–acting neuroleptic • lymphadenopathy

LANC long–arm navicular cast

Lang, lang language

L ANT left anterior

LANV left atrial neovascularization

LAO left anterior oblique • left anterior occipital • left atrial overloading

LAP laparoscopy *also* lap. • laparotomy *also* lap. • left atrial pressure • leucine aminopeptidase *also* LA • leukocyte alkaline phosphatase (stain) • low atmospheric pressure • lyophilized anterior pituitary (tissue)

lap. laparotomy *also* LAP • laparoscopy *also* LAP

LAPA leukocyte alkaline phosphatase activity

LAPF low–affinity platelet factor

lapid [L. *lapideum*] stony

LAPMS long–arm posterior–molded splint

LAPOCA L–asparaginase, prednisone, Oncovin (vincristine), cytarabine, and Adriamycin (doxorubicin)

LAPSE long–term ambulatory physiological surveillance (vitalsign monitor)

LAPW left atrial posterior wall

LAR laryngology *also* Laryngol • late asthmatic response • left arm, reclining/recumbent (blood pressure, pulse measurement)

lar larynx *also* lx

LARC leukocyte automatic recognition computer

LARS Language–Structured Auditory Retention Span (Test) • leucyl–transfer ribonucleic acid synthetase

laryn laryngeal • laryngitis • laryngoscopy

Laryngol laryngology *also* LAR

LAS laboratory automation system • lateral amyotrophic sclerosis • laxative abuse syndrome • left anterior–superior • left arm, sitting (blood pressure, pulse measurement) • leucine acetylsalicylate • linear alkyl sulfonate • local adaptation syndrome • long–arm splint • lower abdominal surgery • lymphadenopathy syndrome • lymphangio-scintigraphy

LASER, laser light amplification (by) stimulated emission (of) radiation

LASFB left anterior–superior fascicular block

LASH left anterior–superior hemiblock

L–ASP L–asparaginase

LASS labile aggregation–stimulating substance • Linguistic Analysis of Speech Samples

LAST leukocyte–antigen sensitivity testing

LAT latent • lateral *also* lat • latex agglutination test • left anterior thigh

Lat Latin *also* L

lat lateral *also* LAT • latissimus (dorsi) • latitude

LAT–A latrunculin A

lat admov [L. *lateri admoveatum*] let it be applied to the side

LAT–B latrunculin B

LATCH literature attached to charts

lat dol [L. *lateri dolenti*] to the painful side

lat & loc lateralizing and localizing

l·atm liter–atmosphere

lat men lateral meniscectomy

LATP left atrial transmural pressure

lat Rin lactated Ringer (solution) *also* LR

LATS long–acting thyroid–stimulating (hormone) • long–acting thyroid stimulator • long–acting transmural stimulator

LATS–P long–acting thyroid stimulator–protector

LATu lobuloalveolar tumor

LAV lymphadenopathy–associated virus

lav lavoratory

LAW left atrial wall

lax . laxative • laxity

LB laboratory (data) *also* lab • lamellar body • large bowel • lateral bending • Lederer–Brill (syndrome) • left breast • left bundle • left buttock • leiomyoblastoma *also* LMB • lipid body • live birth • liver biopsy • Living Bank • loose body • low back (pain) *also* LBP • low breakage • lung biopsy

L–B Liebermann–Burchard (test for cholesterol)

L&B left and below

Lb pound force

lb [L. *libra*] pound *also* L, lib

LBA left basal artery

lb ap [L. *libra apothecary*] apothecary pound

lb av [L. *libra avoirdupois*] avoirdupois pound

LBB left breast biopsy • left bundle–branch • low back bend

LBBB left bundle–branch block

LBBsB left bundle branch system block

LBBX left breast biopsy examination

LBC lidocaine blood concentration

LBCD left border (of) cardiac dullness

LBCF Laboratory Branch Complement Fixation (test)

LBD large bile duct · left border dullness (of heart to percussion)

LBDQ Leader Behavior Description Questionnaire

LBE long below–elbow (cast)

LBF *Lactobacillus bulgaricus* factor (pantetheine) · limb blood flow · liver blood flow

lbf pound force

lbf–ft pound force foot

lb–ft pound–feet

LBH length, breadth, height

LBI low serum–bound iron

lb/in² pounds per square inch *also* PSI, psi

LBL labeled lymphoblast · lymphoblastic lymphoma *also* LL

LBM last bowel movement · lean body mass · loose bowel movement · lung basement membrane

LBNP lower–body negative pressure

LBO large bowel obstruction

LBP low back pain *also* LB · low blood pressure

LBPQ Low Back Pain Questionnaire

LBRF louse–borne relapsing fever

LBS lactobacillus selector (agar) · low back syndrome

lbs [L. *librae*] pounds

LBSA lipid–bound sialic acid *also* LSA

LBT low back tenderness · low back trouble · lupus band test

lb t [L. *libra troy*] pound troy *also* lb tr

LBTI lima bean trypsin inhibitor

lb tr pound troy *also* lb t

LBV left brachial vein · lung blood volume

LBW lean body weight · low birth weight

LBWI low birth weight infant

LBWR lung–body weight ratio

LC lactation consultant · Laennec cirrhosis · lamina cortex · Langerhans cell · large chromophobe · large cleaved (cell) · late clamped (umbilical cord) · lecithin cholesterol (acyltransferase) · left circumflex (coronary artery) *also* LCCA, LCF, LCX, LCx · left (ear), cold (stimulus) · leisure counseling · lethal concentration · Library of Congress · life care · light chain · light coagulation · linguocervical · lining cell · lipid cytosome · liquid chromatography · liquid crystal · lithocolic (acid) · live clinic · liver cirrhosis · liver clinic · living children · locus ceruleus · long–chain (triglycerides) · longus capitus · low calorie *also* lo cal · lung cancer · lung cell · lymph capillary · lymphocyte count ·

lymphocytotoxin *also* LCT, LT • lymphoma culture

lc [L. *loco citato*] in the place cited

LCA Leber congenital amaurosis • left circumflex artery • left coronary artery • light contact assist • lithocholic acid • lymphocyte chemoattractant activity • lymphocytotoxic antibody *also* LCTA

LCAO linear combination (of) atomic orbitals

LCAO–MO linear combination (of) atomic orbital–molecular orbital

LCAR late cutaneous anaphylactic reaction

LCAT lecithin–cholesterol acyltransferase

LCB Laboratory of Cancer Biology • left costal border

LCBF local cerebral blood flow

LCC lactose coliform count • left coronary cusp • liver cell carcinoma

LCCA late cortical cerebellar atrophy • left circumflex coronary artery *also* LC, LCX, LCX • left common carotid artery • leukoclastic angiitis • leukocytoclastic angiitis

LCCP limited channel–capacity process

LCCS lower cervical cesarean section

LCCSCT large–cell calcifying Sertoli cell tumor

LCD liquid–crystal display • (coal tar solution) liquor carbonis detergens • localized collagen dystrophy • low–calcium diet

LCDD light–chain deposition disease

LCED liquid chromatography (with) electrochemical detection

LCF least common factor • left circumflex (coronary artery) *also* LC, LCCA, LCX, LCx • linear correction factor • low–frequency current field • lymphocyte culture fluid

LCFA long–chain fatty acid

LCFAO long–chain fatty acid oxidation

LCFC linear combination (of) fragment configuration

LCFM left circumflex marginal

LCFU leukocyte colony–forming unit

LCG Langerhans cell granule

LCGU local cerebral glucose utilization

LCH local city hospital

L chain light chain (polypeptides with low molecular weight)

LCI length complexity index • lung clearance index

LCIS lobular carcinoma in situ

LCL lateral collateral ligament • Levinthal–Coles–Lillie (cytoplasmic inclusion body) • lower confidence limit • lymphoblastoid cell line • lymphocytic leukemia *also* LL • lymphocytic lymphosarcoma • lymphoid cell line

LCLC large–cell lung carcinoma

LCM latent cardiomyopathy • left costal margin • leukocyte–conditioned medium • lower costal margin • lowest common multiple • lymphatic choriomeningitis • lymphocytic chorio-meningitis

LCMG long–chain monoglyceride

l/cm H₂O liters per centimeter of water

LCMV lymphocytic choriomeningitis virus

LCN lateral cervical nucleus • left caudate nucleus

LCO low cardiac output

LCOS low cardiac output syndrome

LCP Legg–Calvé–Perthes (disease) • long–chain polysaturated (fatty acid)

LCPD Legg–Calvé–Perthes disease

LCQG left caudal quarter ganglion

LCR late cortical response • late cutaneous reaction • leurocristine (vincristine)

LCS left coronary sinus • Leydig cell stimulation • lichen chronicus simplex •

life care service • liquor cerebrospinalis • low constant/continuous suction

LCSW Licensed Clinical Social Worker

LCT liver cell tumor • long–chain triglyceride • low cervical transverse • lung capillary time • Luscher Color Test • lymphocytotoxicity test • lymphocytotoxin *also* LC, LT

LCTA lymphocytotoxic antibody *also* LCA

LCTD low–calcium test diet

LCU life change unit

LCV lecithovitellin • leucovorin *also* LEU, LV, LVR • low cervical vertical (incision)

LCX, LCx left circumflex (coronary artery) *also* LC, LCCA, LCF

LD labor and delivery *also* L&D • laboratory data • labyrinthine defect • lactate dehydrogenase *also* LDH • lactic (acid) dehydrogenase *also* LDG, LDH • last dose • L-DOPA, l–dopa • learning disability • learning disabled • learning disorder • left deltoid • Legionnaires disease • Leishman–Donovan (body) *also* L–D • lethal dose • levodopa *also* L–DOPA, l-dopa • light–dark • light difference • light differentiation • light duty • limited disease • linear dichroism •

linguodistal · lipodystrophy · lithium diluent · lithium discontinuation · liver disease · living donor · loading dose · Lombard–Dowell (agar) · longitudinal diameter (of heart) · long (time) dialysis · low density · low dose · lung destruction · lymphocyte–defined · lymphocyte depletion · lymphocytically determined

L–D Leishman–Donovan (body) *also* LD

L/D light/dark (ratio)

L&D labor and delivery *also* LD · light and distance (in ophthalmology)

LD$_1$—LD$_5$ lactate dehydrogenase fraction 1 through 5 *also* LDH$_1$-LDH$_5$

LD$_{50}$ median lethal dose (lethal for 50% of test subjects)

LD$_{50/30}$ dose that is lethal dose for 50% of test subjects within 30 days

LD$_{100}$ lethal dose in all exposed subjects

LDA laser Doppler anemometry · left dorsoanterior (fetal position) · linear discriminant analysis · linear displacement analysis · lymphocyte–dependent antibody

LDAR latex direct agglutination reaction

LDB lamb dysentery bacillus · Legionnaires disease bacillus

LDC leukocyte differential count · lymphoid dendritic cell

LDCC lectin–dependent cellular cytotoxicity

LDCT late distal cortical tubule

LDD late dedifferentiation · light–dark discrimination

LDE lauric diethamide

LD–EYA Lombard–Dowell egg yolk agar

LDF limit dilution factor

LDG lactic (acid) dehydrogenase *also* LD, LDH · lingual developmental groove · long–distance group · low–dose group

LDH lactate dehydrogenase *also* LD · lactic (acid) dehydrogenase *also* LD, LDG · low–dose heparin

LDH$_1$—LDH$_5$ lactate dehydrogenase fraction 1 through 5 *also* LD$_1$—LD$_5$

LDHA lactate dehydrogenase A

LDHB lactate dehydrogenase B

LDHI lactate dehydrogenase isoenzyme *also* LDISO

LDIH left direct inguinal hernia

LDISO lactate dehydrogenase isoenzyme *also* LDHI

LDL loudness discomfort level · low–density lipoprotein *also* LDLP · low–density lymphocyte

LDLC low–density lipoprotein cholesterol

LDLP low–density lipoprotein *also* LDL

LDM lactate dehydrogenase, muscle

LD–NEYA Lombard–Dowell neomycin egg yolk agar

L–DOPA, L–dopa levodopa *also* LD

L doses limes doses (toxin/ antitoxin combining power)

LDP left dorsoposterior (fetal position) • lumbodorsal pain

LDRP labor, delivery, recovery, postpartum

LDS ligating and dividing stapler

LDT left dorsotransverse (fetal position)

LDU long double upright (brace) *also* LDUB

LDUB long double upright brace *also* LDU

LDV lactic dehydrogenase virus • large dense–cored vesicle • laser Doppler velocimetry • lateral distant view

LE left ear • left eye • lens extraction • leukocyte elastase • leukocyte esterase *also* LKESTR • leukoerythrogenic • live embryo • Long Evans (rat) • lower extremity *also* L ext, l/ext, lx • lupus erythematosus

Le Leonard (cathode ray unit) • Lewis (number, diffusivity:diffusion coefficient of a fluid)

LEA language experience approach • lower extremity amputation • lower extremity arterial • lumbar epidural anesthesia

LEADS Leadership Evaluation and Development Scale

LEB lupus erythematosus body

LEC leukoencephalitis • low–energy charged (particle)

LE cell lupus erythematosus cell

LECP low–energy charged particle

LED light–emitting diode • lowest effective dose • lupus erythematosus disseminatus

LEED low–energy electron diffraction

LEEDS low–energy electron diffraction spectroscopy

LEEP left end–expiratory pressure

LEER lower extremity equipment related

LEE W Lee White tritium (clotting time) *also* L&W, L/W, LWCT

LEF leukokinesis–enhancing factor • lupus erythematosus factor

leg. legal • legislation • legislative

leg. com legal commitment • legally committed

LEHPZ lower esophageal high–pressure zone

LeIF leukocyte interferon

leio leiomyoma

LEIS low–energy ion scattering

LEJ ligation (of) esophagogastric junction

LEL lowest effect level (of toxicity)

LEM lateral eye movement • Leibovitz–Emory medium • leukocyte endogenous mediator • light electron microscope

LEMO lowest empty molecular orbital

LEMS Lambert–Eaton myasthenic syndrome

lenit [L. *leniter*] gently • lenitive

LEOPARD lentigines, electrocardiographic (conduction abnormalities), ocular (hypertelorism), pulmonary (stenosis), abnormal (genitalia), retardation (of growth), and deafness (syndrome)

LEP leptospirosis: lethal effective phase • lipoprotein electrophoresis *also* LPE • low egg passage (strain of virus) • lower esophageal pressure • lower esophagus

L$_{EPN}$ effective perceived noise level

LE$_{prep}$ lupus erythematosus preparation

LEPT leptocyte

LEPTOS leptospirosis agglutinins

Leq loudness equivalent

LER lysozomal enzyme release

LERG local electroretinogram

L–ERX leukoerythroblastic reaction

LES Lawrence Experimental Station (agar) • Life Experience Survey • local excitatory state • Locke egg serum (medium) • lower esophageal segment/sphincter/stricture • lupus erythematosus, systemic

les lesion • low excitatory state

LESA liposomally entrapped second antibody

LESP lower esophageal sphincter pressure

LESS lateral electrical spine stimulation

LET language enrichment therapy • linear energy transfer • low energy transfer

LETD lowest effective toxic dose

LETS large external transformation–sensitive (fibronectin)

LEU leucine *also* L, Leu • leucovorin *also* LCV, LV, LVR • leukocyte equivalent unit

Leu leucine *also* L, LEU

leuk, leuko leukocyte

LEUKAP leukocyte alkaline phosphatase

LEV Leibovitz–Emory medium • lower extremity venous

lev levator (muscle) • [L. *levis*] light

levit [L. *leviter*] lightly

LEW Lewis (rat)

LEX lactate extraction

L ext, l/ext lower extremity *also* LE, lx

LF labile factor • laryngofissure • Lassa fever • latex fixation • lavage fluid • leaflet • left foot • leucine flux • limit (of) flocculation *also* Lf • low–fat (diet) • low forceps (delivery) *also* LFD • low frequency *also* lf

Lf limes flocculation (unit, dose of toxin per mL) • limit (of) flocculation *also* LF

lf left *also* L, (L), l, laev, lf, LT, lt • low frequency *also* LF

LFA left femoral artery • left forearm • left frontoanterior (fetal position) • leukotactic factor activity • low friction arthroplasty

LFB lingual–facial–buccal • liver, iron, and B complex

LFC left frontal craniotomy • living female child • low fat (and) cholesterol (diet)

LFD lactose–free diet • large for date • late fetal death • lateral facial dysplasia • least fatal dose • low–fat diet • low–fiber diet • low forceps delivery *also* LF

LFECT loose fibroelastic connective tissue

LFER linear free–energy relationship

LFH left femoral hernia

LFL left frontolateral • leukocyte feeder layer

LFN lactoferrin

LFOV large field of view

LFP left frontoposterior (fetal position)

LFPPV low–frequency positive pressure ventilation

LFR lymphoid follicular reticulosis

LF–RF local–regional failure

LFS limbic forebrain structure • liver function series

LFT latex fixation test • latex flocculation test • left frontotransverse (fetal position) • liver function test • low–frequency tetanic (stimulation) • low–frequency tetanus • low–frequency transduction • low–frequency transfer

LFTSW left foot switch

LFU limit flocculation unit • lipid fluidity unit

LFV Lassa fever virus • low–frequency ventilation

L fx linear fracture

LG lactoglobulin • lamellar granule • large *also* lg, lge • laryngectomy • left gluteal • left gluteus • linguogingival • lipoglycopeptide • liver graft • low glucose • lymph gland

lg large *also* LG, lge • leg • long

LGA large (for) gestational age • left gastric artery

LGB Landry–Guillain–Barré (syndrome) *also* LGBS • lateral geniculate body

LGBS Landry–Guillain–Barré syndrome *also* LGB

LGC left giant cell

LGD Leaderless Group Discussion (situational test)

LGd dorsal lateral geniculate (nucleus)

lge large *also* LG, lg;

LGF lateral giant fiber

LGH lactogenic hormone *also* LTH • little growth hormone

LGI large glucagon immunoreactivity • lower gastrointestinal

LGL large granular leukocyte • large granular lymphocyte • lobular glomeru-lonephritis • Lown–Ganong–Levine (syndrome)

LGMD limb–girdle muscular dystrophy

LGN lateral geniculate nucleus • lobular glomerulonephritis

LGP labioglossopharyngeal

LGS large green soft (stool) • limb girdle syndrome

LGT Langat encephalitis • late generalized tuberculosis

Lgt, lgt ligament, ligamentum *also* lig

LGV large granular vesicle • lymphogranuloma venereum

LGVHD lethal graft–versus–host disease

LgX lymphogranulomatosis X

LH late healed • lateral hypothalamic (syndrome) • lateral hypothalamus • left hand • left hemisphere • left hyperphoria • liver homogenate • lower half • lues hereditaria (hereditary syphilis) • lung homogenate • luteinizing hormone • luteotropic hormone *also* LTH

LHA lateral hypothalamic area • left hepatic artery

LHb lateral habenular

LHBV left heart blood volume

LHC left heart catheterization • left hypochondrium

LHCG luteinizing hormone–chorionic gonadotropin (hormone)

LHF left heart failure • ligament (of) head (of) femur

LHFA lung Hageman factor activator

LH/FSH–RF luteinizing hormone/follicle–stimulating hormone–releasing factor

LHG left hand grip • localized hemolysis (in) gel

LHH left homonymous hemianopia

LHI lipid hydrocarbon inclusion

LHL left hemisphere lesion • left hepatic lobe

LHM lisuride hydrogen maleate

LHMP Life Health Monitoring Program

LHN lateral hypothalamic nucleus

LHP left hemiparesis • left hemiplegia

LHPZ lower (esophageal) high–pressure zone

LHR leukocyte histamine release (test) • liquid holding recovery

l–hr lumen–hour (unit quantity of light)

LHRF luteinizing hormone–releasing factor • luteotropin hormone–releasing factor

LHRH, LH–RH luteinizing hormone–releasing hormone

LHS left hand side • left heart strain • left heel strike • lymphatic (and) hematopoietic system

LHT left hypertropia

LI labeling index • lactose intolerance • lamellar ichthyosis • large intestine • learning impaired • left injured • left involved • life island • linguoincisal • lithogenic index • low impulsiveness

L&I liver and iron

Ll labrale inferius • lithium

LIA Laser Institute of America • left iliac artery • leukemia–associated inhibitory activity • lock–in amplifier • lymphocyte–induced angiogenesis • lysine–iron agar

LIAC light–induced absorbance change

LIAF lymphocyte–induced angiogenesis factor

LIAFI late infantile amaurotic familial idiocy

LIB left in bottle

lib [L. *libra*] pound *also* L, lb

LIBC latent iron–binding capacity

LIBR Librium

LIC left iliac crest • left internal carotid • leisure–interest class • limiting isorrheic concentration

LICA left internal carotid artery

LICC lectin–induced cellular cytotoxicity

LICD lower intestinal Crohn disease

LICM left intercostal margin

LICS left intercostal space *also* LIS

LID late immunoglobulin deficiency • lymphocytic infiltrative disease

LIDC low–intensity direct current

LIDO lidocaine *also* L

LIF laser–induced fluorescence • left iliac fossa • left index finger • leukocyte infiltration factor • leukocyte inhibitory factor • leukocytosis–inducing factor • liver (migration) inhibitory factor

LIFE Longitudinal Interval Follow–up Evaluation

LIFO last in, first out (re: computer data)

LIFT lymphocyte immunofluorescence test

lig ligament, ligamentum *also* L, Lgt, lgt • ligate • ligation • ligature *also* ligg

ligg ligamenta • ligaments • ligature *also* lig

LIH left inguinal hernia

LIHA low impulsiveness, high anxiety

LII Leisure Interest Inventory

LIJ left internal jugular

LILA low impulsiveness, low anxiety

LIM [L. *limes*] boundary *also* L

lim limit • limitation

LIMA left internal mammary artery (graft)

lin linear • liniment *also* Linim

LINAC linear accelerator

ling lingual *also* L • lingular

Linim liniment *also* lin

LIO left inferior oblique (muscle)

LIP lithium–induced polydipsia • lymphocytic interstitial pneumonia

Lip lipoate (lipoic acid)

LIPA lysosomal acid lipase A

LIPB lysosomal acid lipase B

LIPHE Life Interpersonal History Enquiry

lipoMM lipomyelo-meningocele

LIP P lipid profile

LIPS Leiter International Performance Scale

LIQ low inner quadrant

LIQ, liq [L. *liquor*] liquid, liquor

liq dr liquid dram

liq oz liquid ounce

liq pt liquid pint

liq qt liquid quart

LIR left iliac region • left inferior rectus

LIRBM liver, iron, red bone marrow

LIS laboratory information system • lateral intercellular space • left intercostal space *also* LICS • lithium salicylate • lobular in situ (carcinoma) • low intermittent suction • low ionic strength

LISP List Processing Language

LISS low ionic strength solution (medium test) • low ionic strength saline

litho lithotripsy

LIV law (of) initial value • left innominate vein • liver (battery test) *also* L

liv live • living *also* L

LIV–BP leucine, isoleucine, and valine–binding protein

LIVC left inferior vena cava

LIVEN linear inflammatory verrucous epidermal nevus

LIVIM lethal intestinal virus (of) infant mice

LIVPRO liver profile

LJ Larsen–Johansson (syndrome) • Löwenstein–Jensen (medium) *also* LJM

LJL lateral joint line

LJM limited joint mobility • Löwenstein–Jensen medium *also* LJ

LK lamellar keratoplasty *also* LKP • Landry–Kussmaul (syndrome) • left kidney *also* LKID • lichenoid keratosis • Löhr–Kindberg (syndrome)

LK⁺ low potassium ion

LKA Lazare–Klerman–Armour (Personality Inventory)

LKESTR leukocyte esterase *also* LE

LKID left kidney *also* LK

LKKS liver, kidneys, (and) spleen *also* LKS

LKM liver–kidney microsome

LKP lamellar keratoplasty *also* LK

LKPD Lillehei–Kaster pivoting disk

LKS liver, kidneys, (and) spleen *also* LKKS

LKSB liver, kidneys, spleen, (and) bladder

LKS non. pal. liver, kidneys, (and) spleen not palpable

LKV laked kanamycin vancomycin (agar) • Lengyeh–Kerman–Vargar (rating)

LL large local • large lymphocyte • lateral lemniscus • left lateral *also* LLAT, L lat, lt lat • left

leg • left lower • left lung • lepromatous leprosy • Lewandowski–Lutz (syndrome) • lid lag • limb head • lines • lingual lipase • lipoprotein lipase *also* LPL • long leg • loudness level • lower (eye)lid • lower limb • lower lip • lower lobe • lumbar length • lung length • lymphloblastic lymphoma *also* LBL • lymphocytic leukemia *also* LCL • lymphocytic lymphoma • lymphoid leukemia • lysolecithin *also* LLT

L&L lids and lashes

LLA lids, lashes, (and) adnexa • limulus lysate assay • lupus–like anticoagulant

L lam lumbar laminectomy

LLAT left lateral *also* LL, L lat, lt lat • lysolecithin acyltransferase

L lat left lateral *also* LL, LLAT, lt lat

LLB left lateral bending • left lateral border • left lower border • long–leg brace • lower lobe bronchus

LLBCD left lower border (of) cardiac dullness

LLBP long–leg brace (with) pelvic (band)

LLC Lewis lung carcinoma • liquid–liquid chromatography • long–leg cast • lower level (of) care • lymphocytic leukemia, chronic

LLCC long–leg cylinder cast

LLD *Lactobacillus lactis,* Dorner (factor) • left lateral decubitus (muscle) • leg length discrepancy • liquid liquid distribution • long–lasting depolarization

LLDF *Lactobacillus lactis* Dorner factor (vitamin B_{12})

LLDH liver lactate dehydrogenase

LLE left lower extremity *also* LLX

LLF Laki–Lorand factor (factor XIII) • left lateral femoral (site of injection) • left lateral flexion

LL–GXT low–level graded exercise test

LLL left liver lobe • left lower leg • left lower (eye)lid • left lower lobe (of lung) • left lower lung

L LL brace left long–leg brace

LLLE lower lid, left eye *also* LLOS

LLLM low liquid level monitor

LLLNR left lower lobe, no rales

LLM localized leukocyte mobilization

LLO *Legionella*–like organism

LLOD lower lid, oculus dexter (right eye) *also* LLRE

LLOS lower lid, oculus sinister (left eye) *also* LLLE

LLP late luteal phase • long–lasting potentiation • long–leg plaster (cast)

LLPMS long–leg posterior molded splint

LLQ left lower quadrant

LLR large local reaction • left lateral rectus (eye muscle) • left lumbar region

LLRE lower lid, right eye *also* LLOD

LLS lateral loop suspensor • lazy leukocyte syndrome • long–leg splint

LLSB left lower scapular border • left lower sternal border

LLT left lateral thigh • lysolecithin *also* LL

LLV lymphatic leukemia virus • lymphoid leukosis virus

LLV–F lymphatic leukemia virus, Friend (virus associated)

LLVP left lateral ventricular pre–excitation

LLW low–level waste

LLWC long–leg walking cast

LLX left lower extremity *also* LLE

LM labiomental • lactic (acid) mineral (medium) • lactose malabsorption • laryngeal muscle • lateral malleolus • left main • left median • legal medicine • lemniscus medialis • Licentiate in Midwifery • light microscope • light microscopy • light minimum • lincomycin • lingual margin • linguomesial • lipid mobilization • liquid membrane • longitudinal muscle • Looser–Milkman (syndrome) · lower motor (neuron) *also* LMN

L/M liters per minute *also* l/min, lpm

lm lumen *also* L

LMA left mentoanterior (fetal position) · limbic midbrain area · liver membrane antibody · liver (cell) membrane autoantibody

LMB Laurence–Moon–Biedl (syndrome) *also* LMBS · left main–stem bronchus · leiomyoblastoma *also* LB

LMBB Laurence–Moon–Bardet–Biedl (syndrome)

LMBS Laurence–Moon–Biedl syndrome *also* LMB

LMC large motile cell · lateral motor column · left main coronary (artery) · left middle cerebral (artery) · living male child · lymphocyte–mediated cytolysis · lymphocyte–mediated cytotoxicity · lymphocyte microcytotoxicity · lymphomyeloid complex

LMCA left main coronary artery · left middle cerebral artery

LMCAD left main coronary artery disease

LMCAT left middle cerebral artery thrombosis

LMCL left midclavicular line

LMCT ligand–to–metal charge transfer

LMD left main disease (cardiology) · lipid–moiety modified derivative · local

medical doctor · low–molecular(–weight) dextran *also* LMDX, LMWD

LMDF lupus miliaris disseminatus faciei

LMDX low–molecular(-weight) dextran *also* LMD, LMWD

LME left mediolateral episiotomy *also* LMLE · leukocyte migration enhancement

LMEE left middle ear exploration

LMF left middle finger · Leukeran (chlorambucil), methotrexate, and 5–fluorouracil · leukocyte mitogenic factor · lymphocyte mitogenic factor

lm/ft² lumen per square foot

LMG lethal midline granuloma · low mobility group

LMH lipid–mobilizing hormone

lm·h lumen hour

LMI leukocyte migration inhibition (assay)

LMIF leukocyte migration inhibition factor

L/min liter per minute *also* L/M, lpm

L/min/m² liter per minute per square meter

LMIR leukocyte migration inhibition reaction

LMIT leukocyte migration inhibition test

LML large (and) medium

lymphocytes · left mediolateral (episiotomy) · left middle lobe · lower midline

LMLE left mediolateral episiotomy *also* LME

LML scar w/h lower midline scar with hernia

LMM *Lactobacillus* maintenance medium · lentigo maligna melanoma · light(-molecular–weight) meromyosin

lm/m² lumen per square meter

LMN lower motor neuron *also* LM

LMNL lower motor neuron lesion

LMO localized molecular orbital

LMP last menstrual period · left mentoposterior (fetal position) · lumbar puncture *also* LP

LMR left medial rectus (eye muscle) · linguo-mandibular reflex · log magnitude ratio

LMS lateral medullary syndrome · leiomyosarcoma *also* LS

lm·s lumen–second

LMSV left maximal spatial voltage

LMT left main trunk · left mentotransverse (fetal position) · leukocyte migration technique · luteomammotrophic (hormone)

LMTA Language Modalities Test for Aphasia

LMV larva migrans visceralis

LMW low molecular weight

lm/W lumen per watt *also* lpw

LMWD low–molecular–weight dextran *also* LMD, LMDX

LMWH low–molecular–weight heparin

LN labionasal · later (onset) nephrotic (syndrome) · Lesch–Nyhan (syndrome) · lipoid nephrosis · lobular neoplasia · lupus nephritis · lymph node

L/N letter/numerical (system)

LN₂ liquid nitrogen

ln logarithm, natural

LNAA large neutral amino acid

LNB lymph node biopsy

LNC lymph node cell

LND Lesch–Nyhan disease · light–near dissociation · lymph node dissection

LNE lymph node enlargement

LNG liquified natural gas

LNH large number hypothesis

LNI logarithm neutralization index

LNL lower normal limit · lymph node lymphocyte

LNLS linear–nonlinear least squares

LNMP last normal menstrual period

LNNB Luria–Nebraska Neuropsychological Battery

LNP large neuronal polypeptide

LNPF lymph node permeability factor

LNR lymph node region

LNS lateral nuclear stratum • Lesch–Nyhan syndrome • lymph node seeking (equivalent)

LO lateral oblique (x–ray view) • leucine oxidation • linguo–occlusal • low *also* L • lumber orthosis

LOA leave of absence • Leber optic atrophy • left occipitoanterior (fetal position) • looseness of associations • lysis of adhesions

LOC laxative of choice *also* LXC • level of care • level of consciousness • liquid organic compound • local *also* loc • locus of control • loss of consciousness

loc local *also* LOC • localized • location

LoCa low calcium *also* lo calc

lo cal low–calorie (diet) *also* LC

lo calc low–calcium (diet) *also* LoCa

LOC–C Locus of Control–Chance

loc cit [L. *loco citato*] in the place cited

loc dol [L. *loco dolenti*] to the painful spot

LOC–E Locus of Control–External

LoCHO low carbohydrate

LoChol low cholesterol

LOC–I Locus of Control–Internal

LOCM low–osmolar–contrast medium

LOC–PO Locus of Control–Powerful Others

LOD, lod logarithm of odds (method of genetics linkage analysis)

log. logarithm

LOH loop of Henle

LOI level of incompetence • level of injury • Leyton Obsessive Inventory • limit of impurities

LOIH left oblique inguinal hernia

LoK low kalium (potassium)

LOL left occipitolateral (fetal position)

LOM left otitis media • limitation of motion • limitation of movement • loss of motion • loss of movement • low–osmolar(–contrast) medium

LOMPT Lincoln–Oseretsky Motor Performance Test

LOMSA left otitis media, suppurative, acute

LOMSC, LOMSCH left otitis media, suppurative, chronic

LoNa low sodium *also* LS

long. longitudinal

LOP leave on pass • left occiput posterior (fetal position)

LoPro low protein *also* LP

LOPS length of patient stay

LOQ Leadership Opinion Questionnaire · lower outer quadrant

LOR lorazepam *also* LRZ · lorcainide

lord lordosis/lordotic

LORS–1 Level of Rehabilitation Scale 1

LOS length of stay · loss of site · lower (o)esophageal sphincter · low (cardiac) output syndrome

LOSP lower (o)esophageal sphincter pressure

LOT lateral olfactory tract · left occipitotransverse (fetal position) · lengthened off time

lot. lotion

LOV large opaque vesicle · loss of vision

LOWBI low–birth–weight infant

lox. liquid oxygen

LOZ lozenge

LP labile peptide · labile protein · laboratory procedure · lactic peroxidase · lamina propria · laryngo-pharyngeal · latency/latent period · lateral plantar · lateral pylorus · (nucleus) lateralis posterior · latex particle · leading pole · leukocyte poor · leukocytic pyrogen · levator palati · lichen planus · ligamentum patella · lightly padded · light perception *also* LPerc ·

linear programming · linguopulpal · lipoprotein · lost privileges · low potency · low power (microscopy) · low pressure · low protein *also* LoPro · lumbar puncture *also* LMP · lumbo-peritoneal · lung parenchyma · lymphocyte predominant · lymphoid plasma · lymphoid predominance · lymphomatoid papulosis

L/P lactate/pyruvate (ratio) · liver/plasma (concentration ratio) · lymphocyte/polymorph (ratio) · lymph/plasma (ratio)

LPA larval photoreceptor axon · latex particle agglutination · left pulmonary artery

LPAM, L–PAM L–phenyl-alanine mustard (melphalan)

LPB lipoprotein B

LPB, LPBP low–profile bioprosthesis

LPC laser photocoagulation · late positive component · leukocyte–poor cell · lysophosphatidyl choline

LP$\bar{\text{c}}$P light perception with projection

LPCM low–placed conus medullaris

LPCT late proximal cortical tubule

LPD low–protein diet · luteal phase defect

LPDF lipoprotein–deficient fraction

LPE lipoprotein electrophoresis *also* LEP

LPerc light perception *also* LP

LPF leukocytosis–promoting factor • leukopenia factor • lipopolysaccharide factor • liver plasma flow • localized plaque formation • low–power field *also* lpf • lymphocytosis–promoting factor

lpf low–power field *also* LPF

LPFB left posterior fascicular block

LPFN low–pass–filtered noise

LPFS low–pass–filtered signal

LPG liquified petroleum gas

LPH left posterior hemiblock *also* LPHB • lipotropic pituitary hormone (lipotropin)

LPHB left posterior hemiblock *also* LPH

LPI laser peripheral irridectomy • left posterior–inferior • long process (of) incus

LPICA left posterior internal carotid artery

LPIFB left posterior–inferior fascicular block

LPIH left posterior–inferior hemiblock

LPK liver pyruvate kinase

LPL lamina propria lymphocyte • lichen planus–like lesion • lipoprotein lipase *also* LL

LPLA lipoprotein lipase activity

LPM lateral pterygoid muscle • left posterior measurement • liver plasma membrane • localized pretibial myxedema • lymphoproliferative malignancy

lpm lines (printed) per minute • liter per minute *also* L/M, L/min

LPN Licensed Practical Nurse

LPO lateral preoptic (area) • left posterior oblique • light perception only • lobus parolfactorius

LPOA lateral preoptic area

L POST left posterior

LPP lateral pterygoid plate

LP&P light perception and projection

LPPH late postpartum hemorrhage

LPR lactate–pyruvate ratio • late–phase response

LPRBC leukocyte–poor red blood cell

LProj light projection

LPS last Pap smear • levator palpebrae superioris (muscle) • linear profile scan • lipase • lipopolysaccharide • London Psychogeriatric Scale

lps liter per second

LPSR lipopolysaccharide receptor

LPT lipotropin

LPV left portal view • left pulmonary vein • lymphopathia venereum

LPVP left posterior ventricular pre–excitation

LPW lateral pharyngeal wall

lpw lumen per watt *also* lm/W

LPX, Lp–X lipoprotein–X

LQ longevity quotient • lordosis quotient • lower quadrant • lowest quadrant

LQTS long QT syndrome

LR labeled release (experiment) • laboratory reference • laboratory report • labor room • lactated Ringer (solution) *also* lat Rin • large reticulocyte • latency reaction • latency relaxation • lateral rectus (eye muscle) • left rotation • ligand receptor • light reaction • light reflex • limit (of) reaction • lymphocyte recruitment

L/R left–to–right (ratio)

L&R left and right

L–R, L→R, L R left to right

Lr lawrencium *also* Lw • limes reacting (dose of diphtheria toxin)

LRA left renal artery • low right atrium

LRC locomotor–respiratory coupling • lower rib cage

LRD living related donor • living renal donor

LRDT living related donor transplant

LRE least restrictive environment • leukemic reticuloendotheliosis • lymphoreticuloendothelial

LREH low renin essential hypertension

LRF latex (and) resorcinol formaldehyde • left rectus femoris • liver residue factor • luteinizing (hormone)–releasing factor

LRH luteinizing (hormone)–releasing hormone

LRI lower respiratory (tract) illness *also* LRT I • lower respiratory (tract) infection *also* LRTI • lymphocyte reactivity index

LRM left radical mastectomy

LRMP last regular menstrual period

LRN lateral reticular nucleus

LRNA low renin, normal aldosterone

LRND left radical neck dissection

LROP lower radicular obstetrical paralysis

LRP lichen ruber planus • long–range planning

LRQ lower right quadrant

LRQG left rostral quarter ganglion

LRR labyrinthine righting reflex • lymphatic return rate

LRS lactated Ringer solution • lateral recess syndrome

LRSF lactating rat serum factor • liver regenerating serum factor

LR–SH left–right shunt

LRSP long–range systems planning

LRSS late respiratory systemic syndrome

LRT local radiation therapy · lower respiratory tract

LRTI lower respiratory tract illness *also* LRI · lower respiratory tract infection *also* LRI

LRV left renal vein

LRZ lorazepam *also* LOR

LS lateral septal · lateral suspensor (ligament) · left sacrum · left septum · left side · legally separated · leiomyosarcoma *also* LMS · length of stay · lesser sac · Letterer–Siwe (disease) · Libman–Sacks (disease) · life science · light sensitive/ sensitivity · light sleep · liminal sensation · liminal sensitivity · linear scleroderma · lipid synthesis · liver (and) spleen *also* L&S · liver scan · lower segment · low–sodium (diet) *also* LoNa · lumbar spine *also* L–sp · lumbosacral *also* L/ S · lung strip · lymphosarcoma *also* LSA, Lyp

L–S lipid–saccharide

L/S lactase/sucrase (ratio) · lecithin/sphingomyelin (ratio) · liver/spleen (ratio) · lumbosacral *also* LS

L&S liver and spleen *also* LS

LSA Language Sampling Analysis · left sacroanterior (fetal position) · left subclavian artery · leukocyte–specific activity · lichen sclerosis (et) atrophicus · lipid– bound sialic acid *also* LBSA · lymphosarcoma *also* LS, Lyp

LSANA leukocyte–specific antinuclear antibody

LSAR lymphosarcoma cell

LSA/RCS lymphosarcoma– reticulum cell sarcoma

LSB least significant bit (binary numbers) · left scapular border · left sternal border · local standby · long spike burst · lumbar sympathetic block

LS BPS laparoscopic bilateral partial salpingectomy

LSC late systolic click · left– sided colon (cancer) · left subclavian (artery) · lichen simplex chronicus · liquid scintillation counting · liquid–solid chromatography · lower segment cesarean (section) *also* LSCS

LSCA, LScA left scapuloanterior (fetal position)

LSCL lymphosarcoma cell leukemia

LSCP, LScP left scapuloposterior (fetal position)

LSCS lower segment cesarean section *also* LSC

LSCV left subclavian vein

LSD least significant difference • least significant digit (computers) • low–salt diet • low–sodium diet • lysergic acid diethylamide *also* LSD–25

LSD–25 lysergic acid diethylamide *also* LSD

LSE left sternal edge • local side effect

LSEP left somatosensory evoked potential

LSF low saturated fat • lymphocyte–stimulating factor

LSG labial salivary gland

LSH lutein–stimulating hormone • lymphocyte–stimulating hormone

LSI large–scale integration • Life Satisfaction Index • light scattering index • lumbar spine index

LSK liver, spleen, and kidneys

LSKM liver–spleen–kidney megaly

LSL left sacrolateral (fetal position) • left short–leg (brace) • lymphosarcoma (cell) leukemia

LSM late systolic murmur • lymphocyte separation medium

LSN left substantia nigra • left sympathetic nerve

LSO lateral superior olive (of brain) • left salpingo-oophorectomy • left

superior oblique • lumbosacral orthosis

LSP left sacroposterior (fetal position) • liver–specific protein

LSp life span

L–sp lumbar spine *also* LS

L–Spar asparaginase (Elspar) *also* Aase, ASP, Asp

L–spine lumbar spine

LSQ least square

LSR lanthanide shift reagent (in magnetic resonance imaging) • left superior rectus

LSRA low–septal right atrium

L/S ratio lecithin/sphingomyelin ratio

LSS Life Span Study • Life Study Sample • life support station • liver-spleen scan • lumbosacral spine

LSSA lipid–soluble secondary antioxidant

LST lateral sinus thrombophlebitis • lateral spinothalamic tract • left sacrotransverse (fetal position)

LSTC laparoscopic tubal cautery • laparoscopic tubal coagulation

LSTL laparoscopic tubal ligation *also* LTL

L's & T's lines and tubes

LSU lactose–saccharose–urea (agar) • life support unit

LSV lateral sacral vein • left subclavian vein

LSVC left superior vena cava

LSW left–sided weakness

LSWA large–amplitude, slow–wave activity (in electroencephalography)

LT (heat–)labile toxin · laminar tomography · left *also* L, (L), l, laev, lf, lt · left thigh · left triceps · less than · lethal time · leukotriene · Levin tube · levothyroxine · light *also* L, lt · light touch · long term · low temperature · low transverse · lues test · lumbar traction · lymphocyte transformation · lymphocyte transitional · lymphocytic thyroiditis · lymphocytotoxin *also* LC, LCT · lymphotoxin

lt left *also* L, (L), l, laev, lf, LT · light *also* L, LT · low tension

LTA leukotriene A · lipoate transacetylase · lipotechoic acid · local tracheal anesthesia · lymphocyte–transforming activity

LTAF local tissue–advancement flap

LTAS lead tetra–acetate Schiff

LTB laparoscopic tubal banding · laryngotracheobronchitis · leukotriene B

LTC large transformed cell · left to count · leukotriene C · lidocaine tissue concentration · long–term care · lysed tumor cell

LTCF long–term care facility

LTCP L–tryptophan–containing product

LTCS low transverse cervical (cesarean) section

LTD largest tumor dimension · Laron–type dwarfism · leukotriene D · limited *also* ltd · long–term disability

ltd limited *also* LTD

LTDA limited quantity (test performed on small specimen)

LTE laryngotracheo-esophageal · leukotriene E

LT–ECG long–term electrocardiography

LTF lipotropic factor · lymphocyte–transforming factor

LTG long–term goal

LTGA left transposition (of) great artery

LTH lactogenic hormone *also* LGH · local tumor hyperthermia · low–temperature holding (pasteurization) · luteotropic hormone *also* LH

LtH left–handed

LTI low temperature isotropic · lupus–type inclusion

LTL laparoscopic tubal ligation *also* LSTL

lt lat left lateral *also* LL, LLAT, L lat

LTM long–term memory

LTOT long–term oxygen therapy

LTP leukocyte thromboplastin • long–term potentiation • L–tryptophan

LTPP lipothiamide pyrophosphate

LTR long terminal repeat • lymphocyte transfer reaction

LTS laparoscopic tubal sterilization • long–term storage • long–term surviving • long tract sign (neurology)

LTT lactose tolerance test • leucine tolerance test • limited treadmill test • lymphoblastic transformation test • lymphocyte transformation test

LTUI low transverse uterine incision

LTV Lucké tumor virus • lung thermal volume

lt vent. BBB left ventricular bundle–branch block

LTW Leydig–cell tumor (in) Wistar (rat)

LTX lophotoxin

LU left uninjured • left uninvolved • left upper (limb) • living unit • loudness unit • lung *also* L, Lu • lytic unit

L&U lower and upper (extremities)

Lu lung *also* L, LU • lutetium

LUA left upper arm

LUC large unstained cell

luc prim [L. *luce prima*] at daybreak

LUE left upper extremity *also* LUX

LUF luteinized unruptured follicle

LUFS luteinized unruptured follicle syndrome

LUIS low–dose urea (in) invert sugar

LUL left upper (eye)lid • left upper limb • left upper lobe (lung) • left upper lung

lum, lumb lumbar

LUMO lowest unoccupied molecular orbital

LUO left ureteral orifice

LUOB left upper outer buttock

LUOQ left upper outer quadrant

LUP left ureteropelvic (junction)

LUQ left upper quadrant

LURD living unrelated donor

LUS lower uterine segment

LUSB left upper scapular border • left upper sternal border

lut [L. *luteum*] yellow

LUTT lower urinary tract tumor

LUV large unilamellar vesicle

LUX left upper extremity *also* LUE

LV lacto–ovo–vegetarian • laryngeal vestibule • lateral ventricle • left ventricle,

left ventricular
(echocardiography images) •
leucovorin *also* LCV, LEU,
LVR • leukemia virus •
live vaccine • live virus •
low vertical • low volume •
lumbar vertebra • lung
volume

lv leave

LVA left ventricular
aneurysm • left ventricular
aneurysmectomy • left
vertebral artery • low
vision aid

LVAD left ventricular assist
device

L–VAM leuprolide acetate,
vinblastine, Adriamycin
(doxorubicin), and
mitomycin

LVAS left ventricular assist
system

LVAT left ventricular
activation time

LVBP left ventricle bypass
pump

LVCS low vertical cesarean
section

LVD left ventricular dimension
also LVDI • left
ventricular dysfunction

LV$_D$, LVd left ventricular
(end–)diastolic (pressure)

LVDd left ventricular
dimension (in end)–diastole

LVDI left ventricular
dimension *also* LVD

LVDP left ventricular diastolic
pressure

LVDT linear variable
differential transformer

LVDV left ventricular diastolic
volume

LVE left ventricular ejection •
left ventricular enlargement

LVED left ventricular end–
diastole

LVEDC left ventricular end–
diastolic circumference

LVEDD left ventricular end–
diastolic diameter • left
ventricular end–diastolic
dimension

LVEDP left ventricular end–
diastolic pressure *also*
LVEP

LVEDV left ventricular end–
diastolic volume

LVEF left ventricular ejection
fraction

LVEndo left ventricular
endocardial half

LVEP left ventricular end–
diastolic pressure *also*
LVEDP

LVER liver fraction elevated

LVESD left ventricular end–
systolic dimension

LVESV left ventricular end–
systolic volume

LVESVI left ventricular end–
systolic volume index

LVET left ventricular ejection
time

LVETI left ventricular ejection
time index

LVF left ventricular failure •
left ventricular function •
left visual field • low–
voltage fast • low–voltage
foci

LVFP left ventricular filling pressure

LVFT₂ left ventricular slow filling time

LVG left ventrogluteal

LVH large vessel hematocrit • left ventricular hypertrophy

LVI left ventricular insufficiency • left ventricular ischemia

LVID left ventricular internal diastolic • left ventricular internal dimension

LVIDd left ventricular internal dimension diastole

LVID(ed) left ventricular internal diameter (end diastole)

LVID(es) left ventricular internal diameter (end systole)

LVIDP left ventricular initial diastolic pressure

LVIDs left ventricular internal dimension systole

LVIV left ventricular infarct volume

LVL left vastus lateralis (muscle)

LVLG left ventrolateral gluteal (injection site)

LVM lateral ventromedial (nucleus) • left ventricular mass

LVMF left ventricular minute flow

LVMM left ventricular muscle mass

LVN lateral ventricular nerve • lateral vestibular nucleus •

Licensed Visiting Nurse • Licensed Vocational Nurse • limiting viscosity number

LVO left ventricular outflow • left ventricular overactivity

LVOA left ventricular overactivity

LVOT left ventricular outflow tract

LVP large volume parenteral (infusion) • left ventricular pressure • levator veli palatini (muscle) • lysine–vasopressin

LVPEP left ventricular pre–ejection period

LVPFR left ventricular peak filling rate

LVPSP left ventricular peak systolic pressure

LVPW left ventricular posterior wall

LVPWT left ventricular posterior wall thickness

LVR leucovorin *also* LCV, LEU, LV • limb vascular resistance

L₁VR, L₂VR, etc first lumbar ventral (nerve) root • second lumbar ventral (nerve) root, etc

LVS left ventricular strain

LVs (mean) left ventricular systolic (pressure)

LVSEMI left ventricular subendocardial myocardial ischemia

LVSI left ventricular systolic index

LVSO left ventricular systolic output

LVSP left ventricular systolic pressure

LVST lateral vestibulospinal tract

LVSV left ventricular stroke volume

LVSW left ventricular septal wall • left ventricular stroke work

LVSWI left ventricular stroke work index

LVT left ventricular tension • lysine vasotonin

LVT₁ left ventricular fast filling time

LVV left ventricular volume • live varicella vaccine

LVW lateral vaginal wall • lateral ventricular width • left ventricular wall • left ventricular work

LVW/HW lateral ventricular width to hemispheric width

LVWI left ventricular work index

LVWM left ventricular wall motion

LVWMA left ventricular wall motion abnormality

LVWMI left ventricular wall motion index

LVWT left ventricular wall thickness

LW lacerating wound • lateral wall • Lee–White (blood–clotting method) • left (ear), warm (stimulus) • Léri–Weill (syndrome) • lung weight • lung width

L&W, L/W Lee and White (clotting time) *also* Lee W, LWCT • living and well

L–10–W levulose (10%) in water

Lw lawrencium *also* Lr

LWBS left without being seen

LWC leave without consent

LWCT Lachar–Wrobel Critical Items • Lee–White clotting time *also* L&W, L/W, Lee W

LWD living with disease

LWP large whirlpool • lateral wall pressure

LX, Lx latex *also* L • local irradiation • lux *also* lx

lx larynx *also* lar • lower extremity *also* LE, L ext, l/ext • lux *also* LX, Lx

LXC laxative of choice *also* LOC

LXT left exotropia

LY lymphocyte *also* lym, lymph. • lyophilization

LYDMA lymphocyte–detected membrane antigen

LYEL lost years (of) expected life

LYG lymphomatoid granulomatosis

LYM lymph

lym, lymph. lymphocyte/lymphocytic *also* LY

LyNeF lytic nephritic factor

LYMPH% percentage of lymphocytes (in differential count)

lyo lyophilized

LYP lactose, yeast, (and) peptone (agar) • lower yield point

Lyp lymphosarcoma *also* LS, LSA

LYS, Lys lysine • lysosome

LySLk lymphoma syndrome leukemia

LYTES, lytes electrolytes *also* elytes

LZM, lzm lysozyme

M blood factor in the MNS blood group system • [L. *mentum*] chin *also* m • concentration in moles per liter • [L. *mors*] death • [L. *mutitas*] dullness (of sound) • [L. *mutitas*] dumbness • [L. *manipulus*] handful *also* m, man., manip • [L. *macerare*] macerate/macerated *also* m • macroglobulin • magnetization • male • malignant *also* MAL, mal, malig • manual • marital • married • masculine • mass • massage *also* mass., MSS, mss • maternal contribution • matrix • matt (dull, slightly granular, bacterial colonies) • mature • maximum • mean *also* m • meatus • media • medial • median *also* m, md • mediator (chemical released in the tissues) • medical • medicine • medium • mega– • megohm • melts at • membrane • memory (associative) • mental • mesial *also* m • meta– • metabolite • metal • metastasis *also* MET, metas, met • meter • methionine • method • methotrexate *also* MTRX, MTX • mexiletin • million • minim • minimum • minute • mitral • mitochondria • mitosis • mix/mixed • mixture • molar (permanent tooth) • molar (solution) • molarity • mole • molecular • molecular weight • moment of force • Monday • monkey • monocyte • month *also* MO, mo, mon • morgan (unit of gene separation) • morphine • mother • motile • mouse • mouth • movement response to human figure • mucoid (colony) • mucous (adjective) • mucus (noun) • multipara • cardiac murmur *also* m, (m) • muscle • muscular response to electrical stimulation of motor nerve • myeloma or macroglobulinemia (component) • myopia • myopic • myosin • [L. *meridies*] noon • [L. *macerare*] soften *also* ma., mac • strength of pole • [L. *mille*] thousand

M1 left mastoid

M₁ mitral first sound (slight dullness) • myeloblast

M² square meter (body surface) *also* m²

M2 right mastoid

M₂ mitral second sound (marked dullness) • promyelocyte

M–2 vincristine, carmustine, cyclophosphamide, melphalan, and prednisone

M₃ mitral third sound (absolute dullness) • myelocyte at third stage of maturation

3–M (syndrome) Miller, McKusick, and Malvaux (who first described the syndrome)

M/3 middle third (long bones)

M₄ myelocyte at fourth stage of maturation

M₅ metamyelocyte

M₆ band form in sixth stage of myelocyte maturation

M₇ polymorphonuclear neutrophil *also* PMN, PMNN

M/10 tenth molar solution

M/100 hundredth molar solution

m by mouth • [L. *mentum*] chin *also* M • electromagnetic moment • electron rest mass • [L. *manipulus*] handful *also* M, man. manip • [L. *mane*] in the morning • [L. *macerare*] macerate *also* M • magnetic moment *also* μ • magnetic quantum number • mass • mean *also* M • median *also* M • melts at *also* M • mesial • meter • milli– • minim • minute • [L. *misce*] mix • [L. *mistura*] mixture • modulus • molality • molar (deciduous tooth) • morphine • motile • mucoid • murmur *also* M, (m) • [L. *meridies*] noon • sample mean • [L. *mitte*] send

(m) by mouth *also* m • murmur *also* M, m

m² square meter (body surface) *also* M²

m³ cubic meter *also* cu m

m₈ spin quantum number

MA machine • mafenide acetate • mandelic acid • manifest achievement • Martin–Albright

(syndrome) • masseter • maternal aunt • mean arterial • medical abbreviation • medical assistance • medical assistant • medical audit • medical authorization • mega–ampere • megaloblastic anemia • megestrol acetate • membrane antigen • menstrual age • mental age • mentum anterior (fetal position) • metatarsus aductus • meter angle • Mexican American • microagglutination • microaneurysm • microscopic agglutination • microcytotoxicity assay • Miller–Abbott (tube) • milliampere • mitochondrial antibody • mitogen activation • mitotic apparatus • mixed agglutination • moderately advanced • monoamine • monoclonal antibody *also* MAB, MAb, MCA, MCAB, MoAb • motorcycle accident *also* MCA • multiple action • muscle activity • mutagenic activity • myelinated axon

M/A male, altered (animal) *also* MALT • mood and/or affect

MA–1 mechanically assisted (Bennett brand of respirator)

Ma mass (of) atom • masurium (technetium)

mA, ma meter–angle • milliampere

mÅ milliangstrom

ma [L. *macera*] soften *also* M, mac

MAA macroaggregated albumin *also* MIAA • Medical Assistance for the Aged • melanoma–associated antigen • monoarticular arthritis

MAAAP macroaggregated albumin arterial perfusion

MAACL Multiple Affect Adjective Check List

MAB, MAb monoclonal antibody *also* MA, MCA, MCAB, MoAb

MABI Mother's Assessment of the Behavior of Her Infant

MABOP Mustargen (nitrogen mustard), Adriamycin (doxorubicin), bleomycin, Oncovin (vincristine), and prednisone

MABP mean arterial blood pressure

MAC MacConkey (agar) • MacIntosh (blade) • macrocytic erythrocyte • macule • malignancy–associated change • maximal acid concentration • maximal allowable concentration • maximal allowable cost • medical alert center • membrane attack complex • methotrexate, actinomycin D, and chlorambucil • methotrexate, actinomycin D, and cyclosphosphamide • midarm circumference • minimal anesthetic concentration • minimal alveolar concentration • minimal antibiotic

concentration • mitral anular calcium • modulator (of) adenylate cyclase • monitored anesthesia care • multidimensional actuarial classification • *Mycobacterium avium* complex

Mac macula

mac maceration *also* macer • [L. *macerare*] soften *also* M, ma

MAC AWAKE minimal alveolar (anesthetic) concentration (patient recovering from general anesthesia able to respond to instructions)

Mac blade Macintosh (laryngoscope) blade

MACC macro–ovalocyte • methotrexate, Adriamycin (doxorubicin), cyclophosphamide, and CCNU (lomustine)

m accur [L. *misce accuratissime*] mix very accurately

MACDP Metropolitan Atlanta Congenital Defects Program

MACE methylchloroform chloroacetophenone

macer maceration *also* mac

mAChR muscarinic acetylcholine receptor

MACR macrocytosin • mean axillary count rate

macro macrocyte/ macrocytic • macroscopic

MAD maximal allowable dose • maximum acid

output • methandriol •
methylandrostenediol •
mind–altering drug •
minimal average dose •
myoadenylate deaminase

mAD, MADA muscle
adenylate deaminase

MADD multiple acyl–CoA
dehydrogenation deficiency

MADRS Montgomery–Asberg
Depression Rating Scale

MAE medical air evacuation •
moves all extremities •
Multilingual Aphasia
Examination

MAEW moves all extremities
well

MAF macrophage activation
factor • macrophage–
agglutinating factor •
minimal audible field •
mouse amniotic fluid •
movement aftereffect

MAFA midarm fat area

MAFAs movement–associated
fetal (heart rate)
accelerations

MAFH macroaggregated
ferrous hydroxide

MAG myelin–associated
glycoprotein

Mag magnesium *also* Mg

mag, magn [L. *magnus*]
large • magnification •
magnify

mag cit magnesium citrate

MAGE mean amplitude (of)
glycerine excursion

MAGF male accessory gland
fluid

MAggF macrophage
agglutination factor

MAGIC microprobe analysis
generalized intensity
correction

MAGS Multidimensional
Assessment of Gains in
School (psychologic test)

mag sulf magnesium sulfate

mAH milliampere–hours

MAHA microangiopathic
hemolytic anemia *also*
MHA • microangiopathic
hemolytic aneurysm

MAHH malignancy–associated
humoral hypercalcemia

MAI maximal aggregation
index • microscopic
aggregation index • minor
acute illness • morbid
anxiety inventory •
movement assessment (of)
infants

MAII Milwaukee Academic
Interest Inventory

MAKA major karyotypic
abnormality

MAL malfunction *also* Mal •
malignant *also* M, mal,
malig • midaxillary line

Mal [L. *malum*] ill • malate •
malfunction *also* MAL

mal [L. *malanandro*] by
blistering • malignant *also*
M, MAL, malig

MALA malarial parasites

MALAR malaria

Mal–BSA maleated bovine
serum albumin

MALG Minnesota
antilymphoblast globulin

malig malignant *also* M, MAL, mal

MALIMET Master List of Medical (Indexing) Terms

MALT male, altered (animal) *also* M/A • mucosa–associated lymphoid tissue

MAM methylazoxymethanol

mam milliampere–minute *also* MA min

M+Am compound myopic astigmatism

MAMA midarm muscle area • monoclonal antimalignin antibody

MAM Ac methylazoxy-methanol acetate

MAMC mean arm muscle circumference • midarm muscle circumference

MAmg medial amygdaloid (nucleus)

MA min, ma–min milli-ampere–minute *also* mam

mammo mammography

m–AMSA amascrine

MAN mannose • magnocellular nucleus (of anterior neostratum)

man. [L. *manipulus*] handful *also* M, m, manip • manipulate • [L. *mane*] morning

mand mandible/mandibular

manip [L. *manipulus*] handful *also* M, m, man. • manipulation

MANOVA multivariate analysis of variance

man pr [L. *mane primo*] first thing in morning

manu manufacture

MAO maximal acid output • medical ankle orthosis • monoamine oxidase

MAOI monoamine oxidase inhibitor

MAP maximal aerobic power • mean airway pressure • mean aortic pressure • mean arterial pressure • Medical Audit Program • megaloblastic anemia (of) pregnancy • mercapturic acid pathway • methyl acceptor protein • methyl-acetoxyprogesterone • methylaminopurine • microlithiasis alveolarum pulmonum • microtubule–associated protein • minimal audible pressure • mitomycin, Adriamycin (doxorubicin), and cisplatin • monophasic action potential • mouse antibody production (test) • muscle–action potential • Musical Aptitude Profile

MAPA muscle adenosine phosphoric acid

MAPC migrating action potential complex

MAPE Multidimensional Assessment of Philosophy of Education

MAPF microatomized protein food

MAPI microbial alkaline protease inhibitor • Millon Adolescent Personality Inventory

MAPS Make A Picture Story (test)

MAR Main Admitting Room • marasmus • marrow • maximal aggregation ratio • medication administration record • microanalytical reagent • minimal angle resolution • mixed antiglobulin reaction

mar margin *also* marg, MG • marker (chromosome)

MARC multifocal and recurrent choroidopathy

MARG (acute) marginal (branch of left circumflex artery)

marg margin *also* mar, MG

MARIA macroaggregated radioiodinated albumin

MARS Mathematics Anxiety Rating Scale • mouse antirat serum

MARS–A Mathematics Anxiety Rating Scale–Adolescents

MARTI mobile advanced real–time image

MAS Management Appraisal Survey • Manifest Anxiety Scale • meconium aspiration syndrome • medical advisory service • mesoatrial shunt • milk–alkali syndrome • milliampere–second *also* Mas, mA–s, mas • minor axis shortening (of left ventricle) • mobile arm support • monoclonal antibodies • Morgagni–Adams–Stokes (syndrome) • motion analysis system

Mas, mA–s, mas milli–ampere–second *also* MAS

masc masculine • mass concentration *also* massc

MASER microwave amplification (by) stimulated emission (of) radiation

MASF Melcher acid–soluble fraction

MASH Mobile Army Surgical Hospital • multiple automated sample harvester

mas pil [L. *massa pilularum*] pill mass

mass . massage *also* M, MSS, mss • massive

massc mass concentration *also* masc

MAST Michigan Alcoholism Screening Test • military antishock trousers

mAST mitochondrial aspartate aminotransferase

mast. mastectomy • mastoid

MAT Manipulative Aptitude Test • manual arts therapist • maternal • maternity • mature *also* M • mean absorption time • medication administration team • methionine adenosyl-transferase • Metropolitan Achievement Tests • microagglutination test • Miller Analogies Test • motivation analysis test • multifocal atrial tachycardia • multiple agent therapy

Mat, mat. material • maternal (origin) • maternity • mature

MATE Maternal Attitudes Evaluation

MATSA Marek associated tumor–specific antigen

matut [L. *matutinus*] in the morning

MAU Meyenburg–Altherr–Uehlinger (syndrome)

MAV mechanical auxiliary ventricle • minimal apparent viscosity • minute alveolar volume • movement arm vector • myeloblastosis–associated virus

MAVA multiple abstract variance analysis

MAVIS mobile artery (and) vein imaging system

MAVR mitral (and) aortic valve replacement

max maxilla/maxillary • maximum

max EP maximal esophageal pressure

MB margin, buccal • isoenzyme of creatine kinase containing M and B subunits • Mallory body • mamillary body • Marsh–Bendall (factor) • mercury bougie • mesiobuccal • methyl bromide • methylene blue *also* MB1, MEB, MeB • microbiologic assay • muscle balance • myocardial band

6MB six–meal bland (diet)

Mb mandible body • mouse brain • myoglobin

mb millibar *also* mbar • [L. *misce bene*] mix well

MBA methylbenzyl alcohol • methylbovine albumin • methylbischloroethylamine (nitrogen mustard)

M–BACOD methotrexate, bleomycin, Adriamycin (doxorubicin), cyclophosphamide, Oncovin (vincristine), and dexamethasone

MBAR myocardial β–adrenergic receptor

mbar millibar *also* mb

MBAS methylene blue active substance

MBB modified barbital buffer

MBC male breast cancer • maximum bladder capacity • maximum breathing capacity • methotrexate, bleomycin, and cisplatin • methylthymol blue complex • microcrystalline bovine collagen • minimal bactericidal concentration

MB–CK creatinine kinase isoenzyme containing M and B subunits

MbCO carbon monoxided myoglobin

MBCU metallic bead–chain urethrocystograph

MBD maximal bactericidal dilution • methotrexate, bleomycin, and diamminedichloroplatinum (cisplatin) • methylene blue dye · minimal brain damage · minimal brain dysfunction · Morquio–Brailsford disease

MBDG mesiobuccal developmental groove

MBE may be elevated · medium below–elbow (cast)

MBEST modulus blipped echo–planar single–pulse technique

MBF meat base formula · medullary blood flow · muscle blood flow · myocardial blood flow

MBFC medial brachial fascial compartment

MBFLB monaural bifrequency loudness balance

MBG mean blood glucose

MBGS Morphine–Benzedrine Group Scale

MBH maximal benefit (from) hospitalization · medial basal hypothalamus

MBH₂ methylene blue, reduced *also* MBR

MBHI Millon Behavioral Health Inventory

MBI methylene blue instillation

MBK methyl butyl ketone

MBL medium brown loose (stool) · menstrual blood loss · minimal bactericidal level

MBl methylene blue *also* MB, MEB, MeB

MBLA methylbenzyl linoleic acid · mouse–specific bone marrow–derived lymphocyte antigen

MBM mineral basal medium · mother's breast milk

MBNW multiple–breath nitrogen washout

MBO mesiobucco–occlusal

MbO₂ oxymyoglobin

MBP melitensis, bovine, porcine (antigen from *Brucella melitensis, B. bovis* and *B. suis*) · major basic protein · maltose–binding protein · mean blood pressure · mesiobuccopulpal · myelin basic protein

MBPS multigated (cardiac) blood pool scanning

MBq megabecquerel

MBR methylene blue, reduced *also* MBH₂

MBRT methylene blue reduction time

MBSA methylated bovine serum albumin

MBSD maple bark stripper disease

MBT mercaptobenzothiazole · mixed bacterial toxin

MBTI Myers–Briggs Type Indicator (psychologic test)

MC macroglobulinemia · mass casualty · mast cell · maximal concentration · Medical Corps · medium–chain (triglyceride) · medullary cavity · medullary cystic (disease) · megacoulomb · megacurie *also* MCi · megacycle · melanoma cell · meningeal carcinomatosis · Merkel

cell • mesenteric collateral •
mesiocervical • mesocaval
(shunt) • metacarpal •
metatarsocuneiform •
methyl cellulose •
methylcholanthrene *also*
MCA • microcephaly •
microciliary clearance •
microcirculation •
midcapillary • midcarpal •
mineralocorticoid *also* M–
C • minimal change •
Minkowski–Chauffard
(syndrome) • mitomycin C
also Mit–C, MITO–C,
MMC, MTC • mitotic
cycle • mitoxantrone (and)
cytarabine • mitral
commissurotomy • mixed
cellularity • mixed
cryoglobulinemia •
molluscum contagiosum •
monkey cell • mononuclear
cell • mouth care •
mycelial phase (of fungi) •
myocarditis

M–C Magovern–Cromie
(prosthesis) •
mineralocorticoid *also* MC

M/C male, castrated (animal)

M&C morphine and cocaine

Mc mandible coronoid

mC millicoulomb

mc millicurie *also* mCi

MCA major coronary artery •
medical care
administration • megestrol,
cyclophosphamide, and
Adriamycin (doxorubicin) •
methylcholanthrene *also*
MC • middle cerebral
aneurysm • middle
cerebral artery •
monocarboxylic acid •

monoclonal antibody *also*
MA, MAB, MAb, MCAB,
MoAb • motorcycle
accident *also* MA •
multichannel analyzer •
multiple congenital
abnormalities • multiple
congenital anomalies

MCAB, MC–Ab monoclonal
antibody *also* MA, MAB,
MAb, MCA, MoAb

MCA/MR multiple congenital
anomalies/mental
retardation (syndrome)

MCAR mixed cell
agglutination reaction

MCAS middle cerebral artery
syndrome

MCAT Medical College
Admission Test • middle
cerebral artery thrombosis

m caute [L. *misce caute*] mix
with caution

MCB membranous cytoplasmic
body • monochloro-
benzidine

McB McBurney (point)

mCBF mean cerebral blood
flow

MCBM muscle capillary
basement membrane

MCBMT muscle capillary
basement membrane
thickening

MCBP melphalan,
cyclophosphamide, BCNU
(bischloroethylnitrosourea),
and prednisone

MCBR minimal concentration
(of) bilirubin

MCC marked cocontraction •

mean corpuscular (hemoglobin) concentration • medial cell column • metacarpal–carpal (joints) • metacerebral cell • metastatic cord compression • microcrystalline collagen • midstream clean catch (urine) • minimal complete–killing concentration • mucocutaneous candidiasis

McC McCarthy (panendoscope) • McCoy (antibody)

MCCD minimal cumulative cardiotoxic dose

MCCNU methylchlorethyl-cyclakexylnitrosourea (semustine)

MCCU mobile coronary care unit

MCD magnetic circular dichroism • margin crease distance • mast–cell degranulation • mean cell diameter • mean corpuscular diameter • mean (of) consecutive differences • medullary collecting duct • medullary cystic disease • metabolic coronary dilation • metacarpal cortical density • minimal cerebral dysfunction • minimal change disease • multicystic disease • multiple carboxylase deficiency • muscle carnitine deficiency

mcD millicuries destroyed

MCDI Minnesota Child Development Inventory

MCDK multiceptic dysplastic kidney

MCDP mast cell degranulating peptide

MCDT mast cell degranulation test • multiple choice discrimination test

MCE medical–care evaluation • Medicare Code Editor • multicystic encephalopathy

MCES multiple cholesterol emboli syndrome

MCF macrophage chemotactic factor • macrophage cytotoxicity factor • median cleft face • medium corpuscular fragility • microcomplement fixation • monocyte (leukotactic) factor • mononuclear cell factor • most comfortable frequency • myocardial contractile force

MCFA medium–chain fatty acid • miniature centrifugal fast analyzer

MCFP mean circulating filling pressure

MCG magnetocardiogram • membrane coating granule • mesencephalic central gray • monoclonal gammopathy *also* MG

mcg microgram *also* μg

MCGC metacerebral giant cell

MCGF mast cell growth factor

MCGN mesangiocapillary glomerulonephritis • minimal–change

glomerulonephritis •
mixed cryoglobulinemia
(with) glomerulonephritis

MCH Maternal and Child
Health • mean cell
hemoglobin • mean
corpuscular hemoglobin
also MCHb, MCHg •
methacholine •
microfibrillar collagen
hemostat • muscle
contraction headache

mc–h, mch, mc–hr
millicurie–hour *also* mchr,
mCi–hr

MCHb mean corpuscular
hemoglobin *also* MCH,
MCHg

MCHbC mean cell hemoglobin
concentration *also* MCHC •
mean corpuscular
hemoglobin concentration
also MCHC • mean
corpuscular hemoglobin
count *also* MCHC

MCHC maternal and child
health care • mean cell
hemoglobin concentration
also MCHbC • mean
corpuscular hemoglobin
concentration *also*
MCHbC • mean
corpuscular hemoglobin
count *also* MCHbC

MCHg mean corpuscular
hemoglobin *also* MCH,
MCHb

mchr millicurie–hour *also* mc–
h, mch, mc–hr, mCi–hr

MCHS Maternal and Child
Health Service

MCI mean cardiac index •
methicillin *also* METH

MCi megacurie *also* MC

mCi millicurie *also* mc

mCid millicuries destroyed

mCi–hr millicurie–hour *also*
mc–h, mch, mc–hr, mchr

MCINS minimal change
idiopathic nephrotic
syndrome

MCK multicystic kidney

MCKD multicystic kidney
disease

MCL maximal comfort level •
maximal containment
laboratory • medial
collateral ligament •
midclavian line •
midclavicular line •
midcostal line • minimal
change lesion • mixed
culture, leukocyte •
modified chest lead • most
comfortable listening (level)
also MCLL • most
comfortable loudness (level)
also MCLL

MCLD *Mycobacterium
chelonei*–like organism

MCLL most comfortable
listening level *also* MCL •
most comfortable loudness
level *also* MCL

MCLNS, MCLS
mucocutaneous lymph node
syndrome

MCMI Millon Clinical
Multiaxial Inventory
(psychiatric battery)

mcmol micromole

MCMV mouse
cytomegalovirus • murine
cytomegalovirus

MCN minimal–change nephropathy

MC–N mixed cell nodular (lymphoma)

MCNS minimal–change nephrotic syndrome

MCO medical care organization

mcoul millicoulomb

MCP maximal closure pressure • melanosis circumscripta precancerosa • melphalan, cyclophosphamide, and prednisone • metacarpal • metacarpophalangeal *also* MCPH • metaclopramide • methyl–accepting chemotaxis protein • mitotic–control protein • mucin clot–prevention (test)

MCPH metacarpophalangeal *also* MCP

MCPJ metacarpal phalangeal joint

MCPS Missouri Children's Picture Series (psychologic test)

Mcps, mcps megacycles per second

MCQ multiple choice question

MCR Medical Corps Reserve • message competition ratio • metabolic clearance rate

MCS malignant carcinoid syndrome • Marlowe–Crown (Social Desirability) Scale *also* MCSDS • mesocaval shunt • methylcholanthrene(-induced) sarcoma • microculture and sensitivity • multiple combined sclerosis • myocardial contractile state

mc/s megacycles per second

MCSA minimal cross–sectional area • Moloney cell surface antigen

M–CSF macrophage colony–stimulating factor

MCSDS Marlow–Crowne Social Desirability Scale *also* MCS

MCT manual cervical traction • mean cell thickness • mean cell threshold • mean circulation time • mean corpuscular thickness • medium–chain triglyceride • medullary (carcinoma) of thyroid • medullary collecting tubule • monocrotaline • multiple compressed tablet

MCTC metrizamide computed tomographic cisternography

MCTD mixed connective tissue disease

MCTF mononuclear cell tissue factor

MCU malaria control unit • maximal care unit • micturating cystourethrography • motor cortex unit

McU microunit

MCV mean cell volume • mean clinical value • mean corpuscular volume • median cell volume • motor conduction velocity

mcv microvolt

MCZ miconazole

MD [L. *Medicinae Doctor*]
Doctor of Medicine •
macula degeneration •
macula densa • magnesium
deficiency • main duct •
maintenance dialysis •
maintenance dose • major
depression • malate
dehydrogenase •
malrotation (of) duodenum •
mammary dysplasia •
mandibular • manic–
depression • manic–
depressive • Mantoux
diameter • Marek disease •
maternal deprivation •
maximal dose • mean
deviation • mean diastolic •
measurable disease •
Meckel diverticulum •
(nucleus) medialis dorsalis •
mediastinal disease •
medical department •
medical doctor •
mediodorsal • medium
dosage • mental
deficiency • mental
depression • mesiodistal •
Minamata disease • minimal
dosage • mitral disease •
mixed diet • moderate
disability • monocular
deprivation • movement
disorder • multiple
deficiency • muscular
dystrophy •
myeloproliferative disease •
myocardial damage •
myocardial disease

Md mendelevium *also* Mv

md [L. *more dicto*] as directed •
median *also* M, m

MDA malondialdehyde •
manual dilatation of anus •
monodehydroascorbate •
motor discriminative
acuity • multivariant

discriminant analysis • [L.
mento–dextra anterior]
right mentoanterior (fetal
position)

MDAD mineral dust airway
disease

MDAP Machover Draw–A–
Person (Test)

MDBDF March of Dimes Birth
Defect Foundation

MDBK Madin–Darby bovine
kidney (cell)

MDBSS Mischell–Dutton
balanced salt solution

MDC major diagnostic
category • medial dorsal
cutaneous (nerve) •
minimal detectable
concentration

MDCK Madin–Darby canine
kidney (cell)

MDD major depressive
disorder • manic–
depressive disorder • mean
daily dose

MDDA Minnesota Differential
Diagnosis of Aphasia

MDE major depressive episode

MDEBP mean daily erect
blood pressure

MDF mean dominant
frequency • myocardial
depressant factor

MDG mean diastolic gradient

MDGF macrophage–derived
growth factor

MDH malate dehydrogenase •
medullary dorsal horn

MDHM malate dehydrogenase,
mitochondrial

MDHR maximum determined heart rate

MDHS malate dehydrogenase, soluble

MDHV Marek disease herpesvirus

MDI manic–depressive illness • metered dose inhaler • multiple daily injection • multiple dosage insulin • Multiscore Depression Inventory

MDIA Mental Development Index, Adjusted

m dict [L. *moro dicto*] as directed

MDII multiple daily insulin injection

MDIT mean disintegration time

MDL Master Drug List

MDM mid–diastolic murmur • minor determinant mix (penicillin)

mdn median

MDNB mean daily nitrogen balance • metadinitrobenzene • methylene diphosphate

MDP mandibular dysostosis and peromelia • manic–depressive psychosis • methylene diphosphate • muramyldipeptide • muscular dystrophy, progressive • [L. *mento–dextra posterior*] right mentoposterior (fetal position)

MDPI maximal daily permissible intake

MDQ memory deviation

quotient • minimal detectable quantity

MDR mammalian diving response • median duration (of) response • minimal daily requirement

MDRH multidisciplinary rehabilitation hospital

MDRS Mattis Dementia Rating Scale

MDS maternal deprivation syndrome • medical data screen • medical data system • microdilution system • microsurgical drill system • milk drinker's syndrome • Miller–Dieker syndrome • multidimensional scaling • myelodysplasia • myelodysplastic syndrome • myocardial depressant substance

MDSBP mean daily supine blood pressure

MDSO mentally disordered sex offender

MDT mast (cell) degeneration test • mean dissolution time • median detection threshold • multidisciplinary team • [L. *mento–dextra transversa*] right mentotransverse (fetal position)

MDTA McDonald Deep Test of Articulation

MDTP multidisciplinary treatment plan

MDTR mean diameter–thickness ratio

MDUO myocardial disease (of) unknown origin

MDV Marek disease virus • mucosal disease virus • multiple dose vial

MDY month, date, year

Mdyn megadyne

ME Mache Einkeit • macular edema • magnitude estimation • male equivalent • malic enzyme • manic episode • maximal effort • median eminence • medical education • Medical Examiner • meningoencephalitis • mercaptoethanol • metabolic (and) electrolyte (disorder) • metabolic energy • metabolism • metabolizable energy • metamyelocyte • methyleugenol • microembolization • middle ear • mouse embryo • mouse epithelial (cell) • muscle examination

M/E myeloid/erythroid (ratio)

ME$_{50}$ 50% maximal effect

2ME 2–mercaptoethanol

Me menton • methyl *also* meth

MEA mercaptoethylamine • multiple endocrine adenomatosis

MEA–I multiple endocrine adenomatosis type I

meas measurement

MEB, MeB Medical Evaluation Board •

methylene blue *also* MB, MBl

MeBSA methylated bovine serum albumin

MEC mecillinam • meconium • median effective concentration • middle ear canal • middle ear cell • minimal effective concentration • myoepithelial cell

Mec, mec meconium

MeCCNU methylchloroethyl-cyclohexylmitrosourea (semustine) *also* methyl–CCNU

MECG maternal electrocardiogram • mixed essential cryoglobulinemia

MeCP methyl–CCNU, cyclophosphamide, and prednisone

MECT maximal extrapolated clotting time

MECTA mobile electroconvulsive therapy apparatus

MECY methyltrexate and cyclophosphamide

MED medial *also* Med, med • median erythrocyte diameter • medical *also* Med, med • medication • medicine *also* Med, med • medium *also* Med, med • minimal effective dose • minimal erythema dose • multiple epiphyseal dysplasia

Med, med medial *also* MED • median • medical *also* MED • medicine *also* MED • medium *also* MED

MEDAC multiple endocrine deficiency, Addison disease, and candidiasis (syndrome) • multiple endocrine deficiency–autoimmune candidiasis

MED–ART Medical Automated Records Technology

MEDEX, Medex [Fr. *médicin extension*] extension of physician (physician assistant program using former military medical corpsmen)

medic [L. *medicus*] military medical corpsman

MEDICO Medical International Cooperation

MEDIHC Military Experience Directed into Health Careers

MEDLARS Medical Literature Analysis and Retrieval System

MEDLINE MEDLARS On–Line

med men medial meniscectomy • medial meniscus

MEDPAR Medical Provider Analysis and Review

MEdREP Medical Education Reinforcement and Enrichment Program

MEDs medications

MEDScD Doctor of Medical Science

MedSurg medicine and surgery

Med Tech Medical Technician/Technologist/Technology

MEE measured energy expenditure • methylethyl ether • middle ear effusion

MEET Multistage Exercise Electrocardiographics Test

MEF maximal expiratory flow • middle ear fluid • midexpiratory flow • migration enhancement factor • mouse embryo fibroblast

MEF$_{50}$ mean maximal expiratory flow

MEFA methyl–CCNU (semustine), 5–fluorouracil, and Adriamycin (doxorubicin)

MEFR maximal expiratory flow rate

MEFSR maximal expiratory flow–static recoil (curve)

MEFV maximal expiratory flow volume

MEFVC maximal expiratory flow volume curve • mechanical expiratory flow volume curve

MEG magnetoenceph-alogram • magnetoenceph-alography • mercaptoethyl-guanidine • multifocal eosinophilic granuloma

mEGF mouse epidermal growth factor

MEGX monoethyl-glycinexylidide

MEK methylethylketone

MEL metabolic equivalent level • mouse erythroleukemia • murine erythroleukemia

mel melena

MELAN melanin

MELC murine erythroleukemia cell

MELDOS meliodosis

MELI met–enkaphalin–like immunoreactivity

MEM macrophage electrophoretic mobility • malic enzyme, mitochondrial *also* MEm • minimal essential medium

MEm malic enzyme, mitochondrial *also* MEM

MEMA methyl methacrylate *also* MMA

memb membrane

MEMR multiple exostoses– mental retardation (syndrome)

MEN methylethylnitrosamine • multiple endocrine neoplasia/neoplasms

men. meningeal • meninges • meningitis

MEND Medical Education for National Defense

menst menstrual/menstruate/ menstruating

MEO malignant external otitis

MeOH methyl alcohol

MEOS microsomal ethanol– oxidizing system

MEP maximal expiratory pressure • mean effective pressure • motor end– plate • multimodality evoked potential

MEP, mep meperidine

MEPC miniature end–plate current

MEPH mephobarbital

MEPP miniature end–plate potential

MePr methylprednisolone

mEQ, mEq, meq milliequivalent

mEq/L milliequivalent per liter

MER mean ejection rate • mersalyl (acid) • methanol extraction residue (of bacille Calmette–Guerin) • molar esterification rate • multimodality evoked response

M/E, M:E ratio myeloid/ erythroid ratio

MERB Medical Examination and Review Board • metenkaphalin receptor binding

MERG macular electroretinogram

MES maintenance electrolyte solution • maximal electroshock • maximal electroshock seizure • mesial • Metrazol– electroshock seizure • morpholinoethanesulfonic acid • muscle (in) elongated state • myoelectric signal

Mes mesencephalic • mesencaphalon

Mesc mescaline

MESCH Multi–Environment Scheme

MESGN mesangial glomerulonephritis

MeSH Medical Subject Heading (in MEDLARS)

MesPGN mesangial proliferative glomerulonephritis

MET medical emergency treatment · metabolic *also* metab · metabolic equivalent (of) task · metabolic equivalent test · metastasis/metastatic *also* M, metas, met · metamyelocyte · methionine · metoprolol · midexpiratory time · multistage exercise test

Met methionine

met metallic (chest sounds) · metastasis/metastasize/ metastasizing *also* M, MET, metas

META metamyelocyte

meta metacarpal · metatarsal

metab metabolic *also* MET · metabolism

metas metastasis/metastatic *also* M, MET, met

METH methicillin *also* MCI

Meth methedrine

meth methyl *also* Me

Met–Hb methemoglobin *also* MHB, MHb

MeTHF methyltetrahydrofolic acid

methyl–CCNU methylchloroethylcyclohexylnitrosourea (semustine) *also* MeCCNU

MetMb metmyoglobin

m et n [L. *mane et nocte*] morning and night

METS metabolic equivalents (multiples of resting oxygen consumption) · metastases

m et sig [L. *misce et signa*] mix and write a label

METT maximal exercise tolerance test

m et v [L. *mane et vespere*] morning and evening

MEV maximal exercise ventilation · million electron volts · murine erythroblastosis virus

MeV, mev megaelectron volt

MEX Mexican · mexiletin

MF masculinity/femininity · mass fragmentography · meat free · medium frequency · megafarad · melamine formaldehyde · merthiolate–formaldehyde (solution) · methanol formaldehyde · methotrexate, fluorouracil, and calcium leucovorin · methoxyflurane · microfibrile · microfilament · microfilia · microscopic factor · midcavity forceps · mitogenic factor · mitomycin–fluorouracil · mitotic figure · mossy fiber · mucosal fluid · multifactorial · multiplication factor · mutation frequency · mycosis fungoides · myelin figure · myelofibrosis · myocardial fibrosis · myofibrillar

M/F male to female (ratio)

M&F male and female · mother and father

Mf maxillofrontal · micropilaria *also* mf

mF millifarad

mf microfilaria *also* mf

MFA methyl fluoracetate • monofluoroacetate • multifocal functional autonomy • multifunctional acrylic • multiple factor analysis

MFAT multifocal atrial tachycardia

MFB medial forebrain bundle • metallic foreign body

MFC mean frequency (of) compensation • minimal fungicidal concentration

m–FC membrane focal coli (broth)

MFD mandibulofacial dysostosis • Memory for Designs • midforceps delivery • milk–free diet • minimal fatal dose

MFEM maximal forced expiratory maneuver

MFG modified heat–degraded gelatin

MFH malignant fibrous histiocytoma • membrane–free hemolysate

MFID multielectrode flame ionization detector

m flac [L. *membrana flaccida*] flaccid membrane (Shrapnell membrane)

MFM millipore filter method

MFO mixed function oxidase

MFP monofluorophosphate • myofascial pain

MFPVC multifocal premature ventricular contraction

MFR mean flow rate •

midforceps rotation • mucus flow rate

MFRL maximal force at rest length

MFS medical fee schedule • merthiolate formaldehyde solution • Minnesota Follow–up Study

MF sol merthiolate–formaldehyde solution

MFSS Medical Field Service School

MFST Medical Field Service Technician

MFT multifocal atrial tachycardia • muscle function test

m ft [L. *mistura fiat*] let a mixture be made

MFU medical follow–up

MFVD midforceps vaginal delivery

MFVNS middle fossa vestibular nerve section

MFVPT Motor–Free Visual Perception Test *also* MVPT

MFW multiple fragment wounds

MG Marcus Gunn (pupil) *also* M–G • margin *also* mar., marg • medial gastrocnemius (muscle) • membranous glomerulonephritis *also* MGN • membranous glomerulopathy • menopausal gonadotropin • mesiogingival • methylglucoside • methylguanidine • Michaelis–Gutmann (bodies) • minigastrin •

monoclonal gammopathy *also* MCG • monoglyceride • mucigen granule • mucous granule • muscle group • myasthenia gravis *also* MyG • myoglobin

M–G Marcus Gunn (pupil) *also* MG

Mg magnesium

mg milligram *also* mgm, mgr

mg % milligrams per deciliter • milligrams per 100 cubic centimeters or per 100 grams • milligrams per 100 milliliters • milligrams percent

MGA medical gas analyzer • melengestrol acetate

mγ micromilligram • milligamma • nanogram

MGB medial geniculate body

MGBG methylglyoxal bisguanylhydrazone

MGC minimal glomerular change

MgC magnocellular neuroendocrine cell

MGD maximal glucose disposal • mixed gonadal dysgenesis

mg/dL milligram per deciliter

mg–el milligram–element

MGES multiple gated equilibrium scintigraphy

MGF macrophage growth factor • maternal grandfather • mother's grandfather

MGG May–Grünwald–Giemsa (staining) • molecular

(and) general genetics • mouse gamma globulin

MGGH methylglyoxal guanylhydrazone

MGH monoglyceride hydrolase

mgh, mg–hr milligram–hour

MGI macrophage (and) granulocyte inducer

mg/kg milligram per kilogram

MGL minor glomerular lesion

mg/L milligram per liter

MGM maternal grandmother • mother's grandmother

mgm milligram *also* mg, mgr

MGN membranous glomerulonephritis *also* MG

MGP Marcus–Gunn pupil • marginal granulocyte pool • marginated granulocyte pool • membranous glomerulonephropathy • methyl green pyronin (dye) • mucin glycoprotein • mucous glycoprotein

MGR modified gain ratio • multiple gas rebreathing • murmurs, gallops, or rubs *also* MRG

mgr milligram *also* mg, mgm

MGS metric gravitational system

MGSA melanoma growth–stimulating activity

MGSD mean gestational sac diameter

mgtis meningitis

MGUS monoclonal gammopathies (of) undetermined significance

MGW magnesium sulfate, glycerin, and water (enema)

MGXT multistage graded exercise test

mGy milligray

MH maleic hydrazide • malignant histiocytosis • malignant hyperpyrexia • malignant hypertension • malignant hyperthermia • mammotropic hormone • mannoheptulose • marital history • medial hypothalamus • medical history • melanophore–stimulating hormone *also* MSH • menstrual history • mental health • mental hygiene • moist heat • monosymptomatic hypochondriasis • multiple handicapped • murine hepatitis • mutant hybrid • myohyoid

M/H microcytic hypochromic (anemia)

M–H Mueller–Hinton (agar) *also* MHA

Mh mandible head

mH millihenry

MHA May–Hegglin anomaly • Mental Health Association • methemalbumin • microangiopathic hemolytic anemia *also* MAHA • microhemagglutination • middle hepatic artery • mixed hermadsorption • Mueller–Hinton agar *also* M–H

MHA–TP microhemag-glutination–*Treponema pallidum*

MHB maximal hospital benefit • mental health (assistance) benefit • methemoglobin *also* Met–Hb, MHb

MHb medial habenular • methemoglobin *also* Met–Hb, MHB • myohemoglobin

MHBSS modified Hank's balanced salt solution

MHC major histocompatibility complex • mental health care • mental health center • mental health counselor • multiphasic health check–up

mhcp mean horizontal candle-power

MHCS Mental Hygiene Consultation Service

m/hct microhematocrit

MHCU mental health care unit

MHD maintenance hemodialysis • maximal human dose • mean hemolytic dose • mental health department • minimal hemolytic dilution • minimal hemolytic dose

MHI malignant histiocytosis (of) intestine • Mental Health Index (information) • Mental Health Institute

MHLC Multidimensional Health Locus of Control

MHLS metabolic heat load stimulator

MH/MR mental health and mental retardation

MHN massive hepatic necrosis • Mohs hardness number • morbus haemolyticus neonatorum

MHNTG multiheteronodular toxic goiter

MHO microsomal heme oxygenase

mho reciprocal ohm • siemens unit (ohm spelled backward)

MHP maternal health program • methoxyhydroxypropane • monosymptomatic hypochondriacal psychosis

MHPA mild hyperphenylalaninemia • Minnesota–Hartford Personality Assay

MHPG methoxyhydroxy-phenylglycol

MHR major histocompatibility region • malignant hyperthermia resistance • maximal heart rate • methemoglobin reductase *also* MR, MR–E

MHRI Mental Health Research Institute

MHS major histocompatibility system • malignant hypothermia susceptibility • multiple health screening

MHSA microaggregated human serum albumin

MHST multiphasic health screen test

MHT multiphasic health testing

MHTI minor hypertensive infant

MHTS Multiphasic Health Testing Services

MHV magnetic heart vector • minimal height velocity • mouse hepatitis virus

MHVD Marek herpesvirus disease

MHW medial heel wedge • mental health worker

MHx medical history

mHz megahertz

MI maturation index • medical inspection • melanophore index • membrane intact • menstruation induction • mental illness • mental institution • mercaptoimidazole • mesioincisal • metabolic index • metaproterenol inhaler • methyl indole • migration index • migration inhibition • mild irritant • mitotic index • mitral incompetence • mitral insufficiency • mononucleosis infectiosa • morphology index • motility index • myocardial infarction • myocardial ischemia • myoinositol

M&I maternal and infant (care)

MI mitomycin *also* MIT

mi mile

MIA medically indigent adult • missing in action • multi–institutional arrangement

MIAA microaggregated albumin *also* MAA

MIAP modified innervated antral pouch

MIB Medical Impairment Bureau

mIBG metaiodo-benzylguanidine

MIBK methylisobutyl ketone

MIC maternal (and) infant care • medical intensive care • Medical Interfraternity Conference • methacholine inhalation challenge • microcytic erythrocyte • microscope • microscopic • minimal inhibitory concentration • minimal isorrheic concentration • mobile intensive care • model immune complex

MIC minocycline

MICG macromolecular insoluble cold globulin

MICN mobile intensive care nurse

mic pan [L. *mica panis*] bread crumb

MICR methacoline inhalation challenge response

micro microcyte/microcytic • microscopic

microbiol microbiology

MICU medical intensive care unit • mobile intensive care unit

MID maximum inhibiting duration • mesioincisodistal • midazolam • minimal infective dose • minimal inhibitory dilution • minimal inhibitory dose • minimal irradiation dose • multi–infarct dementia • multiple ion detection

mid middle

mid/3 middle third (of long bone)

Mid I middle insomnia

MIDS Management Information Decision System

midsag midsagittal

MIE medical improvement expected • methylisoeugenol

MIF macrophage inhibitory factor • melanocyte–inhibiting factor • melanocyte(–stimulating hormone)–inhibiting factor • merthiolate–iodine–formaldehyde (method) • merthiolate–iodine–formalin (solution) • methylene–iodine–formalin • microimmunofluorescence • midinspiratory flow • migration–inhibiting factor • mixed immunofluorescence • mHllerian inhibiting factor

MIFA mitomycin–C, 5–fluoro-uracil, and Adriamycin (doxorubicin)

MIFC merthiolate–iodine–formaldehyde concentration

MIFR maximal inspiratory flow rate • midinspiratory flow rate

MIFT merthiolate–iodine–formaldehyde technique

MIG measles immune globulin

MIg malaria immunoglobulin • measles immunoglobulin • membrane immunoglobulin

MIGW maximal increment in growth and weight

MIH methylhydrazine methylisopropylbenzamide · migraine with interparoxysmal headache · minimal intermittent (dosage of) heparin · monoiodohistidine

MIKA minor karyotype abnormality

MIKE mass–analyzed ion kinetic energy

MIL military · mother–in–law *also* M/L

MILP mitogen–induced lymphocyte proliferation

MILS medication information leaflet (for) seniors

MIME mean indices (of) meal excursions

MIMS Medical Information Management System · Medical Inventory Management System

MIN medial interlaminar nucleus · mineral *also* min · minimum *also* min · minor *also* min · minute *also* min

min mineral *also* MIN · minim · minimum/minimal *also* MIN · minor *also* MIN · minute *also* MIN

MINA monoisonitrosoacetone

MINE medical improvement not expected · mesna uroprotection, ifosfamide, mitoxantrone, and etoposide

MINIA monkey intranuclear inclusion agent

MIO minimal identifiable odor

MIP maximal inspiratory pressure · mean intravascular pressure · medical improvement possible · metacarpointerphalangeal · minimal inspiratory pressure

MIPS myocardial isotopic perfusion scan

MIR multiple isomorphous replacement

MIRD medical internal radiation dose

MIRF macrophage immunogenic antigen–recruiting factor

MIRP myocardial infarction rehabilitation program

MIRU myocardial infarction research unit

MIS management information system · Medical Information Service · meiosis–inducing substance · mitral insufficiency · mHllerian inhibiting substance

Mis Astig mixed astigmatism

misc miscarriage · miscellaneous

MISG modified immune serum globulin

MISO misonidazole

MISS modified injury severity score (scale)

MISSGP mercury in Silastic strain gauge plethysmography

MIST Medical Information Service by Telephone

mist. [L. *mistura*] mixture

MIT Male Impotence Test •
marrow iron turnover •
meconium in trachea •
melodic intonation
therapy • metabolism
inhibition test • migration
inhibition test • miracidial
immobilization test •
mitomycin *also* Mi •
monoiodotyrosine

mit mitral • [L. *mitte*] send

Mit–C mitomycin C *also* MC,
MITO–C, MMC, MTC

Mith mithramycin

mit insuf mitral insufficiency

MITO–C mitomycin C *also*
MC, Mit–C, MMC, MTC

mit sang, mitt sang [L. *mitte
sanguinem* let go the blood]
blood–letting procedure

mitt tal [L. *mitte tales*] send
such

mIU milli–International unit
(one–thousandth of an
International unit)

mix. mixture *also* mixt

mix. mon mixed monitor

mixt mixture *also* mix

MJ marijuana • megajoule

MJA mechanical joint
apparatus

MJL medial joint line

MJT Mead Johnson tube •
Mowlem–Jackson technique

MK main kitchen • marked •
menaquinone (vitamin
K_2) • monkey kidney *also*
MkK • myokinase

MK–6 vitamin K_2

Mk monkey

MKAB may keep at bedside

mkat millikatal

mkat/L millikatal per liter

MKB megakaryoblast

MKC monkey kidney cell

MK–CSF megakaryocyte
colony–stimulating factor

mkg meter–kilogram

MkK monkey kidney *also* MK

MKP monobasic potassium
phosphate

MKS, mks meter–kilogram–
second

MKSAP Medical Knowledge
Self–Assessment Program

MKTC monkey kidney tissue
culture

MKV killed measles vaccine

ML Licentiate in Midwifery •
malignant lymphoma •
marked latency • maximal
left • meningeal
leukemia • mesiolingual •
middle lobe • midline •
molecular layer • motor
latency • mucolipidosis •
multiple lentiginosis •
muscular layer • myeloid
leukemia

M:L maltase to lactase (ratio)

M–L Martin–Lewis (medium)

M/L monocyte/lymphocyte
(ratio) • mother–in–law
also MIL

mL milliliter *also* ml

mL, mLa millilambert

ml midline • milliliter *also* mL

MLA [L. *mento–laeva anterior*] left mentoanterior (fetal position) • Medical Library Association • medium long–acting • mesiolabial *also* MLa • monocytic leukemia, acute • multilanguage aphasia

MLa mesiolabial *also* MLA

MLAB Multilingual Aphasia Battery

MLAI, MLaI mesiolabioincisal

MLAP mean left atrial pressure

MLaP mesiolabiopulpal

MLB monaural loudness balance

MLb macrolymphoblast

MLBP mechanical low back pain

MLC Marginal Line Calculus (Index) • minimal lethal concentration • mixed leukocyte concentration • mixed leukocyte culture • mixed ligand chelate • mixed lymphocyte concentration • mixed lymphocyte culture • morphine–like compound • multilamellar cytosome • multilevel care • multilumen catheter • myelomonocytic leukemia, chronic

MLCK myosin light–chain kinase

MLCN multilocular cystic nephroma

MLCP myosin light–chain phosphatase

MLCR mixed lymphocyte culture reaction

MLCT metal–to–ligand charge transfer

ML–CVP multilumen central venous pressure

MLCW mixed lymphocyte culture, weak

MLD masking level difference • median lethal dose *also* MLD_{50} • metachromatic leukodystrophy • minimal lesion disease • minimal lethal dose

MLD_{50} median lethal dose *also* MLD

mL/dL milliliter per deciliter

MLE maximal likelihood estimation

MLE, MLEpis mediolateral episiotomy • midline episiotomy

MLF medial longitudinal fasciculus • median longitudinal fasciculus • morphine–like factor

MLG mesiolingual groove • mitochondria lipid glucogen

MLGN minimal lesion glomerulonephritis

ML–H malignant lymphoma, histiocytic

MLI mesiolinguoincisal • mixed lymphocyte interaction • motilin–like immunoreactivity

MLL malignant lymphoma, lymphoblastic (type)

mL/L milliliters per liter

MLN membranous lupus nephropathy • mesenteric lymph node

MLNS mucocutaneous lymph node syndrome

MLO mesiolinguo–occlusal

MLP [L. *mento–laeva posterior*] left mentoposterior (fetal position) • mesiolinguopulpal • microsomal lipoprotein

ML–PDL malignant lymphoma, poorly differentiated lymphocytic

MLR middle latency response • mixed leukocyte reaction • mixed leukocyte response • mixed lymphocyte reaction • mixed lymphocyte response

MLS mean life–span • median life–span • median longitudinal section • middle lobe syndrome • mucolipidoses • myelomonocytic leukemia, subacute

MLT [L. *mento–laeva transversa*] left mentotransverse (fetal position) • mean latency time • median lethal time • Medical Laboratory Technician

MLT(ASCP) Medical Laboratory Technician certified by American Society of Clinical Pathologists

MLTC mixed leukocyte–trophoblast culture

MLTI mixed lymphocyte target interaction

MLU mean length (of) utterance

MLV Moloney leukemogenic virus • monitored live voice • mouse leukemia virus • multilaminar vesicle • murine leukemia virus

MLVDP maximal left ventricular developed pressure

mlx millilux

MM macromolecule • major medical (insurance) • malignant melanoma • manubrium (of) malleus • Marshall–Marchetti (procedure for urinary incontinence) • medial malleolus • megamitochondria • melanoma metastasis • meningococcic meningitis • mercaptopurine and methotrexate • metastatic melanoma • methadone maintenance • middle molecule • milk and molasses *also* M&M • millimeter *also* mm • minimal medium • missmatch • morbidity and mortality *also* M&M • motor meal • mucous membrane • Muller maneuver • multiple myeloma • muscles *also* mm • muscularis mucosae • myeloid metaplasia • myelomeningocele

M&M milk and molasses *also*

MM • morbidity and mortality *also* MM

Mm mandible mentum

mM millimolar • millimole

mm methylmalonyl • millimeter *also* MM • murmur • muscles *also* MM

mm² square millimeter

mm³ cubic millimeter *also* cmm, cu mm

MMA mastitis–metritis–agalactia (syndrome) • medical materials account • methylmalonic acid • methylmercuric acetate • methyl methacrylate *also* MEMA

MMAA mini–microaggregated albumin colloid

MMAD mass median aerodynamic diameter

MMATP methadone maintenance (and) aftercare treatment program

MMC migrating motor complex • migrating myoelectric complex • minimal medullary concentration • mitomycin C *also* MC, Mit–C, MITO–C, MTC • mucosal mast cell

MMD mass median diameter (of particles) • mean marrow dose • minimal morbidostatic dose • myotonic muscular dystrophy *also* MyMD

MMDA methyoxymethylene dioxyamphetamine

MME M–mode echocardiography • mouse mammary epithelium

MMECT multiple monitored electroconvulsive therapy

MMEF maximal midexpiratory flow *also* MMF

MMEFR maximal midexpiratory flow rate *also* MMFR

MMF magnetomotive force • maximal midexpiratory flow *also* MMEF • mean maximal flow

MMFG mouse milk fat globule

MMFR maximum midflow rate • maximal midexpiratory flow rate *also* MMEFR

MMFV maximal midexpiratory flow volume

MMG mean maternal glucose

MMH monomethylhydrazine

mmHg millimeters of mercury

mmH₂0 millimeters of water

MMI macrophage migration index • macrophage migration inhibition • methimazole • methylmercaptoimidazole

MMIHS megacystis–microcolon–intestinal hypoperistalsis syndrome

MMIS Medicaid Management Information System

MMK Marshall–Marchetti–Krantz (cystourethropexy)

MML Moloney murine leukemia (virus) *also* MMLV •

monomethyllysine •
myelomonocytic leukemia

mM/L millimoles per liter

MMLV Moloney murine
leukemia virus *also* MML,
MMuLV

MMM microsome–mediated
mutagenesis •
myelofibrosis with myeloid
metaplasia • myeloid
metaplasia (with)
myelofibrosis •
myelosclerosis with
myeloid metaplasia

mmm micromillimeter •
millimicron

MMMF man–made mineral
fiber

MMOA maxillary mandibular
odentectomy alveolectomy

MMMT malignant mixed
mHllerian tumor •
metastatic mixed mHllerian
tumor

MMN morbus maculosus
neonatorum

MMNC marrow mononuclear
cell

MMO methane mono–
oxygenase

MMOA maxillary mandibular
odontectomy alveolectomy

MMoL myelomonoblastic
leukemia

mmol millimole

mmol/L millimoles per liter

MMPI McGill–Melzack Pain
Index • Minnesota
Multiphasic Personality
Inventory

MMPI–D Minnesota
Multiphasic Personality
Inventory Depression Scale

MMPNC Medical Maternal
Program for Nuclear
Casualties

mmpp millimeters partial
pressure

MMPR methylmercaptopurine
riboside

mm–PTH mid–molecule
parathyroid hormone

MMR mass miniature
radiography • mass
miniature
roentgenography •
maternal mortality rate •
measles–mumps–rubella
(vaccine) • midline
malignant reticulosis •
mild mental retardation •
mobile mass x–ray •
monomethylorutin •
myocardial metabolic rate

MMS methyl
methanesulfonate • Mini–
Mental State (examination)

MMSE Mini–Mental State
Examination

mm st muscle strength

MMT manual muscle test •
Mini Mental Test • mouse
mammary tumor

MMTA methylmetatyramine

MMTP methadone
maintenance treatment
program

MMTV mouse mammary tumor
virus

MMU medical maintenance
unit • mercaptomethyl
uracil

mmu millimass unit

mμ millimicron

mμc millimicrocurie

mμg millimicrogram

MMuLV Moloney murine leukemia virus *also* MMLV

mμs millimicrosecond

MMV mandatory minute ventilation • mandatory minute volume

MMWR Morbidity and Mortality Weekly Report

MN blood group in MNSs blood group system • malignant nephrosclerosis • meganewton • melena neonatorum • melanocytic nevus • membranous neuropathy • mesenteric node • metanephrine • midnight *also* M/N, Mn, mn • mononuclear • motor neuron • mucosal neurolysis • multinodular • myoneural

M/N macrocytic/normochronic (anemia) • microcytic/morchromic (anemia) • midnight *also* MN, Mn

M&N morning and night

Mn manganese • midnight *also* MN, M/N, mn

mN micronewton • millinormal

mn midnight *also* MN, Mn

MNA maximal noise area

MNAP mixed nerve action potential

MNB murine neuroblastoma

MNC mononuclear cell • mononuclear leukocyte *also* MNL

MNCV motor nerve conduction velocity

MND minimal necrosing dose • minor neurologic dysfunction • modified neck dissection • motor neuron disease

MNG multinodular goiter

mng morning

MNJ myoneural junction

MNL maximal number of lamellae • mononuclear leukocyte *also* MNC

MN/m² meganewton per square meter

MNMK maximal number of microbes killed

MNMS myonephropathic metabolic syndrome

MNO minocycline

MNP mononuclear phagocyte

MNPA methoxy–naphthyl proprionic acid

MNR marrow neutrophil reserve

MNS medial nuclear stratum • Melnick–Needles syndrome • a minor blood group

MNSER mean normalized systolic ejection rate

Mn–SOD manganese–superoxide dismutase

MNSs blood group system consisting of groups M, N, and MN

MnSSEP median nerve somatosensory evoked potential

MNTB medial nucleus (of) trapezoid body

MNZ metronidazole

MO manually operated • medial oblique (x–ray view) • medical officer • mesio–occlusal • mineral oil • minute output • mitral orifice • molecular orbital • mono–oxygenase • month *also* M, mo, mon • months old *also* mo • morbidly obese • mother • no evidence of distant metastases • sulfamethoxine

MO₂ myocardial oxygen consumption

Mo mode • Moloney (strain) • molybdenum • monoclonal

mo mode • month *also* M, MO, mon • months old *also* MO

MOA mechanism of action • medical office assistant

MoAb monoclonal antibody *also* MA, MAB, MAb, MCA, MCAB

MOAD methotrexate, Oncovin (vincristine), L–asparaginase, and dexamethasone

MOB medical office building • mechlorethamine, Oncovin (vincristine), and bleomycin

mob, mobil mobility • mobilization

MOB–PT mitomycin C, Oncovin (vincristine), bleomycin, and cisplatin

MOC maximal oxygen consumption • mother of child

MOCA methotrexate, Oncovin (vincristine), Cytoxan (cyclophosphamide), and Adriamycin (doxorubicin)

MoCM molybdenum–conditioned medium

MOD maturity–onset diabetes *also* MODM • Medical Officer of the Day • mesio–occlusodistal • moderate *also* mod

mod moderate *also* MOD • moderation • modification • modulation • module

modem modulator/demodulator

MODM maturity–onset diabetes mellitus *also* MOD

mod praesc [L. *modo praescripto*] in the way directed

MODY maturity–onset diabetes (of) youth

MOF marine oxidation/fermentation • methotrexate, Oncovin (vincristine), and 5–fluorouracil • methoxy-flurane • multiple organ failure

MOFS multiple–organ failure syndrome

MOH Medical Officer of Health

MOI maximal oxygen intake • multiplicity of infection

MOJAC mood, orientation, judgment, affect, and content

MOL molecular layer

mol mole · molecule/molecular

molc molar concentration

molfr mole fraction

mol/kg mole per kilogram

moll [L. *mollis*] soft

mol/L, mol/l mole per liter

mol/m³ mole per cubic meter

mol/s mole per second

mol wt molecular weight

MOM milk of magnesia · mucoid otitis media

MoM multiples of the median

MOMA methylhydroxy-mandelic acid

MΩ megohm

mΩ milliohm

MoMSV Moloney murine sarcoma virus

MON mongolian (gerbil) · monitor

mon monocyte *also* mono · month *also* M, MO, mo

MONO, Mono mononucleosis *also* mono

mono monocyte *also* mon · mononucleosis *also* MONO, Mono · monospot

monos monocytes

MOOW Medical Officer of the Watch

MOP major organ profile · medical outpatient · medical outpatient program · methotrexate, Oncovin (vincristine), and prednisone

MOP–BAP Mustargen (mechlorethamine), Oncovin (vincristine), prednisone, bleomycin, Adriamycin (doxorubicin), and procarbazine

MOPP Mustargen (mechlorethamine), Oncovin (vincristine), procarbazine, and prednisone

MOPP Mustargen (mechlorethamine), Oncovin (vincristine), procarbazine, prednisone, Adriamycin (doxorubicin), bleomycin, vinblastine, and decarbazine

MOPV monovalent oral poliovirus vaccine

MOR Medical Officer Report · morphine *also* morph

MORA mandibular orthopedic repositioning appliance

MORC Medical Officers Reserve Corps

MORD magnetic optical rotatory dispersion

mor dict [L. *more dicto*] in the manner directed

morph morphine *also* MOR · morphological/morphology *also* morphal

morphol morphological/morphology *also* morph

mor sol [L. *more solito*] in the usual way

mortal. mortality

MOS medial orbital sulcus · mirror optical system · months · myelofibrosis osteosclerosis

mOs milliosmolal

mos months

MOSFET metal oxide semiconductor field effect transistor

mOsm, MOsm, mOsmol milliosmole

mOsm/kg milliosmoles per kilogram

MOT mini–object test • mouse ovarian tumor • motility examination

MOTT mycobacteria other than tubercle

MOU memorandum of understanding

MOUS multiple occurrence (of) unexplained symptoms

MOV multiple oral vitamin

MOVC membranous obstruction (of inferior) vena cava

MOX moxalactam

MP [L. *modo prescripto*] as directed • macrophage • matrix protein • mean pressure • mechanical percussion • mechanical percussor • medial plantar • melphalan and prednisone • melting point • membrane potential • mentoposterior • menstrual period • mentum posterior • mercaptopurine • mesial pit • mesiopulpal • metacarpophalangeal • metaphalangeal • metatarsophalangeal (joint) *also* MTP, MTPJ • methylprednisolone *also* MPS • modulator protein •

moist pack • monophosphate • mouth piece • mouth pressure • mucopolysaccharide *also* MPS • multiparous • muscle potential • mycoplasmal pneumonia

6–MP 6–mercaptopurine

4MP4 methylpyrazole

mp [L. *modo praescripto*] as directed • [L. *mane primo*] early in the morning • millipond • melting point

MPA main pulmonary artery • medial preoptic area • Medical Procurement Agency • medroxy-progesterone acetate • methylprednisolone acetate • minor physical anomaly • mycophenolic acid

MPa, mPa megapascal

MPAG McGill Pain Assessment Questionnaire

MPAP mean pulmonary arterial pressure

MPB male pattern baldness

MPC marine protein concentrate • maximal permissible concentration • meperidine, promethazine, and chlorpromazine • metallophthalocyanine • minimal mycoplasmacidal concentration • minimal protozoacidal concen-tration • mucopurulent cervicitis • myeloblast–promyelocyte compartment

MPCD minimal perceptible color difference

MPCN microscopically positive, culturally negative

MPCUR maximal permissible concentration of unidentified radionuclides

MPCWP mean pulmonary capillary wedge pressure

MPD main pancreatic duct • maximal permissible dose • mean population doubling • membrane potential difference • minimal perceptible difference • minimal phototoxic dose • minimal popular dose • minimal port diameter • Minnesota Percepto–Diagnostic (Test) *also* MPDT • multiplanar display • multiple personality disorder • myeloproliferative disease • myofascial pain dysfunction

MPDS mandibular pain dysfunction syndrome • myofascial pain dysfunction syndrome

MPDT Minnesota Percepto–Diagnostic Test *also* MPD

MPDW mean percentage (of) desirable weight

MPE maximal possible effect • maximal possible error

MPEC monopolar electrocoagulation

MPED minimal phototoxic erythema dose

MPEH methylphenyl-ethylhydantoin

MPF maturation–promoting factor • mean power frequency

MPFM mini–Wright peak flow meter

MPG magnetopneumography

MPGM monophosphoglycerate mutase

MPGN membranoproliferative glomerulonephritis • mesangioproliferative glomerulonephritis

MPH male pseudohermaphroditism • milk protein hydrolysate

mph miles per hour

M phase phase of mitosis in cell growth cycle

MPHD methoxyhydroxphenolglycerol • multiple pituitary hormone deficiencies

MPHR maximal predicted heart rate

MPI mannose phosphate isomerase • Maudsley Personality Inventory • maximal permitted intake • maximal point of impulse • Multiphasic Personality Inventory • Multivariate Personality Inventory • myocardial perfusion imaging

MPJ metacarpophalangeal joint • metatarsophalangeal joint

mpk milligram per kilogram

MPL maximal permissible level • melphalan • mesiopulpolabial *also* MPSa • mesiopulpolingual

MPLa mesiopulpolabial *also* MPL

MPM malignant papillary mesothelioma · medial pterygoid muscle · Mortality Prediction Model · multiple primary malignancy · multipurpose meal

MPMT Murphy punch maneuver test

MPMV Mason–Pfizer monkey virus

MPN most probable number

MPO maximal power output · minimal perceptible odor · myeloperoxidase

MPOA medial preoptic area

MPOS myeloperoxidase system

MPP massive periretinal proliferation · maximal perfusion pressure · maximal print position · medial pterygoid plate · medical personnel pool · mercaptopyrazide pyrimidine · metacarpo-phalangeal profile

MPPG microphotoelectric plethysmography

MPPN malignant persistent positional nystagmus

MPPT methylprednisolone pulse therapy

MPR marrow production rate · massive preretinal retraction · maximal pulse rate · mercaptopurine riboside · myelo-proliferative reaction

MPRE minimal pure radium equivalent

MPS methylprednisolone *also* MP · microbial profile system · mononuclear phagocyte system · Montreal platelet syndrome · movement–produced stimulus · mucopolysaccharide *also* MP · mucopoly-saccharidosis · multiphasic screening · myocardial perfusion scintigraphy

MPSMT Merrill–Palmer Scale of Mental Tests

MPSRT matched pairs signed rank test

MPSS methylprednisolone sodium succinate

MPSV myeloproliferative sarcomavirus

MPT maximal predicted phonation time · Michigan Picture Test

MPTAH Mallory phosphotungstic acid hemotoxylin

MPTR motor, pain, touch, reflex (deficit)

MPT–R Michigan Picture Test, Revised

MPU Medical Practitioners Union

MPV mean plasma volume · mean platelet volume · metatarsus primus varus · mitral valve prolapse

mpz millipièze

MQ memory quotient · menaquinone

MQC microbiologic quality control

MR Maddox rod • magnetic resonance • mandibular reflex • mannose–resistant • maximal right • may repeat • measles–rubella (vaccine) • medial rectus (muscle) • median raphe • medical record • medical rehabilitation • medication responder • medium range • megaroentgen • mentally retarded • mental retardation • menstrual regulation • mesencephalic raphe • metabolic rate • methemoglobin reductase *also* MHR, MR–E • methyl red • milk ring • milliroentgen *also* mR, mr • mitral reflux • mitral regurgitation • mixed respiratory • moderate resistance • modulation rate • mortality rate • mortality ratio • motivation research • multicentric reticulohistiocytosis • multiplication rate • multiplicity reactivation • muscle receptor • muscle relaxant • myotactic reflex

M$_r$ molecular weight ratio • relative molecular mass

M&R measure and record

MRx1 may repeat one time

Mr mandible ramus

mR, mr milliroentgen *also* MR

MRA main renal artery • marrow repopulation activity • medical records administrator • mid–right atrium • multivariate regression analysis

mrad millirad

MRAN medical resident admitting note

MRAP maximal resting anal pressure • mean right atrial pressure

MRAS main renal artery stenosis • mean renal artery stenosis

MRBC monkey red blood cell • mouse red blood cell

MRBF mean renal blood flow

MRC maximal recycling capacity • Medical Registration Council • Medical Research Council • Medical Reserve Corps • methylrosaniline chloride (gentian violet, crystal violet)

MRD margin reflex distance • medical records department • method of rapid determination • minimal reacting dose • minimal renal disease • minimal residual disease

mrd millirutherford

MRDM malnutrition–related diabetes mellitus

MRE maximal restrictive exercise • maximal risk estimate

MR–E methemoglobin reductase *also* MHR, MR

mrem millirem • milliroentgen equivalent man

mrep milliroentgen equivalent physical

MRF medical record file • melanocyte–releasing factor • melanocyte–

(stimulating hormone)–releasing factor • mesencephalic reticular formation • midbrain reticular formation • mitral regurgitant flow • moderate renal failure • monoclonal rheumatoid factor • mHllerian regression factor

mRF monoclonal rheumatoid factor

MRFC mouse rosette–forming cell

MRFIT Multiple Risk Factor Intervention Trial

MRFT modified rapid fermentation test

MRG murmurs, rubs, and gallops *also* MGR

MRH Maddox rod hyperphoria • melanocyte(-stimulating hormone)-releasing hormone

MRHA mannose–resistant hemagglutination

MRHD maximal recommended human dose

mrhm milliroentgens per hour at one meter

MRHT modified rhyme hearing test

MRI machine–readable identifier • magnetic resonance imaging • medical records information • Medical Research Institute • moderate renal insufficiency

MRIF melanocyte(–stimulating hormone) release–inhibiting factor

MRIH melanocyte(–stimulating hormone) release–inhibiting hormone

MRK Mayer–Rokitansky syndrome

MRL Medical Records Librarian • Medical Research Laboratory • minimal response level

MRM modified radical mastectomy

MRN malignant renal neoplasm

mRNA messenger ribonucleic acid

mRNP messenger ribonucleoprotein

MRO minimal recognizable odor • muscle receptor organ

MROD Medical Research and Operations Directorate

MRP maximal reimbursement point • mean resting potential • medical reimbursement plan

MRPAH mixed reverse passive antiglobulin hemagglutination

MRPN medical resident progress note

MRR marrow release rate • maximal relaxation rate • maximal relation rate

MRS magnetic resonance spectroscopy • mania rating scale • median range score • medical receiving station • Melkersson–Rosenthal syndrome • methicillin–resistant

Stapylococcus (aureus) *also* MRSA

MRSA methicillin–resistant *Staphylococcus aureus also* MRS

MRT major role therapy • mean residence time • median reaction time • median recognition threshold • median relapse time • Medical Records Technician • milk ring test • modified rhyme test • muscle response test

MRU mass radiography unit • measure of resource use • minimal reproductive unit

MRUS maximal rate (of) urea synthesis

MRV minute respiratory volume • mixed respiratory vaccine

MRVP mean right ventricular pressure • methyl red, Voges–Proskauer (medium)

MS main scale • maladjustment score • mannose–sensitive • mass spectrometry • mean score • mechanical stimulation • Meckel syndrome • medical services • medical student • medical supplies • medical–surgical • medical survey • menopausal syndrome • mental status • metaproterenol sulfate • microscope slide • Mikuliez syndrome • milkshake • minimal support • mitral sound • mitral stenosis • mobile surgical (unit) • modal sensitivity • molar solution • mongolian spot • morning stiffness •

morphine sulfate *also* ms • motile sperm • mucosubstance • multilaminated structure • multiple sclerosis • muscle shortening • muscle strength • musculoskeletal *also* Ms, MSK

M&S microculture and sensitivity

MSIII third–year medical student

MS–222 tricaine methane sulfonate

Ms murmurs • musculoskeletal *also* MS, MSK

ms manuscript • millisecond *also* msec • morphine sulfate *also* MS

m/s meters per second *also* m/sec

m/s² meters per second squared

MSA major serologic antigen • male specific antigen • mannitol salt agar • Medical Services Administration • membrane stabilizing action • mouse serum albumin • multichannel signed averager • Multidimensional Scalogram Analysis • multiple system atrophy • multiplication–stimulating activity • muscle sympathetic activity

MSAA multiple sclerosis–associated agent

MSAF meconium–stained amniotic fluid

MSAFP maternal serum α–fetoprotein

MSAP mean systemic arterial pressure

MSB Martius scarlet blue • mid–small bowel • most significant bit

MSBC maximal specific binding capacity

MSBLA mouse–specific B–lymphocyte antigen

MSBOS maximl surgical blood order schedule

MSC Medical Service Corps • multiple sib case

MSCA McCarthy Scales of Children's Abilities

MSCLC mouse stem cell–like cell

MSCP, mscp mean spherical candle–power

MSCU medical special care unit

MSCWP musculoskeletal chest wall pain

MSD mean square deviation • metabolic screening disorder • microsurgical discectomy • midsleep disturbance • mild sickle (cell) disease • most significant digit • multiple sulfatase deficiency

MSDS material safety data sheet

MSE medical support equipment • mental status examination • muscle–specific enolase

mse mean square error

msec millisecond *also* ms

m/sec meters per second *also* m/s

MSEL myasthenic syndrome of Eaton–Lambert

MSER mean systolic ejection rate • Mental Status Examination Record

MSES medical school environmental stress

MSET multistage exercise test

MSF macrophage slowing factor • macrophage spreading factor • meconium–stained fluid • Mediterranean spotted fever • megakaryocyte–stimulating factor • migration–stimulating factor • modified sham feeding

MSG methysergide • monosodium glutamate

MSGV mouse salivary gland virus

MSH medical self–help • melanocyte–stimulating hormone • melanophore–stimulating hormone *also* MH

MSHA mannose–sensitive hemagglutination

MSH–IF melanocyte–stimulating hormone–inhibiting factor

MSHRF melanocyte–stimulating hormone–releasing factor

MSI medium–scale integration

MSIR morphine sulfate immediate–release (tablet)

MSIS multistate information system

MSK medullary sponge kidney • musculoskeletal *also* MS, Ms

MSKP Medical Sciences Knowledge Profile

MSL midsternal line • multiple symmetric lipomatosis

MSLA mouse–specific lymphocyte antigen • multisample Luer adapter

MSLR mixed skin (cell)– leukocyte reaction

MSLT multiple sleep latency test

MSM medial superior olive • mineral salts medium

MSN medial septal nucleus • mildly subnormal

MSOF multiple systems organ failure

MSPGN mesangial proliferative glomerulonephritis

MSPN medical student progress note

MSPS myocardial stress perfusion scintigraphy

MSPU medical short procedure unit

MSR mitral stenoregurgitation • monosynaptic reflex • muscle stretch reflex

MSRPP Multidimensional Scale for Rating Psychiatric Patients

MSRT Minnesota Spatial Relations Test

MSS Marital Satisfaction Scale • massage *also* M, mass., mss • Medicare Statistical System • mental status schedule • Metabolic Support Service • minor surgery suite • motion sickness susceptibility • mucus–stimulating substance • muscular subaortic stenosis • multiple sclerosis susceptibility

mss massage *also* M, mass., MSS

MSSG multiple sclerosis susceptibility gene

MST mean survival time • mean swell time (botulism test) • median survival time

MSTA mumps skin test antigen

MSTh mesothorium

MSTI multiple soft tissue injuries

MSU maple syrup urine • medical studies unit • midstream urine (specimen) • monosodium urate • myocardial substrate uptake

MSUA midstream urinalysis

MSUD maple syrup urine disease

MSUM monosodium urate monohydrate

MSV maximal sustained (level of) ventilation • mean scale value • Moloney sarcoma virus • murine sarcoma virus

MSVC maximal sustained ventilatory capacity

MSVL maximal spatial vector (to) left

MSW Medical Social Worker • multiple stab wounds

MSWYE modified sea water yeast extract (agar)

MT empty • malaria therapy • malignant teratoma • mammary tumor • Martin–Thayer (plate, medium) • mastoid tip • maximal therapy • medial thalamus • medial thickening • mediastinal tube • Medical Technologist • Medical Transcriptionist • medical treatment • melatonin • membrana tympani • membrane thickness • mesangial thickening • metatarsal • methyltyrosine • microtome • microtubule • midtrachea • minimal threshold • Monroe tidal drainage • more than • multiple tics • multitest (plate) • muscles and tendons • muscle test • music therapy • [L. *membrana tympani*] tympanic membrane

M–T macroglobulin–trypsin

M/T masses (of) tenderness • myringotomy (with) tubes

M&T *Monilia* and *Trichomonas* • myringotomy and tubes

3–MT 3–methoxytyramine

MT6 mercaptomerin

Mt megatonne

mt [L. *mitte talis*] send of such

MTA malignant teratoma, anaplastic • mammary tumor agent • Medical Technical Assistant • myoclonic twitch activity

MTAC mass transfer–area coefficient

MTAD [L. *membrana tympana auris dextrae*] tympanic membrane of right ear

MTAL medullary thick ascending limb

MTAS [L. *membrana tympana auris sinistrae*] tympanic membrane of left ear

MT(ASCP) Medical Technologist certified by American Society of Clinical Pathologists

MTAU [L. *membranae tympani aures unitae*] tympanic membranes of both ears

MTB methylthymol blue • *Mycobacterium* tuberculosis

MTBE meningeal tick–borne encephalitis • methyl *tert*–butyl ether

MTBF mean time between (or before) failures

MTC mass transfer coefficient • maximal tolerated concentration • medical test cabinet • medical training center • medullary thyroid carcinoma • metoclopramide • mitomycin C *also* MC, Mit-C, MITO–C, MMC

MTD maximal tolerated dose • mean total dose • metastatic trophoblastic disease • Monroe tidal drainage • multiple tic disorder • [L. *mitte tales doses*] send such doses

MTDDA Minnesota Test for Differential Diagnosis of Aphasis

MTDI maximal tolerable daily intake

MT–DN multitest, dermatophytes, and *Nocardia* (plate)

mtDNA mitochondrial deoxyribonucleic acid

MTDT modified tone decay test

MTE medical toxic environment

MTET modified treadmill exercise testing

MTF maximal terminal flow • medical treatment facility • modulation transfer factor • modulation transfer function • mithramycin

MTG midthigh girth

MTg mouse thyroglobulin

MTHF methyl tetraahydrofolic acid

MTI malignant teratoma, intermediate • minimal time interval

MTLP metabolic toxemia (of) late pregnancy

MTM Thayer–Martin, modified (agar)

MT–M multitest, mycology (plate)

MTO Medical Transport Officer

MTOC microtubule organizing center • mitotic organizing center

MTP master treatment plan • maximal tolerated pressure • medial tibial plateau • medical termination of pregnancy • metatarsophalangeal (joint) *also* MP, MTPJ • microtubule protein

MTPJ metatarsophalangeal joint *also* MP, MTP

MTQ methaqualone

MTR mass, tenderness, rebound (abdominal examination) • Meinicke turbidity reaction • mental treatment rules • metronidazole

MTR–0 no masses, tenderness, or rebound (abdominal examination)

MTRX methotrexate *also* M, MTX

MTS moderate tactile stimulus • multicellular tumor spheroid

MTSO medical transcription service organization

MTST maximal treadmill stress test

MTT malignant teratoma, trophoblastic • maximal treadmill testing • meal tolerance test • mean transit time • monotetrazolium

MTU malignant teratoma, undifferentiated • methylthiouracil

MTV mammary tumor virus (of mice)

MTX methotrexate *also* M, MTRX

MT–Y multitest yeast (plate)

MTZ mitoxantrone

MU Mache unit *also* Mu · maternal uncle · megaunit · mescaline unit · million units · Montevideo unit · motor unit · mouse unit *also* mu

Mu Mache unit *also* MU

mU milliunit

mu micron · mouse unit *also* MU

mu (M, μ) twelfth letter of Greek alphabet

μ chemical potential · dynamic viscosity · electrophoretic mobility · heavy chain of immunoglobulin M · linear attenuation coefficient · magnetic moment *also* m · mean *also* M, m · micro- · micrometer *also* μm · mutation rate · permeability · population mean (statistics)

$μ_o$ permeability of vacuum

μA microampere

MUA middle uterine artery · multiple unit activity

MUAC middle upper–arm circumference

MUAP motor unit action potential

μb microbar *also* μbar

$μ_B$ Bohr magneton

μbar microbar *also* μb

MUC maximal urinary concentration

muc mucilage

μC microcoulomb *also* μcoul

μc microcurie *also* μCi

μch, μ–hr microcurie–hour *also* μCi-hr

μCl microcurie *also* μc

μCl–hr microcurie–hour *also* μch, μC–hr

μcoul microcoulomb *also* μC

MUD minimal urticarial dose

μ Eq microequivalent

μF, μf microfarad

MUG MUMPS Massachusetts General Hospital Utility Multi–Programming System Users' Group

μg microgram *also* mcg

MUGA multigated angiogram · multiple gated acquisition (bloodpool image)

μγ microgamma

MUGEx multiple (blood pool scan (during) exercise *also* MUGX

μg/kg microgram per kilogram

μg/L, μg/l microgram per liter

MUGR multigated (blood pool image at) rest

MUGX multigated (blood pool image during) exercise *also* MUGEX

μGy microgray

μH microhenry

μHg micrometer of mercury *also* μmHg

μIn microinch

μIU one–millionth International Unit

μ**kat** microkatal

μ**L,** μ**l** microliter

mult multiple • multiplication

multip multiparous

MuLV, MuLv murine leukemia virus

μ**M** micromolar

μ**m** micrometer *also* μ • micromilli–

μ**mg** micromilligram (nanogram)

μ**mHg** micrometer of mercury *also* μHg

μ**mm** micromillimeter (nanometer)

μ**m**μ meson

μ**mol** micromole

μ**mol/L** micromolar

MUMPS Massachusetts General Hospital Utility Multi–Programming System

MuMTv murine mammary tumor virus

μμ micromicro–

μμ**C** micromicrocurie (picocurie)

μμ**F** micromicrofarad (picofarad)

μμ**g** micromicrogram (picogram)

MUN(WI) Munich Wistar (rat)

MUO myocardiopathy of unknown origin

μΩ microhm

μ**Osm** micro–osmolar

MUP major urinary protein •

maximal urethral pressure • motor unit potential

μ**R,** μ**r** microroentgen

MURC measurable undesirable respiratory contaminants

μ**/**ρ mass attenuation coefficient

MurNAc *N*–acetylmuramate

μ**s** microsecond *also* μsec

musc muscle • muscular • musculature

mus–lig musculoligamentous

μ**sec** microsecond *also* μs

MUST medical unit, self–contained and transportable

μ**U** microunit

MUU mouse uterine unit

μ**U** microunit

μ**V** microvolt

μ**W** microwatt

MUWU mouse uterine weight unit

MV malignant (rabbit fibroma) virus • measles virus • mechanical ventilation • megavolt • microvilli • millivolt • minute ventilation • minute volume • mitoxantrone and etoposide • mitral valve • mixed venous • multivesicular • multivessel • [L. *Medicus Veterinarius*] veterinary physician

Mv mendelevium *also* Md

mV, mv millivolt

MVA malignant ventricular

arrhythmia • mechanical ventricular assistance • mevalonic acid • mitral valve area • modified vaccine (virus), Ankara • motor vehicle accident

MV·A megavolt–ampere

mV·A millivolt–ampere

M–VAC methotrexate, vinblastine, Adriamycin (doxorubicin), and cisplatin

MVB mixed venous blood • multivesicular body

MVC maximal vital capacity • maximal voluntary contraction • myocardial vascular capacity

MVD Doctor of Veterinary Medicine • Marburg virus disease • microvascular decompression • mitral valve disease • mouse vas deferens • multivessel (coronary) disease

MVE mitral valve echo • mitral valve (leaflet) excursion • Murray Valley encephalitis

MVgrad mitral valve gradient

MVH massive variceal hemorrhage • massive vitreous hemorrhage • methotrexate, VP–16, and hexamethylonelamine

MVI multiple vitamin injection • multivalvular involvement • multivitamin infusion

MVLS mandibular vestibulolingual sulcoplasty • Mecham Verbal Language Scale

MVM microvillose membrane • minute virus (of) mice

MVMT movement

MVN medial ventromedial nucleus

MVO maximal venous outflow

MVO2, MVO$_2$ maximal venous oxygen (consumption) • myocardial ventilation, oxygen (rate) • oxygen content of mixed venous blood

mVO$_2$ minimal venous oxygen (consumption)

MVOA mitral valve orifice area

MVOS mixed venous oxygen saturation

MVP mean venous pressure • microvascular pressure • mitral valve prolapse

MVPP mustine, vinblastine, procarbazine, and prednisone

MVPS mitral valve prolapse syndrome

MVPT Motor–Free Visual Perception Test *also* MFVPT

MVR massive vitreous reaction • massive vitreous retractor (blade) • minimal vascular resistance • mitral valve regurgitation • mitral valve replacement

MVRI mixed vaccine, respiratory infection • mixed virus respiratory infection

MVS mitral valve stenosis • motor, vascular, and sensory

mV–sec, mV•s millivolt–second

MVT maximal ventillation time

MVV maximal ventilatory volume • maximal voluntary ventilation

MVV₁ maximal ventilatory volume

MVVPP Mustargen (nitrogen mustard), vincristine, vinblastine, procarbazine, and prednisone

MW mean weight • megawatt • microwave *also* mw • molecular weight *also* MWt • Munich Wistar (rat)

M–W Mallory–Weiss syndrome • men and women

mW milliwatt

mw microwave *also* MW

mWb milliweber

MWCB manufacturer's working cell bank

MWD microwave diathermy • molecular weight distribution

MWI Medical Walk–In (Clinic)

MWLT Modified Word Learning Test

MWMT Monotic Word Memory Test

MWP mean wedge pressure

MWPC multiwire proportional chamber

MWS Marden–Walker syndrome • Mickety–Wilson syndrome •

Moersch–Woltman syndrome

MWT malpositioned wisdom teeth

MWt molecular weight *also* MW

MX matrix

Mx mastectomy • maxillary • maxwell • MEDEX (q.v.) • multiple • myringotomy

Mₓᵧ transverse magnetization

My myopia • myxedematous

my mayer (unit of heat capacity)

Mycol mycologist • mycology

MYD mydriatic

MyD myotonic (muscular) dystrophy

MYEL multiple myeloma

Myel myelocyte

myel myelin/myelinated

Myelo myelogram/myelography

MyG myasthenia gravis *also* MG

Myg myriagram

MyL, Myl myrialiter

Mym myriameter

MyMD myotonic muscular dystrophy *also* MMD

MYO myoglobin *also* MYOGLB

myo myocardial/myocardium

MYOGLB myoglobin *also* MYO

myop myopia

MYS myasthenia syndrome

MYTGC Miller–Yoder Test of
Grammatical
Comprehension

MZ mantle zone •
mezlocillin • monozygotic

M_z longitudinal magnetization

MZA monozygotic (twins
raised) apart

MZL marginal zone lymphocyte

MZT monozygotic (twins
raised) together

N antigenic determinant of erythrocytes • asparagine *also* ASN, Asn • Avogadro constant/number *also* Na • inherited blood factor in MNS blood group • loudness • nasal *also* n, NAS • nasion • nausea • negative *also* neg • negro • neomycin *also* NE, Neo, NM • neper (unit for comparing magnitude of two powers) • nerve *also* n • neural • neuraminidase • neurology/neurologist *also* neur, neuro, neurol • neuropathy • neutron number • neutrophil • newton • nicotinamide • nitrogen • no • nodal • node • nodule • none • nonmalignant • Nonne (globulin test) • noon • normal (solution) • normal concentration • normality (equivalent/liter) • not • noun • NPH insulin • nucleoside *also* Nuc • nucleus • number *also* n, NO, No, no. • number density (number of moles of substance per unit of volume) • number in sample • number of atoms • number of molecules • number of neutrons in an atomic nucleus • number of observations (in statistics) • numerical aptitude (General Aptitude Test Battery) • population size • radiance • refractive index *also* n • sample size *also* n • spin density • unit of neutron dosage

N-I—N-XII first through twelfth cranial nerves

5'-N 5'-nucleotidase

0.02N fiftieth-normal (solution) *also* N/50

0.1N tenth-normal (solution) *also* N/10

0.5N half-normal (solution) *also* N/2

2N double-normal (solution)

N/2 half-normal (solution) *also* 0.5N

N/10 tenth-normal (solution) *also* 0.1N

N/50 fiftieth-normal (solution) *also* 0.02N

n amount of substance expressed in moles • [L. *natus*] born • haploid chromosome number • index of refraction • nano- (prefix) • nasal *also* N • nerve *also* N • neuter *also* neut • neutron • neutron dosage (unit of) • neutron number density • night • normal *also* NL, nl, NOR • [L. *naris*] nostril • number *also* N, NO, No, no. • number of density of molecule • number of observations • principle quantum number • refractive index • rotational frequency • sample size

n̄ mean value of n for a number of observations (in statistics)

2n diploid chromosome number

3n triploid chromosome number

4n tetraploid

NA nalidixic acid · Narcotics Anonymous · Native American · network administrator · neuraminidase · neurologic age · neutralizing antibody · neutrophil antibody · nicotinamide · nicotinic acid · nitric acid · no abnormality · Nomina Anatomica · nonadherent · non-A (hepatitis) · nonalcoholic · nonamnionic · nonmyelinated axon · noradrenaline · not admitted · not antagonized · not applicable *also* N/A · not attempted · not available · nuclear antibody · nuclear antigen · nucleic acid · nucleus accumbens (septi) · nucleus ambiguus · numeric aperture · nurse anesthetist · nurse's aid · nursing action · nursing assistant

N/A not applicable *also* NA · no alternative

N&A normal and active

Na Avogadro's number (constant) *also* N · noise rating number (in acoustics) · [L. *natrium*] sodium

nA nanoampere

NAA naphthaleneacetic acid · neutral amino acid · neutron activation analysis · neutrophil aggregation activity · nicotinic acid amide · no apparent abnormalities

NAAC no apparent anesthetic complication

NAACP neoplasia, allergy, Addison's (disease), collagen (vascular disease), and parasites

NAAP *N*-acetyl-4-amino-phenazone

NAB novarsenobenzene

NABS normoactive bowel sounds

NAC accessory nucleus (Monakow's nucleus) · *N*-acetyl-L-cysteine · nitrogen mustard, Adriamycin (doxorubicin), and CCNU (lomustine) · nonadherent cell

NACD not acidified

NAC-EDTA *N*-acetyl-L-cysteine ethylenediamine-tetraacetic acid

n-Ach achievement need (in psychology)

NACI National Advisory Committee on Immunization

NAD new antigenic determinant · nicotinamide adenine dinucleotide · nicotinic acid dehydrogenase · no abnormal discovery · no abnormality demonstrable · no active disease · no acute/no apparent/no appreciable disease · normal axis deviation · nothing abnormal detected/discovered

NAD+ oxidized form of

nicotinamide adenine dinucleotide

NaD sodium dialysate

NADA New Animal Drug Application

NADG nicotinamide adenine dinucleotide glycohydrolase

NADH reduced nicotinamide adenine dinucleotide

NaDodSO₄ sodium dodecyl sulfate *also* SDS

NADP nicotinamide adenine dinucleotide phosphate

NADP⁺ oxidized form of nicotinamide adenine dinucleotide phosphate

NADPH reduced nicotinamide adenine dinucleotide phosphate

NADSIC no apparent disease seen in chest

NAE net acid excretion

Na$_e$ exchangeable body sodium (natrium)

NAF nafcillin *also* NF • net acid flux

NAG narrow angle glaucoma • nonagglutinable (vibrios) • nonagglutinating

NAGO neuraminidase and galactose oxidase

NAHI National Athletic Health Institute

NAI net acid input (urinary) • neuraminidase inhibition *also* NI • no acute inflammation • nonaccidental injury • nonadherence index

NAIR nonadrenergic inhibitory response

NaI(T) thallium-activated sodium iodide (sodium iodide crystal)

NaI(TI) thallium-activated sodium iodide crystal (in gamma-ray detectors)

NaK ATPase sodium- and potassium-activated adenosine triphosphate

Na&K sodium and potassium (in urine)

Na&KSP sodium and potassium spot (urine test)

NAL nonadherent leukocyte

NALD neonatal adrenoleukodystrophy

NALL null (cell line of) acute lymphocytic leukemia

NALP neuroadenolysis (of) pituitary

NAM natural actomyosin

NAMCS National Ambulatory Medical Care Survey

NAME nevi, atrial myxoma, myxoid neurofibroma, ephelides (syndrome)

NAMN nicotinic acid mononucleotide

NAMRU Navy Medical Reserve Unit

NANB non-A, non-B (hepatitis)

NANBH non-A, non-B hepatitis

NANBV non-A, non-B (hepatitis) virus

NAND not-and (result is false

only if all arguments are true— otherwise, result is true)

N ant/post anterior and posterior "zones" (nerve cell groups—nuclei) of hypothalamus

NAP narrative, assessment, (and) plan • nasion pogonion (angle of convexity in craniometrics) • nerve action potential • neutrophil alkaline phosphatase • nonacute profile • nucleic acid phosphatase

NAPA *N*-acetylprocainamide

NAPD no active pulmonary disease

Na Pent Pentothal Sodium

NaPG sodium pregnanediol glucuronide

NAPH naphthyl

NAR nasal airway resistance • no action required • not at risk

NARA Narcotics Addict Rehabilitation Act

NARC, narc narcotic *also* narco • narcotics (officer, slang) *also* NO

Narc nucleus arcuatus (nucleus infundibularis)

narco narcotic *also* NARC • narcotics (hospital, officer, treatment center—slang) • narcotic addict (slang)

NARMC Naval Aerospace and Regional Medical Center

NAS nasal *also* N, n • neonatal abstinence syndrome • neonatal airleak syndrome • neuroallergic syndrome • no added salt • normalized alignment score

Na-Spt sodium spot (urine test)

NAS-NRC National Academy of Science-National Research Council

NAT *N*-acetyltransferase • natal • neonatal alloimmune thrombocytopenia • no action taken • nonaccidental trauma

Nat native *also* nat • natural *also* nat

nat national • native *also* Nat • nature/natural *also* Nat

NATB Nonreading Aptitude Test Battery

NATM sodium aurothiomalate

NATP neonatal autoimmune thrombocytopenic purpura

NB nail bed • needle biopsy • Negri bodies • nervus buccalis • neurometric (test) battery • newborn *also* nb • nitrogen balance • nitrous oxide-barbiturate • non-B (hepatitis) • normoblast • [L. *nota bene*] note well *also* nb • novobiocin • nuclear bag (certain intrafusal muscle fiber nuclei of a neuromuscular spindle) • nutrient broth

N/B neopterin to biopterin (ratio)

Nb niobium

nb newborn *also* NB • [L. *nota bene*] note well *also* NB

NBC nonbattle casualty • nonbed care • nuclear, biologic, chemical

NBCC nevoid basal cell carcinoma

NBCCS nevoid basal cell carcinoma syndrome

NBD neurogenic bladder dysfunction • neurologic bladder dysfunction • no brain damage

NBE northern bean extract

NBEI non–butanol-extractable iodine (syndrome)

NBF not breast fed

NBI neutrophil bactericidal index • no bone injury • nonbattle injury

NBICU newborn intensive care unit *also* NICU

NBIL neonatal bilirubin

NB Int newborn intensive (care unit)

nbl normoblast

NBM no bowel movement • normal bone marrow • normal bowel movement • nothing by mouth *also* NPO • nucleus basalis (of) Meynert

nbM newborn mouse

nbMb newborn mouse brain

NBME National Board of Medical Examiners • normal bone marrow extract

NBN narrow band noise • newborn nursery

NBO nonbed occupancy

NBP needle biopsy (of) prostate • neoplastic brachial plexopathy

NBQC narrow base quad cane

NBS National Bureau of Standards • Neri-Barré syndrome • nevoid basal (cell carcinoma) syndrome • newborn screen (serum thyroxine and phenylketonuria) • Nijmegen breakage syndrome • no bacteria seen • normal blood serum • normal bowel sounds • normal brain stem • normal burro serum • nystagmus blockage syndrome

NBT nitroblue tetrazolium • normal breast tissue

NBTE nonbacterial thrombotic endocarditis

NBTG nitrobenzylthioguanosine

NBTNF newborn, term, normal, female

NBTNM newborn, term, normal, male

NBTS National Blood Transfusion Service

NBW normal birth weight

NC nabothian cyst • nasal cannula • nasal clearance • natural cytotoxicity • neck complaint • neonatal cholestasis • nerve conduction • neural crest • neurologic check • neurologic control • nevus comedonicus • nitrocellulose •

nitrosocarbazole • no casualty • no change *also* N/C • no charge • no complaints *also* N/C • noise criterion • noncirrhotic • noncontributory • normal control • normocephalic • noseclip • nose cone • not classified • not completed • not cultured • nucleocapsid • Nurse Corps • nursing coordination

N:C nuclear-cytoplasmic (ratio) *also* NCR

N/C nerves and circulation *also* N&C • neurocirculatory • no change *also* NC • no complaints *also* NC • nuclear/cytoplasmic (ratio)

N&C nerves and circulation *also* N/C

nC nanocoulomb

nc nanocurie *also* nCi

NCA neurocirculatory asthenia • neutrophil chemotactic activity • no congenital abnormalities • nodulocystic acne • noncontractile area • nonspecific cross-reacting antigen • nuclear cerebral angiogram

N-CAM nerve cell adhesion molecule

NcAMP nephrogenous cyclic adenosine monophosphate

NCAS neocarzinostatin (zinostatin) *also* NCS

NCAT, NC/AT normal cephalic (and) atraumatic

NCB no code blue

NCC no concentrated carbohydrates • noncoronary cusp • nucleus caudalis centralis • nursing care continuity

NCCLS National Committee for Clinical Laboratory Standards

NCCU newborn convalescent care unit

NCD neurocirculatory dystonia • nitrogen clearance delay • no congenital deformities • normal childhood diseases • normal childhood disorders • not considered disabling

NCDV National Communicable Disease Center • Nebraska calf diarrhea virus

NCE negative contrast echocardiography • new chemical entity • nonconvulsive epilepsy

NCF (polymorphonuclear) neutrophil chemotactic factor • night care facility • no cold fluids

NCF(C) neutrophil chemotactic factor (complement)

NCGL nucleus corporis geniculati lateralis

NCI naphthalene creosote, iodoform • National Cancer Institute • nuclear contour index • nucleus colliculi inferioris • nursing care integration

nCi nanocurie *also* nc

NCJ needle catheter jejunostomy

NCL neuronal ceroid lipofuscinosis • nuclear cardiology laboratory

NCLEX-RN National Council Licensure Examination for Registered Nurses

NCM nailfold capillary microscope

N/cm² newton per square centimeter

NCMC natural cell-mediated cytotoxicity

NCME Network for Continuing Medical Education

NCMHI National Clearinghouse for Mental Health Information

NCNC normochromic normocytic (erythrocyte)

NCNCA normochromic normocytic anemia

NCO no complaints offered

NCP no caffeine (or) pepper • nonclonogenic proliferating (cells) • noncollagen protein • nursing care plan

n-CPAP nasal continuous positive airway pressure

NCPE noncardiogenic pulmonary edema

NCPR no cardiopulmonary resuscitation

NCR neurologic/circulatory/ range of motion • neutrophil chemotactic response • nuclear-cytoplasmic ratio *also* N:C

NCRC non–child-resistant container

NCRP National Council on Radiation Protection (and Measurements)

NCS neocarzinostatin (zinostatin) *also* NCAS • nerve conduction study • newborn calf serum • no concentrated sweets • noncircumferential stenosis • noncoronary sinus • noncured sarcoidosis • noncurrent serum

NCT neural crest tumor • neutron capture therapy • noncontact tonometry • number connection test

NCTC National Cancer Tissue Culture • National Collection of Type Cultures

NCV nerve conduction velocity (study) • no commercial value • noncholera vibrio

NCVS nerve conduction velocity studies

NCYC National Collection of Yeast Cultures

ND Doctor of Naturopathy • nasal deformity • nasolacrimal duct • natural death • Naval Dispensary • neonatal death *also* NND • neoplastic disease • nervous debility • neurologic development • neuropsychologic deficit • neurotic depression • neutral density • Newcastle disease • new drug • nifedipine *also* NIF • no data • no date • no

disease • nondetectable •
nondetermined •
nondiabetic • nondi-
sabling • none detectable •
normal delivery • normal
deposition • normal
development • normal
dose • nose drops • not
nondetectable • not
determined • not
diagnosed • not done •
nothing done • nucleus of
Darkschewitsch • nurse's
diagnosis • nutritionally
deprived

N/D no defects

N&D nodular and diffuse
(lymphoma)

N$_D$, n$_D$ refractive index

Nd neodymium • number (of)
dissimilar (matches)

NDA New Drug Application •
no data available • no
demonstrable antibodies •
no detectable activity • no
detectable antibody

NDC National Data
Communications •
National Drug Code •
Naval Dental Clinic •
nondifferentiated cell •
nuclear dehydrogenating
clostridia

NDCD National Drug Code
Directory

NDD no-dialysis days

NDDG National Diabetes Data
Group

NDE near-death experience •
nondiabetic extremity

NDEA no deviation of
electrical axis

NDF neutral detergent fiber •
neutrophil diffraction
factor • new dosage form •
Nicolas-Durand-Favre
(disease) • no disease
found

NDGA nordihydroguaiaretic
acid

NDI naphthalene
diisocyanate • nephrogenic
diabetes insipidus

NDIR nondispersive infrared
(analyzer)

NDMA nitrosodimethylamine

N dm/vm nucleus
dorsomedialis-
ventromedialis

nDNA native deoxyribonucleic
acid

N/D NHL nodular/diffuse non-
Hodgkin lymphoma

Nd/NT nondistended/nontender

NDP net dietary protein

NDR neonatal death rate •
neurotic depressive
reaction • normal detrusor
reflex • nucleus dorsalis
raphe

NDS Naval Dental School •
New Drug Submission •
normal dog serum

NDSB Narcotic Drugs
Supervisory Board

NDT neurodevelopmental
treatment (physical
therapy) • noise detection
threshold • nondestructive
testing

NDTI National Disease and
Therapeutic Index

NDV Newcastle disease virus

NDx nondiagnostic

Nd:YAG neodymium:yttrium-aluminum garnet (surgical laser)

NE national emergency • necrotic enteritis • neomycin *also* N, Neo, NM • nephropathia epidemica • nerve ending • nerve excitability (test) • neural excitation • neuroendocrine • neuroepithelium • neurologic examination • neutrophil elastase • never exposed • no ectopia • no effect • no enlargement • nonelastic • nonendogenous • norepinephrine *also* NOR-EPI • not elevated • not enlarged • not equal • not evaluated • not examined • nutcracker esophagus

Ne neon

NEA neoplasm embryonic antigen • no evidence (of) abnormality

NEB neuroendocrine body

nebul [L. *nebula*] cloud (as a nebulizer) • spray

NEC necrotizing enterocolitis • neuroendocrine cell • no essential change • nonesterified cholesterol • not elsewhere classified/classifiable • not elsewhere coded • not enough cells

nec necessary

NECHI Northeastern Consortium for Health Information

NECT non-enhanced computed tomography

NED no evidence (of) disease • no expiration date • normal equivalent deviation

NEEE Near East equine encephalomyelitis

NEEP negative end-expiratory pressure

NEF nephritic factor *also* NF • negative expiratory force

NEFA nonesterified fatty acid

NEFG normal external female genitalia

NEG neglect

neg negative *also* N

NEI National Eye Institute

NEISS National Electronic Injury Surveillance System

NEJ neuroeffector junction

NEM no evidence (of) malignancy • nonspecific esophageal motility (disorder)

nem [Ger. *Nährungs Einheit Milch*] nutritional milk unit

nema nematode (threadworm)

Nemb Nembutal

NEMD nonspecific esophageal motility disorder • nonspecific esophageal motor dysfunction

neo neoarsphenamine • neomycin *also* N, NE, NM • neonatal *also* neonat • neovascularity

NEOH neonatal/high (risk)

NEOM neonatal/medium (risk)

neonat neonatal *also* neo

NEP negative expiratory pressure • nephrology *also* NEPH • no evidence (of) pathology • noise equivalent power

nep nephrectomy

NEPD no evidence of pulmonary disease

NEPH nephrology *also* NEP

neph nephritis

NEPHGE nonequilibrium pH (gradient) gel electrophoresis

NEPHRO nephrogram

NER no evidence (of) recurrence • nonionizing electromagnetic radiation

ner nervous • nervousness

NERD no evidence (of) recurrent disease

NERO noninvasive evaluation of radiation output

nerv nervous • nervousness

NES not elsewhere specified

NET nasoendotracheal tube • nerve excitability test • netilmicin • norethisterone

NETEN norethisterone enanthate

n et m [L. *nocte et mane*] night and morning

ne tr s num [L. *ne tradas sine nummo*] do not deliver unless paid

NETT nasal endotracheal tube

neu neurilemma

neur, neuro, neurol neurology/neurologic/ neurologist *also* N

neuropath neuropathology *also* NP

neurosurg neurosurgeon/ neurosurgery *also* NS, Nsurg

neut neuter *also* n • neutral • neutralize • neutrophil

NEX nose to ear to xiphoid

NEY neomycin egg yolk (agar)

NEYA neomycin egg yolk agar

NF nafcillin *also* NAF • nasopharyngeal fibroma • National Formulary • nephritic factor *also* NEF • neurofibromatosis • neurofilament • neutral fraction • noise factor • none found • nonfiltered • nonfluent • nonfront • nonfunction • Nonne-Froin (syndrome) • nonwhite female • normal flow • not filtered • not found • nursed fair • nylon fiber

nF nanofarad

NFAR no further action required

NFB National Foundation for the Blind • nonfermenting bacteria

NFC not favorably considered

NFCC neighborhood family care center

NFD neurofibrillary degeneration • no family doctor

NFDR neurofacial-digitorenal (syndrome)

NFE nonferrous extract

NFH nonfamilial hematuria

NFL nerve fiber layer

NFLD nerve-fiber-layer defect

NFM northern fowl mite

NFP natural family planning • no family physician

NFS National Fertility Study • non-fire setter

NFT neurofibrillary tangle • Nitrazine fern test

NFTD normal full-term delivery

NFTSD normal, full-term, spontaneous delivery

NFTT nonorganic failure to thrive

NFW nursed fairly well

NG nasogastric *also* N-G • new growth • nitroglycerin *also* Nitro, NTG, NTZ • nodose ganglion • no good • no growth • nongenetic • nongroupable

N-G nasogastric *also* NG

ng nanogram

NGA nutrient gelatin agar

NGB neurogenic bladder

NGC nucleus (reticularis) gigantocellularis

N-Ger neurologic geriatrics

NGF nerve growth factor

NG fdgs nasogastric feedings

NGGR nonglucogenic/ glucogenic ratio

NGI nuclear globulin inclusion • nurse's global impressions

n giv not given

ng/mL nanogram per mL

NGR narrow gauze roll • nasogastric replacement

NGS normal goat serum

NGSA nerve growth stimulating activity

NGSF non–genital skin fibroblast

NGT nasogastric tube • normal glucose tolerance

NGU nongonococcal urethritis

NH natriuretic hormone • Naval Hospital • neonatal hepatitis • neurologically handicapped • nodular (and) histiocytic • nonhuman • nursing home

NHA nonspecific hepatocellular abnormality

NHAIS Naylor-Harwood Adult Intelligence Scale

NHANES National Health and Nutrition Examination Survey

NHC neighborhood health center • neonatal hypocalcemia • nonhistone chromatin • nonhistone chromosomal (protein) • nursing home care

NHCP nonhistone chromosomal protein

NHCV nursing home care unit

NHD normal hair distribution

NHDF normal human diploid fibroblast

NHDL non–high-density lipoprotein

NHDS National Hospital Discharge Survey

NHG normal human globulin

NHGJ normal human gastric juice

NHH neurohypophyseal hormone

NHI National Health Insurance

NHIS National Health Interview Survey

NHK normal human kidney

NHL nodular histiocytic lymphoma · non-Hodgkin lymphoma

nHL normalized hearing level

NHML non-Hodgkin malignant lymphoma

NHP nonhemoglobin protein · nonhistone protein · normal human (pooled) plasma · nursing home placement

NHPF National Health Policy Forum

NHPP normal human pooled plasma

NHPPN National Health Professions Placement Network

NHR net histocompatibility ratio

NHS National Health Service (British) · normal horse serum · normal human serum

NHSR National Hospital Service Reserve

NHWM normal human white matter

NI neuraminidase inhibition *also* NAI · neurologic improvement · neutralization index · nitroxoline · no information · noise index · not identified · not isolated · nucleus intercalatus

NI nickel

NIA nephelometric inhibition assay · neutrophil-inducing activity · niacin · no information available

NIAL not in active labor

NIB noninvolved bone

NIBS nearly ideal binary solvent

NIC neurogenic intermittent claudication · Nomarsky interference contrast · noninvasive carotid (study)

Nic nicotinyl alcohol

NICC neonatal intensive care center

NICE noninvasive carotid examination

NICU neonatal intensive care unit · neurologic intensive care unit · neurosurgical intensive care unit · newborn intensive care unit *also* NBICU · nonimmunologic contact urticaria

NIDDM non–insulin-dependent diabetes mellitus

NIDS nonionic detergent soluble

NIF negative inspiratory force *also* Nif · neutrophil

immobilizing factor •
nifedipine *also* N •
nifuroquine • nonintestinal
fibroblast • not in file

NIF negative inspiratory force
also NIF

nif genes nitrogen fixation
(genes for)

NIG NSAIA (nonsteroidal anti-
inflammatory agent)-
induced gastropathy

Nig nonimmunoglobulin

nig [L. *niger*] black

NIH National Institutes of
Health

NIHD noise-induced hearing
damage

NIHL noise-induced hearing
loss

NIIC National Injury
Information Clearinghouse

NIL noise interference level •
nothing in light • not in
labor

nil [L. *nihil*] nothing

NIMH National Institute of
Mental Health

NIMH-DIS National Institute
for Mental Health
Diagnostic Interview
Schedule

NINU neurointermediate
nursing unit

NINVS noninvasive
neurovascular studies

NIP National Inpatient
Profile • nipple •
nitroiodophenyl • no
infection present • no
inflammation present

NIPS noninvolved psoriatic
skin

NIPTS noise-induced
permanent threshold shift

NIR near infrared

NIRA nitrite reductase

NIRD nonimmune renal
disease

NIRMP National Intern and
Resident Matching Program

NIRR non–insulin-requiring
remission

NIRS normal inactivated rabbit
serum

NIS no inflammatory signs •
nonimmune sheep (serum)

NISM (bed) nucleus of stria
medullaris

NIST (bed) nucleus of stria
terminalis

NIT nasointestinal tube •
National Intelligence Test •
neonatal isoimmune
thrombocytopenia

NITD non–insulin-treated
disease

nit. ox. nitrous oxide *also* NO

nitro nitroglycerin *also* NG,
NTG, NTZ

NITTS noise-induced
temporary threshold shift

NIV nodule-inducing virus

NJ nasojejunal

NK natural killer (cell) • not
known *also* N/K

N/K not known *also* NK

NKA no known allergies

nkat nanokatal

NKC nonketotic coma

NKDA no known drug allergies

NKFA no known food allergies

NKH nonketotic hyperglycemia *also* NKHG • nonketotic hyperosmolar • nonketotic hyperosmotic

NKHA nonketotic hyperosmolar acidosis

NKHG nonketotic hyperglycemia *also* NKH

NKHS nonketotic hyperosmolar syndrome • normal Krebs-Henseleit solution

NKMA no known medication allergies

NKR normal rat kidney

NKTS natural killer target structure

NL nasolacrimal • neural lobe • neutral lipid • nodular lymphoma • normal *also* n, nl, NOR, norm • normal libido • normal limits • normolipemic • Nyhan-Lesch (syndrome)

nL nanoliter *also* nl

nl [L. *non liquet*] it is not clear • [L. *non licet*] it is not permitted • nanoliter *also* nL • normal (value) *also* n, NL, NOR, norm • normal limits

NLA neuroleptanalgesia • neuroleptanesthesia • normal lactase activity

NLAA naphthoxylactic acid

NLAL nodule-like alveolar lesion

NLB needle liver biopsy

NLC&C, NL C/Cl normal libido, coitus, and climax

NLD nasolacrimal duct • necrobiosis lipoidica diabeticorum

NLDL normal low-density lipoprotein

NLE neonatal lupus erythematosus • nurse's late entry

Nle norleucine

NLF nasolabial fold • neonatal lung fibroblast • nonlactose fermentation

NLM National Library of Medicine • noise level monitor

NLMC nocturnal leg muscle cramp

NLN no longer needed

NLP neurolinguistic program • nodular liquefying panniculitis • no light perception • normal light perception • normal luteal phase

NLPD nodular lymphocytic, poorly differentiated

NLS neonatal lupus syndrome • nonlinear least squares (method) • normal lymphocyte supernatant

NLSD normal life-span (for) dogs

NLT Names Learning Test • normal lymphocyte transfer (test) • not later than *also*

nlt · not less than *also*
nlt · nucleus lateralis
tuberis

nlt not later than *also* NLT ·
not less than *also* NLT

NLX naloxone *also* Nx

NM neomycin *also* N, NE,
Neo · neuromedical ·
neuromuscular · [L.
nictitare to wink] nictitating
membrane · night (and)
morning *also* N&M ·
nitrogen mustard · nodular
melanoma · nodular mixed
(lymphocytic-histiocystic) ·
nonmalignant · nonmotile
(bacteria) · nonwhite
male · normetadrenaline ·
normetanephrine · not
measurable/measured · not
mentioned · not motile ·
nuclear medicine · nuclear
membrane

N/M newton per meter

N&M nerves and muscles ·
night and morning *also* NM

Nm newton-meter

Nm, nm nux moschata
(nutmeg)

N x m newton by meter

N/m² newton per square meter

nM nanomolar

nm nanometer · [L. *nocte et
mane*] night and morning ·
nonmetallic

NMA neurogenic muscular
atrophy

NMAC National Medical
Audio-Visual Center

NM(ASCP) Technologist in
Nuclear Medicine certified

by American Society of
Clinical Pathologists

NMATWT New Mexico
Attitude Toward Work Test

NMBA nitrosomethyl-
benzylamine

NMC National Medical Care ·
neuromuscular control ·
nodular, mixed-cell
(lymphoma) · nucleus
reticularis
magnocellularis · nurse-
managed center

NMCD nephrophthisis-
medullary cystic disease

NMCPT New Mexico Career
Planning Test

NMCUES National Medical
Care Utilization and
Expenditure Survey

NMD normal muscle
development

NMF nonmigrating fraction (of
spermatozoa)

NMFI National Master Facility
Inventory

NMI no mental illness · no
middle initial · normal
male infant

NMJ neuromuscular junction

NMJAPT New Mexico Job
Application Procedures Test

NMKOT New Mexico
Knowledge of Occupations
Test

NML National Medical
Library · nodular mixed
lymphoma

NMM nodular malignant
melanoma · Nonne-
Milroy-Meige (syndrome)

NMN nicotinamide mononucleotide • no middle name • normetanephrine

NMN+ nicotinamide mononucleotide (reduced form)

NMNRU National Medical Neuropsychiatric Research Unit

NMO nitrogen mustard oxide

nmol nanomole

nmol/L millimicromolar • nanomole per liter

NMOS N-type metal oxide semiconductor

NMP neutral metallopeptidase • normal menstrual period • nucleoside 5'-monophosphate

NMPCA nonmetric principal component analysis

NMR Neill-Mooser reaction • neonatal mortality rate • nictitating membrane response • nuclear magnetic resonance

NMRDC Naval Medical Research and Development Command

NMRI nuclear magnetic resonance imaging

NMRL Naval Medical Research Laboratory

NMRU Naval Medical Research Unit

NMS Naval Medical School • neuroleptic malignant syndrome • neuromuscular spindle • normal mouse serum

N·m/s newton meter per second

NMSE normalized mean square root

NMSIDS near-miss sudden infant death syndrome

NMT nebulized mist treatment • neuromuscular tension • neuromuscular transmission • no more than • nuclear medicine technology

NMTB neuromuscular transmission blockade

NMTD nonmetastatic trophoblastic disease

NMTS neuromuscular tension state

NMU neuromuscular unit

NMUT nitrosomethylurethane

NN neonatal • nevocellular nevus • normally nourished • normal nursery • nurse's notes *also* N/N

N/N negative/negative • nurse's notes *also* NN

N:N azo group (chemical group with two nitrogen atoms)

N-N nurse to nurse (orders)

nn nerves • [L. *nomen novum*] new name *also* n nov, nom nov, nov n

NNA normochromic normocytic anemia

NNAS neonatal narcotic abstinence syndrome

NNC National Nutrition Consortium

NND neonatal death *also* ND • New and Nonofficial Drugs • nonspecific nonerosive duodenitis

NNDC National Naval Dental Center

NNE neonatal necrotizing enterocolitis • nonneuronal enolase

NNG nonspecific nonerosive gastritis

NNHS National Nursing Home Survey

NNI noise and number index

NNL no new laboratory (test orders)

NNM neonatal mortality • Nicolle-Novy-MacNeal (medium) *also* NNN

NNN nitrosonornicotine • Novy-MacNeal-Nicolle (medium) *also* NNM

NNO no new orders

n nov [L. *nomen novum*] new name *also* nn, nom nov, nov m

NNP neonatal nurse practitioner • nerve net pulse

NNR New and Nonofficial Remedies • not necessary to return

NNS neonatal screen (hematocrit, total bilirubin, and total protein) • nonneoplastic syndrome • nonnutritive sucking

NNT neonatally tolerant • nuclei nervi trigemini

NNU net nitrogen utilization

NNWI Neonatal Narcotic Withdrawal Index

NO narcotics officer • nasal oxygen • nitric oxide • nitroso- • nitrous oxide *also* nit. ox. • none obtained • nonobese • number *also* N, n, No, no. • nursing office

No nobelium

No, no. [L. *numero*] number *also* N, n, NO

NOA nurse obstetric assistant

NOBT nonoperative biopsy technique

noc, noct nocturia • [L. *noctis* of the night] nocturnal

NO-CCE no clubbing, cyanosis, or edema

noc maneq [L. *nocte maneque*] at night and in the morning

NOCTI National Occupation Competency Testing (Program)

NOD nodular (melanoma) • nondefinitive (pattern) • nonobese diabetic • notify of death

NOEL no observed effect level (of toxin)

no ess abn no essential abnormalities

NOFT nonorganic failure-to-thrive

NOGM no gammopathy (detected)

NOII nonocclusive intestinal ischemia

NOK next of kin

NOM nonsuppurative otitis media • normal extraocular movements

nom dub [L. *nomen dubium*] a doubtful name

NOMI nonocclusive mesenteric infarction

nom nov [L. *nomen novum*] new name *also* nn, n nov, nov m

nom nud [L. *nomen nudum*] name without designation

NOND none detected

NONF nonfasting

non pal not palpable

non reb nonrebreathing (mask)

non-REM nonrapid eye movement (sleep) *also* NREM

non rep, non repetat [L. *non repetatur*] do not repeat (no refills) *also* NR

NONS nonspecific

nonsegs nonsegmented (neutrophils)

nonvis, nonviz nonvisualized

NOOB not out of bed

NOP national outpatient profile • not otherwise provided (for) *also* NP

NOR noradrenaline *also* Noradr • normal *also* n, NL, nl, norm • nortriptyline • nucleolar organizing region (cytogenetics)

Noradr noradrenaline *also* NOR

NORC normal curve

NOR-EPI norepinephrine *also* NE

norleu norleucine

norm normal *also* n, NL, nl, NOR

normet normetanephrine

NOS network operating system • not on staff • not otherwise specified

nos numbers

NOSAC nonsteroidal anti-inflammatory compound

NOSIE Nurses' Observation Scale for Inpatient Evaluation

NOSTA Naval Ophthalmic Support and Training Activity

NOT nocturnal oxygen therapy • nucleus (of) optic tract

NOTT nocturnal oxygen therapy trial

Nov novobiocin

nov [L. *novum*] new

nov n [L. *novum nomen*] new name *also* nn, n nov, nom nov

NOVS National Office of Vital Statistics

nov sp [L. *novum species*] new species

NOW negotiable order (of) withdrawal

NP nasal prongs • nasopharynx/nasopharyngeal *also* NPhx • near point (ophthalmology) • neonatal-

perinatal • nerve palsy •
neuritic plaque •
neuropathology *also*
neuropath • neuropeptide •
neurophysin *also* Np •
neuropsychiatry • newly
presented • new patient •
Niemann-Pick (disease) •
nitrogen-phosphorus
(detector in gas
chromatography) •
nitrophenide • nitrophenol •
nitroprusside •
nonpalpable •
nonpathologic •
nonpaying •
nonphagocytic •
nonpracticing • nonproducer
(cell) • no pain • no
phone • no progression •
normal plasma • normal
pressure • not palpable •
not perceptible • not
performed • not practiced •
not pregnant • not present •
not (otherwise) provided
(for) *also* NOP • nuclear
pharmacist/pharmacy •
nucleoplasmic (index) •
nucleoprotein • nucleoside
phosphorylase • nursed
poorly • Nurse
Practitioner • nursing
practice • nursing
procedure • [L. *nomen
proprium*] proper name *also*
np

N-P need-persistence

Np neper (unit for comparing
magnitude of two powers,
ususally electrical or
acoustic) • neptunium •
neurophysin *also* NP

np nucleotide pair • [L.
nomen proprium] proper
name *also* NP

NPA nasal pharyngeal
airway • near-point
accomodation • no
previous admission •
nucleus of pretectal area

NPa nail patella

Np-AVP neurophysin
associated with vasopressin

NPAT nonparoxysmal atrial
tachycardia

NPB nodal premature beat •
non–protein bound

NPBF nonplacental blood flow

NPC nasopharyngeal cancer •
nasopharyngeal
carcinoma • near point of
convergence • nodal
premature contractions •
nonparenchymal (liver)
cell • nonpatient contact •
nonproductive cough •
nonprotein calorie • no
prenatal care *also* NPNC •
no previous complaint •
nucleus of posterior
commissure

NPCa nasopharyngeal
carcinoma

NPD narcissistic personality
disorder • natriuretic
plasma dialysate • negative
pressure device •
Niemann-Pick disease •
nitrogen-phosphorus
detector • no pathologic
diagnosis • nonprescription
drugs

NPDL nodular poorly
differentiated lymphocytic
(lymphoma)

NPDR nonproliferative
diabetic retinopathy

NPE neurogenic pulmonary edema · neuropsychologic examination · no palpable enlargement · normal pelvic examination

N periv nuclei periventriculares

NPEV nonpolio enterovirus

NPF nasopharyngeal fiberscope · no predisposing factor

NPFT Neurotic Personality Factor Test

NPG nonpregnant

NPGS neopentyl glycol succinate

NPH neutral protamine Hagedorn (insulin) · no previous history · normal pressure hydrocephalus · nucleus pulposus herniation

NPHI neutral protamine Hagedorn insulin

NPhx nasopharynx *also* NP

NPI Narcissistic Personality Inventory · neonatal perception inventory · neuropsychiatric institute · no present illness · nucleoplasmic index

NPIC neurogenic peripheral intermittent claudication

NPII Neonatal Pulmonary Insufficiency Index

NPJT nonparoxysmal (atrioventricular) junctional tachycardia

NPL neoproteolipid · nodular poorly differentiated lymphoma

NPM nothing per mouth

NPN nonprotein nitrogen

NPNC no prenatal care *also* NPC

NPO [L. *non per os*] nothing by mouth *also* NBM · nucleus preopticus

NPO/HS [L. *nulla per os hora somni*] nothing by mouth at bedtime

NPOS nitrite positive

Np-OT oxytocin-associated neurophysin

NPP nitrophenylphosphate · normal pool plasma · normal postpartum

NPPNG nonpenicillinase-producing *Neisseria gonorrheae*

NP polio nonparalytic poliomyelitis

NPR net protein ratio · normal pulse rate · nothing per rectum · nucleoside phosphoribosyl

NPRM notice (of) proposed rule-making

Nps nitrophenylsulfenyl

NPSA nonphysician surgical assistant · normal pilosebaceous apparatus

NPSG nocturnal polysomnogram

NPSH nonprotein sulhydryl (group)

NPT neoprecipitin test · nocturnal penile tumescence · normal pressure (and) temperature

NPU net protein utilization

NPV negative pressure ventilation • nuclear polyhidrosis virus • nucleus paraventricularis • nutritive

NQA nursing quality assurance

NQMI non–Q wave myocardial infarction

NQR nuclear quadruple resonance

NR [L. *non repetatur*] do not repeat (no refills) *also* non rep, non repetat • nerve root • neural retina • neutral red • noise reduction • nonreactive • nonrebreathing • nonreimbursable • no radiation • no reaction • no recurrence • no refill • no rehearsal • no report • no response • no return • normal *also* n, NL, nl, norm • normal range • normal reaction • normal record • normotensive rat *also* NTR • not reached • not readable • not recorded • not reported • not resolved • nurse • nutrition ratio • Reynold's number *also* N_R

N_R Reynold's number *also* NR

N/R not remarkable

nr [L. *non repetatur*] do not repeat • near • no refills

NRA nitrate reductase • nucleus raphe alatus • nucleus retroambigualis

NRAF nonrheumatic atrial fibrillation

NRB nonrejoining (DNA strand) break

NRBC normal red blood cell • nucleated red blood cell (mass) *also* NRbc

NRbc nucleated red blood cell (mass) *also* NRBC

NRBS nonrebreathing system

NRC National Research Council • noise reduction coefficient • normal retinal correspondence • not routine care • Nuclear Regulatory Commission

NRCL nonrenal clearance

NRD nonrenal death

NREH normal renin essential hypertension

NREM nonrapid eye movement (sleep) *also* non-REM

NREMS nonrapid eye movement sleep

NRF normal renal function

NRFC nonrosette-forming cell

NRGC nucleus reticularis gigantocellularis

NRH nodular regenerative hyperplasia (of liver)

NRI nerve root involvement • nerve root irritation • neutral regular insulin • nonrespiratory infection

NRK normal rat kidney

NRL nucleus reticularis lateralis

NRM normal range (of) motion *also* NROM • normal retinal movement • nucleus raphe magnus • nucleus reticularis magnocellularis

NRMP National Residency Matching Plan

NRN no return necessary

nRNA nuclear ribonucleic acid

nRNP nuclear ribonucleoprotein

NROM normal range of motion *also* NRM

NRP nucleus reticularis parvocellularis

NRPAT net revenue, patient

NRPC nucleus reticularis pontis caudalis

NRPG nucleus reticularis paragigantocellularis

NRR net reproduction rate • Noise Reduction Rating • note, record, report

NRS nonimmunized rabbit serum • normal rabbit serum • normal reference serum • numerical rating scale

NRSCC National Reference System in Clinical Chemistry

NRSFPS National Reporting System for Family Planning Services

nrsng nursing *also* NSG, ngs

NRT neuromuscular re-education technique

NRTOT net revenue, total

NRV nucleus reticularis ventralis

NS natural science • needle shower • nephrosclerosis •

nephrotic syndrome • nervous system • neurologic sign • neurologic surgery • neurologic survey • neurosecretory • neurosurgery *also* neurosurg, NSurg • neurosyphilis • neurotic score • nipple stimulation • nodular sclerosis • nonsmoker *also* NSM • nonsnorer • nonspecific • non-stimulation • nonstructural (protein) • nonstutterer • nonsymptomatic • Noonan syndrome • normal saline *also* N/S • normal serum • normal sodium (diet) • normal study • Norwegian scabies • no sample • no sequelae *also* ns • no specimen *also* ns • not seen • not significant *also* ns • not specified *also* NSP • not stated • not symptomatic • not suf-ficient • nuclear sclerosis • nursing services • nylon suture *also* ns

N/S normal saline *also* NS

Ns nasopinale • nerves

ns nanosecond *also* nsec • no sequelae *also* NS • no specimen *also* NS • not significant *also* NS • nylon suture *also* NS

NSA normal serum albumin • no salt added *also* nsa • no serious abnormality • no significant abnormality • no significant anomaly • nutritional status assessment

nsa no salt added *also* NSA

NSAD no signs (of) acute disease

NSAE nonsupported arm exercise

NSAIA nonsteroidal anti-inflammatory agent

NSAID nonsteroidal anti-inflammatory drug

NSC neurosecretory cell • non-service connected (disability) *also* NSCD • nonspecific suppressor cell • no significant change

NSCD non-service-connected disability *also* NSC

NSCLC non–small-cell lung cancer

NSD Nairobi sheep disease • neonatal staphyloccal disease • night sleep deprivation • nitrogen-specific detector • nominal single dose • nominal standard dose • no significant defect • no significant deficiency • no significant deviation • no significant difference • no significant disease • normal spontaneous delivery

NSDA non–steroid-dependent asthmatic

NSE neuron-specific enolase • nonspecific esterase • normal saline enema

NS̄E [Fr. *sans*] nausea without emesis

nsec nanosecond *also* ns

NSED nonsurgeon, emergency department

NSF nodular subepidermal fibrosis • no significant findings

NSFTD normal spontaneous full-term delivery

NSG neurosecretory granule • nursing *also* nrsng, nsg

nsg nursing *also* nrsng, NSG

NSGCT nonseminomatous germ cell tumor

NSG STA nursing station

NSGCTT nonseminomatous germ cell testicular tumor

NSHD nodular sclerosing Hodgkin disease

NSI negative self-image • no sign (of) infection • no sign (of) inflammation

NSIDS near–sudden infant death syndrome

NSILA nonsuppressible insulin-like activity

NSILP nonsuppressible insulin-like protein

NSL nonsalt loser

NSLF normal sheep lung fibroblast

NSM neurosecretory material • neurosecretory motor neuron • nonantigenic specific mediator • nonsmoker *also* NS • nutrient sporulation medium

N·s/m² newton-second per square meter

NSN nephrotoxic serum nephritis • nicotine-stimulated neurophysin • number (of) similar negatives

NSND nonsymptomatic (and) not disabling

NSO Neosporin ointment • nucleus supraopticus

NSol nerve to soleus

NSP neck (and) shoulder pain • neuron-specific protein • not specified *also* NS • number (of) similar positives

NSPE no specimen (obtainable)

NSPVT nonsustained polymorphic ventricular tachycardia

NSQ Neuroticism Scale Questionnaire • not sufficient quantity

NSR nasoseptal repair/ reconstruction • nonspecific reaction • nonsystemic reaction • normal sinus rhythm • not seen regularly

nSRBC normal sheep red blood cell

NSS normal saline solution • normal size (and) shape • not statistically significant • nutritional support service

NSSC normal size, shape, (and) consistency

NSSL normal size, shape, (and) location

NSSP normal size, shape, (and) position

NSSPAVAF normalsize, shape, (and) position, anteverted (and) anteflexed (uterus)

NSST nonspecific ST (wave) segment changes (on electroencephalogram) • Northwestern Syntax Screening Test

NSSTT nonspecific ST and T (wave)

NST neospinothalamic (tract) • nonshivering thermogenesis • nonstress test (fetal monitoring) • not sooner than • nutritional status type • nutritional support team

NSTT nonseminomatous testicular tumor

NSU neurosurgical unit • nonspecific urethritis

NSurg neurosurgery/ neurosurgeon *also* neurosurg, NS

NSV nonspecific vaginitis

NSVD normal spontaneous vaginal delivery

NSVT nonsustained ventricular tachycardia

NSX neurosurgical examination

NSY nursery

NT nasotracheal • neotetrazolium • neurotensin • neutralization technique • neutralization test • neutralizing • nicotine tartrate • normal temperature • normal tissue • normotensive • nortriptyline • no test • not tender • not tested • nourishment taken

N&T, N+T nose and throat

5′-NT 5′-nucleotidase

Nt amino terminal

NTA natural thymocytotoxic autoantibody •

nitrilotriacetic acid • Nurse Training Act

NTAB nephrotoxic antibody

N/TBC nontuberculous

NTBR not to be resuscitated

NTC neurotrauma center

NTD neural tube defect • nitroblue tetrazolium dye • noise tone difference

NTE neurotoxic esterase • nontest ear • not to exceed • nuclear track emulsion

NTF normal throat flora

NTG nitroglycerin *also* NG, Nitro, NTZ • nontoxic goiter • nontreatment group • normal triglyceridemia

NTGO nitroglycerin ointment

NTHH nontumorous hypergastrinemic hyperchlorhydria

NTI nonthyroid illness • nonthyroid index • no treatment indicated

NTIS National Technical Information Service

NTLI neurotensin-like immunoreactivity

NTM Neuman-Tytell medium • nocturnal tumescence monitor • nontuberculous mycobacteria *also* NTMB

NTMB nontuberculous myobacteria *also* NTM

NTMI nontransmural myocardial infarction

NTMNG nontoxic multinodular goiter

NTN nephrotoxic nephritis

NTND not tender, not distended (abdomen)

NTP National Toxicology Program • nitropaste • normal temperature (and) pressure • nucleoside triphosphate • sodium nitroprusside

NTR negative therapeutic reaction • normotensive rat *also* NR • nutrition

NTS nasotracheal suction • nephrotoxic serum • nonturning (against) self (psychology) • nucleus tractus solitarius

NTT nasotracheal tube

NTV nervous tissue vaccine

NTX naltrexone

NTZ nitroglycerin *also* NG, Nitro, NTG • normal transformation zone (colposcopy)

NU name unknown

Nu nucleolus • nucleus

nU nanounit *also* nu

nu nanounit *also* nU • neurilemma • nude (mouse)

nu (N, ν) 13th letter of Greek alphabet

ν frequency • kinematic viscosity • neutrino • number of degrees of freedom

NUC nuclear *also* nucl • nuclear medicine • sodium urate crystal

Nuc nucleoside *also* N

nuc nucleated

nucl nuclear *also* NUC

NUD nonulcer dyspepsia

NUG necrotizing ulcerative gingivitis

NUI number user identification

nullip nulliparous

num numerator

numc number concentration

NUN nonurea nitrogen

NURB Neville upper reservoir buffer

NUV near-ultraviolet

NV naked vision *also* Nv • nausea and vomiting *also* N/V, N&V • near vision • negative variation • neurovascular • new vessel • next visit • nonvegetarian • nonveteran • normal value • normal volunteer • norverapamil • not vaccinated • not venereal • not verified • not volatile

N/V, N&V nausea and vomiting *also* NV

Nv naked vision *also* NV

nv nonvolatile

NVA near visual acuity • normal visual acuity

NVAF nonvalvular atrial fibrillation

NVB neurovascular bundle

NVC nonvalved conduit

NVD nausea, vomiting, (and) diarrhea • neck vein

distention • neovascularization (of optic) disc • neurovesicle dysfunction • Newcastle virus disease • nonvalvular (heart) disease • no venereal disease • no venous distention

NVE neovascularization elsewhere • new vessels elsewhere

NVG neovascular glaucoma • neoviridogrisein • nonventilated group

NVL neurovascular laboratory

NVM nonvolatile matter

NVS neurologic vital signs • nonvaccine serotype

NVSS normal variant short stature

NVWSC nonvolatile whole-smoke condensate

NW naked weight • nasal wash • nonwithdrawn • not weighed

NWB non-weight-bearing • no weight bearing

NWC number (of) words chosen

NWD neuroleptic withdrawal

NWF new working formulation

NWm nitrogen washout, multiple (breath)

NWs nitrogen washout, single (breath)

NWSM *Nocardia* water-soluble nitrogen

NWR normotensive Wistar rat

NX, Nx naloxone *also* NLX • nephrectomy

NY nystatin

NYC New York City (medium)

NYD not yet diagnosed • not yet discovered

NYHA New York Heart Association (classification)

NYP not yet published

nyst nystagmus

NZ normal zone

NZB New Zealand black (mouse)

NZO New Zealand obese (mouse)

NZR New Zealand red (rabbit)

NZW New Zealand white (mouse)

O absence of sex chromosone • blood type in ABO blood group • [L. *oculus*] eye • [Ger. *ohne Hauch* no film] nonmotile microorganisms and their somatic antigens, antibodies, and agglutinative reactions • no special preparation necessary (for test) • obese *also* OB, ob • objective (findings) *also* Obj • observation *also* OBS, Obs • obstetrics • obvious • occipital • occiput *also* Occ • occlusal • often • old • open/opening *also* o, opg • operator • operon (genetics) • opium • oral/orally *also* (o) • orange (indicator color) • orbit • orderly *also* ord • Oriental • orthopedic *also* OR, Orth, ortho • osteocyte • other • output • oxidative • oxygen *also* O$_2$, OXY, oxy • [L. *octarius*] pint *also* $\bar{\text{O}}$, oct • respirations (on anesthesia chart)

O, Ø negative • nil • no • none • without *also* $\bar{\text{o}}$

$\bar{\text{O}}$ [L. *octarius*] pint *also* O, oct

(O) oral/orally *also* O

O2, O$_2$ both eyes • oxygen (symbol for the diatomic gas) *also* O, OXY, oxy

O$_3$ ozone

o opening *also* O, opg • ovary transplant

$\bar{\text{o}}$ negative • none • without *also* O, Q

o– ortho– (chemical symbol)

OA object assembly

(psychology) • obstructive apnea • occipital artery • occipitoanterior (fetal position) • ocular albinism • old age • oleic acid • opiate analgesia • opsonic activity • optic atrophy • oral airway *also* OAW • oral alimentation • orotic acid *also* Oro • orthopedic assistant • orthophonic acid • osteoarthritis *also* osteo • ovalbumin *also* OVA, OV • overall assessment • oxalic acid • oxolinic acid

O–A Objective–Analytic (Anxiety Battery)

O&A observation and assessment • odontectomy and alveoloplasty

O$_2$a oxygen availability

OAA Old Age Assistance • oxaloacetic acid (test)

OAAD ovarian ascorbic acid depletion (test)

OAB old age benefits

OABP organic anion–binding protein

OAC oral anticoagulant • overaction

OAD obstructive airway disease • occlusive arterial disease • organic anionic dye

OADC oleic acid, albumin, dextrose, and catalase (medium)

OADMT Oliphant Auditory Discrimination Memory Test

OAE otoacoustic emission

OAF open air factor • osteoclast–activating factor

OAG open–angle glaucoma

OAH ovarian androgenic hyperfunction

OAJ open apophyseal joint

OALF organic acid–labile fluoride

OALL ossification (of) anterior longitudinal ligament

o alt hor [L. *omnibus alternis horis*] every other hour

OAM outer acrosomal membrane • oxyacetate malonate

OAP old age pension/ pensioner • Oncovin (vincristine), araC (cytarabine), and prednisone • ophthalmic artery pressure • osteoarthropathy • oxygen (at) atmospheric pressure

OAPs Occupational Ability Patterns (psychologic test)

OAR orientation/alertness remediation • other administrative reasons

OARSA oxacillin aminoglycoside–resistant *Staphylococcus aureus*

OAS old–age security • osmotically active substance

OASDHI Old Age, Survivors, Disability, and Health Insurance

OASDI Old Age, Survivors, and Disability Insurance

OASI Old Age and Survivors Insurance

OASO overactive superior oblique

OASP organic acid–soluble phosphorus

OASR overactive superior rectus

OAST Oliphant Auditory Synthesizing Test

OAT ornithine aminotransferase

OAV oculoauriculovertebral (dysplasia, syndrome)

OAW oral airway *also* OA

OB [L. *obiit*] he/she died *also* ob • obese *also* O, ob • objective benefit • obstetrics *also* OBS, Obs, Obst • obstetrician • occult bleeding • occult blood • olfactory bulb *also* OLB

OB+ occult blood positive

O&B opium and belladonna

ob [L. *obiit*] he/she died *also* OB • obese *also* O, OB

OBB own bed bath

OBD organic brain disease

OBE out–of–body experience

OBF organ blood flow

OBG, ObG obstetrics (and) gynecology/obstetrician– gynecologist *also* OB– GYN, ObGyn, OG, O&G

OBGS obstetric (and) gynecologic surgery

OB–GYN, OB/GYN,ObGyn, OB obstetrics (and) gynecology/obstetrician–gynecologist *also* OBG, ObG, O&G

Obj, obj objective *also* O

obj object

obl oblique

OBP ova, blood, (and) parasites (stool exam)

OBRR obstetric recovery room

OBS observation *also* O, Obs • obstetrical service/obstetrics *also* OB, Obs, Obst • organic brain syndrome

Obs observation/observed *also* O, OBS • obstetrics/obstetrician *also* OB, OBS, Obst

obs obsolete

obsd observed

Obst obstetrics/obstetrician *also* OB, OBS, Obs

obst obstipation • obstructed/obstruction

obstet obstetric

obt obtained

OB–US obstetrical ultrasound

OC obstetrical conjugate • occlusocervical • office call • on call • only child • optic chiasm *also* OX • oral care • oral cavity • oral contraceptive • organ culture • original claim • outer canthal (distance) • ovarian cancer • oxygen consumed

O&C, O+C onset and course (of disease)

Oc ochre (suppressor)

OCA oculocutaneous albinism • open care area • operant conditioning audiometry • oral contraceptive agent

OCA olivopontocerebellar atrophy *also* OPCA

OCAD occlusive carotid artery disease

O₂ cap. oxygen capacity

OCBF outer cortical blood flow

Occ occasional • occipital/occiput *also* O • occlusion/occlusive *also* occl

occ occupation *also* occup • occurrence

occ, occas occasional/occasionally

OCCC open–chest cardiac compression

occip occipital • occiput

occip F occipitofrontal *also* OF

occip–F HA occipitofrontal headache *also* O–FHA, OF-HA

occl occlusion *also* Occ

OCCPR open–chest cardiopulmonary resuscitation

OccTh occupational therapist/therapy *also* Occup Rx, OT

occup occupation/occupational *also* occ • occupies/occupying

Occup Rx occupational therapy *also* OccTh, OT

OCD obsessive–compulsive disorder • Office of Child Development • Office of Civil Defense • osteochondritis dissecans • ovarian cholesterol depletion (test)

OCG omnicardiogram • oral cholecystogram

OCH oral contraceptive hormone

OCHS Office of Cooperative Health Statistics

OCIS Oncology Center Information System

OCL Occupational Check List (psychologic test) • oral colonic lavage

OCM oral contraceptive medication

OCN oculomotor nucleus *also* OMN • Oncology Certified Nurse

OCP octacalcium phosphate • oral contraceptive pill • ova, cysts, and parasites (stool exam)

OCR ocular counterrolling • ocular countertorsion reflex • oculocardiac reflex • oculocerebrorenal

oCRF ovine corticotropin–releasing factor

OCRS oculocerebrorenal syndrome

OCS open canalicular system (of platelets) • oral contraceptive steroid • outpatient clinic

substation • oxycorticosteroid

OCT Object Classification Test • optimal cutting temperature (medium) • oral contraceptive therapy • ornithine carbamoyl-transferase • oxytocin challenge test

O₂CT oxygen content

oct [L. *octarius*] pint *also* O, ō

OCTD ornithine carbamoyltransferase deficiency

octup [L. *octuplus*] eightfold

OCU observation care unit

OCV ordinary conversational voice

OCVM occult vascular malformation

OD Doctor of Optometry • occipital dysplasia • occupational dermatitis • occupational disease • on duty • open drop (anesthesia) • open duct • optical density • optic disk • optimal dose • organization development • originally derived • outdoor • out–of–date • outside diameter • (drug) overdose/overdosage • [L. *oculus dexter*] right eye

O–D obstacle–dominance • original–derived

od [L. *omni die*] every day • daily

ODA osmotic driving agent • [L. *occipitodextra anterior*] right occipitoanterior (fetal position)

ODAC on–demand analgesia computer

ODAP Oncovin (vincristine), dianhydrogalactitol, Adriamycin (doxorubicin), and Platinol (cisplatin)

ODAT one day at a time

ODB opiate–directed behavior

ODC orotidylate decarboxylase (deficiency) • outpatient diagnostic center • oxygen dissociation curve

ODCH ordinary disease (of) childhood

ODD oculodentodigital (dysplasia, syndrome)

OD'd (drug) overdosed

ODE *o*–desmethylencainide

ODM, ODm ophthalmodyn-amometer/ophthalmo-dyamometry

ODOD oculodento–osseous dysplasia

Odont odontology

odont odontogenic

ODP offspring (of) diabetic parents • [L. *occipitodextra posterior*] right occipitoposterior (fetal position)

ODQ on direct questioning • opponens digiti quinti (muscle)

ODSG ophthalmic Doppler sonogram

ODT oculodynamic test • [L. *occipitodextra transversa*] right occipitotransverse (fetal position)

ODTS organic dust toxic syndrome

ODU optical density unit

OE on examination *also* O/E • orthopedic examination *also* OX • otitis externa

O/E (ratio of) observed to expected • on examination *also* OE

O&E observation and examination

Oe oersted (centimeter–gram–second unit of magnetic field strength)

OEC outer ear canal

OEE osmotic erythrocyte enrichment • outer enamel epithelium

OEF oil emersion field • oxygen extraction fraction

OEM open–end marriage • opposite ear masked • original equipment manufacturer (computers)

OER osmotic erythrocyte (enrichment) • oxygen enhancement ratio

O₂ER oxygen extraction ratio

OES optical emission spectroscopy • oral esophageal stethoscope

oesoph esophagus (oesophagus) *also* E, ES, ESO, esoph

OESP orthopedic examination, special

OET oral esophageal tube • oral endotracheal tube *also* OETT

OETT oral endotracheal tube *also* OET

OF occipitofrontal *also* occip F • optic fundi • orbitofrontal • osmotic fragility (test) • osteitis fibrosa • Ostrum–Furst (syndrome) • other (medical/surgical) facility • oxidation–fermentation (medium) *also* O–F, O/F

O–F, O/F oxidation–fermentation (medium) *also* OF

OFA oncofetal antigen

OFBM oxidation–fermentation basal medium

OFC occipitofrontal circumference • orbitofacial cleft • osteitis fibrosa cystica

ofc office *also* off.

OFD object–film distance (radiology) *also* ofd • occipitofrontal diameter • orofaciodigital (dysostosis, syndrome)

ofd object–film distance (radiology) *also* OFD

Off, off. official

off. office *also* ofc

O–FHA, OF–HA occipitofrontal headache *also* occip–F HA

OFM orofacial malformation

OFPF optic fundi (and) peripheral fields

OF rad occipitofrontal radiation

OFTT organic failure to thrive

OG obstetrics (and) gynecology *also* OBG,

ObG, OB–GYN, ObGyn, O&G • occlusogingival • oligodendrocyte • optic ganglion • orange green (stain) • orogastric (feeding)

O&G obstetrics and gynecology *also* OBG, ObG, OB/GYN, ObGyn, OG

OGA orogastric gonococcal aspirate

OGD old granulomatous disease

OGF ovarian growth factor • oxygen gain factor

OGH ovine growth hormone

OGM outgrowth medium

OGS oxygenic steroid

OGT oral glucose tolerance

OGTT oral glucose tolerance test

OH hydroxycorticosteroid *also* HCS, OHCS • hydroxyl group • hydroxyl radical • obstructive hypopnea • occipital horn • occupational health • occupational history • on hand • open–heart (surgery) • oral hygiene • orthostatic hypotension • osteopathic hospital • out (of) hospital • outpatient hospital

o.h. [L. *omni hora*] every hour *also* omn hor

OHA oral hypoglycemic agent

OHB₁₂ hydroxocobalamin (vitamin B_{12}) *also* OH–Cbl

O₂Hb oxyhemoglobin

OHC hydroxycholecalciferol *also* OHD · occupational health center · outer hair cell

OH–Cbl hydroxocobalamin *also* OHB$_{12}$

OHCS hydroxycorticosteroid *also* HCS, OH

OHD hydroxycholecalciferol *also* OHC · organic heart disease

OHDA hydroxydopamine *also* HD, HDA

OH–DOC hydroxydeoxy-corticosterone

OHF Omsk hemorrhagic fever · overhead frame

OHFA hydroxy fatty acid

OHFT overhead frame trapeze

OHG oral hypoglycemic

OHI ocular hypertension indicator · oral hygiene index

OH–IAA hydroxyindoleacetic acid *also* HIAA

OHI–S Oral Hygiene Index—Simplified

OHL oral hairy leukoplakia

ohm–cm ohm–centimeter

OHN Occupational Health Nurse

OHP hydroxyproline · orthogonal–hole test pattern · oxygen (under) high pressure

17–OHP 17α–hydroxy-progesterone

OHRR open heart recovery room

OHS obesity hypoventilation syndrome · ocular hypoperfusion syndrome · open–heart surgery · ovarian hyperstimulation syndrome · Overcontrolled Hostility Scale

OHSS ovarian hyperstimulation syndrome

OHT Occupational Health Technician · ocular hypertensive (glaucoma suspect)

OHU hydroxyurea

OI objective improvement · obturator internus · occipitoiliacus · opportunistic infection · opsonic index · orgasmic impairment · Orientation Inventory (psychologic test) · orthoiodohippurate *also* OIH · osteogenesis imperfecta · otitis interna · ouabain insensitive · oxygen income · oxygen intake

O–I outer–to–inner

OID optimal immunomodu-lating dose · organism identification (number)

OIF observed intrinsic frequency · oil immersion field

OIH orthoiodohippurate *also* OI · ovulation–inducing hormone

OIHA orthoidobippurate · orthoiodohippuric acid

oint ointment

OIP organizing interstitial pneumonia

OIT (Tien) organic integrity test (psychiatry)

OJ, oj orange juice *also* OrJ

OK, ok all right • approved • correct

OKAN optokinetic after nystagmus

OKN optokinetic nystagmus

OKT Ollier–Klippel–Trenaunay (syndrome) • ornithine–ketoacid transaminase • Ortho–Kung T (cell)

OL [L. *oculus laevus*] left eye • other location

Ol, ol [L. *oleum*] oil

OLA [L. *occipitolaeva anterior*] left occipitoanterior (fetal position)

OLB olfactory bulb *also* OB • open–liver biopsy

OLD obstructive lung disease

OLH ovine lactogenic hormone • ovine leuteinizing hormone *also* oLH

oLH ovine leuteinizing hormone *also* OLH

OLIB osmiophilic lamellar inclusion body

OLIDS open–loop insulin delivery system

OLMAT Otis–Lennon Mental Ability Test

ol oliv [L. *oleum olivarium*] olive oil

OLP [L. *occipitolaeva posterior*] left occipitoposterior (fetal position)

OLR otology, laryngology, (and) rhinology

ol res oleoresin

OLSIST Oral Language Sentence Imitation Screening Test

OLT [L. *occipitolaeva posterior*] left occipitotransverse (fetal position)

OLT, Olt orthoptic liver transplantation

OM obtuse marginal (coronary artery) • occipitomental • occupational medicine • oculomotor • Osborn–Mendel (rat) • osteomalacia • osteomyelitis *also* osteo • osteopathic manipulation • otitis media • outer membrane • ovulation method (birth control)

om [L. *omni mane*] every morning *also* omn man.

OMAC otitis media, acute, catarrhal

OMAD Oncovin (vincristine), methotrexate, Adriamycin (doxorubicin), and dactinomycin

OMAS occupational maladjustment syndrome • otitis media, acute, suppurating

OMC open mitral commissurotomy

OMCA otitis media, catarrhal, acute

OMCC, OMCCH otitis media, catarrhal, chronic

OMChS otitis media, chronic, suppurating

OMD ocular muscle dystrophy • oculomandibulodyscephaly • organic mental disorder

OME Office of Medical Examiner • otitis media (with) effusion

omega (Ω, ω) 24th and last letter of Greek alphabet

Ω ohm

ω angular frequency • angular velocity • carbon atom farthest from principal functioning group

om 1/4 h [L. *omni quadranta hora*] every quarter hour/ every 15 minutes *also* omn quad hor, om quad hor

OMI old myocardial infarction

omicron (O, o) 15th letter of Greek alphabet

OML orbitomeatal line

OMM ophthalmomandibulo-melic (dysplasia, syndrome) • outer mitochondrial membrane

om mane vel noc [L. *omni mane vel nocte*] every morning or night

OMN oculomotor nerve • oculomotor nucleus *also* OCN

omn bid. [L. *omni bidendis*] every two days

omn bih [L. *omni bihora*] every two hours

omn hor [L. *omni hora*] every hour

omn 2 hor [L. *omni secunda hora*] every second hour

omn man. [L. *omni mane*] every morning *also* o.m.

omn noct [L. *omni nocte*] every night *also* ON, o.n.

omn quad hor [L. *omni quadrante hora*] every quarter hour *also* om 1/4 h, om quad hor

omn sec hor [L. *imni secunda hora*] every second hour

OMP olfactory marker protein • outer membrane protein

OMPA octamethyl pyrophosphoramide • otitis media, purulent, acute

OMPC, OMPCh otitis media, purulent, chronic

om quad hor [L. *omni quadrante hora*] every quarter hour *also* om 1/4 h, omn quad hor

OMR operative mortality rate

OMS offshore medical school • organic mental syndrome • otomandibular syndrome

OM&S osteopathic medicine and surgery

OMSA otitis media, suppurative, acute

OMSC, OMSCh otitis media, secretory, chronic • otitis media, suppurative, chronic

OMT, OM/T osteopathic manipulation treatment

OMVC open mitral valve commissurotomy

OMVI operating motor vehicle (while) intoxicated

ON [L. *omni nocte*] every night *also* omn noct, o.n. • occipitonuchal • office nurse • onlay • optic nerve • optic neuritis • optic neuropathy • oronasal • orthopedic nurse *also* ORN • osteonecrosis • overnight

o.n. [L. *omni nocte*] every night *also* omn noct, ON

ONC oncology *also* onco, oncol • Orthopedic Nursing Certificate • over–the–needle catheter

ONCG–A oncogenic virus battery–acute

onco, oncol oncology *also* ONC

ONCORNA oncogene ribonucleic acid

OND orbitonasal dislocation • other neurologic disorder/disease

ONDS Oriental nocturnal death syndrome

ONH optic nerve head • optic nerve hypoplasia

ONP operating nursing procedure

ONPG, ONP–GAL *o*–nitro-phenyl–β–galactosidase

ONTG oral nitroglycerin

ONTR orders not to resuscitate

OO oophorectomy • oral order(s)

O–O outer–to–outer

O&O off and on

o/o on account of

OOA outer optic anlage

OOB out of bed • out–of–body (experience)

OOBBRP out of bed (with) bathroom privileges

OOC onset of contractions • out of cast • out of control

OOH&NS ophthalmology, otorhinolaryngology, and head and neck surgery

OOL onset of labor

OOLR ophthalmology, otology, laryngology, (and) rhinology

OOP out of pelvis • out of plaster (cast) • out on pass

OOR out of room

OOS out of stock *also* OS

OOT out of town

OOW out of wedlock *also* OW

OP oblique presentation • occipitoparietal • occipitoposterior • old patient (previously seen) • olfactory penduncle • opening pressure • operation *also* op • operative • operative procedure • ophthalmology • opponens pollicis • original package • oropharynx • orthostatic proteinuria • oscillatory potential • osmotic pressure • osteoporosis • other (than) psychotic • outpatient *also* O/P, OPT • overproof • ovine prolactin

O/P outpatient *also* OP, OPT

O&P ova and parasites (stool exam)

Op opisthocranion

op operation/operational/ operator *also* OP • opposite • [L. *opus*] work

OPA oral pharyngeal airway • outpatient anesthesia

OPAL Oncovin (vincristine), prednisone, and L-aspar-aginase

OPB outpatient basis

OPC outpatient clinic

OPCA olivopontocerebellar atrophy *also* OCA

op clt [L. *opere citato*] in the work cited

OPD obstetric prediabetes • optical path difference • otopalatodigital (syndrome) • outpatient department • outpatient dispensary

OpDent operative dentistry

OPDG ocular plethysmodynamography

OPE outpatient evaluation

OPG ocular plethysmography • oculoplethysmograph • oculopneumoplethysmography *also* OPPG • ophthalmoplethysmograph • oxypolygelatin (plasma volume extender)

opg opening *also* O, o

OPH, Oph obliterative pulmonary hypotension • ophthalmia • ophthal-mologist • ophthalmology • ophthalmoscopy • ophthalmoscope *also* Ophth

oph ophthalmic • ophthalmologic

OphD Doctor of Ophthalmology

Ophth ophthalmologist • ophthalmology • ophthalmoscope • ophthalmoscopy *also* OPH

OPI oculoparalytic illusion • Omnibus Personality Inventory

OPK optokinetic

OPL osmotic pressure (of proteins in) lymph • outer plexiform layer • ovine placental lactogen

OPLL ossification (of) posterior longitudinal ligament

OPM occult primary malignancy • ophthalmoplegic migraine

OPN ophthalmic nurse

OPP Oncovin (vincristine), procarbazine, and prednisone • osmotic pressure (of) plasma • ovine pancreatic polypeptide • oxygen partial pressure

opp opposing • opposite

OPPES oil–associated pneumoparalytic eosinophilic syndrome

OPPG oculopneumo-plethysmography *also* OPG

op reg operative region

oprg operating

OPRT orotate phosphoribosyltransferase

OPS operations • outpatient service • outpatient surgery

OPSA ovarian papillary serous (cyst)adenocarcinoma

OpScan optical scanning

OPSI overwhelming postsplenectomy infection

OPSR Office of Professional Standards Review

OPST–BQA Office of Professional Standards Review—Bureau of Quality Assurance

OPT outpatient *also* OP, O/P • outpatient treatment

Opt optometrist

opt. [L. *optimus*] best • optical • optician • optics • optimal • optimum • optional

OPT c̄ CA Ohio pediatric tent with compressed air

OPT c̄ O$_2$ Ohio pediatric tent with oxygen

OPV oral poliovaccine • oral (attenuated) poliovirus vaccine • out–patient visit

OPW, OPWL opiate withdrawal

OQSMAT Otis Quick Scoring Mental Abilities Test

OR odds ratio • oil retention (enema) • open reduction • operating room • optic radiation • oral rehydration • organ recovery • orienting reflex • orienting response • orthopedic *also* O, Orth, ortho • orthopedic research • own recognizance • oxidized– reduced

O–R, o/r oxidation–reduction

Or outflow rate

ORA occiput right anterior (fetal position) • opiate receptor agonist

ORAN orthopedic resident admit note

ORBC ox red blood cell

ORC ox red cell • order/ results communication

ORCH orchiectomy

orch orchitis

ORD optical rotatory dispersion • oral radiation death

Ord orotidine

ord orderly *also* O • ordinate

OREF open reduction (and) external fixation

OR en oil–retention enema

OR&F open reduction and fixation

org organ • organic • organism

ORIF open reduction (with) internal fixation

orig origin • original

OrJ orange juice *also* OJ, oj

ORL otorhinolaryngology

ORN operating room nurse • orthopedic nurse *also* ON

Orn ornithine

ORO oil red O

Oro orotic acid *also* OA • orotate

OROS oral osmotic

ORP occiput right posterior (fetal position) • oxidation–reduction potential

ORPM orthorhythmic pacemaker

ORS olfactory reference syndrome • oral rehydration salt • oral rehydration solution • oral surgeon • oral surgery *also* OS • orthopedic surgeon *also* OS • orthopedic surgery

ORT operating room technician • oral rehydration therapy • Registered Occupational Therapist

OR tech operating room technician

Orth, ortho orthopedic *also* O, OR • orthopedics

orthot orthotonus

ORx oriented

OR x1 oriented to time

OR x2 oriented to time and place

OR x3 oriented to time, place, and person

OS [L. *oculus sinister*] left eye • occipitosacral (fetal position) • occupational safety • opening snap (heart sound) • operating suite • oral surgery *also* ORS • orthopedic

surgery • orthopedic surgeon *also* ORS • Osgood–Schlatter (disease) • osteogenic sarcoma • osteoid surface • osteosarcoma • osteosclerosis • ouabain sensitive • out (of) stock *also* OOS • overall survival • oxygen saturation *also* O_2 sat., SaO_2, SO_2

Os osmium

os [L. pl. *ossa*] bone • [L. pl. *ora*] mouth

OSA obstructive sleep apnea

OSAS obstructive sleep apnea syndrome

O_2 sat. oxygen saturation *also* OS, SaO_2, SO_2

OSBCL Ottawa School Behavior Check List

osc oscillate

OSCE objective structural clinical examination

OSCJ original squamocolumnar junction

OSD outside doctor • overside drainage

OSF outer spiral fibers (of cochlea) • overgrowth–stimulating factor

OSFT outstretched fingertips

OSHA Occupational Safety and Health Administration

OSIQ Offer Self–Image Questionnaire (for Adolescents)

OSL Osgood–Schlatter lesion

OSM osmolarity • ovine submaxillary mucin • oxygen saturation meter

Osm osmole *also* osmol

osM osmolar

osm osmosis • osmotic

OSMF oral submucous fibrosis

Osm/kg osmole per kilogram (osmolality)

Osm/L, Osm/l osmole per liter (osmolarity)

osmo osmolality

osmol osmole *also* Osm

OSM S osmolarity serum

OSM U osmolarity urine

OSN off–service note

OSS Object Sorting Scales (psychologic test) • osseous • over–shoulder strap

OS–SPT osmodality urine spot (test)

OST object–sorting test

Ost osteotomy

Osteo osteopathologist *also* osteopath • osteopathy

osteo osteoarthritis *also* OA • osteomyelitis *also* OM • osteopathology

osteocart osteocartilaginous

osteopath osteopathologist *also* Osteo

OT objective test • oblique talus • occiput transverse • occlusion time • occupational therapy/therapist *also*

OccTh, Occup Rx • ocular tension • Oesterreicher–Turner (syndrome) • office treatment • old term • old terminology (anatomy) • (Koch's) old tuberculin • olfactory threshold • olfactory tubercle *also* OTU • optic tract • orientation test • original tuberculin • orotracheal (tube) • orthopedic treatment • otolaryngology *also* Ot, OTO, Oto, Otolar • otology *also* OTO, Oto, Otol • oxytocin *also* OX, OXT, OXY, oxy

O/T oral temperature

Ot otolaryngology *also* OT, OTO, Oto, Otolar

OTA open to air • Opinions toward Adolescents (psychologic test) • ornithine transaminase • orthotoluidine arsenite

OTC ornithine transcarbamylase (deficiency) • oval target cell • over–the–counter (nonprescription drug) *also* OTCD • oxytetracycline

OTc heart–rate–corrected OT interval

OTCD over–the–counter drug (nonprescription) *also* OTC

OTC Rx over–the–counter prescription

OTD oral temperature device • organ tolerance dose • out the door

OTE optically transparent electrode

OTF oral transfer factor

OTH other

OTI ovomucoid trypsin inhibitor

OTM orthotoluidine manganese (sulfate)

OTO, Oto otolaryngology *also* OT, Ot, Otolar • otology *also* OT, Otol

Otol otologist/otology *also* OT, OTO, Oto

Otolar otolaryngology *also* OT, Ot, OTO, Oto

OTR Ovarian Tumor Registry • Occupational Therapist, Registered

OT/RT Occupational Therapy/ Recreational Therapy

OTS occipital temporal sulcus • orotracheal suction

OTSG Office of the Surgeon General

OTT, OT(T) orotracheal tube

OTU olfactory tubercle *also* OT • operational taxonomic unit

OU [L. *oculi unitas*] both eyes (together) • [L. *oculi uterque*] each eye • Observation Unit • Oppenheim–Urbach (syndrome)

OULQ outer upper left quadrant

OURQ outer upper right quadrant

OV oculovestibular • office visit • Osler–Vaquez (disease) • osteoid volume • outflow volume:

ovalbumin *also* OA, OVA • overventilation • ovulating/ovulation

O₂V oxygen ventilation equivalent

Ov ovary

Oᵥ outflow volume

ov [L. *ovum*] egg • ovarian

OVA ovalbumin *also* OA, OV

OVAL ovalocyte

OVD occlusal vertical dimension

OvDF ovarian dysfunction

OVDQ Organizational Value Dimensions Questionnaire

OVIS Ohio Vocational Interest Survey

OVIT Oral Verbal Intelligence Test

OVLT organum vasculosum (of) lamina terminalis

OVX ovariectomized

OW off work • once weekly • open wedge (osteotomy) • ordinary warfare • outer wall • out (of) wedlock *also* OOW • oval window

O/W oil in water (emulsion) • oil–water (ratio)

o/w otherwise

OWA organics–in–water analyzer

OWNK out of wedlock (and) not keeping (child)

OWR ovarian wedge resection

OWS overwear syndrome

OWVI Ohio Work Values Inventory

OX optic chiasm *also* OC •
orthopedic examination *also*
OE • oxacillin • oxymel
(honey, water, and
vinegar) • oxytocin *also*
OT, OXT, OXY, oxy

Ox oxygen

OXLAT oxalate

OXEA ox erythrocyte antibody

OxI oximeter • oximetry

OXP oxypressin

OXT oxytocin *also* OT, OX,
OXY, oxy

OXY, oxy oxygen *also* O,
O_2 • oxytocin *also* OT,
OX, OXT

OYE old yellow enzyme

oz ounce

oz ap apothecary's ounce

oz t ounce troy

P [L. *post*] after *also* p • [L. *pondere*] by weight • [L. *pater*] father • form perception (in General Aptitude Test Battery) • gas partial pressure • [L. *pugillus*] handful • [L. *proximum*] near • [L. *punctum proximum*] near point (of vision) *also* PP, pp • page • pain • para (parity) • parent • parenteral • parietal electrode placement in electroencephalography • parity • parous • part *also* pt • partial pressure *also* p, PP • passive • paternal • paternally contributing • patient *also* PNT, Pnt, PT, Pt, pt • pelvis • penicillin *also* PCN, Pen, pen., PN, PNC • per • percent • percentile • perceptual speed • percussion • perforation *also* perf • peripheral • permeability • peta– • peyote • pharmacopoeia • phenacetin • phenolph-thalein • phenylalanine *also* PA, PHA, PHE, Phe • phon (unit of loudness) • phosphate (group) • phosphorus • physiology *also* PHY, PHYS • pico– • pig • pilocarpine • pin • pink (indicator color) • pint *also* p, PT, pt • placebo *also* PBO, PL • plan • plasma • point • poise (unit of dynamic viscosity) • poison/ poisoning • polarity • polarization • pole • polymyxin • pons • poor • popular response • population • porcelain • porcine • porphyrin • position *also* pos • positive

also POS, pos • posterior *also* post. • postpartum • power • precipitin • prednisone *also* PDN, PRED • premolar • presbyopia *also* PR, Pr • pressure *also* p, PR, press. • primary • primipara *also* I–para, primip, PRIMP • primitive (hemoglobin) • private (patient, room) • probable error • probability • product • progesterone • prolactin *also* P, PR, Pr, PRL, Prl • proline *also* Pro • properdin • propionate • protein *also* PR, Pr, PRO, pro, prot • Protestant • proximal • psoralen • psychiatry *also* PS, Psy, psychiat • psychosis • pulmonary *also* P, PUL, pul, pulm • pulse • pupil • P wave (in electrocardi-ography) • pyroplasty • radiant flux • radiant power • significance probability (value) • sound power • [L. *pondus*] weight

P/ partial upper denture

/P partial lower denture

P₁ first parental generation

P₂, P–2 pulmonic second (heart) sound

P₃ luminous flux • proximal third (of bone) *also* P/3

P/3 proximal third (of bone)

P₄ progesterone

³²p radioisotope of phosphorus

P–50 oxygen half–saturation pressure of hemoglobin

P–55 hydroxypregnanedione

P$_{700}$ chloroplast pigment bleached by 700 nm

P$_{870}$ bacterial chromatophore pigment bleached by 870 nm

p after *also* P • atomic orbital with angular momentum quantum number 1 • freeze preservation • frequency of the more common allele of a pair • momentum • optic papilla • page • papilla • para • partial pressure *also* P, PP • peripheral • phosphate • pico– • pint *also* P, PT, pt • pond • pressure *also* P, PR, press. • probability • probable error • proton • pupil • sample proportion (in statistics) • short arm of chromosome • sound pressure

p̄ [L. *post*] after • mean pressure (gas)

p– *para–* (chemical prefix for two symmetrical sub-stitutions in benzene ring)

PA panic attack • pantothenic acid • paralysis agitans • paranoia • parietal (cell) antibody • passive aggressive • paternal aunt • pathology • pentemoic acid • periarteritis • peridural artery • periodic acid • periodontal abscess • permeability area • pernicious anemia • peroxidatic activity • phakic–aphakic • phenol alcohol • phenylalanine *also*

P, PHA, PHE, Phe • phosphatidic acid • phosphoarginine • photo–allergy • phthalic anhydride • physical assistance • Physician Assistant • Picture Arrangement (psychology) • pineapple (test for butyric acid in stomach) • pituitary–adrenal • plasma aldosterone • plasminogen activator • platelet adhesiveness • platelet aggregation • platelet associated • polyacrylamide • polyarteritis • polyarthritis • postaural • posteroanterior • prealbumin • predictive accuracy • pregnancy associated • presents again • primary aldosteronism • primary amenorrhea • primary anemia • prior to admission • proactivator • proanthocyanidin • procainamide • professional association • proinsulin antibody • prolonged action • prophylactic antibiotic • propionic acid • prostate antigen • proteolytic activity • prothrombin activity • protrusio acetabuli • psychiatric aide • psychoanalysis *also* PYA • psychogenic aspermia • pulmonary artery • pulmonary atresia • pulpoaxial • puromycin aminonucleoside • pyrophosphate arthropathy • pyrrolizidine alkaloid • [L. *per annum*] yearly

PA alveolar pressure

PA partial pressure

P/A percussion (and) auscultation • position (and) alignment

P–A posteroanterior *also* PA

P&A percussion and auscultation • position and alignment • present and active (reflex)

P$_2$>A$_2$ pulmonic second heart sound greater than aortic second heart sound

P$_2$=A$_2$ pulmonic second heart sound equal to aortic second heart sounds

P$_2$<A$_2$ pulmonic heart sound less than aortic second heart sound

Pa arterial pressure • pascal • protactinium • pulmonary arterial (pressure) • pulmonary artery (line)

pA picoampere

pA$_2$ affinity constant (binding drug to drug receptor)

p.a. [L. *post applicationem*] after application • [L. *pro anno*] for the year

PAA partial agonist activity • phenylacetic acid • physical abilities analysis • plasma angiotensinase activity • polyacrylamide • polyacrylic acid • poly(amino acid) • premarket approval application • pyridineacetic acid

paa [L. *parti affectase applicetur*] let it be applied to the affected area

P(A–aDO$_2$), P(A–a)O$_2$ alveolar–arterial oxygen tension difference

PAB *para*–aminobenzoate • polyacrylamide bead • Positive Attention Behavior • premature atrial beat • purple agar base (medium)

PABA *para*–aminobenzoic acid

PAC papular acrodermatitis (of) childhood • *para*–aminoclonidine • parent–adult–child (in transactional analysis) • phenacetin (acetophenetidin), aspirin, and caffeine • plasma aldosterone concentration • Platinol (cisplatin), Adriamycin (doxorubicin), and cyclophosphamide *also* PAC–V • preadmission certification • premature atrial contraction • premature auricular contraction • Progress Assessment Chart of Social and Personal Development

PACC protein A (immobilized in) colodion charcoal

PACE Pacing and Clinical Electrophysiology • performance and cost efficiency • Personal Assessment for Continuing Education • personalized aerobics for cardiovascular enhancement • promoting aphasics' communicative effectiveness • pulmonary angiotensin I converting enzyme

PaCO$_2$, Pa$_{CO2}$ partial pressure of carbon dioxide in arterial gas

PACP pulmonary artery counterpulsation

PACS picture archiving and communications

PACT precordial acceleration tracing

PAC–V Platinol (cisplatin), Adriamycin (doxorubicin), and cyclophosphamide *also* PAC

PACU postanesthesia care unit

PAD per adjusted discharge • percutaneous abscess drainage • phenacetin, aspirin, and desoxyephedrine • phonologic-acquisition device • photon absorption densitometry • pre–aid to the disabled • primary affective disorder • psychoaffective disorder • pulmonary artery diastolic *also* PAd • pulsatile assist device

PAd pulmonary artery diastolic *also* PAD

PADDS photon–activated drug delivery system

PADP pulmonary artery diastolic pressure

PAE postanoxic encephalopathy • postantibiotic effect • progressive assistive exercise

p ae [L. *partes aequales*] equal parts

paed paediatrics/paediatric *also* PD, PED, ped, Peds

PAEDP pulmonary artery end–diastolic pressure

PAF paroxysmal atrial fibrillation *also* PAFIB • paroxysmal auricular fibrillation • phosphodi-esterase–activating factor • platelet–activating factor • platelet–aggregating factor *also* PAgF • platelet aggregation factor • pollen adherence factor • premenstrual assessment form • pseudoamniotic fluid • pulmonary arteriovenous fistula

PA&F percussion, ausculation, and fremitus

PAF–A platelet–activating factor of anaphylaxis

PAFD pulmonary artery filling defect

PAFG picric acid formaldehyde–glutaraldehyde

PAFI platelet–aggregation factor inhibitor

PAFIB paroxysmal atrial fibrillation *also* PAF

PAFP pre–Achilles fat pad

PAG periaqueductal gray (matter) • phenylacetylglutamine • polyacrylamide gel • pregnancy–associated globulin

pAg protein A–gold (technique)

PAGE polyacrylamide gel electrophoresis

PAgF platelet–aggregating factor

PAGG pentaacetylglucopyranosyl guanine

PAGIF polyacrylamide gel isoelectric focusing

PAGMK primary African green monkey kidney

PAH *para*–aminohippurate · phenylalamine hydroxylase · phenylalanine hydroxylase · polycyclic aromatic hydrocarbon · pulmonary artery hypertension · pulmonary artery hypotension

PAHA *para*–aminohippuric acid

PAHVC pulmonary alveolar hypoxic vasoconstriction

PAI Pair Attraction Inventory · plasminogen activator inhibitor · platelet accumulation index

PAIDS pediatric acquired immunodeficiency syndrome

PAIgG platelet–associated immunoglobulin G

PAIR Personal Assessment of Intimacy in Relationships

PAIS Psychosocial Adjustment to Illness Scale

PAIVS pulmonary atresia with intact ventricular septum

PAJ paralysis agitans juvenilis

PAL pathology laboratory · phenylalanine ammonia lyase · posterior axillary line · product (of) activated lymphocyte · pyogenic abscess (of) liver

pal. palate

PA&Lat posteroanterior and lateral

PALN para–aortic lymph node

palp palpable · palpate · palpation · palpitation *also* palpi

palpi palpitation *also* palp

PALS Paired Associate Learning Subtest · pediatric advanced life support · periarteriolar lymphocyte sheath · prison–acquired lymphoproliferative syndrome

PA–LS–ID pernicious anemia– like syndrome (and) immunoglobulin deficiency

PALST Picture Articulation and Language Screening Test

Palv alveolar pressure

PAM crystalline penicillin G in 2% aluminum monostearate · pancreatic acinor mass · penicillin aluminum monostearate · phenylalanine mustard · postauricular myogenic · potential acuity meter · pralidoxime · primary amebic meningoencephalitis · pulmonary alveolar macrophage · pulmonary alveolar microlithiasis · pyridine aldoxime methiodide

PAMC pterygoarthro- myodysplasia congenital

PAME primary amebic meningoencephalitis

PAMP pulmonary artery mean pressure

PAN periarteritis nodosa *also* PN · periodic alternating nystagmus • peroxyacetyl nitrate • polyacrilonitryl • polyarteritis nodosa *also* PN • positional alcohol nystagmus • puromycin aminonucleoside *also* PANS

pan. pancreas • pancreatectomy • pancreatic

PAND primary adrenocortical nodular dysplasia

PANESS physical and neurologic examination (for) soft signs

PANS puromycin aminonucleoside *also* PAN

PAO peak acid output • peripheral airway obstruction • plasma amine oxidase • polyamine oxidase

PaO$_2$ partial pressure of arterial oxygen

PAO$_2$ partial pressure of oxygen in alvedi

PAO$_2$—PaO$_2$ alveolar–arterial difference in partial pressure of oxygen

PAo pulmonary artery occlusion (pressure)

Pao ascending aortic pressure

P$_{ao}$ airway opening pressure

PAOD peripheral arterial occlusive disease • peripheral arteriosclerotic occlusive disease

PAOI peak acid output insulin-induced

PAOP pulmonary artery occlusion pressure

PAOx phenylacetone oxime

PAP Papanicolaou (smear, test) *also* Pap • papaverine • *para–*aminophenol • passive aggressive personality • Patient Assessment Program • peak airway pressure • peroxidase antibody (to) peroxidase • peroxidase–antiperoxidase (technique) • placental acid phosphatase • placental alkaline phosphatase • positive airway pressure • primary atypical pneumonia • prostatic acid phosphatase • pulmonary alveolar proteinosis • pulmonary arterial pressure *also* Ppa • purified alternate pathway

Pap Papanicolaou (smear, test) *also* PAP • papillary

pap. papilla

PAPF platelet adhesiveness plasma factor

Pap in. canthus papilloma, inner canthus

papova papilloma–polyoma–vacuolating agent (virus)

PAPP Pappenheimer bodies • pregnancy–associated plasma protein

PAPPC pregnancy–associated plasma protein C

PA/PS pulmonary atresia/pulmonary stenosis

Paps papillomas

Pap sm Papanicolaou smear

PAPUFA physiologically active polyunsaturated fatty acid

Pa–Pv pulmonary arterial pressure–pulmonary venous pressure

PAPVC partial anomalous pulmonary venous connection

PAPVR partial anomalous pulmonary venous return

PAPW posterior aspect (of the) pharyngeal wall

PAQ Personal Attributes Questionnaire • Position Analysis Questionnaire (job analysis)

PAR paraffin • parallel *also* par. • passive avoidance reaction • perennial allergic rhinitis • photosynthetically active radiation • physiologic aging rate • platelet aggregate ratio • positive attention received • postanesthesia recovery (room) *also* PARR • probable allergic rhinitis • problem–analysis report • Program for Alcohol Recovery • proximal alveolar region • pulmonary arteriolar resistance

PAr polyarteritis

Par paranoid

par. paraffin • parallel *also* PAR • paralysis

Para, para paraplegic • parous (having borne one or more children)

para number of pregnancies producing viable offspring • paraparesis • paraplegia/paraplegic *also* Para • parathyroid *also* PT,

PTH • parathyroidectomy • woman who has given birth

para 0 nullipara (no child borne)

para I unipara (having borne one child)

para II bipara (having borne two children)

para III tripara (having borne three children)

para IV quadripara (having borne four children)

I–para primipara (first pregnancy) *also* P, primip

II–para secundipara (second pregnancy)

III–para tertipara (third pregnancy)

para C, para c paracervical

par. aff [L. *pars affecta*] to the part affected

para L paralumbar

parapsych parapsychology

parasit parasite/parasitic • parasitology

parasym parasympathetic (division of antonomic nervous system) *also* PS

para T parathoracic

PARD platelet aggregation (as a) risk (of) diabetes

parent. parenteral/parenterally

PARH plasminogen activator–releasing hormone

parox paroxysm/paroxysmal

PARR postanesthesia recovery room *also* PAR

PARS Personal Adjustment and Role Skills (Scale)

PaRS pararectal space

part. [L. *partis*] of a part • [L. *partim*] partly • parturition

part. aeq [L. *partes aequales*] equal parts

part. dolent [L. *partes dolentes*] painful parts

part. vic [L. *partitis vicibus*] in divided doses

PARU postanesthetic recovery unit

parv [L. *parvus*] small

PAS *para*–aminosalicylate • Parent Attitude Scale • patient appointments (and) scheduling • periodic acid–Schiff (stain) • peripheral anterior synechia • persistent atrial standstill • personality assessment system • phosphatase acid serum • photoacoustic spectroscopy • Physician's Activity Study • pneumatic antiembolic stocking • postanesthesia score • posterior airway space • preadmission screening • pregnancy advisory service • premature atrial stimulus • premature auricular systole • Professional Activities Study • progressive accumulated stress • pseudoachievement syndrome • pulmonary arterial stenosis • pulmonary artery systolic

Pas pascal (unit of pressure)

Pa·s pascal–second

Pa x s pascal per second

PASA *para*–aminosalicylic acid

PaSat saturation of oxygen in arterial blood

PAS–C *para*–aminosalicylic acid crystallized (with ascorbic acid)

PASD after diastase digestion

P'ase alkaline phosphatase

Pas Ex passive exercise

PASG pneumatic antishock garment

PASH periodic acid–Schiff hematoxylin

PASI psoriasis area sensitivity index

PASM periodic acid–silver methenamine

PAS/MAP Professional Activities Study Medical Audit Program (medical records)

PASP pulmonary artery systolic pressure

pass. [L. *passim*] here and there • passive

PAST periodic acid–Schiff technique

PASVR pulmonary anomalous superior venous return

PAT Pain Apperception Test • paroxysmal atrial tachycardia • paroxysmal auricular tachycardia • patella • patient • percentage of acceleration time • Photo Articulation Test (psychology) • physical abilities test •

picric acid turbidity •
platelet aggregation test •
polyamine acetyltrans-
ferase • preadmission
(screening and) assessment
team • preadmission
testing • Predictive Ability
Test (psychology) •
pregnancy at term • prism
adaptation test •
psychoacoustic testing •
pulmonary artery trunk

pat. patella • patent •
paternal origin

PATCO prednisone, araC,
thioguanine,
cyclophosphamide, and
Oncovin (vincristine)

PATE psychodynamic and
therapeutic education •
pulmonary artery
thromboembolism •
pulmonary artery
thromboendarterectomy

PATH Partnership Approach to
Health • pathology/
pathologic • pituitary
adrenotropic hormone

path. pathogen/pathogenesis/
pathogenic • pathology/
pathologic/pathologist

path. fx pathologic fracture

PATLC Progressive
Achievement Tests of
Listening Comprehension

pat. med patent medicine

PA–T–SP periodic acid–
thiocarbohydrazide–silver
proteinate

pat. T patellar tenderness

PAT/TM patient's time

p aur [L. *post aurem*] behind
the ear

PAV partial atrioventricular •
Pavulon (pancuronium
bromide) • poikiloderma
atrophicans vasculare •
posterior arch vein

Pa Va Ex passive vascular (or
venoarterial) exercise (a
negative pressure)

PAVe procarbazine, Alkeran
(melphalan), and Velban
(vinblastine sulfate)

PA–VF pulmonary
arteriovenous fistula

PAVM pulmonary
arteriovenous malformation

PAVN paraventricular nucleus

PAW peak airway pressure •
peripheral airways •
pulmonary artery wedge

Paw mean airway pressure

Pawo pressure at airway
opening

PAWP pulmonary arterial
wedge pressure

PB [*Pharmacopoeia Britannica*]
British Pharmacopeia *also*
BP • pancreaticobiliary •
paraffin bath • Paul–Bunnell
(antibodies, test) •
pentobarbital • perineal
body • periodic breathing •
peripheral blood •
phenobarbital • phonetically
balanced (word lists) • pinch
biopsy • pinealoblastoma •
piperonyl butoxide •
polymyxin B • posterior
baffle • powder bed •
powder board • power
building • premature beat •
pressure balanced • pressure
breathing • protein
binding • protein bound •

Pudendal block • punch biopsy

PB% phonetically balanced percentage (of word lists)

P&B pain and burning • phenobarbital and belladonna

PB barometric pressure

Pb [L. *plumbum*] lead • phenobarbital • presbyopia • probenecid

PBA percutaneous bladder aspiration • polyclonal B-cell activity • pressure breathing assister • prolactin–binding assay • prune belly anomaly • pulpobuccoaxial

P$_{BA}$ brachial arterial pressure

PBB polybromated biphenyl(s)

Pb–B lead level in blood

PBC peripheral blood cell • point of basal convergence • prebed care • pregnancy and birth complications • primary biliary cirrhosis • progestin–binding complement

PBD percutaneous biliary drainage • postburn day

PBE partial breech extraction • [Ger. *Perlsucht Bacillenemulsion*] tuberculin from *Mycobacterium tuberculosis bovis*

PBF peripheral blood flow • phosphate–buffered formalin • placental blood flow • pulmonary blood flow *also* Qp

PB–Fe protein–bound iron

PBG Penassay broth plus glucose • porphobilinogen

PBGM Penassay broth plus glucose plus menadione

PGG–Q porphobilinogen—quantitative

PBG–S porphobilinogen synthase

PBI parental bonding instrument • partial bony impaction • penile–brachial index • phenformin • protein–bound iodine

PbI lead intoxication

PBK phosphorylase *b* kinase • pseudophakic bullous keratopathy

PBL peripheral blood leukocyte • peripheral blood lymphocyte

PBLI premature birth, live infant

PBLT peripheral blood lymphocyte transformation

PBM peripheral basement membrane • peripheral blood mononuclear (cell) *also* PBMC

PBMC peripheral blood mononuclear cell *also* PBM

PBMV pulmonary blood mixing volume

PBN paralytic brachial neuritis • peripheral benign neoplasm • polymyxin B sulfate, bacitracin, and neomycin

PBNA partial body neutron activation

PBO penicillin in beeswax and oil • placebo *also* P, PL

PbO lead monoxide

PBP peak blood pressure • penicillin–binding protein • porphyrin biosynthetic pathway • progressive bulbar palsy • prostate–binding protein • pseudobulbar palsy • purified *Brucella* protein

PBPI penile–brachial pulse index

PBQ phenylbenzoquinone • Preschool Behavior Questionnaire

PBRT phonetically balanced rhyme test

PBS peripheral–blood smear • phenobarbital sodium • phosphate–buffered saline • phosphate–buffered sodium • polybrominated salicylanilide • prune belly syndrome • pulmonary branch stenosis

PBSP prognostically bad signs (during) pregnancy

PBT Paul Bunnell test • phenacetin breath test • profile–based therapy

PBT₄ protein–bound thyroxine

PBV percutaneous balloon valvuloplasty • Platinol (cisplatin), bleomycin, and vinblastine • predicted blood volume • pulmonary blood volume

PBW posterior bite wing

PBZ phenoxybenzamine • phenylbutazone • Pyribenzamine (tripelennanine)

PC [L. *pondus civile*] avoirdupois weight • packed cells • palmitoyl carnitine • paper chromatography • parent cell • parent to child • particulate component • partition coefficient • pelvic cramp • penicillin • pentose cycle • peritoneal cell • pharmacology • phosphate cycle • phosphatidylcholine (lecithin) • phosphocreatine • phosphorylcholine • photoconductive • phrase construction • Physicians' Corporation • picryl chloride • picture completion • pill counter • piriform cortex • plasma concentration • plasma cortisol • plasmacytoma • platelet concentrate • platelet count • pneumotaxic center • polycentric • polyposis coli • poor condition • popliteal cyst • portacaval (shunt) • portal cirrhosis • postcoital • posterior cervical • posterior chamber • posterior column • posterior commissure • posterior cortex • precordial • prepiriform cortex • present complaint • primary cleavage • primary closure • printed circuit • procollagen • producing cell • productive cough • professional corporation • proliferative capacity • prostatic carcinoma • provisional cortex • proximal colon • pseudocyst • pubococcygeus (muscle) *also*

PCG • pulmonary capillary • pulmonic closure • Purkinje cell • pyloric canal • pyruvate carboxylase

P–C phlogistic corticoid

P&C prism and (alternative) cover–test (cross–over test, screen and cover test in ophthalmology)

Pc penicillin *also* PC

pc [L. *post cibum*] after a meal • parsec • percent • picocurie *also* pCi

pc1 platelet count pretransfusion

pc2 platelet count posttransfusion

PCA *para*–chloramphetamine • parietal cell antibody • passive cutaneous anaphylaxis • patient care assistant/aide • patient–controlled analgesia • perchloric acid • percutaneous carotid arteriogram • percutaneous coronary angioplasty • percutaneous coronary angioplasty • personal care attendant • phenylcarboxylic acid • photocontact allergic • plasma catecholamine concentration • portacaval anastomosis • postconceptional age • posterior cerebral artery • posterior communicating aneurysm • posterior communicating artery • posterior cricoarytenoid • precoronary care area • President's Council on

Aging • principal components analysis • procainamide • procoagulant activity • prostatic carcinoma • pyrrolidone carboxylic acid

PCAS Psychotherapy Competence Assessment Schedule

PCAVC persistent complete atrioventricular canal

PCB pancuronium bromide • paracervical block • polychlorinated biphenyl • portacaval bypass • prepared childbirth • procarbazine

Pcb, PcB (L. *punctum convergens basalis*) near point of convergence to intercentral baseline

PC–BMP phosphorylcholine–binding myeloma protein

PCC Pasteur Culture Collection • pheochromocytoma • phosphate carrier compound • plasma catecholamine concentration • Poison Control Center • precoronary care • premature chromosome condensation • primary care clinic • prothrombin–complex concentration

PCc periscopic concave

PCCC pediatric critical care center

PCCP percutaneous cord cyst puncture

PCCS parent–child communication schedule

PCCU post–coronary care unit

PCD papillary collecting duct • paroxysmal cerebral dysrhythmia • phosphate–citrate–dextrose • plasma cell dyscrasia • polycystic disease • posterior corneal deposits • postmortem cesarean delivery • primary ciliary dyskinesia • prolonged contractile duration • pulmonary clearance delay

PCDC plasma clot diffusion chamber

PCDF polychlorinated dibenzofuran

PCDUS plasma cell dyscrasia of unknown significance

PCE physical capacity evaluation • pseudo-cholinesterase *also* PCHE • pulmocutaneous exchange

PCF peripheral circulatory failure • pharyngocon-junctival fever • posterior cranial fossa • prothrombin conversion factor

pcf pound per cubic foot

PCFT platelet complement fixation test

PCG paracervical ganglion • phonocardiogram • Planning Career Goals (psychologic test) • pneumocardiogram • primate chorionic gonadotropin • pubococcygeus (muscle) *also* PC

PCGG percutaneous coagulation (of) gasserian ganglion

PCH paroxysmal cold hemoglobinuria • polycyclic hydrocarbon

PCHE pseudocholinesterase *also* PCE

PC&HS aftermeals and at bedtime

PCI pneumatosis cystoides intestinalis • posterior curve intermediate (cornea) • Premarital Communication Inventory • prophylactic cranial irradiation • prothrombin consumption index

pCi picocurie

PCIC Poison Control Information Center

PCIOL posterior chamber intraocular lens

PC–IRV pressure–controlled inverted ratio ventilation

PCIS Patient–Care Information System • post–cardiac injury syndrome

PCK polycystic kidney

PCKD polycystic kidney disease

PCL pacing cycle length • persistent corpus luteum • plasma cell leukemia • posterior chamber lens • posterior cruciate ligament

P closure plastic closure

PCM primary cutaneous melanoma • protein–calorie malnutrition • protein carboxymethylase • pulse code modulation

p–CMB *para*–chloromercuri-benzoate

PCMC Primary Children's Medical Center

PCMBSA *para*–chloromer-curibenzine sulfonic acid

PCMF perceptual cognitive motor function

PCMO Principal Clinical Medical Officer

PCMX chloroxylenol • *para*–chloro–*m*–xylenol

PCN penicillin *also* P, PEN, pen., PN, PNC • percutaneous nephrostomy • pregnenolone carbonitril • primary care network • primary care nursing

PCNA proliferating cell nuclear antigen

PCNB pentachloronitro-benzene

PCNV postchemotherapy nausea (and) vomiting

PCO patient complains of • polycystic ovary • predicted cardiac output • procytoxid

Pco, P$_{CO}$ carbon monoxide pressure or tension

Pco, P$_{CO2}$ partial pressure of carbon dioxide

PCoA posterior communicating artery

PCOD polycystic ovarian disease

PCom posterior communicating artery

PCOS polycystic ovary syndrome *also* POS

PCP parachlorophenate • patient care plan • pentachlorophenol • peripheral coronary pressure • persistent cough (and) phlegm • phencyclidine • pneumocystic pneumonia • *Pneumocystis carinii* pneumonia • primary care physician • prochlorperazine • procollagen peptide • psilocybin • pulmonary capillary pressure • pulse cytophotometry

PCPA *para*–chlorophenyl-alanine

PCPL pulmonary capillary protein leakage

pcpn precipitation *also* pcpt, precip

PCPS phosphatidylcholine–phosphatidylserine

pcpt perception • precipitate/precipitation *also* pcpn, precip

PCR patient contact record • phosphocreatine • plasma clearance rate • polymerase chain reaction • probable causal relationship • protein catabolic rate

PCr phosphocreatine

PCS palliative care service • Patient Care System • patterns of care study • pharmacogenic confusional syndrome • portable cervical spine • portacaval shunt • post–cardiac surgery • postcardiotomy syndrome • postchole-cystectomy syndrome • postconcussion syndrome • precordial stethoscope •

primary cancer site •
primary cesarian section •
Priority Counseling
Survey • proportional
counter spectrometry •
proximal coronary sinus •
pseudotumor cerebri
syndrome

Pcs, pcs preconscious

P c/s primary cesarian section

PCSM percutaneous stone
manipulation

PCT Physiognomic Cue Test
(psychology) • plasma
clotting time • plasmacrit
test (for syphilis) •
plasmacytoma • platelet
hematocrit •
polychlorinated triphenyl •
porcine calcitonin •
porphyria cutanea tarda •
portacaval transportation •
portacaval transposition •
positron computed
tomography • postcoital •
postcoital test • progestin
challenge test •
prothrombin consumption
time • proximal convoluted
tubule • pulmonary care
team

pct percent

PCTA percutaneous coronary
transluminal angioplasty

PCU pain control unit •
palliative care unit •
patient care unit • primary
care unit • progressive care
unit • protective care
unit • protein–calorie
undernutrition • pulmonary
care unit

p cut percutaneous

PCV packed cell volume •
parietal cell vagotomy •
polycythemia vera •
postcapillary venule •
premature ventricular
contraction

PCV–M polycythemia vera
(with myeloid) metaplasia

PCW pulmonary capillary
wedge (pressure) *also*
PCWP • purified cell walls

PCWP pulmonary capillary
wedge pressure *also* PCW

PCX paracervical

PCx periscopic convex

PCXR portable chest
radiograph • portable chest
x–ray

PCZ procarbazine •
prochlorperazine

PD [L. *per diem*] by the day •
Doctor of Pharmacy •
Paget disease • pancreatic
duct • papilla diameter •
paralyzing dose • Parkinson
disease • parkinsonian
dementia • paroxysmal
discharge • pars distalis
(pituitary) • patent
ductus • patient day •
patient demonstration •
pediatrics/pediatric *also*
paed, PED, ped, Peds •
percutaneous drain •
peritoneal dialysis •
personality disorder •
pharmacodynamics •
phenyldichlorarsine •
phosphate dehydrogenase •
photosensitivity
dermatitis • Pick disease •
plasma defect • poorly
differentiated • Porak–
Durante (syndrome) •

porphobilinogen deaminase • posterior division • postnasal drainage • postural drainage • potential difference • present disease • pressor dose • primary dendrite • prism diopter • problem drinker • progression (of) disease • protein degradation • protein deprived • protein diet • provocation dose • psychopathic deviate • psychotic dementia • psychotic depression • pulmonary disease *also* PUD, PuD • pulpodistal • pulse duration • (inter)pupillary distance • pyloric dilator

P(D+) probability of having disease

P(D–) probability of not having disease

P/D packs per day (cigarettes) *also* p/d, PPD

PD$_{50}$ median paralyzing dose

Pd palladium • pediatrics

pd [L. *per diem*] by the day • [L. *pro die*] for the day • papilla diameter • period

p/d packs per day (cigarettes) *also* P/D, PPD

PDA parenteral drug abuser • patent ductus arteriosus • patient distress alarm • pediatric allergy *also* PdA • posterior descending (coronary) artery • predialyzed human albumin • pulmonary disease anemia

PdA pediatric allergy *also* PDA

PDAB *para*–dimethylamino-benzaldehyde

PDB Paget disease of bone • *para*–dichlorobenzene *also* PDCB • phosphorus–dissolving bacteria • preventive dental (health) behavior

PDC pediatric cardiology • pentadecylcatechol • physical dependence capacity • plasma digoxin concentration • plasma disappearance curve • postdecapitation convulsion • preliminary diagnostic clinic • private diagnostic clinic • pyrindinol carbamate

PD&C postural drainage and clapping

PdC pediatric cardiology

PDCB *para*–dichlorobenzene *also* PDB

PDCD primary degenerative cerebral disease

PDD pervasive developmental disorder • platinum diamminodichloride (cisplatin) • primary degenerative dementia • pyridoxine–deficient diet

PDDB phenododecinium bromide

PDE paroxysmal dyspnea (on) exertion • phospho-diesterase • progressive dialysis encephalopathy • pulsed Doppler echocardiography

PdE pediatric endocrinology

PDF peritoneal dialysis fluid • probability density function

PDFC premature dead female child

PDG parkinsonism–dementia (complex of) Guam • phosphogluconate dehydrogenase • phosphate–dependent glutaminase

PDGA pteroyldiglutamic acid

PDGF platelet–derived growth factor

PDGXT predischarge graded exercise test

PDH past dental history • phosphate dehydrogenase • pyruvate dehydrogenase

PDHC pyruvate dehydrogenase complex

PdHO pediatric hematology–oncology

PDI periodontal disease index • plan–do integration • Psychomotor Development Index

Pdi transdiaphragmatic pressure

PDIE phosphodiesterase

P–diol pregnanediol

PDL periodontal ligament • poorly differentiated lymphocyte • population doubling level • primary dysfunctional labor • progressively diffused leukoencephalopathy

Pdl, pdl poundal (force of acceleration) • pudendal

PDLC poorly differentiated lung cancer

PDLD poorly differentiated lymphocytic–diffuse

PDLL poorly differentiated lymphocytic lymphoma

PDLN poorly differentiated (lymphocytic) lymphoma–nodular

PDLP predigested liquid protein

PDM polymyositis (and) dermatomyositis

PDMC premature dead male child

PDMEA phosphoryldimethyl-ethanolamine

PDMS Patient Data Management Systems • pharmacokinetic drug–monitoring service

PDN prednisone *also* P, PRED • private day nurse • private duty nurse

PdNEO pediatric neonatology

PdNEP pediatric nephrology

PDP pattern disruption point • piperidinopyrimidine • platelet–depleted plasma • primer–dependent deoxynucleic acid polymerase • Product Development Protocol

PD&P postural drainage and percussion

PDPD prolonged dwell peritoneal dialysis

PDPI primer–dependent deoxynucleic acid polymerase index

PDQ pretty damn quick (slang) • parental development questionnaire • Prescreening Development

Questionnaire • protocol data query

PDR pandevelopmental retardation • pediatric radiology • peripheral diabetic retinopathy • *Physician's Desk Reference* • pleiotropic drug resistance • postdelivery room • primary drug resistance • proliferative diabetic retinopathy

PdR pediatric radiology

pdr powder *also* powd, pwd

PDRB Permanent Disability Rating Board

PDRc̄VH proliferative diabetic retinopathy (with) vitreous hemorrhage

PDS pain–dysfunction syndrome • paroxysmal depolarizing shift • patient data system • pediatric surgery *also* PdS, PS • peritoneal dialysis system • predialyzed (human) serum • primary dependence study

PdS pediatric surgery *also* PDS, PS • psychiatric deviate, subtle

PDT phenyldimethyltriazine • photodynamic therapy • population doubling time

PDU pulsed Doppler ultrasonography

PDUF pulsed Doppler ultrasonic flowmeter

PDUR Predischarge Utilization Review

PDV peak diastolic velocity

PDW platelet distribution width

PDWHF platelet–derived wound healing factor

PE pancreatic extract • paper electrophoresis • parallel elastic (component of muscle) • partial epilepsy • Pel–Ebstein (disease) • pelvic examination • penile erection • pericardial effusion • peritoneal exudate • phakoemulsification • pharyngoesophageal • phenylephrine • phosphatidylethanolamine • photographic effect • phycoerythrin • physical education *also* PE, PED, PEd, Phys Ed • physical evaluation • physical examination *also* PX, Px • physical exercise • physiologic ecology • pigmented epithelium • plasma exchange • plating efficiency • Platinol (cisplatin) and etoposide • pleural effusion • point of entry • polyethylene • polynuclear eosinophil • potential energy • powdered extract • pre–eclampsia • pre–excitation • present examination • pressure equalization • prior to exposure • probable error • probe excision • protein excretion • pulmonary edema • pulmonary embolism • pyramidal eminence • pyroelectric • pyrogenic exotoxin

PE, P$_E$ expiratory pressure

Pe Peclet number •

perylene • pregnenolone •
pressure (on) expiration

pe [L. *per exemplum*] for
example

PE2 secondary plating
efficiency

PEA pelvic examination
(under) anesthesia •
phenylethel alcohol (agar) •
phenylethyl alcohol •
phenylethylamine •
polysaccharide egg antigen

PE↓A pelvic examination
under anesthesia

PEACH Preschool Evaluation
and Assessment for
Children with Handicaps

PEAO phenylethylamine
oxidase

PEAQ Personal Experience
and Attitude Questionnaire

PEARLA pupils equal and
react to light and
accommodation

PEB Platinol (cisplatin),
etoposide, and bleomycin

PEBG phenethylbiguanide

PEC parallel elastic
component • patient
evaluation center •
peduncle (of) cerebrum •
peritoneal exudate cell •
pulmonary ejection click •
pyrogenic exotoxin C

PECHO, Pecho prostatic
echogram

PECO₂ mixed expired carbon
dioxide tension

PECT positron emission
computed tomography

PED pediatrics *also* paed, PD,
ped, Peds • peduncle
(cerebral) • pharyngo-
esophageal diverticulum •
pollution (and)
environmental degradation •
postentry day •
postexertional dyspnea

PEd, P Ed physical education
also PE, Phys Ed

ped pedangle • pedestrian •
pediatrics *also* paed, PED

ped ed pedal edema

PEDG phenylethyldiguanide

PED/MVA pedestrian hit by
motor vehicle

PeDS Pediatric Drug
Surveillance

Peds pediatrics

PEE parallel elastic element

PEEP peak end–expiratory
pressure • positive end–
expiratory pressure

PEER Pediatric Examination
of Educational Readiness

PEF peak expiratory flow •
pharyngoepiglottic fold •
Psychiatric Evaluation
Form • pulmonary edema
fluid

PEFR peak expiratory flow
rate

PEFSR partial expiratory
flow–static recoil (curve)

PEFT peak expiratory flow
time

PEFV partial expiratory flow
volume

PEG Patient Evaluation Grid •
percutaneous endoscopic

gastrostomy ·
pneumoencephalogram/
pneumonencephalography ·
polyethylene glycol

PEG–ELS polyethylene glycol
(and iso–osmolar)
electrolyte solution

PEI phosphate excretion
index · phosphorus
excretion index · physical
efficiency index

PEJ percutaneous endoscopic
jejunostomy

PEL peritoneal exudate
lymphocyte · permissible
exposure limit

Pel elastic recoil pressure of
lung

PELISA paper enzyme–linked
immunosorbent assay

PEM peritoneal exudate
macrophage · precordial
electrocardiographic
mapping · prescription
event monitoring · primary
enrichment medium ·
probable error (of)
measurement · protein
energy malnutrition ·
pulmonary endothelial
membrane

PEMA phenylethylmalonamide

PEMF pulsating
electromagnetic field

PEMS physical, emotional,
mental, and safety

PEN parenteral (and) enteral
nutrition

Pen, pen. penicillin *also* P,
PCN, PN, PNC

pen. penetrating

PENG photoelectric
nystagmography

PENS percutaneous epidural
nerve stimulator

Pent pentothal

PEO progressive external
ophthalmoplegia

PEP peptidase · performance
evaluation procedure ·
phosphoenolpyruvate ·
polyestradiol phosphate ·
positive expiratory
pressure · postencephalitic
parkinsonism · pre–
ejection period · protein
electrophoresis ·
Psychiatric Evaluation
Profile

Pep peptidase

PEPA peptidase A · protected
environment (units and)
prophylactic antibiotics

PEPC peptidase C

PEPc corrected pre–ejection
period

PEPCK, PEPK phosphoenolpyruvate carboxykinase

PEPD peptidase D

PEPI pre–ejection period index

PEP/LVET pre–ejection
period/left ventricular
ejection time

PEPP positive expiratory
pressure plateau

PEPR precision encoder (and)
pattern recognizer

PEPS peptidase S

PER peak ejection rate ·
pediatric emergency room ·
periodic evaluation record ·

protein efficiency ratio • pudendal evoked response

per perineal • periodic • periodicity • person • [L. *per*] through, by

per bid. [L. *per bidum*] for a period of two days

PERC perceptual • percutaneous • potential erythropoietin–responsive cell

percus, PERCUSS percussion

PERD photoelectric registration device

PERF peak expiratory flow rate

perf perfect • perforation *also* P

PERI peritoneal fluid • Psychiatric Epidemiology Research Interview

perl perineal

periap periapical

perim perimeter

Perio periodontics

PERK prospective evaluation (of) radial keratomy

PERL pupils equal (and) react (to) light

PERLA pupils equal (and) react (to) light (and) accommodation

perm permanent • permutation

per op emet [L. *peracta operatione emetici*] when action of emetic is over

perp perpendicular

Per pad perineal pad

PERR pattern evoked retinal response

PERRLA pupils equal, round, react (to) light (and) accommodation

PERS patient evaluation rating scale

pers personal

PERT program evaluation and review technique

PES photoelectron spectroscopy • postextrasystolic • pre–epiglottic space • pre–excitation syndrome • programmed electrical stimulation • pseudo-exfoliation syndrome

PESP postextrasystolic potentiation

pe SPL peak equivalent sound pressure level

Pess pessary

PEST point estimation (by) sequential testing

PET parent effectiveness training • peak ejection time • pear–shaped extension tube • poly-ethylene tube • poor exercise tolerance • positron emission tomography • pre–eclamptic toxemia • pressure equalizing tube • progressive exercise test • Psychiatric Emergency Team

PETA pentaerythritol triacrylate

PETH pink–eyed, tan–hooded (rat)

PETN pentaerythritol tetranitrate

petr petroleum

PETT pendular eye–tracking test • positron emission transverse/transaxial tomography

PEU plasma equivalent unit • polyether urethane

PEV pulmonary extravascular (fluid) volume

PeV, PV peripheral vein

pev, peV peak electron volt

PEVN periventricular nucleus

PEWV pulmonary extravascular water volume

PEx physical examination

PF parafasicular (nucleus) • parallel fiber • parotid fluid • partially follicular • patellofemoral (joint) • peak flow • pericardial fluid • peripheral field • peritoneal fluid • permeability factor • personality factor • phenol formaldehyde • physicians' forum • picture–frustration (study, test) *also* P–F • plantar flexion • plasma factor • plasma fibronectin • platelet factor • pleural fluid • power factor • precursor fluid • preservative free • proflavin • prostatic fluid • protection factor • pterygoid fossa • pulmonary factor • pulmonary function • Purkinje fiber • purpura fulminans • push fluids

P–F picture–frustration (study, test) *also* PF

P/F pass/fail (system)

PF$_{1-4}$ platelet factors 1 through 4

pF picofarad

PFA phosphonoformatic acid • profunda femoris artery

PFAGH penalty, frustration, anxiety, guilt, hostility

PFAS performic acid–Schiff (reaction)

PFB properdin factor B • pseudofolliculitis barbae

PFC pelvic flexion contracture • perfluorocarbon • pericardial fluid culture • persistent fetal circulation • plaque–forming cell

pFc noncovalently bonded dimer of C–terminal immunoglobulin of Fc fragment

PFCPH persistent fetal circulation (with) pulmonary hypertension

PFD polyostotic fibrous dysplasia • primary flash distillate

PFEAAC posterior fossa extra–axial arachnoid cyst

PFFD proximal femur focal deficiency

PFFFP Pall–filtered fresh–frozen plasma

PFG peak–flow gauge

PFIB perfluoroisobutylene

PFJS patellofemoral joint syndrome

PFK phosphofructoaldolase • phosphofructokinase

PFKL phosphofructokinase, liver (type)

PFKM phosphofructokinase, muscle (type)

PFKP phosphofructokinase, platelet (type)

PFL profibrinolysin

PFM peak flow meter • porcelain fused (to) metal

PFN partially functional neutrophil

PFO patent foramen ovale

PFP pentafluoropropionyl • platelet–free plasma • preceding foreperiod

PFPC Pall–filtered packed cells

PFQ personality factor questionnaire

PFR parotid flow rate • peak filling rate • peak flow rate • pericardial friction rub

PFRC plasma–free red cell • predicted functional residual capacity

PFS penile flow study • primary fibromyalgia syndrome • protein–free supernatant • pulmonary function score

PFST positional feedback stimulation trainer

PFT pancreatic function test • posterior fossa tumor • prednisone, fluorouracil, and tamoxifen • pulmonary function test

PFT$_4$ proportion free thyroxin

PFTBE progressive form of tick–borne encephalitis

PFU plaque–forming unit • pock–forming unit

PFUO prolonged fever (of) unknown origin

PFV physiologic full value

PFW peak flow whistle

PFWB Pall–filtered whole blood

PG parapsoriasis guttata • paregoric • parotid gland • pentagastrin • pepsinogen • peptidoglycan • pergolide • *Pharmacopoeia Germanica* also PhG • phosphate glutamate • phosphatidyl-glycerol • phosphatidyl glycine • phosphoglu-conate • phosphoglycerate • pigment granule • pituitary gonadotropin • plasma gastrin • plasma glucose • plasma triglyceride • polygalacturonate • postgraduate • postgraft • pregnanediol glucuronide • pregnant • propylene glycol • prostaglandin • proteoglycan • pyoderma gangrenosum

P$_G$ plasma glucose

Pg gastric pressure • nasopharyngeal electrode placement in electroencephalography • pogonion • pregnancy • pregnant • pregnenolone

pg page • picogram

PGA phosphoglyceric acid • polyglandular autoimmune (syndrome) • polyglycolic acid • prostaglandin A • pteroylglutamic acid

PGAC phenylglycine acid chloride

PGAS persisting galactorrhea–amenorrhea syndrome

PGB prostaglandin B

PGC percentage (of) goblet cells • primordial germ cell • prostaglandin C

PGD phosphogluconate dehydrogenase • phosphoglyceraldehyde dehydrogenase • prostaglandin D

PGDH phosphogluconate dehydrogenase

PGDR plasma glucose disappearance rate

PGE platelet granule extract • posterior gastroenterostomy • primary generalized epilepsy • prostaglandin E

PGEM prostaglandin E metabolite

PGF paternal grandfather *also* pgf • prostaglandin F

pgf paternal grandfather *also* PGF

PGG polyclonal gamma globulin • prostaglandin G

PGH pituitary growth hormone • plasma growth hormone • porcine growth hormone • prostaglandin H

PGI pepsinogen I • phosphoglucose isomerase • potassium, glucose, and insulin • prostaglandin I

PGK phosphoglycerate kinase • phosphoglycerokinase

PGL persistent generalized lymphadenopathy • phosphoglycolipid

PGlyM phosphoglyceromutase

PGM paternal grandmother *also* pgm • phosphoglucomutase

pgm paternal grandmother *also* PGM

PGMA polyglycerol methacrylate

PGN proliferative glomerulonephritis

PGO pontogeniculo–occipital (spike)

PGP postgamma proteinuria • prepaid group practice

PGR progesterone receptor *also* PgR • psychogalvanic response

PgR progesterone receptor *also* PGR

P–GRN prograrnnlocyte

PGS pineal gonadal syndrome • plant growth substance • prostaglandin synthetase • proteoglycan subunit

PGSR psychogalvanic skin response

PGT playgroup therapy

PGTR plasma glucose tolerance rate

PGTT prednisolone glucose tolerance test

PGU peripheral glucose uptake • postgonococcal urethritis

PGUT phosphogalactose uridyl transferase

PGV proximal gastric vagotomy

PGX prostaglandin X

PGY postgraduate year

PGYE peptone, glucose, and yeast extract (medium)

PH parathyroid hormone *also* PTH • partial hepatectomy • passive hemagglutination • past history *also* Px • peliosis hepatitis • perianal herpes • persistent hepatitis • personal history • pharmacopeia • phenethicillin • phenylalanine hydroxylase • pinhole • polycythemia hypertonica • poor health • porphyria hepatica • posterior hypothalamus • post history • previous history • primary hyperparathyroidism • prolyl hydroxylase • prostatic hypertrophy • pseudohermaphroditism • pubic hair • public health • pulmonary hypertension • punctate hemorrhage

Ph pharmacopeia • phenanthrene • phenyl • phosphate

pH hydrogen ion concentration

Ph¹ Philadelphia chromosome

pH₁ isoelectric point

ph phase • phial • phote (unit of surface illumination)

PHA passive hemagglutination • peripheral hyperalimentation • phenylalanine *also* P, PA, PHE, Phe • phytohemagglutinin activation • phytohemagglutinin antigen • pseudohypoaldosteronism • pulse–height analyzer

pH_A arterial blood hydrogen tension

pHa arterial pH

PHAL phytohemagglutinin–stimulated lymphocyte

PHAlb polymerized human albumin

PHA–m phytohemagglutinin–mucopolysaccharide (fraction)

PHA–P phytohemagglutinin–protein (fraction)

PHAR, phar pharmaceutical • pharmacopeia • pharmacy • pharynx

Phar G Graduate in Pharmacy

PHARM pharmacy *also* pharm

pharm pharmacopeia • pharmacy *also* PHARM

Pharm D [L. *Pharmaciae Doctor*] Doctor of Pharmacy *also* PhD

PHB preventive health behavior

PHBB propylhydroxybenzyl benzimidazole

PHC personal health cost • posthospital care • premolar aplasia, hyperhidrosis, and (premature) canities • premolar hypodontia, hyperhidrosis, and canities prematura (Böök syndrome) • primary health care • primary hepatic carcinoma • primary hepatocellular carcinoma • proliferative helper cell

PhC pharmaceutical chemist

PHCC primary hepatocellular carcinoma

PHD photoelectron diffraction • pulmonary heart disease

PhD [L. *Pharmaciae Doctor*] Doctor of Pharmacy *also* Pharm D • [L. *Philosophiae Doctor*] Doctor of Philosophy

PHDD personal history (of) depressive disorders

PHDPE porous high–density polyethylene

PHE periodic health examination • phenylalanine *also* P, PA, PHA, Phe • postheparin esterase • proliferative hemorrhagic enteropathy

Phe phenylalanine *also* P, PA, PHA, PHE

PhEEM photoemission electron microscopy

Phen phenformin

Pheo, pheo pheochromo-cytoma

PHF paired helical filaments • personal hygiene facility

PHFG primary human fetal glia

PhG Graduate in Pharmacy • *Pharmacopoeia Germanica* *also* PG

Phgly, phgly phenylglycine

PHH posthemorrhagic hydrocephalus

PHI passive hemagglutination inhibition • peptide histidine isoleucine • phosphohexose isomerase • physiologic hyaluronidase inhibitor • prehospital index

PhI *Pharmacopoeia Internationalis also* PI

phi (Φ, φ) twenty–first letter of Greek alphabet

φ ability continuum • magnetic flux • osmotic coefficient • phi coefficient (statistics)

PHIM posthypoxic intention myoclonus

PHIS post–head injury syndrome

PHK platelet phosphohexokinase • postmortem human kidney

PHKC postmortem human kidney cell

PHLA postheparin lipolytic activity

PHLS Public Health Laboratory Service

PHM psyllium hydrophilic mucilloid

PhM pharyngeal musculature

PHN paroxysmal noctural hemoglobinuria • passive Heymann nephritis • postherpetic neuralgia • public health nursing/nurse

PhNCS phenyl isothiocyanate

PHO public health official

PH₂O partial pressure of water vapor

phos phosphatase • phosphate • phosphorus *also* PHP

PHP passive hyperpolarizing potential • persistent hyperphenylalaninemia • phosphorus *also* phos • postheparin phospholipase •

prehospital program •
prepaid health plan •
primary
hyperparathyroidism •
pseudohypoparathyroidism

PHPP, *p*–HPPO *p*–hydroxyphenyl pyruvate oxidase

pHPT primary
hyperparathyroidism

PHPV persistent hyperplastic
primary vitreous

PHR peak heart rate •
photoreactivity

PHRT procarbazine,
hydroxyurea, and
radiotherapy (protocol)

PHS partial hospitalization
program • patient–heated
serum • phenylalanine
hydroxylase stimulator •
pooled human serum •
posthypnotic suggestion •
Public Health Service

PHSC pluripotent hemopoietic
stem cell

pH–stat apparatus for
maintaining pH of solution

PHT peroxide hemolysis test •
phentolamine • phenytoin •
portal hypertension •
primary hyperthyroidism •
pulmonary hypertension

PhTD Doctor of Physical
Therapy

PHTN portal hypertension

PHV persistent hypertrophic
vitreous

PHx past history

Phx pharynx

PHY pharyngitis • physical •
physiology *also* P, PHYS

PHY, phy phytohemagglutinin

PHYS physiology *also* P, PHY

PhyS physiologic saline
(solution)

phys physical • physician

phys dis physical disability

Phys Ed physical education
also PE, PED, PEd

physio physiologic •
physiotherapy

Physiol physiology

Phys Med physical medicine

Phys Ther physical therapy
also PT

PI international protocol •
isoelectric point • pacing
impulse • package insert •
pancreatic insufficiency •
parainfluenza (virus) • pars
intermedia • paternity
index • patient's interest •
performance index •
performance intensity •
perinatal injury •
periodontal index •
peripheral iridectomy •
permanent incidence •
permeability index •
personal injury •
personality inventory •
phagocytic index •
*Pharmacopoeia
Internationalis also* PhI •
phosphatidylinositol •
physically impaired •
pineal body • plaque
index • pneumatosis
intestinalis • poison ivy •
ponderal index • postictal
immobility • postinfection •
postinjury • postinocula-
tion • preinduction
(examination) • premature

infant • prematurity index • preparatory interval • present illness • pressure (on) inspiration • primary infarction • primary infection • proactive inhibition • proactive interference • programmed instruction • proinsulin • prolactin inhibitor • protamine insulin • protease inhibitor • proximal intestine • pulmonary incompetence • pulmonary infarction

P_i inorganic phosphate *also* Pi

PI inorganic phosphate *also* P_i • parental generation • pressure in inspiration • protease inhibitor

pI isoelectric point • platelet count increment *also* pi

pi platelet count increment *also* pI

pi (Π, π) sixteenth letter of Greek alphabet

Π product of a sequence (math)

π ratio of circumference to diameter (3.1415926536)

PIA peripheral interface adapter • phenylisopropyl-adenosine • photoelectronic intravenous angiography • plasma insulin activity • porcine intestinal adenoma-tosis • preinfarction angina

PIAT Peabody Individual Achievement Test

PIB psi–interactive biomolecules

PIC peripherally inserted

catheter • Personality Inventory for Children • postinflammatory corticoid • postintercourse

PICA Porch Index of Communicative Ability • posterior inferior cerebellar artery • posterior inferior communicating artery

PICC peripherally inserted central catheter

PICD primary irritant contact dermatitis

PICU pediatric intensive care unit • pulmonary intensive care unit

PID pain intensity difference (score) • pelvic inflammatory disease • photoionization detector • plasma iron disappearance • prolapsed intervertebral disk • proportional–integral–derivative • protruded intervertebral disk

PIDRA portable insulin dosage–regulating apparatus

PIDT plasma iron disappearance time

PIE postinfectious encephalomyelitis • preimplantation embryo • prosthetic infectious endocarditis • pulmonary infiltration with eosinophilia • pulmonary interstitial edema • pulmonary interstitial emphysema

PIEF isoelectric focusing in polyarylamide

PIF peak inspiratory flow • pigment inspiratory factor •

point of identical flow • premorbid inferiority feeling • proinsulin–free • prolactin–inhibiting factor • proliferation–inhibiting factor • prostatic interstitial fluid

PIFG poor intrauterine fetal growth

PIFR peak inspiratory flow rate

PIFT platelet immuno-fluorescence test

PIG pertussis immune globulin

PIg pigmentation

PIGI pregnancy–induced glucose intolerance

pigm pigment/pigmented

PIGPA pyruvate, inosine, glucose phosphate, adenine

PIH pregnancy–induced hypertension • prolactin–inhibiting hormone

PIHH postinfluenza–like hyposmia and hypogeusia

PII plasma inorganic iodine • primary irritation index

pil [L. *pilula*] pill

PIIP portable insulin infusion pump

PIIS posterior inferior iliac spine

PIM penicillamine–induced myasthenia

PIMS programmable implantable medication system

PIN personal identification number

PINN proposed international nonproprietary name

PINS person in need of supervision

PINV postimperative negative variation

PIO progesterone in oil

PIO₂ inspired oxygen tension • intra–alveolar oxygen tension • partial pressure of inspiratory oxygen

PIOK poikilocytosis

PIP paralytic infantile paralysis • peak inflation pressure • peak inspiratory pressure • personal injury protection • piperacillin • postinflammatory polyposis • postinfusion phlebitis • postinspiratory pressure • proximal interphalangeal (joint) • Psychotic Inpatient Profile

PIPA platelet ^{125}I–labeled (staphylococcal) protein A

PI–PB performance versus intensity function for phonetically balanced words

PIPIDA paraisoprophyimino-diacetic acid (scan)

PIPJ proximal interphalangeal joint

PIQ Performance Intelligence Quotient

PIR piriform • postinhibition rebound

P–IRI plasma immunoreactive insulin

PIRS plasma immunoreactive secretion

PIS primary immunodeficiency syndrome • Provisional International Standard

pls isoelectric point

PISA phase–invariant signature algorithm

PISCES percutaneously inserted spinal cord electrical stimulation

PIT pacing–induced tachycardia • perceived illness threat • picture identification test • plasma iron turnover

PIt patellar inhibition test

pit. pituitary

PITC phenylisothiocyanate

PITP pseudoidiopathic thrombocytopenic purpura

PITR plasma iron turnover rate

PITS parent–infant traumatic stress

PIU polymerase–inducing unit

PIV parainfluenza virus • peripheral intravenous

PIVD protruded intervertebral disk

PIVH peripheral intravenous hyperalimentation

PIVKA protein in vitamin K absence

PIWT partially impacted wisdom teeth

PIXE particle–induced x–ray emission • proton–induced x–ray emission *also* PIXIE

pixel picture element

PIXIE proton–induced x–ray emission *also* PIXE

PJ pancreatic juice

PJB premature junctional beat

PJC premature junctional contraction

PJP pancreatic juice protein

PJS peritoneojugular shunt • Peutz–Jeghers syndrome

PJT paroxysmal junctional tachycardia

PJVT paroxysmal junctional–ventricular tachycardia

PK pack (cigarette) • penetrating keratoplasty • pericardial knock • pharmacokinetic • pig kidney • Prausnitz–Küstner (reaction) • protein kinase • psychokinesis • pyruvate kinase

P$_K$ plasma potassium

pK ionization constant of acid • negative logarithm of dissociation constant *also* pK'

pK' apparent value of pK • negative logarithm of dissociation constant of acid *also* pk

pk peck

PKA prekallikrein activator • prokininogenase

pKa measure of acid strength

pK$_a$ negative logarithm of acid ionization constant

PKAR protein kinase activation ratio

PKase protein kinase

PKB prone knee bend

PKD polycystic kidney disease

PKF phagocytosis (and) killing function

PKI potato kallikrein inhibitor

PKK plasma prekallikrein • prekallikrein

PKN parkinsonism

PKP penetrating keratoplasty

PKR phased knee rehabilitation

PKT Prausnitz–Küstner test

PKU phenylketonuria

PKV killed poliomyelitis vaccine

pkV peak kilovoltage

PL palmaris longus • pancreatic lipase • perception (of) light • phospholipase • phospholipid *also* PPL • photoluminescence • place • placebo *also* P, PBO • placental lactogen • plantar • plasma lemma • plastic surgery • platelet • platelet antigen • platelet lactogen • plural • polymer (of) lactic (acid) • posterior lip (of acetabulum) • preleukemia platelet *also* PLT, Plt • premature labor • problem list • procaine (and) lactic acid • psychosocial–labile • pulpolingual • pulpolinguoaxial • Purkinje layer • trans-pulmonary pressure *also* P_L

P_L pulmonary venous pressure • transpulmonary pressure *also* PL

PL/1 programming language 1 (one)

Pl plasma • poiseuille

pL, pl picoliter

pl place • pleural • plural

PLA peroxidase–labeled antibodies (test) • phospholipase A • platelet antigen • polylactic acid • potentially lethal arrhythmia • pulpolinguoaxial

PLa pulpolabial

Pla left atrial pressure

PLAP placental alkaline phosphatase

Plat platelet

PLAX parasternal long axis

PLB parietal lobe battery • phospholipase B • porous layer bead

PLBO placebo

PLC personal locus (of) control • phospholipase C • primary liver cell • proinsulin–like component • protein–lipid complex • pseudolymphocytic choriomeningitis

PLCC primary liver cell cancer

PLCL polyclonal gammopathy identified

PLCO postoperative low cardiac output

PL–CLP platelet clumps

PLD peripheral light detection • phospholipase D • platelet defect • posterior latissimus dorsi (muscle) • postlaser day • potentially lethal damage

PLDH plasma lactic dehydrogenase

PLDR potentially lethal damage repair

PLE panlobular emphysema •
pleura • polymorphous
light eruption *also* PMLE •
protein–losing
enteropathy • pseudolupus
erythematosus syndrome

PLED periodic lateralizing
epileptiform discharge

PLES parallel–line equal
spacing

PLET polymyxin, lysozyme,
EDTA, and thallous acetate
(in heart infusion agar)

PLEU pleural (fluid)

PLEVA pityriasis lichenoides
et varioliformis

PLF perilymphatic fistula

PLFC premature living female
child

PLG plasminogen

P–LGV psittacosis–lymphogranuloma venereum

PLH paroxysmal localized
hyperhidrosis • placental
lactogenic hormone

PLIF posterior lumbar
interbody fusion

PLISSIT permission, limited
information, specific
suggestions, intensive
therapy

PLL peripheral light loss •
poly–L–lysine • posterior
longitudinal ligament •
pressure length loop •
prolymphocytic leukemia

PLM percentage of labeled
mitoses • plasma level
monitoring • polarized
light microscopy

PLMC premature living male
child

PLMT plasmacytoid
lymphocyte

PLMV posterior–leaf mitral
valve

PLN pelvic lymph node •
peripheral lymph node •
popliteal lymph node •
posterior lip nerve

PLND pelvic lymph node
dissection

PLO polycystic lipomem-
branous osteodysplasia

PLP paraformaldehyde–
lysine–periodate • plasma
leukopheresis •
polystyrene latex particle •
pyridoxal phosphate

PLPD pseudoperiodic
lateralized paroxysmal
discharge

PLR pronation–lateral rotation
(fracture) • pupillary light
reflex

PLS Papillon–Lefevre
syndrome • plastic
surgery • preleukemic
syndrome • Preschool
Language Scale • primary
lateral sclerosis • prostaglandin–like substance

pls please

PLSO posterior leafspring
orthosis

PLT pancreatic lymphocytic
infiltration • platelet *also*
PL, Plt • primed
lymphocyte test • primed
lymphocyte typing •
psittacosis–
lymphogranuloma
venereum–trachoma (group)

Plt   platelet *also* PL, PLT

PLT EST   platelet estimate

PLT–G   giant platelet

plumb.   [L. *plumbum*] lead

PLUT   Plutchnik (geriatric rating scale)

PLV   live poliomyelitis vaccine • panleukopenia virus • phenylalanine, lysine, and vasopressin • posterior left ventricular

PLWS   Prader–Labhart–Willi syndrome

plx   plexus

PLYM   prolymphocyte

PM   [L. *post mortem*] after death • [L. *post meridiem*] afternoon *also* pm • evening • pacemaker • papilla mammae • papillary muscle • papular mucinosis • paromycin • partially muscular • partial meniscectomy • perinatal mortality • peritoneal macrophage • petit mal (epilepsy) • photomulti-plier • physical medicine • plasma membrane • platelet membrane • platelet microsome • pneumomediastinum • poliomyelitis • polymorph • polymorpho-nuclear • polymyositis • poor metabolizer • porokeratosis (of) Mibelli • posterior mitral • post-menopausal • postmortem *also* post. • premamillary nucleus • premarketing (approval) • premolar • presents mainly • presystolic murmur •

pretibial myxedema • preventive medicine *also* PRM, PrM, PVMed • primary motivation • prostatic massage • protein methylesterase • pterygoid muscle • puberal macromastia • pulmonary macrophage • pulpomesial

P/M   parent–metabolite ratio

Pm   promethium

pM   picomolar

pm   picometer • [L. *post meridiem*] afternoon *also* PM

PMA   papillary, marginal, attached (gingiva) • *para–*methoxyamphetamine • phenylmercuric acetate • phorbol myristate acetate • phosphomolybdic acid • premenstrual asthma • primary mental abilities • Prinzmetal angina • pro-gressive muscular atrophy • psychomotor agitation • pyridylmercuric acetate

PMAC   phenylmercuric acetate

PMB   papillomacular bundle • *para–*hydroxymercuri-benzoate • polychrome methylene blue • polymorphonuclear basophil • polymyxin B • postmenopausal bleeding

PMC   phenylmercuric chloride • pleural mesothelial cell • premature mitral closure • pseudomembranous colitis

PMCP   *para–*monochloro-phenol

PMD   perceptual motor development • posterior mandibular depth •

primary myocardial disease • private medical doctor • programmed multiple development • progressive muscular dystrophy

PM/DM polymyositis/ dermatomyositis

PMDS primary myelodysplastic syndrome

PME polymorphonuclear eosinophil • postmenopausal estrogen • progressive myoclonus epilepsy

PMEC pseudomembranous enterocolitis

PMF progressive massive fibrosis • pterygomaxillary fossa

PMF, pmf proton motive force

PMH past medical history • posteromedial hypothalamus • programmed medical history

PMHR predicted maximal heart rate

PMHx past medical history

PMI past medical illness • patient medical instructions • patient medication instruction • perioperative myocardial infarction • phosphomannose isomerase • plea (of) mental incompetence • point of maximal impulse • point of maximal intensity • posterior myocardial infarction • postmyocardial infarction • present medical illness • previous medical illness

PMIS postmyocardial infarction syndrome • PSRO (Professional Standards Review Organization) Management Information System

PMK primary monkey kidney

PML polymorphonuclear leukocyte *also* PMNL, POLY • posterior mitral leaflet • progressive multifocal leukodystrophy • progressive multifocal leukoencephalopathy • pulmonary microlithiasis

pML posterior mitral valve leaflet

PMLE polymorphous light eruption *also* PLE

PMM protoplast maintenance medium

PMMA polymethylmethacrylate

PMMF pectoralis major myocutaneous flap

PMN polymorphonuclear *also* POLY • polymorphonuclear neutrophil *also* M_7, PMNN • polymorphonuclear neutrophilic (leukocyte)

PMNC percentage (of) multinucleated cells • peripheral blood mononuclear cell

PMNG polymorphonuclear granulocyte

PMNL polymorphonuclear leukocyte *also* PML, POLY

PMNN polymorphonuclear neutrophil *also* M_7, PMN

PMNR periadenitis mucosa necrotica recurrens

PMO postmenopausal osteoporosis • Principal Medical Officer

pmol picomole

PMP pain management program • past menstrual period • patient management problem • patient medication profile • persistent mentoposterior (fetal position) • previous menstrual period • psychotropic medication plan

PMPO postmenopausal palpable ovary

PMQ phytylmenaquinone (vitamin K)

PMR perinatal morbidity rate • perinatal mortality rate • periodic medical review • physical medicine (and) rehabilitation • polymorphic reticulosis • polymyalgia rheumatica • prior medical record • proportional morbidity ratio • proportionate mortality ratio • proton magnetic resonance • psychomotor retardation

PM&R physical medicine and rehabilitation

PMRS physical medicine (and) rehabilitation service

PMS patient management system • phenazine methosulfate • postmarketing surveillance • postmenopausal syndrome • postmenstrual stress • postmitochondrial supernatant • pregnant mare serum • premenstrual symptoms • premenstrual syndrome • pureed, mechanical, soft (diet)

PMSC pluripotent myeloid stem cell

PMSF phenylmethyl sulfonyl fluoride

PMSG pregnant mare serum gonadotropin

PMT photoelectric multiplier tube • photomultiplier tube • Porteus maze test • premenstrual tension

PMTS premenstrual tension syndrome

PMTT pulmonary mean transit time

PMV paralyzed (and) mechanically ventilated • prolapse (of) mitral valve

PMVL, pMVL posterior mitral–valve leaflet

PMW pacemaker wire(s)

PMZ pentamethylenetetrazol

PN [L. *pavor nocturnus*] nightmare • papillary necrosis • parenteral nutrition • penicillin *also* P, PCN, Pen, pen., PNC • perceived noise • percussion note • percutaneous nephrostogram • periarteritis nodosa *also* PAN • peripheral nerve • peripheral neuropathy *also* PNP • peripheral node • phrenic nerve • plaque neutralization • pneumonia *also* Pn, pneu, PNM • polyarteritis nodosa *also* PAN • polynephritis • polyneuritis • pontine nucleus • poorly nourished • positional nystagmus • posterior nares • postnasal • postnatal • Practical Nurse • predicted normal • premie nipple • primary nurse • progress note • propoxyphene napsylate • psychiatry (and) neurology • psychoneurotic • pulmonary disease • pyelonephritis • pyridine nucleotide • pyrrolinitrin

P/N positive to negative (ratio)

P&N psychiatry and neurology

P$_{N2}$ partial pressure of nitrogen

Pn pneumonia *also* PN, pneu

PNA Paris Nomina Anatomica • peanut agglutinin • pediatric nurse associate • pentosenucleic acid

P$_{Na}$ plasma sodium

PNAB percutaneous needle aspiration biopsy

PNAH polynuclear aromatic hydrocarbon

PNAS prudent no–salt–added (diet)

PNAvQ positive–negative ambivalent quotient

PNB percutaneous needle biopsy • polymyxin, neomycin, bacitracin • premature newborn • premature nodal beat

PNBT *para*–nitroblue tetrozolium

PNC penicillin *also* P, PCN, Pen, pen., PN • peripheral

nerve conduction • peripheral nucleated cell • pneumotaxic center • postnecrotic cirrhosis • premature nodal contraction • prenatal care • purine nucleotide cycle

PND paroxysmal nocturnal dyspnea • pelvic node dissection • postnasal drainage • postnasal drip • postneonatal death • pregnancy, not delivered

pnd pound *also* L, lb, lib

PNdb perceived noise decibel

PNE plasma norepinephrine

PNET permeative neuroectodermal tumor

PNET–MB permeative neuroectodermal tumor–medulloblastoma

pneu pneumonia *also* PN, Pn, PNM

PNF prenatal fluoride • proprioceptive neuromuscular fasciculation (reaction)

PNG penicillin G • pneumogram

PNH paroxysmal nocturnal hemoglobinuria

PNI peripheral nerve injury • postnatal infection • prognostic nutrition index • pseudoneointimal • psychoneuroimmunology

PNID Peer Nomination Inventory for Depression

PNK polynucleotide kinase

PNL percutaneous nephrostolithotomy •

peripheral nerve lesion •
polymorphonuclear
neutrophilic leukocyte

PNLA percutaneous needle
lung aspiration

PNM perinatal mortality •
peripheral nerve myelin •
pneumonia *also* PN, Pn,
pneu • postneonatal
mortality

PNMG persistent neonatal
myasthenia gravis

PNO Principal Nursing Officer

PNP *para*–nitrophenol *also* P–
NP • peak negative
pressure • Pediatric Nurse
Practitioner • peripheral
neuropathy *also* PN •
platelet neutralization
procedure •
polyneuropathy •
progressive nuclear palsy •
psychogenic nocturnal
polydipsia • purine
nucleoside phosphorylase

P–NP *para*–nitrophenol *also*
PNP

PNPB positive–negative
pressure breathing

PNPG *para*–nitrophenyl–β–
galactoside

pNPP, *p*NPP *para*–nitro–
phenylphosphate

PNPR positive–negative
pressure respiration

PNPS *para*–nitrophenylsulfate

PNRS premature nursery

PNS parasympathetic nervous
system • partial
nonprogressive stroke •
peripheral nervous
stimulator • peripheral

nervous system • posterior
nasal spine

PNT partial nodular transformation • percutaneous
nephrostomy tube

PNT, Pnt patient *also* P, PT,
Pt, pt

PNU protein nitrogen unit

PNV prenatal vitamins

Pnx pneumonectomy •
pneumothorax *also* PT,
PTX, Px

PNZ posterior necrotic zone

PO [L. *per os*] by mouth *also*
po • parapineal organ •
parietal operculum •
parieto–occipital •
perceptual organization •
period (of) onset •
perioperative • phone order
also P/O • physician
only • posterior •
postoperative *also* postop,
post–op • predominating
organism

P–O postoperative

P/O oxidative phosphorylation
ratio • phone order *also*
PO • protein to osmolar
(ratio)

P&O parasites and ova

PO$_2$, P$_{o2}$ partial pressure of
oxygen

Po polonium • porion •
position response •
progesterone

po [L. *per os*] by mouth, orally
also PO

POA pancreatic oncofetal
antigen • phalangeal
osteoarthritis • point of

application · preoptic area · primary optic atrophy

POAG primary open–angle glaucoma

POA–HA preoptic anterior hypothalamic area

POB penicillin, oil, beeswax · phenoxybenzamine · place of birth

POBE Profile of Out–of–Body Experiences

POC particulate organic carbon · postoperative care · procarbazine, Oncovin (vincristine), and CCNU (lomustine) · products of conception

Po/C ocular pressure

POCC procarbazine, Oncovin (vincristine), CCNU (lomustine), and Cytoxan (cyclophosphamide)

pocill [L. *pocillum*] small cup

pocul [L. *poculum*] cup

POCY postoperative chronologic year

POD pacing on demand · peroxidase · place of death · polycystic ovary disease · podiatry *also* Pod · postoperative day · postovulatory day

Pod podiatry *also* POD

Pod D Doctor of Podiatry

PODx preoperative diagnosis

POE port of entry · position of ease · postoperative endophthalmitis · proof of eligibility

POEMS polyneuropathy, organomegaly, endocrinopathy, M protein, skin changes (syndrome)

POET pulse oximeter/end tidal (carbon dioxide)

POEx postoperative exercise

POF position of function · primary ovarian failure · pyruvate oxidation factor

PofE portal of entry

POG pediatric oncology group · polymyositis ossificans generalisata · products of gestation

Pog pogonion

pOH hydroxide ion concentration in a concentration/solution

POHI physically (or) otherwise health–impaired

POHS presumed ocular histoplasmosis syndrome

POI Personal Orientation Inventory

poik poikilocyte/poikilocytosis

pois poison/poisoning/ poisoned

POL premature onset (of) labor

pol polish/polishing

polio poliomyelitis

POLY polymorphonuclear *also* PMN · polymorphonuclear leukocyte *also* PML, PMNL

poly–A, poly(A) polyadenylic (acid)

poly–C, poly(C) poly-cytidylic (acid)

POLY–CHR poly-chromatophilia

poly–G, poly(G) poly-guanylic (acid)

poly–I, poly(I) polyinosinic (acid)

poly–LC, poly–L:C copolymer of polyinosinic and polycytidylic acids • synthetic RNA polymer

% POLPS percent of polymorphonuclear leukocytes

polys polymorphonuclear leukocytes

polys(segs) polymorpho-nuclear segmented neutrophils

poly–T, poly(T) poly-thymidylic (acid)

poly–U, poly(U) polyuridylic (acid)

POM pain on motion • polyoximethylene • prescription only medicine

POMC propiomelanocortin

POMP principal outer material protein • prednisone, Oncovin (vincristine), methotrexate, and Purinethol (mercaptopurine)

POMR problem–oriented medical record *also* POR

POMS Profile of Mood States

PON paraxonase • particulate organic nitrogen

pond. [L. *pondere*] by weight

PONI postoperative narcotic infusion

POOH postoperative open–heart (surgery)

POOR poor clot

POP diphosphate group • pain on palpation • par-oxypropione • persistent occipitoposterior (fetal position) • pituitary opioid peptide • plasma oncotic pressure • plasma osmotic pressure • plaster of Paris *also* PP • polymyositis ossificans progressiva • popliteal *also* Pop., poplit • postoperative *also* POp

POp postoperative *also* POP

Pop. popliteal *also* POP, poplit • population

poplit popliteal *also* POP, Pop.

POR physician of record • postocclusive oscillatory response • problem–oriented (medical) record *also* POMR

PORH postocclusive reactive hyperemia

PORK porkilocytosis

PORP partial ossicular replacement prosthesis

Porph porphyrin(s)

PORT perioperative respiratory therapy • post-operative respiratory therapy

port portable

POS paraosteal osteosarcoma • polycystic ovary syndrome *also* PCOS • positive *also* P • psychoorganic syndrome

pos position *also* P • positive *also* P, POS

POSC problem–oriented
system (of) charting

POSM patient–operated
selector mechanism

Pos pr positive pressure

POSS percutaneous on–
surface stimulation •
proximal over–shoulder
strap

poss possible

post. posterior *also* P •
postmortem *also* PM

postgangl postganglionic

postop, post–op post-
operative *also* PO

post prand [L. *post prandium*]
after dinner *also* pp

POSTS positive occipital
sharp transients of sleep

post sag D posterior sagittal
diameter

post sing sed liq [L. *post
singulas sedes liquidas*]
after very loose stool

POT periostitis ossificans
toxica • postoperative
treatment • purulent otitis
media

pot. [L. *potus*] a drink •
potassium *also* potass •
potential *also* poten •
potash • potassa • potion

potass potassium *also* pot.

PotAGT potential abnormality
(of) glucose tolerance

poten potential *also* pot.

POU placenta, ovary, uterus

PoV portal vein

POVT puerperal ovarian vein
thrombophlebitis

POW Powassan (encephalitis) •
prisoner of war

powd powder *also* pdr, pwd

PP diphosphate group • [L.
punctum proximum] near
point of accomodation *also*
P, pp • pacesetter potential
also PCP • pancreatic
polypeptide • paradoxical
pulse • parietal pleura •
partial pressure *also* P, p •
pathology point • pedal
pulse • pellagra
preventive • pentose
pathway • perfusion
pressure • peripheral
pulse • peritoneal
pseudomyxoma •
permanent partial •
persisting proteinuria •
Peyer patch • phosphorylase
phosphatase • pink puffer
(sign of emphysema) •
pinpoint • pinprick •
placental protein • plane
polarization • planned
parenthood • plasma
pepsinogen • plasma-
pheresis • plasma protein •
plaster (of) Paris *also*
POP • polypeptide •
polystyrene agglutination
plate • poor person •
population planning •
porcine pancreatic •
posterior papillary •
posterior pituitary •
postpartum *also* pp •
postprandial *also* pp, PPD •
preferred provider •
presenting part • private
practice • private patient •
prothrombin–proconvertin •
protoporphyria •

protoporphyrin • proximal phalanx • pseudomyxoma peritonei • pterygoid process • pulse pressure • pulsus paradoxus • purulent pericarditis • push pills • pyrophosphate *also* PYP, Pyro

P&P pins and plaster • policy and procedure • prothrombin and proconvertin (test)

PP₁ free pyrophosphate

PP5 placental protein 5

pp [L. *post prandial*] after meals *also* p̄p̄, post prand • [L. *punctum proximum*] near point of accomodation *also* P, PP • polyphosphate • postpartum *also* PP • postpill (amenorrhea) • postprandial *also* PP, PPD • private patient

p̄p̄ [L. *post prandial*] after meals *also* pp, post prand

PPA [L. *phiala prius agitata*] first shake well • palpitation, percussion, and auscultation *also* PP&A, pp&a • pepsin A • phenylpropanolamine • phenylpyruvic acid • Pittsburgh pneumonia agent • polyphosphoric acid • postpartum amenorrhea • postpill amenorrhea • pure pulmonary atresia

PP&A, pp&a palpation, percussion, and auscultation *also* PPA

PPA pulmonary arterial pressure *also* PAP

ppa [L. *phiala prius agitata*] shake well

PPAS peripheral pulmonary artery stenosis • postpolio atrophy syndrome

PPB platelet–poor blood • positive pressure breathing

PPB, ppb parts per billion

PPBE postpartum breast engorgement • proteose–peptone beef extract

PPBS postprandial blood sugar

PPC pentose phosphate cycle • plasma prothrombin conversion • plaster of paris cast • pneumopericardium • pooled platelet concentrate • progressive patient care • proximal palmar crease

PPCA plasma prothrombin conversion accelerator • proserum prothrombin conversion accelerator

PPCF peripartum cardiac failure • plasma prothrombin conversion factor

PPCH piperazinylmethyl cyclohexanone

PPCM postpartum cardiomyopathy

PPD packs per day (cigarettes) *also* P/D, p/d • paraphenyl-enediamine • percussion (and) postural drainage • permanent partial disability • phenyldi-phenyloxadiazole • posterior polymorphous dystrophy • postpartum day • postprandial *also* PP, pp • primary physical dependence • progressive perceptive deafness • purified protein derivative • (Siebert) purified protein derivative (of tuberculin)

P&PD percussion and postural drainage

ppd prepared

PPD–B purified protein derivative–Battey

PPDR preproliferative diabetic retinopathy

PPD–S purified protein derivative–standard

PPE partial plasma exchange • permeability pulmonary edema • polyphosphoric ester • porcine pancreatic elastase • programmed physical examination

PPF pellagra preventive factor • phagocytosis promoting factor • plasma protein fraction

PPFA Planned Parenthood Federation of America

PPG photoplethysmography • polymorphonuclear (cells) per glomerulus • polyurethane–polyvinyl graphite • postprandial glucose • pretragal parotid gland

ppg picopicogram

PPGA postpill galactorrhea/ amenorrhea

PPGF polypeptide growth factor

PPGI psychophysiologic gastrointestinal (reaction)

PPGP prepaid group practice

PPH persistent pulmonary hypertension • postpartum hemorrhage • primary pulmonary hypertension • protocollagen proline hydroxylase

pphm parts per hundred million

PPHN persistent pulmonary hypertension (of) newborn

PPHP pseudopseudohypo-parathyroidism

ppht parts per hundred thousand

PPHx previous psychiatric history

PPI partial permanent impair-ment • patient package insert • Plan–Position–Indication • preceding preparatory interval • present pain intensity • purified porcine insulin

PPI, PP$_i$ inorganic pyrophosphate *also* IPP

PPID peak pain intensity difference (score)

PPIM postperinatal infant mortality

PPK palmoplantar keratosis • partial penetrating keratoplasty

PPL pars plana lensectomy • penicilloylpolylysine • phospholipid *also* PL • protein polysaccharide

Ppl intrapleural pressure

PPLF postperfusion low flow

PPLO pleuropneumonia–like organism

PPM parts per million *also*
ppm • permanent
pacemaker • phospho-
pentomutase • pigmented
pupillary membrane •
posterior papillary muscle

ppm parts per million *also*
PPM • pulses per minute

PPMA postpoliomyelitis
muscular atrophy •
progressive postmyelitis
muscular atrophy

PPMD posterior polymorphous
dystrophy (of cornea)

PPMM postpolycythemia
myeloid metaplasia

PPMS psychophysiologic
musculoskeletal (reaction)

PPN partial parenteral
nutrition • pedunculo-
pontine nucleus

PPNA peak phrenic nerve
activity

PPNAD primary pigmented
nodular adrenocortical
disease

PPNG penicillinase–producing
Neisseria gonorrhoeae

PPO diphenyloxazole • peak
pepsin output • platelet
peroxidase • pleuro-
pneumonia organism •
preferred provider
organization • prepatient
periods to oocyst

PPP palatopharyngoplasty •
palmoplantar pustulosis •
passage, power, and
passenger (progress of
labor) • pedal pulse
present • pentosephosphate
pathway • peripheral pulse
palpable • Pickford

projective pictures • plasma
protamine precipitating •
platelet–poor plasma •
polyphoretic phosphate •
porcine pancreatic
polypeptide • postpartum
psychosis • protamine
paracoagulation pheno-
menon • purified placental
protein • pustulosis
palmaris et plantaris

PPPBL peripheral pulses
palpable both legs

PPPG postprandial plasma
glucose

PPPH purified placental
protein, human

PPPI primary private practice
insurance

PPPPP pain, pallor, pulse loss,
paresthesia, paralysis

PPR patient–physician
relationship • patient
progress record •
photopalpebral reflex •
poor partial response •
Price precipitation reaction

PPr paraprosthetic

PPRF paramedian pontine
reticular formation •
postpartum renal failure

PPROM prolonged premature
rupture of membranes

PPRP phosphoribosyl
pyrophosphate

PPRWP poor precordial R–
wave progression

PPS pepsin A • peripheral
pulmonary stenosis •
Personal Preference Scale •
phosphoribosylpyrophosphate
synthetase • polyvalent
pneumococcal

polysaccharide • postpartum sterilization • postperfusion syndrome • postpericardiotomy syndrome • postpolio syndrome • postpump syndrome • primary acquired pre-leukemic syndrome • prospective payment system • prospective pricing system • protein plasma substitute

PPSB prothrombin, proconvertin, Stuart factor, antihemophilic B factor

PPSH pseudovaginal perineoscrotal hypospadias

PPT partial prothrombin time • peak–to–peak threshold • plant protease test • potassium phophotungstate • pulmonary platelet trapping

ppt precipitate • precipitation *also* pptn • [L. *praeparatus*] prepared

pptd precipitated

PPTL postpartum tubal ligation

pptn precipitation *also* ppt

PPTT postpartum painless thyroiditis (with transient) thyrotoxicosis

PPU perforated peptic ulcer

PPV porcine parvovirus • positive predictive value • positive pressure ventilation • progressive pneumonia virus

PPVT Peabody Picture Vocabulary Test

PPVT–R Peabody Picture Vocabulary Test, Revised

Ppw pulmonary wedge pressure *also* PWP

PPZ perphenazine

PPZSO perphanazine sulfoxide

PQ paraquat • permeability quotient • plastoquinone • pronator quadratus • pyrimethamine–quinine

PQD protocol data query

PQNS protein, quantity not sufficient

PR [L. *per rectum*] by way of rectum *also* pr, p rec • [L. *punctum remotum*] far point (of accommodation) • Panama red (variety of marijuana) • parallax (and) refraction • pars recta • partial reinforcement • partial remission • partial response • patient relations • peer review • percentile rank • peripheral resistance • phenol red • photoreaction • photoreactivation • physical rehabilitation • physician reviewer • pityriasis rosea • polymyalgia rheumatica • posterior root • postural reflex • potency ratio • potential relation • preference record • pregnancy *also* preg, pregn • pregnancy rate • premature *also* Pr, prem • presbyopia *also* P, Pr • pressoreceptor • pressure *also* P, P, press. • prevention • Preyer reflex • proctology • production rate • professional relations • profile • progesterone receptor • progressive relaxation •

progressive resistance · prolactin *also* P, Pr, PRL, Prl · prolonged remission · propicillin · propranolol · prosthion · protein *also* P, Pr, PRO, pro, prot · psychotherapy responder · public relations · Puerto Rican · pulmonary regurgitation · pulmonary rehabilitation · pulse rate · pulse repetition · pyramidal response

P–R time between P wave and beginning of QRS complex in electrocardiography

P/R productivity to respiration (ratio)

P&R pelvic and rectal (examination) · pulse and respiration

Pr praseodymium · premature *also* PR, prem · presbyopia *also* P, PR · primary · prism · proctologist · production rate (of steroid hormones) · prolactin *also* P, PR, PRL, Prl · propyl · protein *also* P, PR, PRO, pro, prot

pr [L. *punctum remotum*] far point of accomodation · pair · [L. *per rectum*] by way of rectum *also* PR, p rec

PRA phonation, respiration, articulation–resonance · phosphoribosylamine · plasma renin activity · progesterone receptor assay

prac, pract practice · practitioner

PrA–HPA protein A hemolytic plaque assay

prand [L. *prandium*] dinner

PRAS prereduced anaerobically sterilized (medium)

PRAT platelet radioactive antiglobulin test

p rat aetat [L. *pro ratione aetatis*] in proportion to age

PRB Prosthetics Research Board

PRBC packed red blood cells *also* PRC

PRBV placental residual blood volume

PRC packed red blood cells *also* PRBC · peer review committee · phase response curve · plasma renin concentration

PRCA pure red cell agenesis · pure red cell aplasia

PRD partial reaction (of) degeneration · phosphate restricted diet · polycystic renal disease · postradiation dysplasia

PRE passive resistance exercise · photoreacting enzyme · physical reconditioning exercise · pigmented retina epithelial (cell) · progressive resistive exercise

pre preliminary

pre–AIDS pre–acquired immune deficiency syndrome

p rec [L. *per rectum*] by way of rectum *also* PR, pr

precip precipitate/precipitated/precipitation *also* pcpn

PRED prednisone *also* P, PDN

pred predicted

PREE partial reinforcement extinction effect

prefd preferred

PREG pregnelone

preg, pregn pregnancy/ pregnant *also* PR

prelim preliminary

prem premature *also* PR, Pr • prematurity

premie premature (infant)

preop, pre–op preoperative

prep preparation • prepare (for surgery) • preposition

prepd, prepped prepared (for surgery)

PRERLA pupils round, equal, react to light (and) accommodation

PREs progressive resistive exercises (ophthalmology)

preserv preservation • preserve

press. pressure *also* P, p, PR

prev prevention/preventive • previous

PrevAGT previous abnormality (of) glucose tolerance

PREVMEDU preventive medicine unit

PRF partial reinforcement • patient report form • pontine reticular formation • progressive renal failure • prolactin–releasing factor • pyrogen–releasing factor

pRF polyclonal rheumatoid factor

PRFA plasma–recognition– factor activity

PRFM premature rupture (of) fetal membranes *also* PROM • prolonged rupture (of) fetal membranes *also* PROM

PRFN percutaneous radiofrequency

PRFR pressure–retaining flow–relieving

PRG phleborheogram/ phleborheography • phleborheography • purge

PRGI percutaneous retrogasserian glycerol injection

PRH past relevant history • preretinal hemorrhage • prolactin–releasing hormone

PRHBF peak reactive hyperemia blood flow

PRI Pain Rating Index • phosphate reabsorption index • phosphoribose isomerase • plexus rectales inferiores

PRIAS Packard radioimmuno- assay system

PRIH prolactin release– inhibiting hormone

prim primary

PRIME Prematriculation Program in Medical Education • procarbazine, iglosamide, and methotrexate

primip primipara *also* I–para, P, PRIMP

prim luc [L. *prima luce* at first light] early in morning

prim m [L. *primo mane*] first thing in morning

PRIMP primipara *also* I–para, P, primip

PRIND prolonged reversible ischemic neurologic deficit

PRISM Pediatric Risk of Mortality Score

PRIST paper radioimmunosorbent technique · paper radioimmunosorbent test

priv private

PRK primary rabbit kidney

PRL, Prl prolactin *also* P, PR, Pr

PRLA pupils react to light and accommodation

PRM phosphoribomutase · photoreceptor membrane · prematurely ruptured membrane · preventive medicine *also* PM, PrM, PVMed · Primary Reference Material · primidone

PrM preventive medicine *also* PM, PRM, PVMed

PRM–SDX, PRM–SOX pyrimethamine sulfadoxine

PRN, prn [L. *pro re nata*] as required

PRNT plaque reduction neutralization test

PRO peer review organization · projection · prolapse · pronation *also* pron · protein *also* P, PR, Pr, pro, prot

Pro proline *also* P · prophylactic *also* prop. · prothrombin

pro protein *also* P, PR, Pr, PRO, prot

prob probable · probability · problem

proc procedure · proceedings · process

Procarb procarbazine

Proct proctology

procto proctoscopy

prod. production/product

pro dos [L. *pro dose*] for a dose

Pro El protein electrophoresis

PROG progesterone · prognathism · program · progressive

prog, progn prognosis *also* Px

progr progress

prolong. prolongation · prolonged

PROM passive range of motion · premature rupture of (fetal) membranes *also* PRFM · programmable read–only memory · prolonged rupture of (fetal) membranes *also* PRFM

PROMIN programmable multiple ion monitor

PROMIS Problem–oriented Medical Information System

Promy promyelocyte

pron pronator/pronation *also* PRO

PROP propranolol

prop. prophylaxis/prophylactic *also* Pro

ProPac Prospective Payment Assessment Commission

proph, prophy prophylactic

PROPLA prophospholipase A

pro rat. aet [L. *pro ratione aetatis*] according to age

PROSO protamine sulfate

pros, prostat prostate/ prostatic

prosth prosthesis/prosthetic

prot protein *also* P, PR, Pr, PRO, pro

proTime prothrombin time *also* PT

PROTO protoporphyrin

pro us. ext [L. *pro usum externum*] for external use

prov provisional (diagnosis)

PROVIMI proteins, vitamins, and minerals

prox proximal

prox luc [L. *proxima luce*] the day before

PRP panretinal photocoagulation • penicillinase–resistant penicillin • physiologic rest position • pityriasis rubra pilaris • platelet–rich plasma • polymer (of) ribose phosphate • polyribophosphate • polyribosyl ribitol phosphate • postreplication repair • postural rest position • pressure rate product • problem reporting program • progressive rubella panencephalitis • proliferative retinopathy photocoagulation •

Psychotic Reaction Profile • pulse repetition frequency

PRPP phosphoribosyl pyrophosphate

PRR proton relaxation rate

PRRE pupils round, regular, (and) equal

PR–RSV Prague Rous sarcoma virus

PRS parent's rating scale • Personality Rating Scale • plasma renin substrate • positive rolandic spike • pupil rating scale

PRSA plasma renin substrate activity

PRSIS Prospective Rate Setting Information System

PRSM peripheral smear

PRSM peripheral smear

PRSP penicillinase–resistant synthetic penicillin

PRT *Penicillium roqueforti* toxin • pharmaceutical research (and) testing • phosphoribosyltransferase *also* PRTase • photoradiation therapy • postoperative respiratory treatment

PRTase phosphoribosyltransferase *also* PRT

PRTH–C prothrombin (time) control *also* PT–C

PRU peripheral resistance unit

PRV polycythemia rubra vera • pseudorabies virus

PRVA peripheral vein renin activity

PRVEP pattern reversal visual evoked potential(s)

PRVR peak–to–resting–
velocity ratio

PrVS prevesicle space

PRW polymerized ragweed

PRWP poor R–wave pro-
gression (electrocardiogram)

PRZ prazepam

PRZF pyrazofurin

PS chloropicrin • paired
stimulation • paradoxical
sleep • paralaryngeal
space • paranoid
schizophrenia • para-
septal • parasternal •
parasympathetic (division of
autonomic nervous system)
also parasym • partial
shoulder • pathologic
stage • patient's serum •
pediatric surgery *also*
PDS • performance
status • performing scale
(IQ) • periodic syndrome •
peripheral smear •
permeability surface •
phosphate saline (buffer) •
phosphatidyl serine •
photosynthesis • phrenic
(nerve) stimulation •
physical status • pigeon
serum • plastic surgery
also PSurg • point (of)
symmetry • poly-
saccharide • polystyrene •
population sample •
Porter–Silber (chromogen)
also P–S • postmaturity
syndrome • pregnancy
serum • prescription •
pressure support •
prestimulus • principal
sulcus • programmed
symbols • prostatic
secretion • protamine
sulfate • protective

services • protein
synthesis • psychiatric *also*
psychiat • pulmonary
stenosis • pulse sequence •
pyloric stenosis

P–S pancreozymin–secretin •
Porter–Silber (chromogen)
also PS • pyramid surface

P/S polisher–stimulator •
polyunsaturated/saturated
(fatty acid ratio)

P&S pain and suffering •
paracentesis and suction •
permanent and stationary •
pharmacy and supply

Ps prescription • pseudocyst

ps per second • picosecond
also psec

PSA picryl sulfonic acid •
polyethylene sulfonic acid •
product selection allowed •
progressive spinal ataxia •
prolonged sleep apnea •
prostate specific antigen •
public service announcement

PsA psoriatic arthritis

Psa systemic blood pressure
also SBP

PSAGN poststreptococcal
acute glomerulonephritis

PSAn psychoanalysis/
psychoanalytic

PSAP prostate–specific acid
phosphatase

PSAX parasternal short axis

PSB protected specimen brush

PSBO partial small bowel
obstruction

PSC partial subligamentous
calcification • patient

services coordination • physiologic squamocolumnar • pluripotential stem cell • Porter–Silber chromogen • posterior semicircular canal • posterior subcapsular cataract *also* PSCC • primary sclerosing cholangitis • pulse–synchronized contractions

PSCC posterior subcapsular cataract *also* PSC

PSCE presurgical coagulation evaluation

PsChE pseudocholinesterase

Pscl pressure at slow component intercept

PSCM pokeweed activated spleen conditioned medium

PSCP posterior subscapular cataractous plague

PSCT peripheral stem cell transplant

P/score pressure score

PSD particle size distribution • peptone, starch, dextrose • periodic synchronous discharge • phosphate supplemental diet • photon–stimulated desorption • posterior sagittal diameter • poststenotic dilation • postsynaptic density

PSDES primary symptomatic diffuse esophageal spasm

PSE paradoxical systolic expansion • partial splenic embolization • penicillin–sensitive enzyme • point (of) subjective equality • portal systemic

encephalopathy • postshunt encephalopathy • purified spleen extract

PSEC poststress ethanol (alcohol) consumption

psec picosecond *also* ps

PSF peak scatter factor • point spread function • posterior spinal fusion • prostacyclin production–stimulating factor • pseudosarcomatous faciitis

psf pound per square foot

PSG peak systolic gradient • phosphate, saline, glucose • polysomnogram • presystolic gallop

PSGN poststreptococcal glomerulonephritis

PSH past surgical history • postspinal (anesthetic) headache

PsHD pseudoheart disease

PSI personal security index • physiologic stability index • posterior sagittal index • posterior superior iliac (spine) *also* PSIS • problem solving infor-mation • prostaglandin synthetic inhibitor • psychologic screening inventory • psychosomatic inventory

PSI, psi pound per square inch *also* lb/in²

psi (Ψ, ψ) twenty–third letter of Greek alphabet

ψ wave function

psia pounds per square inch absolute

PSIFT platelet suspension immunofluorescence test

pslg pounds per square inch gauge

PSIL preferred frequency speech interference level

PSIS posterior superior iliac spine *also* PSI

PSL parasternal line • percent stroke length • potassium, sodium chloride, and sodium lactate (solution)

PSLT Picture–Story Language Test

PSM presystolic murmur

PSMA progressive spinal muscular atrophy • proximal spinal muscular atrophy

PSMed psychosomatic medicine *also* PsychosMed

PSMF protein–sparing modified fast

PSMT psychiatric services management team

PSNS parasympathetic nervous system

PSO physostigmine salicylate ophthalmic • proximal subungual onychomycosis

Psol partly soluble

PSOR psoralen

P/sore pressure sore

PSP pacesetter potential *also* PP • pancreatic spasmolytic peptide • paralytic shellfish poisoning • parathyroid secretory protein • periodic short pulse • phenolsul-

fonphthalein (phenol red) • positive spike pattern • postsynaptic potential • professional simulated patient • progressive supranuclear palsy • pseudopregnancy

psp posterior subscapular plague

PSPF prostacyclin synthesis–stimulating plasma factor

PSQ Parent Symptom Questionnaire • patient satisfaction questionnaire

PSR pain sensitivity range • (extrahepatic) portal–systemic resistance • problem status report • proliferative sickle retinopathy • pulmonary stretch receptor

PSRBOW premature spontaneous rupture (of) bag of waters

PSRC Plastic Surgery Research Council

PSRO Professional Standards Review Organization

PSS painful shoulder syndrome • physiologic saline solution • progressive systemic scleroderma • progressive systemic sclerosis • psoriasis severity scale • Psychiatric Status Schedule

PST pancreatic suppression test • paroxysmal supra-ventricular tachycardia • Pascal–Suttle Test (psychiatry) • penicillin, streptomycin, tetracycline • perceptual span time • peristimulus time •

phenolsulfotransferase • phonemic segmentation test • platelet survival time • poststenotic • poststimulus time • prefrontal sonic treatment • protein–sparing therapy • proximal straight tubule

PSTH poststimulus time histograph

PSTI pancreatic secretory trypsin inhibitor

PSTP pentasodium triphosphate

PSTV potato spindle tuber viroid

PSU photosynthetic unit • postsurgical unit • primary sampling unit

PSurg, P–Surg plastic surgery *also* PS

PSV pressure supported ventilation • psychological, social, and vocational (adjustment factors)

PSVER pattern–shift visual evoked response

PSVT paroxysmal supraventricular tachycardia

PSW past sleepwalker • primary surgical ward

PSY, Psy psychiatry *also* P, PS, psychiat • psychology

Psych, psych psychology/ psychologic *also* psychol

psychiat psychiatry/ psychiatric *also* P, PS, Psy

psychoan psychoanalysis/ psychoanalytical

psychol psychology/ psychologic *also* psych

psychopath. psycho-pathology/psychopathologic *also* psy–path

PsychosMed psychosomatic medicine *also* PSMed

psychother psycho-therapeutic/psychotherapy

psy–path psychopathic *also* psychopath.

PT parathormone *also* PTH • parathyroid *also* para, PTH • paroxysmal tachycardia • patient *also* P, PNT, Pnt, Pt, pt • pericardial tamponade • permanent (and) total • pharmacy (and) thera-peutics • phenytoin • phonation time • photo-phobia • phototoxicity • physical therapy/therapist *also* PT • physical training • physiotherapy • pine tar • pint *also* P, p, pt • plasma thrombo-plastin • pneumothorax *also* Pnx, PTX, Px • polyvalent tolerance • posterior tibial (artery pulse) • posttransplanta-tion • preterm • propyl-thiouracil • prothrombin time *also* proTime • protriptyline • pulmonary thrombosis • pulmonary toilet • pulmonary trunk • pulmonary tuberculosis *also* PTB • pure tone (audiometry) • pyramidal tract • temporal plane

P&T paracentesis and tubing (of ears) • peak and trough • permanent and total • pharmacy and therapeutics

Pt [L. *perstetur*] let it be continued • patient *also* P, PNT, Pnt, PT, pt • platinum • psychoasthenia

pt part *also* P • patient *also* P, PNT, Pnt, PT, Pt • pint *also* P, p, PT • point

PTA parathyroid adenoma • percutaneous transluminal angioplasty • persistent trigeminal artery • persistent truncus arteriosus • phosphotungstic acid • physical therapy asistant • plasma thromboplastin antecedent • platelet thromboplastin antecedent • posttraumatic amnesia • pretreatment anxiety • prior to admission • prior to arrival • prothrombin activity • pure tone acuity • pure tone average *also* PT(A)

PT(A) pure tone average *also* PTA

PTAF policy target adjustment factor

P–TAG target–attaching globulin precursor

PTAH phosphotungstic acid hematoxylin

PTAP purified (diphtheria) toxoid (precipitated by) aluminum phosphate

PTB patellar tendon–bearing (cast prosthesis) • prior to birth • pulmonary tuberculosis *also* PT

PTBA percutaneous transluminal balloon angioplasty

PTBD percutaneous transhepatic biliary drainage

PTBD–EF percutaneous transhepatic biliary drainage–enteric feeding

PTBE pyretic tick–borne encephalitis

PTBP *para*–tertiary butylphenol

PTBS posttraumatic brain syndrome

PTC patient to call • percutaneous transhepatic cholangiography • phase transfer catalyst • phenylthiocarbamide • phenylthiocarbamoyl • pheochromocytoma, thyroid carcinoma (syndrome) • plasma thromboplastin component • premature tricuspid closure • prior to conception • prothrombin complex • pseudotumor cerebri

PT–C prothrombin time control *also* PRTH–C

PTCA percutaneous transluminal coronary angioplasty

PTCL peripheral T–cell lymphoma

PtcCO$_2$ transcutaneous carbon dioxide tension

PTCP pseudothrombo-cytopenia

PTCR percutaneous transluminal coronary recanalization

PT–CT prothrombin time control

PTD *para*–toluenediamine • percutaneous transluminal dilatation • period to discharge • permanent total disability • prior to delivery

Ptd phosphatidyl

PtdCho phosphatidylcholine

PtdEtn phosphatidyl-ethanolamine

PtdIns phosphatidylinositol

PTDP permanent transvenous demand pacemaker

PtdSer phosphatidylserine

PTE parathyroid extract • posttraumatic endophthalmitis • pretibial edema • proximal tibial epiphysis • pulmonary thromboembolism

PTED pulmonary thromboembolic disease

PteGlu pteroylglutamic (acid)

PTEN pentaerythritol tetranitrate

pter end of short arm of chromosome

PTF patient treatment file • plasma thromboplastin factor

PTFA prothrombin time fixing agent

PTFE polytetrafluoroethylene

PTG parathyroid gland

PTGA pteroyltriglutamic acid

PTH parathormone *also* PT • parathyroid *also* para, PT • parathyroid hormone *also* PH • phenylthiohydan-toin • plasma thrombo-plastin (component) • posttransfusion hepatitis • prior to hospitalization

PTh primary thrombocythemia

PTHBD percutaneous transhepatic biliary drain(age)

PTHC percutaneous transhepatic cholangiography

PTHS parathyroid hormone secretion (rate)

PTI pancreatic trypsin inhibitor • persistent tolerant infection • Pictorial Test of Intelligence • pressure time index

PTJV percutaneous transtracheal jet ventilation

PTL perinatal telencephalic leukoencephalopathy • pharyngeotracheal lumen • posterior tricuspid (valve) leaflet *also* pTL • preterm labor • protriptyline • (Sodium) Pentothal

pTL posterior tricuspid (valve) leaflet *also* PTL

PTLC precipitation thin–layer chromatography

PTM posterior trabecular meshwork • posttransfusion mononucleosis • posttraumatic meningitis • pressure time (per) minute • preterm milk

Ptm pterygomaxillary (fissure) • transmural pressure (airway, blood vessel)

PTMA phenyltrimethyl-ammonium

PTMDF pupils, tension, media, disc, fundus

PTN pain transmission neuron

pTNM postsurgical, tumor, nodes, metastases (postsurgical staging of cancer)

PTO [Ger. *Perlsucht Tuberculin Original*] Klemperer tuberculin • percutaneous transhepatic obliteration • personal time off • please turn over

PTP percutaneous transhepatic portography • posterior tibial pulse • posttetanic potentiation • posttransfusion purpura • prior to program • prothrombin–procovertin • proximal tubular pressure • prothrombin–proconvertin

Ptp transpulmonary pressure

PTPI posttraumatic pulmonary insufficiency

PTPM posttraumatic progressive myelopathy

PTPN peripheral (vein) total parenteral nutrition

PTR patella tendon reflex • patient termination record • patient to return • peripheral total resistance • prothrombin time ratio • psychotic trigger reaction • [Ger. *Perlsucht Tuberculin Rest*] tuberculin *Mycobacterium tuberculosis bovis*

PTr porcine trypsin

PTRA percutaneous transluminal renal angioplasty

PTRIA polystyrene–tube radioimmunoassay

PTS painful tonic seizure • *para*–toluenesulfonic (acid) • patella tendon socket • patellar tendon suspension • permanent threshold shift • phospho-transferase system • postthrombotic syndrome • prior to surgery

Pts, pts patients

PTSD posttraumatic stress disorder

PTSH poststimulus time histogram

PTT partial thromboplastin time • particle transport time • platelet transfusion therapy • posterior tibial transfer • pulmonary transit time • pulse transmission time

PTT–CT partial thromboplastin time control

PTU pain treatment unit • propylthiouracil

PTV posterior tibial vein

PTWTKG patient's weight (in) kilograms

PTX parathyroidectomy *also* PTx • pelvic traction • phototoxic reaction • picrotoxinin • pneumothorax *also* Pnx, PT, Px

PTx parathyroidectomy *also* PTX

PTXA parathyroidectomy and antotransplantation

PTZ pentamethylenetetrazole • pentylenetetrazol • phenothiazine

PU [L. *per urethra*] by way of urethra • passed urine •

paternal uncle • pelvic–ureteric • pepsin unit • peptic ulcer • posterior urethra • precursor uptake • pregnancy urine

Pu plutonium • purple (indicator color) *also* Pur • putrescine *also* PUT

pub, publ public

PUBS percutaneous umbilical blood sampling

PUC pediatric urine collector

PUD peptic ulcer disease • pulmonary disease *also* PD, PuD

PuD pulmonary disease *also* PD, PUD

PUE pyrexia (of) unknown etiology

PUFA polyunsaturated fatty acid

PUH pregnancy urine hormone

PUL pubourethral ligament

PUL, pul pulmonary *also* P, pulm

pulm [L. *pulmentum*] gruel • pulmonary *also* P, PUL, pul • pulmonic

PULSES general physical, upper extremities, lower extremities, sensory, excretory, social support (physical profile)

pulv [L. *pulvis*] powder

pulv gros [L. *pulvis grossus*] coarse powder

pulv subtil [L. *pulvis subtilis*] smooth powder

pulv tenu [L. *pulvis tenuis*] very fine powder

PUN plasma urea nitrogen

PUNL percutaneous ultrasonic nephrolithotripsy

PUO pyrexia (of) un-determined/unknown origin

PUP percutaneous ultrasonic pyelolithotomy

PU–PC polyunsaturated phosphatidylcholine

PUPPP pruritic urticarial papules and plaques of pregnancy

PUR polyurethane

Pur purple *also* Pu

purg purgative

PUT putamen • putrescine *also* Pu

PUVA psoralen plus ultraviolet light of A wavelength • pulsed ultraviolet actinotherapy

PUVD pulsed ultrasonic (blood) velocity detector

PUW pick–up walker

PV [L. *per vaginam*] by way of vagina • pancreatic vein • papillomavirus • paraventricular • pemphigus vulgaris • peripheral vascular • peripheral vein • peripheral vessel(s) • phonation volume • photovoltaic • pinocytotic vesicle • pityriasis versicolor • plasma viscosity • plasma volume • pneumococcus vaccine • polio vaccine • polycythemia vera • polyoma virus • polyvinyl • popliteal vein • portal vein • postvasectomy •

postvoiding • predictive value • pressure–volume • pulmonary vein • pure vegetarian

P–V Paton–Valentine (leukocidin) *also* RVL • pressure–volume (curve)

P/V pressure to volume (ratio)

P&V peak and valley • percuss and vibrate • pyloroplasty and vagotomy

Pv venous pressure *also* VP

PVA partial villous atrophy • polyvinyl alcohol (fixative) • Prinzmental variant angina

PVAc polyvinyl acetate

PVAS postvasectomy (specimen)

PVB Platinol (cisplatin), vinblastine, and bleomycin • premature ventricular beat

PVBS possible vertebral–basilar system

PVC persistent vaginal cornification • polyvinyl chloride • postvoiding cystogram • predicted vital capacity • premature ventricular complex • premature ventricular contraction • primary visual cortex • pulmonary venous capillary • pulmonary venous congestion

PVCM paradoxical vocal cord motion

Pv$_{CO2}$ partial pressure of carbon dioxide in mixed venous blood

PVD patient very disturbed • peripheral vascular disease • postural vertical dimension • portal vein dilation • posterior vitreous detachment • postvagotomy diarrhea • premature ventricular depolarization • pulmonary vascular disease

PVE perivenous encephalo-myelitis • periventricular echogenicity • premature ventricular extrasystole • prosthetic valve endocarditis

PVEP pattern visual evoked potential

PVF peripheral visual field • portal venous flow • primary ventricular fibrillation

PVFS postviral fatigue syndrome

PVH periventricular hemorrhage • pulmonary vascular hypertension

PVI peripheral vascular insufficiency • periventricular inhibitor

PVK penicillin V potassium

PVL periventricular leukomalacia

P–VL Panton–Valentine leukocidin *also* P–V

PVM pneumonia virus (of) mice • proteins, vitamins, (and) minerals

PVMed preventive medicine *also* PM, PRM, PrM

PVN paraventricular nucleus • predictive value (of a) negative test

PVNPS post–Viet Nam psychiatric syndrome

PVNS pigmented villonodular synovitis

PVO peripheral vascular occlusion • pulmonary venous obstruction • pulmonary venous occlusion

Pv$_{O2}$ partial oxygen pressure in mixed venous blood

PVOD peripheral vascular occlusive disease • pulmonary vascular obstructive disease • pulmonary veno–occlusive disease

PVP penicillin V potassium • peripheral vein plasma • peripheral venous pressure • polyvinyl-pyrrolidone (povidone) • portal venous pressure • predictive value (of a) positive (test) • pulmonary venous pressure

PVP–I polyvinylpyrrolidone (povidone)–iodine

PVR paraventricular nuclear stratum • peripheral vascular resistance • postvoiding residual • proliferative vitreoretinopathy • pulmonary vascular resistance • pulmonary venous redistribution • pulse–volume recording

PVRI peripheral vascular resistance index

PVS paravesicle space • percussion, vibration, and suction • peritoneovenous shunt • persistent vegetative state • pigmented villonodular synovitis • Plummer–Vinson syndrome • poliovirus sensitivity • polyvinyl sponge • premature ventricular systole • programmed ventricular stimulation • pulmonary vein stenosis • pulmonic valve stenosis

PVT paroxysmal ventricular tachycardia • physical volume test • portal vein thrombosis • pressure, volume, temperature • private (patient) *also* pvt

pvt private (patient) *also* PVT

PVW posterior vaginal wall

PW pacing wire • patient waiting • peristaltic wave • posterior wall (of heart) • Prader–Willi (syndrome) *also* P–W • pulmonary wedge (pressure) • pulsed wave • puncture wound

P–W Prader–Willi (syndrome) *also* PW

P&W pressures and waves

Pw progesterone withdrawal

PWA people with acquired immunodeficiency syndrome

PWB partial weight bearing • psychologic well–being

PWBC peripheral white blood cell(s)

PWBRT prophylactic whole brain radiation therapy

PWC peak work capacity • physical work capacity

PWD precipitated withdrawal diarrhea • pulsed–wave Doppler

pwd powder *also* pdr, powd

PWE posterior wall excursion

PWI posterior wall infarct

PWLV posterior wall (of) left ventricle

PWM pokeweed mitogen

PWP pulmonary wedge pressure *also* Ppw

PWS port wine stain • Prader–Willi syndrome • pulse–wave speed

pwt pennyweight

PWV peak weight velocity • polistes wasp venom • posterior wall velocity • pulse wave velocity

PX pancreatectomized • peroxidase • physical examination *also* PE, Px

Px past history *also* PH • physical examination *also* PE, PX • pneumothorax *also* Pnx, PT, PTX • prognosis *also* prog, progn

PXE pseudoxanthoma elasticum

PXM projection x–ray microscopy

PY, P/Y pack–year (cigarettes) • person–year

Py phosphopyridoxal • polyoma (virus) • pyrene • pyridine

PYA psychoanalysis *also* PA

PYC proteose–yeast castione (medium)

PyC pyogenic culture

PYE peptone yeast extract

PYG peptone–yeast (extract)–glucose (broth)

PYGM peptone–yeast–glucose–maltose (broth)

PYLL potential years (of) life lost

PYM psychosomatic

PYP pyrophosphate *also* PP, Pyro

PYR person–year rad

Pyr pyridine • pyruvate

Pyro pyrophosphate *also* PP, PYP

PyrP pyridoxal phosphate

PYS pyriform sinus

PZ pancreozymin • peripheral zone • prazosin • pregnancy zone • proliferative zone

Pz parietal midline (zero) electrode placement in electroencephalography

pz pieze (unit of pressure)

PZA pyrazinamide

PzB parenzyme, buccal

PZ–CCK pancreozymin–cholecystokinin

PZD piperazinedione

PZE piezoelectric

PZI protamine zinc insulin

PZP pregnancy zone protein

Q cardiac output *also* CO, QT • clerical perception (General Aptitude Test Battery) • coenzyme Q (ubiquinone) *also* CoQ • coulomb *also* C • [L. *quaque*] each, every *also* q, qq • electrocardiographic wave • 1,4–glucan branching enzyme • glutamine *also* Gln • perfusion (flow) • quantitative *also* qt, quant • quantity *also* q, qt, qty, quant • quantity of heat • quart *also* q, qt • quarter *also* q, qr • quartile • query (fever) • question *also* quest. • quinacrine (fluorescent method) • quinidine • quinone • quotient *also* quot • radiant energy • reaction energy • reactive power • volume of blood flow

Q°, q° every hour

Q1° every hour around the clock

Q2° every two hours around the clock

Q–6, Q₆ ubiquinone–6 • ubiquinone–Q_6

Q₉ ubichromanol–9 • ubichromenol–9

Q₁₀ temperature coefficient • ubiquinone–50

q [L. *quaque*] each, every *also* Q, qq • electric charge • [L. *quattuor*] four *also* Quat, quat • frequency of rarer allele of a gene pair • long arm of chromosome • quantity *also* Q, qt, qty, quant • quart *also* Q, qt •

quarter *also* Q, qr • quintal • volume *also* V, vol

QA quality assessment • quality assurance • quinaldic acid • quisqualic acid

QAC quaternary ammonium compound

QALE quality–adjusted life expectancy

QALY quality–adjusted life years

QAM quality assurance monitor

Qa m, qAM, qam [L. *quaque ante meridiem*] every morning *also* qm

Q angle Quatrefages angle (parietal angle)

QAP quality assurance program • quinine, Atabrine (quinacrine hydrochloride), and pamaquine

QAR quality assurance reagent • quantitative autoradiographic

QA/RM quality assurance/risk management

QAS quality assurance standards

QAT quality assurance technical (material)

QAUR quality assurance (and) utilization review

QB Quantitative

(Electrophysiological) Battery • whole blood *also* WB, W Bld

Q_B blood flow *also* BF • total body clearance *also* TBC

QBC quality buffy coat

QBCA quantitative buffy–coat analysis

QBV whole blood volume

QC quality control • quick catheter • quinine (and) colchicine

Qc pulmonary capillary blood flow (perfusion)

QCA quantitative coronary angiography

QCD quantum chromodynamics

Q_{CO2} microliters of carbon dioxide given off per mg of dry weight of tissue per hour

Q_{CSF} rate of bulk flow of cerebrospinal fluid from cerebrospinal space by arachnoid villi uptake

QCT quantitative computed tomography

qd [L. *quaque die*] every day *also* qqd

qds [L. *quater die sumendum*] to be taken four times a day

QED quantum electrodynamics • [L. *quod erat demonstrandum*] that which is to be demonstrated *also* qed

qed [L. *quod erat demonstrandum*] that which is to be demonstrated *also* QED

QEE quadriceps extension exercise

QET Quality Extinction Test

QEW quick early warning

QF quality factor (relative biologic effectiveness) • query fever *also* Q fever • quick freeze

Q fever (Australian) query fever *also* QF

Q fract quick fraction

qh [L. *quaque hora*] every hour *also* qq hor

q2h [L. *quaque secunda hora*] every two hours

q3h [L. *quaque tertia hora*] every three hours

q4h [L. *quaque quarta hora*] every four hours *also* qqh

qhs [L. *quaque hora somni* every hour of sleep] each bedtime, every night

qid [L. *quater in die*] four times daily

QIg quantitative immunoglobulin

QJ quadriceps jerk

ql [L. *quantum libet*] as much as desired

QLS Quality of Life Scale

qlty quality

QM Quénu–Muret (sign) • quinacrine mustard

qm [L. *quaque mane*] every morning *also* Qa m, qAM, qam

QMI Q–wave myocardial infarction

QMT quantitative muscle testing

QMWS quasi–morphine withdrawal syndrome

qn [L. *quaque nocte*] every night

QNB quinuclidinyl benzilate

QNS, qns quantity not sufficient

Qo oxygen consumption *also* Q_{o2}

Q_{o2} oxygen consumption *also* Qo • oxygen quotient • oxygen utilization

QOC Quality of Contact

qod [L. *quaque altera die*] every other day

qoh [L. *quaque altera hora*] every other hour

qon [L. *quaque altera nocte*] every other night

QP quadrant pain • quanti–Pirquet (reaction)

Qp pulmonary blood flow *also* PBF

qp [L. *quantum placeat*] as much as desired

QPC quadrigeminal plate cistern • quality of patient care

Qpc pulmonary capillary blood flow

QPEEG quantitative pharmacoelectroencephalography

Qpm, qPM, qpm [L. *quaque post meridiem*] each evening

QP/QS ratio of pulmonary to systemic circulation

Qp/Qs left–to–right shunt ratio (electrocardiography)

QPVT Quick Picture Vocabulary Test

qq [L. *quoque*] also • [L. *quaque*] each or every *also* Q, q

qqd [L. *quoque die*] every day *also* qd

qqh [L. *quaque quarta hora*] every four hours *also* q4h

qq hor [L. *quaque hora*] every hour *also* qh

QR quality review • quadriradial • [L. *quantum rectum*] quantity is correct *also* qr • quieting reflex • Quick Recovery (Defibrillator) • quieting response • quiet room • quinaldine red

qr [L. *quantum rectum*] quantity is correct *also* QR • quarter *also* Q, q

QRB Quality Review Bulletin

Q–RB electrocardiographic time–wave interval

QRN quasiresonant nucleus

QRS electrocardiographic wave complex or interval

QRS–ST electrocardiographic junction between QRS complex and ST segment

QRS–T electrocardiographic angle between QRS and T vectors

QRZ [Ger. *Quaddel Reaktion Zeit*] wheal reaction time

QS quantity sufficient • quiet sleep

QS2 total electromechanical systole

Qs systemic blood flow

qs [L. *quantum sufficiat*] as much as may suffice · [L. *quantum satis*] sufficient quantity *also* q sat

qs ad [L. *quantum sufficiat ad*] sufficient quantity to make · [L. *quantum satis ad*] to a sufficient quantity

QSAR quantitative structure–activity relationship

q sat [L. *quantum satis*] sufficient quantity *also* qs

QSC quasistatic compliance

QS₂I shortened electrochemical systole

Qsp physiologic shunt flow

QSPV quasistatic pressure volume

Qs/Qt intrapulmonary shunt fraction · right–to–left shunt ratio

Qsrel relative shunt flow

QSS quantitative sacroiliac scintigraphy

Q's sign Quant's sign

Q–S test Queckenstedt–Stookey test

q suff [L. *quantum sufficit*] as much as suffices

QT blood volume (quantity) per unit time · cardiac output *also* CO, Q · qualification test · Queckenstedt test · Quick Test (psychology, pregnancy, prothrombin) *also* Q–T

Q–T electrocardiographic interval from the beginning of QRS complex to end of the T wave · Quick Test (psychology, pregnancy, prothrombin) *also* QT

Qt quiet *also* qt

qt quantitative *also* Q, quant · quantity *also* Q, q, qty, quant · quart *also* Q, qt · quiet *also* Qt

QTC quantitative tip culture

QT_c QT interval corrected for heart rate

qter end of long arm of chromosome

qty quantity *also* Q, q, qt, quant

quad quadrant · quadriceps · quadrilateral · quadriplegia

quad ex quadriceps exercise

quadrupl [L. *quadruplicato*] four times as much

qual qualitative · quality

qual anal qualitative analysis

quant quantitative *also* Q, qt · quantity *also* Q, q, qt, qty

quar quarantine

quart. [L. *quartus*] fourth · quadrantectomy, axillary dissection, and radiotherapy · quarterly

Quat, quat [L. *quattuor*] four *also* q

quats quaternary ammonium compounds

quer querulous

QUEST Quality, Utilization, Effectiveness, Statistically Tabulated

quest. question *also* Q • questionable

QuF (Australian) Q (Queensland) fever

QUICHA quantitative inhalation challenge apparatus

quinq [L. *quinque*] five

quint [L. *quintus*] fifth

quor [L. *quorum*] of which

quot [L. *quoties*] as often as necessary • [L. *quotidie*] daily *also* quotid • quotient *also* Q

quotid [L. *quotidie*] daily *also* quot

quot op sit, quot o s [L. *quoties opus sit*] as often as necessary

qv [L. *quantum vis*] as much as you desire • [L. *quod vide*] which see (literature citation)

QW quality of working (life) *also* QWL

qwk once a week

QWL quality of working life *also* QW

R arginine *also* ARG, Arg • Behnken's unit (of roentgen–ray exposure) • Broadbent registration point • drug–resistant plasmid • electrocardiographic wave in QRS complex • [L. *remotum*] far point *also* r • gas constant (8.315 joules) • metabolic respiratory quotient • organic radical • race • racemic • rad • radioactive *also* RA • radiology • radius *also* r, Ra, rad • ramus • range • Rankine • rare • rate • ratio • rationale • raw • reaction • reading • Réaumur • recessive • rectal • rectified average • rectum *also* rect • red (indicator color) *also* rub. • reference *also* ref • regimen • registered (trademark) *also* Reg • regression coefficient • regular *also* reg • regulator (gene) • rejection (factor) • relapse • relaxation • release (factor) • remission • remote point of convergence • repressor • resazurin • Resident • residuum • resistance (electrical) *also* RES • resistance determinant (plasmid) • resistance unit (in cardiovascular system) *also* RU • resistant • respiration *also* Resp, resp • respiratory exchange ratio *also* R$_E$, RER • response *also* resp • rest (cell cycle) • resting • restricted • reticulocyte *also* RET, RETIC, retic • reverse (banding) *also*

REV • review *also* REV • rhythm • rib • ribose *also* r, Rib • right *also* (R), RT, Rt, rt • Rinne (hearing test) • roentgen *also* r • rough (bacterial colony) • routine • rub • side chain in amino acid formula • [G. *Reiz*] stimulus *also* S, ST • [L. *recipe*] take • total response *also* TR

+R Rinne test positive

–R Rinne test negative

(R) rectal • right *also* R, RT, Rt rt

°R (degree) Rankine • (degree) Réaumur

R#1 good risk (for anesthesia)

R#2 fairly good risk (for anesthesia)

R#3 poor risk (for anesthesia)

R#4 very poor risk (for anesthesia)

r angle of refraction • correlation coefficient • [L. *remotum*] far point *also* R • radius *also* R, Ra, rad • reproductive potential • ribose *also* R, Rib • ring chromosome • roentgen *also* R • round • sample correlation coefficient

r^2 coefficient of determination

RA radioactive *also* R • radionuclide angiography *also* RNA • radium *also* Ra, Rad • ragocyte (cell) • ragweed antigen • rales • Raynaud (phenomenon) •

reading age • reciprocal asymmetrical • refractory anemia • refractory ascites • remittance advice • renal artery • renin activity • renin–angiotensin • repeat action (drugs) • residual air • retinoic acid • rheumatic arthritis • rheumatoid agglutinin *also* Rh agglut • rheumatoid arthritis • rifampicin • right angle • right arm • right atrial (pressure) • right atrium • right auricle • Rokintansky–Aschoff (sinues) • room air

R$_A$ airway resistance *also* AR

Ra radial *also* rad • radium *also* RA, Rad • radius *also* R, r, rad • Rayleigh number

rA riboadenylate

RAA renin–angiotensin–aldosterone (system) • right atrial abnormality

RAAGG rheumatoid arthritis agglutinin

RAAS renin–angiotensin–aldosterone system

RAB rice, applesauce, and bannana (diet) • remote afterload brachy therapy

Rab rabbit

RABA rabbit antibladder antibody

RABBI Rapid Access Blood Bank Information

RABCa rabbit antibladder cancer

RABG room air blood gas

RAbody right atrium body

RABP retinoic acid–binding protein

RAC radial artery catheter • right atrial contraction

rac racemate/racemic

RACCO right anterior caudocranial oblique

RACT recalcified (whole–blood)–activated clotting time

RAD radiation absorbed dose *also* rad • radical *also* rad • radiology *also* Rad, Radiol • reactive airway disease • right anterior descending • right atrial diameter • right axis deviation • roentgen administered dose

Rad radiologist *also* Radiol • radiology *also* RAD, Radiol • radiotherapist • radiotherapy *also* RADIO, Rad, Ther, RT, Rx • radium *also* RA, Ra

rad radial *also* Ra • radian • radiation absorbed dose *also* RAD • radical *also* RAD • radiculitis • radius *also* R, r, Ra • [L. *radix*] root

RADA right acromiodorso-anterior (fetal position)

RADCA right anterior descending coronary artery

rad imp radium implant

RADIO radiotherapy *also* Rad, Rad Ther, RT, Rx

Radiol radiologist *also* Rad • radiology *also* RAD, Rad

RAD ISO VENO BILAT
radioactive isotopic
venagram, bilateral

RADISH rheumatoid arthritis
diffuse idiopathic skeletal
hyperostosis

RadLV radiation leukemia
virus

RADP right acromiodorso-
posterior (fetal position)

RADS reactive airway disease
syndrome • retrospective
assessment (of) drug safety

rad/s radian per second

Rad Ther radiotherapy *also*
Rad, RADIO, RT, Rx

RADTS rabbit anti–dog–
thymus serum

Rad UI radius–ulna

RADWASTE radioactive
waste

RAE right atrial enlargement

RaE rabbit erythrocyte

RAEB refractory anemia,
erythroblastic • refractory
anemia with excess blasts

RAEB–T refractory anemia
with excess of blasts in
transformation

RAEM refractory anemia with
excess myeloblasts

RAF rheumatoid arthritis factor

Ra–F radium–F

RAG ragweed • room air gas

Ragg rheumatoid agglutinator

RAH radioactive Hippuran
(test) • regressing atypical
histiocytosis • right

anterior hemiblock *also*
RAHB • right atrial
hypertrophy

RAHB right anterior
hemiblock *also* RAH

RAHO rabbit antibody to
human ovary

RAHTG rabbit anti–human–
thymocyte globulin

RAI radioactive iodine •
resting ankle index • right
atrial involvement

RAID radioimmunodetection
also RID

RAIS reflection–absorption
infrared spectroscopy

RAIU radioactive iodine uptake
also RIU

RAL resorcylic acid lactone

RALT Riley Articulation and
Language Test • routine
admission laboratory tests

RAM radioactive material •
random–access memory •
rapid alternating
movements • research
aviation medicine • right
anterior measurement

RAMI Risk–adjusted Mortality
Index

RAMP radioactive antigen
microprecipitin • right
atrial mean pressure

RAMT rabbit anti–mouse
thymocyte

RAN resident's admission
notes

RANA rheumatoid arthritis
nuclear antigen

RAND random (sample,
specimen)

RANT right anterior

RAO right anterior oblique • right anterior occipital

RaONC radiation oncology

RAP recurrent abdominal pain • regression–associated protein • renal artery pressure • rheumatoid arthritis precipitin • right atrial pressure

RAPD relative afferent pupillary defect

RAPE right atrial pressure elevation

RAPM refractory anemia with partial myeloblastosis

RAPO rabbit antibody to pig ovary

RAQ right anterior quadrant

RAR rat insulin receptor • right arm reclining • right arm recumbent

RARLS rabbit anti–rat–lymphocyte serum

RARTS rabbit anti–rat–thymocyte serum

RAS recurrent aphthous stomatitis • reflex–activating stimulus • renal artery stenosis • renin–angiotensin system • reticular activating system • rheumatoid arthritis serum (factor)

ras [L. *rasurae*] scrapings, filings

RASP rapidly alternating speech

RASS rheumatoid arthritis (and) Sjögren syndrome

RAST radioallergosorbent test

RASV recovered avian sarcoma virus

RAT rat aortic tissue • repeat action tablet • rheumatoid arthritis (factor) test • right anterior thigh

RATA radioimmunologic assay antithyroid antibody

RATG rabbit antithymocyte globulin

RATHAS rat thymus antiserum

RATS rabbit antithymocyte serum

RATx radiation therapy

RAU radioactive uptake

RAUC raw area under curve

RAV Rouse–associated virus

RAW, R(AW), R_{AW} airway resistance

RAZ razoxane

RB rating board • rebreathing • Renaut body • respiratory bronchiole • respiratory burst • reticulate body • retinoblastoma • retrobulbar • right bundle • right buttock • round body

R&B right and below

Rb rubidium

RBA relative binding affinity • rescue breathing apparatus • right basilar artery • right brachial artery • rose bengal antigen

RBAF rheumatoid biologically active factor

RBAP repetitive bursts (of) action potential

RBB right breast biopsy • right bundle–branch

RBBB right bundle–branch block

RBBsB right bundle branch system block

RBBX right breast biopsy examination

RBC red blood cell • red blood corpuscle • red blood (cell) count

RBC–ADA red blood cell adenosine deaminase

RBCD right border cardiac dullness

RBC FO red blood cell fallout

RBC frag red blood cell fragility

RBC/hpf red blood cells per high power field

RBCM red blood cell mass

RBC/P red blood cell to plasma (ratio)

RBC s/f red blood cells spun filtration

RBCV red blood cell volume

RBD right border of dullness (percussion of heart)

RBE relative biologic effectiveness

RBF regional blood flow • renal blood flow • riboflavin

RBG random blood glucose

Rb Imp rubber base impression

RBL rat basophilic leukemia • Reid baseline

RBM Raji (cell)–binding material • regional bone mass

RBME regenerating bone marrow extract

RBN retrobulbar neuritis

RBOW rupture of bag of waters

RBP resting blood pressure • retinol–binding protein • riboflavin–binding protein

RBR radiation bowel reaction

RBS random blood sugar • Rutherford backscattering

RbSA rabbit serum albumin *also* RSA

RBU Raji (cell)–binding unit

RBV right brachial vein

RB–V right bundle ventricular

RBW relative body weight

RBZ rubidazone (zorubicin)

RC radiocarpal • reaction center • receptor–chemo-effector (complex) *also* RCC • recrystallized • red cell • red (cell) cast *also* RCC • red corpuscle • Red Cross • referred care • reflection coefficient • regenerated cellulose • resistance (and) capacitance • respiration cease • respiratory care • respiratory center • response, conditioned *also* Rc • rest cure • retention catheter *also* ret cath • retrograde cystogram • rib cage • right ear, cold stimulus • Roman Catholic • root canal • rotator cuff • Roussy–Cornil (syndrome) • routine cholecystectomy

R/C reclining chair

Rc response, conditioned *also* RC • receptor

RCA radionuclide cerebral angiogram • Raji cell assay • red cell adherence • red cell agglutination • relative chemotactic activity • renal cell carcinoma • retrograde to the atria • right carotid artery • right coronary artery

rCBF regional cerebral blood flow

RCBV regional cerebral blood volume

RCC radiographic coronary calcification • radiologic control center • rape crisis center • ratio of cost to charges • receptor–chemoeffector complex *also* RC • red cell cast *also* RC • red cell concentrate • red cell count • renal cell carcinoma • right common carotid • right coronary cusp

Rcc radiochemical

RCCA right common carotid artery

RCCT randomized controlled clinical trial • results (of) clinical controlled trial

RCD relative (area of) cardiac dullness

RCDR relative corrected death rate

RCE reasonable compensation equivalent

RCF red cell filterability • red cell folate • Reiter complement fixation • relative centrifugal field/force • ristocetin cofactor *also* RCoF

RCFS reticulocyte cell–free system

RCG radioelectrocardiography *also* RECG

RCH rectocolic hemorrhage

RCHF right–sided congestive heart failure

RCI rate change induced • respiratory control index

RCIA red cell immune adherence

RCIT red cell iron turnover

RCITR red cell iron turnover rate

RCL range of comfortable loudness • renal clearance

RCLAAR red cell–linked antigen–antiglobulin reaction

RCM radiocontrast material • radiographic contrast medium • red cell mass • reinforced clostridial medium • replacement culture medium • retinal capillary microaneurysm • rheumatoid cervical myelopathy • right costal margin • Roux conditioned medium

RCMI red cell morphology index

rCMRO$_2$ regional cerebral metabolic rate for oxygen

RCN right caudate nucleus

RCoF ristocetin cofactor *also* RCF

RCP random chemistry profile • retrocorneal pigmentation • riboflavin carrier protein

rcp reciprocal (translocation)

RCPH red cell peroxide hemolysis

RCPM Raven Colored Progressive Matrix

RCQG right caudal quarter ganglion

RCR relative consumption rate • respiratory control ratio

RCRS Rehabilitation Client Rating Scale

RCS rabbit (aorta)–contracting substance • red cell suspension • repeat cesarean section *also* R/CS • reticulum cell sarcoma • right coronary sinus

R/CS repeat cesarean section *also* RCS

RCT randomized clinical trial • red colloidal test • retrograde conduction time • root canal therapy • Rorschach content test

RC TNTC red cells too numerous to count

RCU respiratory care unit

RCV red cell volume

RD radial deviation • rate difference • Raynaud disease • reaction of degeneration • reaction of

denervation • reflex decay • Registered Dietician • Reiter disease • renal disease • Rénon–Delille (syndrome) • resistance determinant • respiratory disease • respiratory distress • retinal detachment • Reye disease • rheumatoid disease • right deltoid • right dorsoanterior • Riley–Day (syndrome) • rubber dam • ruptured disk

R&D research and development

Rd reading • rutherford (unit of radioactivity) *also* rd

rd reading • rutherford *also* Rd

RDA recommended daily allowance • recommended dietary allowance • Registered Dental Assistant • right dorsoanterior (fetal position) • rubidium dihydrogen arsenate

RdA reading age

RDB randomized double–blind (trial) • research and development board

RDC research diagnostic criteria

RDDA recommended daily dietary allowance

RDDP ribonucleic acid–dependent deoxynucleic acid polymerase *also* RDPase • ribonucleic acid–directed deoxynucleic acid polymerase

RDE receptor–destroying enzyme

RDEB recessive dystrophic epidermolysis bullosa

RDES remote data entry system

RDFC recurring digital fibroma (of) childhood

RDFS ratio (of) decayed (and) filled surfaces (teeth)

RDFT ratio (of) decayed (and) filled teeth

RDG Research Discussion Group · right dorsogluteal

RDH Registered Dental Hygienist

RDHBF regional distribution (of) hepatic blood flow

RDI recommended daily intake · recommended dietary intake · rupture–delivery interval

RDIH right direct inguinal hernia

RDLBBB rate–dependent left bundle–branch block

RDLS Reynell Development Language Scales (psychologic test)

RDM readmission *also* Rdm · rod disk membrane

Rdm readmission *also* RDM

RDMS Registered Diagnostic Medical Sonographer

rDNA recombinant deoxyribonucleic acid · ribosomal deoxyribonucleic acid

RDOD retinal detachment, oculus dexter (right eye)

RDOS retinal detachment, oculas sinister (left eye)

RDP radiopharmaceutical drug product · right dorsoposterior (fetal positon)

RDPase ribonucleic acid–dependent deoxyribonucleic acid polymerase *also* RDDP

RDPE reticular degeneration of pigment epithelium

RDQ respiratory disease questionnaire

RdQ reading quotient *also* RG

RDRC radioactive drug research committee

RDRV rhesus diploid (cell strain) rabies vaccine

RDS research diagnostic (criteria) · respiratory distress syndrome · reticuloendothelial depressing substance

RDT regular (hemo)dialysis treatment · retinal damage threshold · routine dialysis therapy

RDTD referral, diagnosis, treatment, and discharge

RDVT recurrent deep vein thrombosis

RDW red (blood cell) distribution width (index)

RE concerning *also* re · racemic epinephrine · radium emanation · readmission · rectal examination · reflux esophagitis · regional enteritis · regular education · renal (and) electrolyte · renal excretion · resting energy · reticuloendothelial · retinol

equivalent • right ear •
right eye • ring
enhancement • rostral end

R_E repiratory exchange ratio
also R, RER

R&E research and education •
rest and exercise • round
and equal

R↑E right upper extremity

RE√ recheck

Re rhenium

R_e Reynold number

re concerning *also* RE •
regarding

REA radiation emergency
area • radioenzymatic
assay • renal anastomosis •
right ear advantage

REACH Reassurance to Each
(assistance to family of
mentally ill)

readm readmission

REAS reasonably expected as
safe

REAT radiologic emergency
assistance team

REB roentgen–equivalent
biologic

R–EBD–HS recessive
epidermolysis bullosa
dystrophica–Hallopeau–
Siemen (syndrome)

REC radioelectrocomplexing •
rear end collision •
receptor • recommend •
record *also* rec • recovery •
recreation *also* rec • recur •
right external carotid

rec reactive • [L. *recens*]
fresh • recent •

recombinant chromosome •
recommendation • record
also REC • recreation *also*
REC • recurrent/recurrence
also recur

RECA right external carotid
artery

recd, rec'd received

RE CEL reticulum cell(s)

RECG radioelectro-
cardiography *also* RCG

recip recipient • reciprocal

recon [recombination + Ger.
on quantum] smallest unit
of DNA capable of
recombination

recond reconditioning/
reconditioned

reconstr reconstruction

recryst recrystallization

rect rectification/rectified •
rectum/rectal *also* R •
rectus (muscle)

recur recurrence/recurrent *also*
rec

RED radiation experience
data • rapid erythrocyte
degeneration

Re–D re–evaluation deadline

red. reduce/reducing •
reduction *also* redn

redig in pulv [L. *redigatur in
pulverem*] let it be reduced
to powder

red in pulv [L. *reductus in
pulverem*] reduced to
powder

redn reduction *also* red.

redox oxidation–reduction

REE rapid extinction effect · rare earth element · resting energy expenditure

re–ed re–education

REEDS retention (of tears), ectrodactyly, ectodermal dysplasia, (and) strange (hair, skin, and teeth syndrome)

REEG radioelectro-encephalography

R–EEG resting electroencephalogram

REELS Receptive–Expressive Emergent Language Scale

REEP right end–expiratory pressure · role exchange/education–practice

ReEND reproductive endocrinology

REF ejection fraction at rest · referred · refused · renal erythropoietic factor

ref reference *also* R · reflex *also* Refl

Ref Doc referring doctor

REFI regional ejection fraction image

ref ind refractive index *also* RI

Refl reflect · reflection · reflex *also* ref

REFMS Recreation and Education for Multiple Sclerosis (Victims)

Ref Phys referring physician

REFRAD released from active duty

REG radiation exposure guide · radioen-cephalogram/radioen-cephalography · rheoencephalography

Reg registered *also* R

reg regarding · region · regular *also* R · regulation

regen regenerate · regeneration

reg rhy regular rhythm

reg R&R regular rate and rhythm

reg umb [L. *regio umbilici*] umbilical region

regurg regurgitation

REH renin essential hypertension

REHAB, rehab rehabilitation/rehabilitated

REL rate of energy loss · relative · religion · resting expiratory level

rel related · relation · relative

RELE resistive exercises, lower extremities

reliq [L. *reliquus*] remainder

REM radiation–equivalent–man · rapid eye movement (sleep) · recent event memory · reticular erythematous mucinosis · return electrode monitor · roentgen–equivalent–man *also* rem

Rem, rem removal

rem removal *also* Rem · roentgen–equivalent–man *also* REM

REMA repetitive excess mixed anhydride (method)

REMAB radiation–equivalent–manikin absorption

REMCAL radiation–equivalent–manikin calibration

REMP roentgen–equivalent–man period

REMS rapid eye movement sleep

REN, ren renal *also* RN

ren [L. *renoveatur*] renew

ren sem [L. *renovetum semel*] renew only once

REO respiratory enteric orphan (virus)

REP (surgical) repair • repeat *also* rept • report *also* rep, rept • rest–exercise program • retrograde pyelogram *also* RP • roentgen equivalent–physical *also* rep

rep [L. *repetatur*] let it be repeated • replication • report *also* REP, rept • roentgen equivalent–physical *also* REP

rep B&S repetitive bending and stooping

REPC reticuloendothelial phagocytic capacity

repet [L. *repetatur*] to be repeated

repol repolarization

REPS reactive extensor postural synergy • repetitions

rept repeat *also* REP • report *also* REP, rep

req requested • required

REQF wrong test requested—floor error

RER renal excretion rate • respiratory exchange ratio *also* R, R_E • rough endoplasmic reticulum

RES (electrical) resistance *also* R • resection • resident • reticuloendothelial system

Res research *also* res

res research *also* Res • reserve • residence • resident • residue

RESC, resc resuscitation *also* resus

resist. ex. resistive exercise

Resp respectively *also* resp • respiration/respiratory *also* R, resp

resp respiration/respiratory *also* R, Resp • respective/respectively *also* Resp • response *also* R • responsible

RESP–A respiratory battery, acute

REST Raynaud (phenomenon), esophageal (motor dysfunction), sclerodactyly, (and) telangiectasia (syndrome) • regressive electric shock therapy • restoration • reticulospinal tract

resus resuscitation *also* RESC, resc

RET rational–emotive therapy • retention • reticulocyte *also* R, RETIC, retic • retina • retired *also* ret • return • right esotropia

ret rad equivalent therapeutic • retired *also* RET

RETC rat embryo tissue culture

ret cath retention catheter *also* RC

RETIC, retic reticulocyte *also* R, RET

Retro Pyelo retrograde pyelogram

RETUL reticulum cell(s)

REUE resistive exercises to upper extremities

REV reticuloendotheliosis virus • reversal • reverse *also* R • review *also* R • revolution *also* rev

REV, rev reverse • review • revolution

REVL to be reviewed by laboratory (pathologist)

rev/min revolution per minute

Rev of Sym review of symptoms

Rev of Sys review of systems

re-x re-examination

RF radial fiber (of cochlea) • radiofrequency *also* rf • rate of flow (chromatography) *also* R_F • receptive field (of visual cortex) • recognition factor • reflecting (platelet) • regurgitant fraction • Reitland–Franklin (unit) • relative flow • relative fluorescence • release factor • renal failure • replicative form • resistance factor • resorcinol formaldehyde • respiratory failure •

respiratory frequency *also* Rf • retardation factor *also* Rf • reticular formation • retroflexed • retroperitoneal fibromatosis • rheumatic fever • rheumatoid factor • riboflavin • Riga–Fede (syndrome) • risk factor • root (canal) filling • rosette formation • Rundles–Falls (syndrome)

R&F radiographic and fluoroscopic

R_F rate of flow *also* RF

Rf respiratory frequency *also* RF • retardation factor *also* RF • rutherfordium

rf radiofrequency *also* RF

RFA right femoral artery • right forearm • right frontoanterior (fetal position)

RFB retained foreign body • rheumatoid factor binding

RFC retrograde femoral catheter • right frontal craniotomy • rosette–forming cell

RFE relative fluorescence efficiency

RFFIT rapid fluorescent focus inhibition test

RFI recurrence–free interval • renal failure index

RFL right frontolateral (fetal position)

RFLA rheumatoid–factor–like activity

RFLC resistant Friend leukemia cell

RFLP restriction fragment length polymorphism

RFLS rheumatoid–factor–like substance

RFM, Rfm rifampin

RFOL results to follow

RFP request for payment • request for proposals • right frontoposterior (fetal position)

RFR rapid filling rate • refraction

RFS rapid frozen section • relapse–free survival • renal function study

RFT right fibrous trigone • right frontotransverse (fetal position) • rod–and–frame test • routine fever therapy

RFTB riboflavin tetrabutyrate

RFTSW right foot switch

RFV right femoralvein

RFW rapid filling wave

RG retrograde • right gluteal

R/G red/green

Rg Rodgers antibodies

RGAS retained gastric antrum syndrome

RGBMT renal glomerular basement membrane thickness

RGC radio–gas chromatography • remnant gastric cancer • retinal ganglion cell • right giant cell

RGD range–gated Doppler

RGE relative gas expansion • respiratory gas equation

RGH rat growth hormone

RGM right gluteus maximus

RGMT reciprocal geometric mean titer

RGN Registered General Nurse

RGO reciprocating gait orthosis

RGP retrograde pyelogram • rural general practitioner

RGR relative growth rate

RGT reversed gastric tube

RH radial hemolysis • radiant heat • radiologic health • reactive hyperemia • recurrent herpes • reduced haloperidol • regional heparinization • regulatory hormone • relative humidity • releasing hormone • rest home • retinal hemorrhage • Richner–Hanhart (syndrome) • right hand • right hemisphere • right hyperphoria • room humidifier

Rh Rhesus (blood factor) • rhinion (craniometric point) • rhodium • rhonchi *also* rh

Rh+ Rhesus positive

Rh– Rhesus negative

rh rheumatic • rhonchi *also* Rh

r/h roentgen per hour

RHA right hepatic artery

RhA rheumatoid arthritis

Rh agglut rheumatoid agglutinins *also* RA

RHB raise head (of) bed •
right heart bypass

RHBF reactive hyperemia
blood flow

RHBV right–heart blood
volume

RHC resin hemoperfusion
column • respiration has
ceased • right heart
catheterization • right
hypochondrium

RHD radial head dislocation •
radiologic health data •
relative hepatic dullness •
renal hypertensive disease •
rheumatic heart disease •
round heart disease

RhD Rhesus (hemolytic)
disease

RHE respiratory heat exchange

RHEED reflection high–energy
electron diffraction

rheo rheostat

rheu, rheum rheumatic •
rheumatoid

rheu ht dis rheumatic heart
disease

RHF right heart failure

RHG radial hemolysis (in)
gel • relative hemoglobin •
right hand grip

RHH right homonymous
hemianopia

Rhi, Rhin rhinology

RhIG Rhesus immune globulin

Rhin rhinologist • rhinology

rhin rhinitis

rhino rhinoplasty

RHL recurrent herpes labialis •

right hemisphere lesion •
right hepatic lobe

RHLN right hilar lymph node

rhm roentgen per hour at one
meter

rHm EPO recombinant human
erythropoietin

RhMK, RhMk, RhMkK
Rhesus monkey kidney *also*
RMK

RHMV right heart mixing
volume

RHN Rockwell hardness
number

Rh$_{null}$ Rhesus factor null (all
Rh factors are lacking)

RHO right heeloff

rho (P, ρ) seventeenth letter of
Greek alphabet

ρ electrical resistivity •
electric charge density •
mass density • population
correlation coefficient •
reactivity

rhom rhomboid (muscle)

RHP right hemiparesis • right
hemiplegia

RHPA reverse hemolytic
plaque assay

RHR resting heart rate

r/hr roentgens per hour

RHS right hand side • right
heelstrike • rough hard
sphere

RHT renal homotransplan-
tation • right hypertropia

RHU Registered Health
Underwriter •
rheumatology

RHW radiant heat warmer

RI input resistor • radiation intensity • radioimmunology • radioisotope • recession index • recombinant inbred (strain) • refractive index *also* ref ind • regenerative index • regional ileitis • regular insulin • relative intensity • release inhibition • remission induced/induction • renal insufficiency • replicative intermediate • respiratory illness • respiratory index • reticulocyte index • retroactive inhibition • retroactive interference • ribosome • right iliac (crest) • rooming in • rosette inhibition

R/I rule in

RIA radioimmune assay • radioimmunoassay • reversible ischemic attack • right iliac artery

RIA–DA radioimmunoassay double antibody (test)

RIAST Reitan Indiana Aphasic Screening Test

RIAT radioimmune antiglobulin test

Rib ribose *also* R, r

RIBS rutherford ion backscattering

RIC renomedullary interstitial cell • right iliac crest • right internal capsule • right internal carotid

RICA reverse immune cytoadhesion • right internal carotid artery

RICE rest, ice, compression, elevation

RICM right intercostal margin

RICS right intercostal space

RICU respiratory intensive care unit

RID radial immunodiffusion • radioimmunodetection *also* RAID • radioimmuno-diffusion • remission–inducing drug • remove intoxicated driver • right (ventricular) internal diameter • ruptured intervertebral disk

RIDCSF radial immuno-diffusion cerebrospinal fluid

RIE, RIEP rocket immunoelectrophoresis

RIF release–inhibiting factor • rifampin • right iliac fossa • right index finger • rigid internal fixation • rosette inhibitory factor

RIFA radioiodinated fatty acid

RIFC rat intrinsic factor concentrate

RIG rabies immune globulin

RIGH rabies immune globulin, human

RIH right inguinal hernia

RIHSA radioactive iodinated human serum albumin

RIJ right internal jugular (vein or catheter)

RILT rabbit ileal loop test

RIM radioisotope medicine • recurrent induced malaria • relative–intensity measure •

RIMA right internal mammary anastomosis • right internal mammary artery

RIMS resonance ionization mass spectrometry

RIN rat insulinoma

RIND resolving ischemic neurologic deficit • reversible ischemic neurologic deficit

RINN recommended international nonproprietary name

RIOJ recurrent intrahepatic obstructive jaundice

RIP radioimmunoprecipin (test) • rapid infusion pump • reflex–inhibiting pattern • respiratory inductance plethysmography

RIPA radioimmunoprecipitation assay

RIR right iliac region • right inferior rectus

RIRB radioiodinated rose bengal (dye)

RIS rapid immunofluorescence staining • resonance ionization spectroscopy

RISA radioiodinated serum albumin • radioimmunosorbent assay

RIST radioimmunosorbent test

RIT radioiodinated triolein • Rorschack Inkblot Test *also* Ror • rosette inhibition titer

RITC rhodamine isothiocyanate • rhodamine isothiocyanate conjugated

RIU radioactive iodine uptake *also* RAIU

RIV ramus interventricularis • right innominate vein

RIVC radionuclide (imaging of) inferior vena cava • right inferior vena cava

RIVD ruptured intervertebral disk

RIVS ruptured interventricular septum

RJ radial jerk (reflex)

RJI radionuclide joint imaging

RK rabbit kidney • radial keratotomy • right kidney

RKG radio(electro)cardiogram

RKH Rokitansky–Kuster–Hauser (syndrome)

RKID right kidney (urine sample)

RKS renal kidney stone • retrograde kidney study

RKV rabbit kidney vacuolating (virus)

RKW renal kalium (potassium) wasting

RKY roentgen kymography

RL coarse rales • radiation laboratory • reduction level • resistive load • reticular lamina • right lateral *also* R LAT, R Lat • right leg • right lower • right lung • Ringer lactate (solution) *also* RLS

R L, R–L, R/L, R→L right to left (shunt)

R$_L$ pulmonary resistance *also* R$_L$R$_P$

RL$_3$ numerous coarse rales

Rl medium rales

RI$_2$ moderate number of medium rales

rl fine rales

rl$_1$ few fine rales

RLA radiographic lung area

R Lat, R LAT right lateral *also* RL

RLBCD right lower border of cardiac dullness

RLC rectus (and) longus capitus • residual lung capacity • rhodopsin–lipid complex

RLD related living donor • resistive load detection • right lateral decubitus (position) • ruptured lumbar disk

RLE Recent Life Events • right lower extremity

RLF retained lung fluid • retrolental fibroplasia • right lateral femoral

RLL right liver lobe • right lower lobe

RLMD rat liver mitochondria (and submitochondrial particles derived by) digitonin (treatment)

RLN recurrent laryngeal nerve • regional lymph node

RLNC regional lymph node cell

RLND regional lymph node dissection • retroperitoneal lymph node dissection

RLO residual lymphocyte output

RLP radiation leukemia protection • ribosome–like particle

RLQ right lower quadrant (of abdomen)

RLR right lateral rectus (muscle)

R$_L$R$_P$ pulmonary resistance *also* R$_L$

RLS person who stammers having difficulty in enunciating R, L, and S • rat lung strip • restless leg syndrome • Ringer lactate solution *also* RL

RLSB right lower scapular border • right lower sternal border

rl–sh right–left shunt

RLT right lateral thigh

RLTCS repeat low transverse cesarean section

RLV Rauscher leukemia virus

RLWD routine laboratory work done

RLX right lower extremity

RM radical mastectomy • random migration • range of movement • red marrow • reference material • regional myocardial • rehabilitation medicine • repetition maximum • resistive movement • respiratory metabolism • respiratory movement • right median • risk management • room • Rosenthal–Melkersson (syndrome) • Rothmann–Makai (syndrome) • ruptured membranes

R&M routine and microscopic

Rm relative mobility • remission

rm room

RMA Registered Medical Assistant • relative medullary area (of kidney) • right mentoanterior (fetal position)

RMB right main–stem bronchus

RMBF regional myocardial blood flow

RMC right middle cerebral (artery)

RMCA right main coronary artery • right middle cerebral artery

RMCAT right middle cerebral artery thrombosis

RMCL right midclavicular line

RMCP rat mast cell protease

RMCT rat mast cell technique

RMD rapid movement disorder • ratio (of) midsagittal diameters • retromanubrial dullness • right manubrial dullness

RME rapid maxillary expansion • resting metabolic expenditure • right mediolateral episiotomy *also* RMLE

RMEE right middle ear exploration

RMF right middle finger

RMI Reading Miscue Inventory

RMK Rhesus monkey kidney *also* RhMK, RhLMk, RhMkK

RML radiation myeloid leukemia • right mediolateral • right

mentolateral • right middle lobe (of lung)

RMLB right middle lobe bronchus

RMLE right mediolateral episiotomy *also* RME

RMLS right middle lobe syndrome

RMLV Rauscher murine leukemia virus *also* RMuLV

RMM rapid micromedia method

RMO Resident Medical Officer

RMP rapidly miscible pool • resting membrane potential • rifampin • right mento-posterior (fetal position)

RMR resting metabolic rate • right medial rectus (muscle)

RMS rectal morphine sulfate (suppository) • repetitive motion syndrome • respiratory muscle strength • rheumatic mitral stenosis • rhodomyosarcoma

RMS, rms root–mean–square

RMSD root–mean–square deviation

RMSE root mean square error

RMSF Rocky Mountain spotted fever

RMT Registered Music Therapist • relative medullary thickness • retromolar trigone • right mentotransverse (fetal position)

RMUI relief medication unit index

RMuLV Rauscher murine leukemia virus *also* RMLV

RMV respiratory minute volume

RN radionuclide • red nucleus • reflex nephropathy • Registered Nurse • renal (disease) *also* REN, ren • reticular nucleus

Rn radon

RNA radionuclide angiography *also* RA • Registered Nurse Anesthetist • ribonucleic acid • rough, noncapsulated, avirulent (bacterial culture)

RNAA radiochemical neutron activation analysis

RNAse, RNase ribonuclease

RND radical neck dissection • reactive neurotic depression

RNEF resting (radio)nuclide ejection fraction

RNG radionuclide angiography

RNICU regional neonatal intensive care unit

RNL renal laboratory profile

RNMT Registered Nuclear Medicine Technologist

RNP Registered Nurse Practitioner • ribonucleoprotein

RNR ribonucleotide reductase

RNS reference normal serum

RNSC radionuclide superior cavography

RNT radioassayable neurotensin

Rnt roentgenology *also* roent

RNTC rat nephroma tissue culture

RNV radionuclide venography • radionuclide ventriculography *also* RNVG

RNVG radionuclide ventriculography *also* RNV

RO reality orientation • relative odds • reverse osmosis • Ritter–Oleson (technique) • routine order • rule out *also* R/O

R/O rule out *also* RO

R$_o$ resting radium

ROA right occipitoanterior (fetal position)

ROAC repeated oral (doses of) activated charcoal

ROAD reversible obstructive airway disease

ROATS rabbit ovarian antitumor serum

rob. robertsonian (translocation)

ROC receiver operating characteristic • relative operating characteristic • resident on call • residual organic carbon

roc reciprocal ohm centimeter

RODAC replicate organism detection and counting

ROE return on equity • roentgen *also* roent

roent roentgen *also* ROE • roentgenology *also* Rnt

ROH rat ovarian hyperemia (test)

ROI region of interest

ROIDS hemorrhoids

ROIH right oblique inguinal hernia

ROL right occipitolateral (fetal position)

ROM range of motion · range of movement · read–only memory · right otitis media · rupture of membranes

Rom, Romb Romberg (sign)

rom reciprocal ohm meter

ROM C P range of motion complete (and) pain–free

ROMI rule out myocardial infarction

ROMSA right otitis media, suppurative, acute

ROMSC right otitis media, suppurative, chronic

ROM WNL range of motion within normal limits

ROP retinopathy of prematurity · right occipito-posterior (fetal position)

Ror Rorschach (Inkblot Test) *also* RIT

ROS review of symptoms *also* RS · review of systems *also* RS · rod outer segment

RoS rostral sulcus

ROSC restoration of spontaneous circulation

ROSS review of subjective symptoms · review other subjective symptoms

ROT real oxygen transport · remedial occupational therapy · right occipito-transverse (fetal position) · rotating *also* Rot, rot. · rotator · rule of thumb

Rot, rot. rotating/rotation *also* ROT

rot. ny rotatory nystagmus

ROU recurrent oral ulcer

rout routine

ROW rat ovarian weight · Rendu–Osler–Weber (syndrome)

RP radial pulse · radiographic planimetry · radiopharmaceutical · rapid processing (of film) · Raynaud phenomenon · reaction product · reactive protein · readiness potential · rectal prolapse · re–entrant pathway · refractory period · regulatory protein · relapsing polychondritis · relative potency · respiratory rate:pulse rate (index) · resting potential · resting pressure · rest pain · retinitis pigmentosa · retinitis proliferans *also* R Pr · retrograde pyelogram *also* REP · retroperitoneal · reverse phase · rheumatoid polyarthritis · ribose phosphate

R$_p$ pulmonary resistance

RPA radial photon absorptiometry · resultant physiologic acceleration · reverse passive anaphylaxis · right pulmonary artery

RPAW right pulmonary artery withdrawal

rPBF regional pulmonary blood flow

RPC relapsing polychondritis · relative proliferative capacity

RPCF, RPCFT Reiter protein complement fixation test

RPCGN rapidly progressive crescenting glomerulonephritis

RPCV retropubic cytourethropexy

RPD removable partial denture

RPE rate (of) perceived exertion • recurrent pulmonary emboli • retinal pigment epithelium

RPF relaxed pelvic floor • renal plasma flow • retroperitoneal fibrosis

RPF^a arterial renal plasma flow

RPF^V venous renal plasma flow

RPG radiation protection guide • retrograde pyelogram • rheoplethysmography

RPGG retroplacental gamma globulin

RPGN rapidly progressive glomerulonephritis

RPH retroperitoneal hemorrhage

RPh Registered Pharmacist

RPHA reversed passive hemagglutination

RPHAMCFA reversed passive hemagglutination by miniature centrifugal fast analysis

RP–HPLC reversed phase high–performance liquid chromatography

RPI reticulocyte production index

RPICA right posterior internal carotid artery

RPICCE round pupil intracapsular cataract extraction

RPIPP reversed phase ion–pair partition

RPL, RPLAD retroperitoneal lymphadenectomy

RPLC reversed–phase liquid chromatography

RPLD repair of potentially lethal damage

RPLND retroperitoneal lymph node dissection

RPM, rpm radical pair mechanism • rapid processing mode • revolutions per minute

RPMD rheumatic pain modulation disorder

RPN renal papillary necrosis • resident's progress note

RPO right posterior oblique (radiologic view)

RPP (heart) rate–(systolic blood) pressure product • retropubic prostatectomy

RPPC regional pediatric pulmonary center

RPPI role perception picture inventory

RPPR red (cell) precursor production rate

RPR rapid plasma reagent (test) • Reiter protein reagin

R Pr retinitis proliferans *also* RP

RPRCF rapid plasma reagin complement fixation

RPRCT rapid plasma reagin card test

RPS renal pressor substance

RPS, rps revolutions per second

RPT rapid pull–through • refractory period of transmission • Registered Physical Therapist

rpt repeat • report

RPTA renal percutaneous transluminal angioplasty

Rptd ruptured

RPU retropubic urethropexy

RPV right portal vein • right pulmonary vein

RPVP right posterior ventricular pre–excitation

RQ reading quotient *also* RdQ • recovery quotient • respiratory quotient

RR radial rate • radiation reaction • radiation response • rapid radiometric • rate ratio • reading retarded • recovery room • red reflex • regular rate • regular respiration • relative response • relative risk • renin release • respiratory rate • respiratory reserve • response rate • retinal reflex • rheumatoid rosette • right rotation • risk ratio • Riva–Rocci (sphygmomanometer) *also* RRS • road rash • roentgenographic pelvimetry • ruthenium red

R/R rales/ronchi

R&R rate and rhythm • recent and remote • recession and resection • rest and recuperation

Rr rami

RRA radioreceptor activity • radioreceptor assay • Registered Record Administrator • right renal artery

RRAM rapid rhythmic alternating movements

RRBC rabbit red blood cell

RRC residency review committee • risk reduction component • routine respiratory care

RRCT no(m) regular rate, clear tones, no murmurs

RRE radiation–related eosinophilia • regressive resistive exercise

RRE, RR&E round, regular, and equal (pupils)

RREF resting radionuclide ejection fraction

RRF residual renal function

RR–HPO rapid recompression–high pressure oxygen

RRI reflex relaxation index • relative response index

RRL Registered Record Librarian

rRNA ribosomal ribonucleic acid

RRND right radical neck dissection

RROM resistive range of motion

RRP relative refractory period

RRQG right rostal quarter ganglion

RRR regular rhythm and rate • renin–release ratio • risk rescue rating

RRRN round, regular, react normally (pupils)

RRS retrorectal space • Richards–Rundle syndrome • Riva–Rocci sphygmomanometer *also* RR

RRT randomized response technique • Registered Respiratory Therapist • relative retention time • resazurin reduction time

RRU respiratory resistance unit

RRV right renal vein

RS random sample • rapid smoking • rating schedule • Raynaud syndrome • reading (of) standard • recipient's serum • rectal sinus • rectosigmoid • Reed–Sternberg (cell) • reinforcing stimulus • Reiter syndrome • relative survival • remnant stomach • renal specialist • Repression–Sensitization (Scale) • reproductive success • resolved sarcoidosis • resorcinol–sulfur • respiratory syncytial (virus) • respiratory system • response (to) stimulus (ratio) • reticulated siderocyte *also* R–S • review (of) symptoms *also*

ROS • review (of) systems *also* ROS • Reye syndrome • rhythm strip • right sacrum • right septum • right side • right stellate (ganglion) • right subclavian • Ringer solution • Ritchie sedimentation • Roberts syndrome

R–S reticulated siderocyte *also* RS • rough–smooth (variation)

R/S rest stress • rupture spontaneous

R&S restraint and seclusion

Rs respond/response • (total) systemic resistance

R/s roentgen per second

r_s rank correlation coefficient

RSA rabbit serum albumin *also* RbSA • rat serum albumin • regular spiking activity • relative specific activity • relative standard accuracy • respiratory sinus arrhythmia • reticulum (cell) sarcoma • right sacro-anterior (fetal position) • right subclavian artery

Rsa (total) systemic arterial resistance

RSB reticulocyte standard buffer • right sternal border

RSBT rhythmic sensory bombardment therapy

RSC rat spleen cell • rested–state contraction • reversible sickle cell • right side colon (cancer)

RScA right scapuloanterior (fetal position)

RSCN Registered Sick Children's Nurse

RScP right scapuloposterior (fetal position)

rscu–PA recombinant, single–chain, urokinase–type plasminogen activator

RSD reflex sympathetic dystrophy • relative sagittal depth • relative standard deviation

RSDS reflex sympathetic dystrophy syndrome

RSE rat synaptic ending • reverse sutured eye • right sternal edge

RSEP right somatosensory evoked potential

RSES Rosenberg Self–Esteem Scale

RSF raw soybean flour

RSG Reitan Strength of Grip

RSI repetition strain injury

R–SICU respiratory–surgical intensive care unit

RSIVP rapid–sequence intravenous pyelography

RSL right sacrolateral (fetal position)

R SL brace right short–leg brace

RSLD repair of sublethal damage

RSM risk–screening model

RSMR relative standardized mortality ratio

RSN right substantia nigra

RSO Resident Surgical Officer • right salpingo–oophorectomy • right superior oblique (muscle)

RSP recirculating single pass • removable silicone plug • rhinoseptoplasty • right sacroposterior (fetal position)

RSPK recurrent spontaneous psychokinesis

RSR regular sinus rhythm • relative survival rate • response–stimulus ratio • right superior rectus (muscle)

RSS rat stomach strip • rectosigmoidoscope • Russian spring–summer (encephalitis)

RSSE Russian spring–summer encephalitis

RSSR relatively slow sinus rate

RST radiosensitivity test • rapid surfactant test • reagin screen test • right sacro–transverse (fetal position) • rubrospinal tract

RSTL relaxed skin tension lines

RSTs Rodney Smith tubes

RSV respiratory syncytial virus • right subclavian vein • Rous sarcoma virus

RSVC right superior vena cava

RSW right–sided weakness

RT rabbit trachia • radiation therapy *also* RXT • Radiologic Technologist/technology • radio–telemetry • radiotherapy *also* Rad, RADIO, Rad Ther, Rx • radium

therapy • random
transfusion • raphe
transection • reaction
time • reading task •
reading test • reading
time • receptor
transforming •
reciprocating tachycardia •
recreational therapy •
rectal temperature *also* R/
T • red tetrazolium •
reduction time • Registered
Technologist • relaxation
time • renal transplant •
repetition time • Reporter's
Test • reptilase time •
resistance transfer •
respiratory technology •
Respiratory Therapist/
therapy • rest tremor •
retransformation • right
also R, (R), Rt, rt • right
thigh • right triceps •
room temperature •
running total

R/T rectal temperature *also*
RT • related to *also* R/t

R_T total pulmonary resistance

RT_3 (serum) resin
triiodothyronine (uptake)

rT_3 reverse triiodothyronine

RT_4 resin thyroxin

Rt, rt right *also* R, (R), RT

R/t related to *also* R/T

rT ribothymidine

RTA renal tubular acidosis •
renal tubular antigen • road
traffic accident

RT(ARRT) Registered
Technologist certified by
American Registry of
Radiologic Technologists

RTC randomized trial,

controlled • renal tubular
cell • research (and)
training center • residential
treatment center • return to
clinic • (a)round the clock

RTD resubmission turnaround
document • routine test
dilution

Rtd retarded • retired

RTE rabbit thymus extract

RTECS Registry of Toxic
Effects of Chemical
Substances

RTER return to emergency
room

RTF replication (and) transfer •
resistance transfer factor •
respiratory tract fluid •
return to flow

RTI respiratory tract infection

RtH right–handed

Rtl tissue resistance

RTKP radiothermokeratoplasty

RTL reactive to light (pupils)

rtl rectal

RT LAT, rt lat right lateral

RTM routine medical care

R_{tmf} total matrix formation rate

RTN renal tubular necrosis •
routine

RT(N) Registered Technologist
in Nuclear Medicine

rtn return

RT(N)(AART) Registered
Technologist in Nuclear
Medicine certified by
American Registry of
Radiologic Technologists

RTNM retreatment (staging of cancer)

RTO return to office • right toe off

RTOG radiation therapy oncology group

RTP renal transplant patient • reverse transcriptase-producing (agent)

RTPA, rt PA recombinant tissue–type plasminogen activator

RTPS radiation therapy planning system

RTR Recreational Therapist, Registered • red (blood cell) turnover rate • retention time ratio • return to room

RT(R)(ARRT) Registered Technologist in Radiography certified by American Registry of Radiologic Technologists

RTRR return to recovery room

RTS real time scan • relative tumor size • return to sender • right toestrike

rTSAB rodent thyroid–stimulating antibody

rt scap bord right scapular border

RT(T)(AART) Radiologic Technologist in Radiation Therapy certified by American Registry of Radiologic Technologists

r$_{tt}$ obtained coefficient • reliability coefficient

RTU ready to use • real–time ultrasonography *also* RTUS • relative time unit

RT$_3$U resin triiodothyronine uptake

rTU ribosomal ribonucleic acid transcription unit

RTUS real–time ultrasonography *also* RTU

RTV room temperature vulcanization

RTW return to work *also* R/W

RTWD return to work determination

RTx radiation therapy

RU radioactive uptake • radioulnar • rat unit • reading of unknown • reading unknown • recto-urethral • recurrent ulcer • residual urine • resin uptake • resistance unit *also* R • retrograde uro-gram • retroverted uterus • right uninjured • right uninvolved • right upper • rodent ulcer • roentgen unit • routine urinalysis

RU–1 human embryonic lung fibroblast

Ru ruthenium

RUA routine urine analysis

rub. [L. *ruber*] red *also* R

RuBP ribulose bisphophate

RUE right upper extremity

RUG resource utilization group • retrograde urethrogram

RUL right upper lateral • right upper (eye)lid • right upper limb • right upper lobe • right upper lung

RUM right upper medial

RUO right ureteral orifice

RUOQ right upper outer quadrant

RUP right upper pole

rupt ruptured

RUQ right upper quadrant

RUR resin uptake ratio

RURTI recurrent upper respiratory tract infection

RUS radioulnar synostosis • recurrent ulcerative stomatitis

RUSB right upper sternal border

RUSS recurrent ulcerative scarifying stomatitis

RUV residual urine volume

RUX right upper extremity

RV random variable • rat virus • Rauscher virus • rectal vault • recto-vaginal • reinforcement value • renal venous • reovirus • reserve volume • residual volume • respiratory volume • retinal vasculitis • retrovaginal • retroversion • return visit • rheumatoid vasculitis • rhinovirus • right ventricle, right ventricular • rubella vaccine • rubella virus • Russell viper

R$_V$ radius of view

RVA rabies vaccine adsorbed • re-entrant ventricular arrhythmia • right ventricular activation • right ventricular apical • right vertebral artery

RVAD right ventricular assist device

RVAW right ventricle anterior wall

RVB red venous blood

RVC radioactivity (of) vegetative cells • respond to verbal command

RVD relative vertebral density • relative volume decrease • right ventricular dimension • right vertebral density

RVDO right ventricular diastolic overload

RVDV right ventricular diastolic volume

RVE right ventricular enlargement

RVECP right ventricular endocardial potential

RVEDD right ventricular end-diastolic diameter

RVEDV right ventricular end-diastolic volume

RVEF right ventricular ejection fraction • right ventricular end-flow

RVESVI right ventricular end-systolic volume index

RVET right ventricular ejection time

RVF Rift Valley fever • right ventricular failure • right visual field

RVFP right ventricular filling pressure

RVG radionuclide ventricu-logram/ventriculography • relative value guide • right ventrogluteal • right visceral ganglion

RVH renovascular hypertension • right ventricular hypertrophy

RVHD rheumatic valvular heart disease

RVI relative value index • right ventricle infarction

RVID right ventricular internal dimension

RVIDd right ventricle internal dimension diastole

RVIDP right ventricular initial diastolic pressure

RVIT right ventricular inflow tract (view)

RVL right vastus lateralis

RVLG right ventrolateral gluteal

RVO relaxed vaginal outlet • retinal vein occlusion • right ventricular outflow • right ventricular overactivity

RVOT right ventricular outflow tract

RVP red veterinary petrolatum • renovascular pressure • resting venous pressure • right ventricular pressure

RVPFR right ventricular peak filling rate

RVPRA renal vein plasma renin activity

RVR rapid ventricular response • reduced vascular response • reduced vestibular response • renal vascular resistance • renal

vein renin • repetitive ventricular response • resistance (to) venous return

RVRA renal vein renin activity • renal venous renin assay

RV/RA renal vein/renal activity (ratio)

RVRC renal vein renin concentration

RV/RF retroverted/retroflexed

RVS rabies vaccine, adsorbed • relative value scale • relative value schedule • relative value study • reported visual sensation • retrovaginal space • Rokeach Value Survey (psychologic test)

RVSO right ventricle stroke output

RVSW right ventricular stroke work

RVSWI right ventricular stroke work index

RVT renal vein thrombosis • Russell viper (venom) time *also* RV time, RVVT

RVTE recurring venous thromboembolism

RV time Russell viper (venom) time *also* RVT, RVVT

RV/TLC residual volume to total lung capacity (ratio)

RVU relative value unit

RVV rubella vaccine–like virus • Russell viper venom

RVVT Russell viper venom time *also* RVT, RV time

RVWD right ventricular wall device

RW radiologic warfare • ragweed • respiratory work • right (ear), warm (stimulus) • Romano–Ward (syndrome) • round window

R–W Rideal–Walker (coefficient)

R/W return to work *also* RTW

RWAGE ragweed antigen E

RWIS restraint (and) water immersion stress

RWM regional wall motion

RWP ragweed pollen • R-wave progression (electrocardiography)

RWS ragweed sensitivity

RWT R–wave threshold (electrocardiography)

Rx drug • medication • pharmacy • prescribe/ prescription • prescription drug • radiotherapy *also* Rad, RADIO, Rad Ther, RT • [L. *recipe*] take • therapy • treatment

r(X) right X (chromosome)

Rxd treated

Rx'd US, diath, trx treated with ultrasound, diathermy, traction

RXLI recessive X–linked ichthyosis

RXN reaction

Rx Phys treating physician

RXT radiation therapy *also* RT • right exotropia

R–Y Roux–en–Y (anastomosis)

S apparent power • area *also* A, a • entropy (in thermodynamics) • [L. *semis*] half *also* HF, hf, s, sem, semi, ss • exposure time (radiology) • [L. *signa* mark, write on] label *also* s, sig • [L. *sinister*] left *also* s • mean dose per unit cumulated activity • midpoint of sella turcica (point) • relative storage capacity • response to white space • sacral • saline *also* SA, Sa, SAL, sal • same • saturated • saturation (of hemoglobin) • schizophrenia • screen–containing cassette • second *also* s, sec • section *also* s, SEC, sec, sect • sedimentation coefficient • sella (turcica) • semilente (insulin) • senility/senile • sensation *also* s • sensitivity • sensory • septum • sequential (analysis) • series *also* s, ser • serine *also* Ser • serum • sick • siderocyte • siemens • sign/signed *also* /S/, /s/, s • signature (prescription) *also* /S/, /s/ • silicate • single (marital status) • singular • sinus • sister • small *also* Sm, sm • smooth (bacterial colony) • soft • soil • solid • soluble • solute • son • sone (unit of loudness) • space • spasm • spatial aptitude (in General Aptitude Test Battery) • specific activity *also* SA • spherical • spherical (lens) • spleen • sporadic • standard normal deviation • stem (cell) • stimulus *also* R, ST • storage • streptomycin *also* SM • subject •

subjective (findings) • substrate • suction • sulcus • sulfur • sum of arithmetic series • supervision • supravergence • surface • surgery *also* SURG, surg • suture • Svedberg (unit) • swine • Swiss (mouse) • symmetrical • sympathetic • synthesis (phase in cell cycle) • systole • [L. *sine*, Fr. *sans*] without *also* WO, w/o, s, $\overline{s}$ • [L. *signa*] write, let it be written

S, /S/ signature • signed *also* /s/

S1—S5 first to fifth sacral nerves or vertebrae

S$_1$, S$_2$, S$_3$, S$_4$ suicide risk classification

S$_1$—S$_4$ first to fourth heart sounds

s atomic orbital with angular momentum quantum number zero • distance • [L. *semis*] half *also* HF, hf, S, sem, semi, ss • [L. *signa*] label *also* S, sig • left *also* S • length of path • sample standard deviation • sample variance *also* s^2 • satellite (chromosome) • scruple • second *also* S • section *also* S, SEC, sec, sect • sensation *also* S • series *also* S, ser • signed *also* S • steady state • suckling • [L. *sine*, Fr.*sans*] without *also* S, $\overline{s}$

s^2 sample variance *also* s

s̄ [L. *sine,* Fr. sans] without *also* S, s • without spectacles

/s/ signed *also* S, /S/

SA [L. *secundum artem*] according to art • salicylamide • salicylic acid • saline *also* S, Sa, SAL, sal • salt added • sarcoma *also* sarc • second antibody • secondary amenorrhea • secondary anemia • secondary arrest • self–agglutinating • self–analysis • semen analysis • sensitizing antibody • serum albumin *also* SAB • serum aldolase • short acting • sialic acid • sialoadenectomy • siblings (raised) apart • simian adenovirus • sinoatrial *also* S–A • sinus arrest • sinus arrhythmia • skeletal age • sleep apnea • slightly active • social acquiescence • soluble (in) alkaline (medium) • Spanish–American • spatial average • specific activity *also* S • spectrum analysis • sperm abnormality • spermagglutinin • spiking activity • splenic artery • standard accuracy • stimulus artifact • Stokes–Adams • suicide alert • suicide attempt • surface antigen • surface area • surgeon's assistant • surgical assistant • sustained action • sympathetic activity • systemic artery • systemic aspergillosis

S–A sinoatrial *also* SA • sinoauricular

S/A same as • sugar (and) acetone *also* S&A

S&A sickness and accident (insurance) • sugar and acetone *also* S/A

Sa most anterior point of anterior contour of the sella turcica (point) • saline *also* S, SA, SAL, sal • samarium

sa [L. *secumdum artem* according to art] by skill *also* sec a

sA statampere

SAA same as above • serum amyloid–A • severe aplastic anemia • Stokes–Adams attack

SAARD slow–acting antirheumatic drug

SAAST self–administered alcohol screening test

SAB serum albumin *also* SA • significant asymptomatic bacteriuria • sinoatrial block • spontaneous abortion • subarachnoid bleed • subarachnoid block

SABP spontaneous acute bacterial peritonitis

SAC saccharin • screening (and) acute care • short–arm cast • splenic adherent cell • subarea advisory council • substance abuse counselor

SACC short–arm cylinder cast

sacc [Fr. *saccades* to jerk] cogwheel respiration

SACD subacute combined degeneration *also* SCD

SACE serum angiotensin–converting enzyme (activity)

SACH small animal care hospital • solid ankle, cushion heel (orthopedic appliance)

SACHT serum antichromotrypsin

sac–Il sacroiliac *also* SI

SACS secondary anticoagulation system

SACSF subarachnoid cerebrospinal fluid

SACT sinoatrial conduction time

SAD seasonal affective disorder • Self–Assessment Depression (Scale) • separation anxiety disorder • small airway dysfunction • social avoidance (and) distress • source–to–axis distance • subacute dialysis • sugar, acetone, diacetic acid (test) • suppressor–activating determinant

SADBE squaric acid dibutylester

SADD Standardized Assessment of Depressive Disorders • Students Against Drunk Driving

SADL simulated activities of daily living

SADQ Self–Administered Dependency Questionnaire

SADR suspected adverse drug reaction

SADS Schedule for Affective Disorders and Schizophrenia • Shipman Anxiety Depression Scale

SADS–C Schedule for Affective Disorders and Schizophrenia—Change

SADS–L Schedule for Affective Disorders and Schizophrenia—Lifetime (Version)

SADT Stetson Auditory Discrimination Test

SAE short above–elbow (cast) • specific action exercise • subcortical atherosclerotic encephalopathy • supported arm exercise

SAEB sinoatrial entrance block

SAEP *Salmonella abortus equi* pyrogen

SAF self–articulating femoral (hip prosthesis) • serum accelerator factor • simultaneous auditory feedback • Spanish–American female

SAFA soluble antigen fluorescent antibody (test)

SAFE simulated aircraft fire (and) emergency

SAG Swiss(–type) agammaglobulinemia

sag sagittal

Sag D sagittal diameter

SAGM sodium chloride, adenine, glucose, mannitol

SAH *S*–adenosyl–L–homo-cysterine • subarachnoid hemorrhage • systemic arterial hypertension

SAHS sleep apnea–hypersomnolence syndrome

SAI Self–Analysis Inventory • Sexual Arousability Inventory • Social Adequacy Index • Sodium Amytal interview • systemic active immunotherapy • [L. *sine altera indicatione*] without other qualification

SAICAR succinoaminoimidazole carboxamide (ribonucleotide)

SAID sexually acquired immunodeficiency (syndrome)

SAIDS simian acquired immunodeficiency syndrome

SAL [L. *secundum artis legis*] according to the rules of the art *also* sal • salbutamol • salicylate • saline *also* S, SA, Sa, sal • sensorineural acuity level • specified antilymphocytic • suction–assisted lipectomy

SAL 12 sequential analysis of twelve chemistry constituents

Sal salicylate/salicylic *also* sal

sal [L. *secundum artis legis*] according to the rules of the art *also* SAL • salicylate/salicylic *also* Sal • saline *also* S, SA, Sa, SAL • saliva • salt

SAM *S*–adenosyl–L–methionine • salicylamide • scanning acoustic microscope • self–administered medication • sex arousal mechanism • Spanish–American male • sulfated acid mucopolysaccharide •

surface–active material • synthetic, adhesive, moisture (vapor permeable) • systolic anterior motion (of mitral valve)

SAMF single antibody millipore filtration

SAMI socially acceptable monitoring instrument

SAMO Senior Administrative Medical Officer

S–AMY serum amylase

SAN side–arm nebulizer • sinoatrial node • sinoauricular node • slept all night • solitary autonomous nodule

SANA sinoatrial node artery

Sanat sanatorium

SANC short–arm navicular cast

SANDR sinoatrial nodal re–entry

sang. sanguinous

sanit sanitarium • sanitary • sanitation

SANS Scale for the Assessment of Negative Symptoms

SAO small airway obstruction • splanchnic artery occlusion

SaO$_2$, S$_{Ao2}$ oxygen saturation *also* OS, O$_2$ sat., SO$_2$

SAP sensory action potential • serum acid phosphatase • serum alkaline phosphatase • serum amyloid P (component) • situs ambiguus (with) polysplenia • *Staphylococcus aureus*

protease • systemic arterial pressure

sap. saponify/saponification

SAPD self–administration (of) psychotropic drug

SAPH saphenous

SAPMS short–arm posterior–molded splint

sapon saponification

SAPP sodium acid pyrophosphate

SAPS short–arm plaster splint • Simplified Acute Physiology Score

SAQ short–arc quadriceps (test)

SAQC statistical analysis (and) quality control

SAR seasonal allergic rhinitis • sexual attitude reassessment • sexual attitude restructuring • structure–activity relationship

Sar sulfarsphenamine

SARA sexually acquired reactive arthritis • system (for) anesthetic (and) respiratory administration

sarc sarcoma *also* SA

SART sinoatrial recovery time

SAS saline, agent, and saline • self–rating anxiety scale • short–arm splint • Sklar Aphasia Scale • sleep apnea syndrome • small animal surgery • small aorta syndrome • sodium amylosulfate • space–adaptation syndrome • statistical analysis system •

sterile aqueous solution/suspension • subaortic stenosis • subarachnoid space • sulfasalazine • supravalvular aortic stenosis • surface–active substance

SASH saline, agent, saline, and heparin

SASP salazosulfapyridine • salicylazosulfapyridine

SAT satellite • saturated/saturation *also* Sat, sat. • Scholastic Aptitude Test • School Ability Test • School Attitude Test • Senior Apperception Technique • serum antitrypsin • Shapes Analysis Test • single–agent (chemo)therapy • slide agglutination test • specific antithymocytic • speech awareness threshold • spermatogenic activity test • spontaneous activity test • spontaneous autoimmune thyroiditis • Stanford Achievement Test • structural atypia • subacute thyroiditis • symptomless autoimmune thyroiditis • systematized assertive therapy • systemic assertive therapy

Sat, sat. saturation/saturated *also* SAT

sat. satisfactory

s.a.t. [L. *sine acido thymonucleinico*] without thymonucleic acid

SATA spatial average/temporal average

SATB Special Aptitude Test Battery

sat. cond satisfactory condition

sat'd saturated *also* std

SATL surgical Achilles tendon lengthening

SATM sodium aurothiomalate

satn saturation

SATP spatial average temporal peak

sat. sol saturated solution

SAU statistical analysis unit

SAV sequential atrioventricular (pacing) • streptavidin • supra–anular valve

SAVD spontaneous assisted vaginal delivery

SAZ sulfasalazine

SB safety belt • sandbag • Schwartz–Bartter (syndrome) • scleral buckle • Sengstaken–Blakemore (tube) *also* S–B • serum bilirubin • shortness (of) breath • sick bay (Navy) • sideroblast • Silvestroni–Bianco (syndrome) • single blind • single breath • sinus bradycardia • small bowel • sodium balance • soybean • spina bifida • spontaneous blastogenesis • spontaneously breathing • stand by *also* ST BY • Stanford–Binet (Intelligence Scale) *also* S–B • stereotyped behavior • sternal border • stillbirth • stillborn *also* Stb, stillb • suction biopsy • surface binding (protein)

SB– not wearing seat belt

+SB wearing seat belt

S–B Sengstaken–Blakemore (tube) *also* SB • Stanford–Binet (Intelligence Scale) *also* SB

S/B seen by • side bending

Sb [L. *stibium*] antimony • strabismus *also* strab

sb stilb (unit of luminous intensity)

SBA serum bactericidal activity • serum bile acid • soybean agglutinin • spina bifida aperta • stand–by assistance

SBB simultaneous binaural bithermal • small bowel biopsy • stimulation–bound behavior

SBC serum bactericidal concentration • standard bicarbonate • strict bed confinement • sunburn cell

SBD straight bag drainage • suggested brain dysfunction

S–BD seizure–brain damage

SbDH sorbitol dehydrogenase

SBE breast self–examination • short below–elbow (cast) • shortness (of) breath (on) exertion • subacute bacterial endocarditis

SBEP somatosensory brainstem evoked potential(s)

S/β sickle cell beta

SBF serologic–blocking factor • serum blocking factor • specific blocking factor • splanchnic blood flow • splenic blood flow

SBFT small bowel follow–through *also* SMBFT

SBG selenite brilliant green •
stand–by guard

SBGM self blood–glucose
monitoring

SBH sea–blue histiocyte

SBI soybean trypsin inhibitor •
systemic bacterial infection

SBIS Stanford–Binet
Intelligence Scale

SBJ skin, bones, joints

SBL serum bactericidal level •
soybean lecithin

SBMPL simultaneous binaural
midplace localization

SBN$_2$, SB$_{N2}$ single–breath
nitrogen (test)

SBNT single–breath nitrogen
test

SBNW single–breath nitrogen
washout

SBO small bowel obstruction •
spina bifida occulta

SBOD scleral buckle, right eye
(oculus dexter)

SBOM soybean oil meal

SBOS scleral buckle, left eye
(oculus sinister)

SBP school breakfast
program • scleral buckling
procedure • serotonin–
binding protein •
spontaneous bacterial
peritonitis • steroid–
binding plasma (protein) •
sulfobromophthalein •
systemic blood pressure
also Psa • systolic blood
pressure *also* SYS BP

SBPC sulfobenzyl penicillin

SBQC small–based quad cane

SBR spleen–to–body (weight)
ratio • stillbirth rate •
strict bed rest • styrene–
butadiene rubber

SBS shaken baby syndrome •
short bowel syndrome •
side to back to side • small
bowel series • social
breakdown syndrome •
staff burn–out scale •
straight back syndrome

SBSM self–blood sugar
monitoring

SBSRT Spreen–Benton
Sentence Repetition Test

SBSS Seligmann buffered salt
solution

SBT serum bactericidal test •
serum bacteriologic titer •
single–breath test •
sulbactam

SBTI soybean trypsin inhibitor
also STI

SBTPE State Boards Test Pool
Examination

SBTT small bowel transit time

SC sacrococcygeal • Sanitary
Corps • schedule change •
schizophrenia • SchHller–
Christian (disease) •
Schwann cell • Scianna
(blood group) • sciatic
(nerve) • science • scruple
also scr • secondary
cleavage • secretory coil •
secretory component •
self–care • self–control •
semicircular • semiclosed •
semilunar–valve closure •
serum complement • serum
creatinine *also* SCr •
service connected • sex
chromatin • Sezary cell •
shallow compartment •

short circuit · sick call · sickle cell *also* S–C · silicone coated · single chemical · skin conduction · slow component · Smeloff–Cutter · Snellen chart · sodium citrate · soluble complex · special care · specific characteristic · spinal cord · spleen cell *also* SPC · squamous carcinoma · statistical control · stellate cell · stepped care · sternoclavicular · stimulus, conditioned · stratum corneum · stroke count · subcellular · subclavian · subcorneal · subcortical · subcoastal (view) · subcutaneous *also* sc, SQ, subcu, subcut, subq · succinylcholine *also* SCH · sugar coated · sulfur colloid · sulfur containing · superior colliculus · superior constrictor (muscles of pharynx) · superior cornu · supportive care · supressor cell · surface colony · surgical cone · systemic candidiasis · systolic click · [L. *sine correctione*] without correction (without glasses) *also* s̄ gl

S–C sickle cell *also* SC

S&C sclerae and conjunctivae · singly and consensually

Sc scandium · scapula · science/scientific *also* Sci

sC statcoulomb

sc [L. *scilicet*] one may know (certainly, evidently, of course) · scant · sclera ·

subcutaneously *also* SC, SQ, subcu, subcut, subq

SCA School and College Ability (tests) · self–care agency · severe congenital anomaly · sickle–cell anemia · single–channel analyzer · sperm–coating antigen · spleen colony assay · steroidal–cell antibody · subclavian artery · subcutaneous abdominal (block) · superior cerebellar artery · suppressor cell activity

SCa, S$_{Ca}$ serum calcium

SCAb autoantibody to stratum corneum

SCABG single coronary artery bypass graft

SCAG single coronary artery graft

SCAN suspected child abuse (and) neglect · systolic coronary artery narrowing

SCAS semicontinuous activated sludge

SCAT sheep cell agglutination test · sickle cell anemia test

scat. [L. *scatula*] box

scat. orig [L. *scatula originalis*] original package

SCB sedative cabinet bath · stratum corneum basic · strictly confined (to) bed

SCBC small cell bronchogenic carcinoma

SCBE single–contrast barium enema

SCBF spinal cord blood flow

SCBG symmetrical calcification (of) basal (cerebral) ganglia

SCBH systemic cutaneous basophil hypersensitivity

SCBP stratum corneum basic protein

SCBU special care baby unit

ScBU screening bacteriuria

SCC sequential combination chemotherapy • Services for Crippled Children • short circuit current • short course chemotherapy • sickle cell crisis • small–cell carcinoma • small cleaved cell • squamous carcinoma (of) cervix • squamous cell carcinoma *also* SCCA, SqCCA, sq cell ca

SCCA semiclosed circle absorber system • squamous cell carcinoma *also* SCC, SqCCA, sq cell ca

SCCB small cell carcinoma (of) bronchus

SCCH sternocostoclavicular hyperostosis

SCCHN squamous cell carcinoma (of) head (and) neck

SCCL small cell carcinoma (of) lung

SCCM Sertoli cell culture medium

SCD sequential compression device • service–connected disability • sickle–cell disease • spinal cord disease • spinocerebellar degeneration • subacute combined degeneration *also*

SACD • sudden cardiac death • sudden coronary death • sulfur–carbon drug • systemic carnitine deficiency

ScD Doctor of Science

ScDA [L. *scapulodextra anterior*] right scapulo-anterior (fetal position)

ScDP [L. *scapulodextra posterior*] right scapulo-posterior (fetal position)

SCE saturated calomel electrode • secretory carcinoma (of the) endometrium • sister chromatid exchange • subcutaneous emphysema

SCEP sandwich counterelectrophoresis • somatosensory cortical evoked potential

SCER sister chromatid exchange rate

SCF supercritical fluid

SCFA short–chain fatty acid

SCFE slipped capital femoral epiphysis

SCFI specific clotting factor (and) inhibitor

SCG serum chemistry graft • serum chemogram • sodium cromoglycate • superior cervical ganglion

SCH Schirmer (test) • sole community hospital • succinylcholine *also* SC • suprachiasmatic

SCh succinylcholine chloride

SChE serum cholinesterase

sched schedule

SCHISTO, SCHIZ schizocyte

schiz schizophrenia

SCHL subcapsular hematoma (of) liver

SCHLP supracricoid hemi-laryngopharyngectomy

SCI Science Citation Index • short crus of incus • spinal cord injury • structured clinical interview

Sci science/scientific *also* Sc

SCIBTA stem cell indicated by transplantation assay

SCID severe combined immunodeficiency disease

SCII Strong–Campbell Interest Inventory

SCIPP sacrococcygeal to inferior pubic point

SCIS severe combined immunodeficiency syndrome

SCIU spinal cord injury unit

SCIV subclavian intravenous • subcutaneous intravenous

SCJ squamocolumnar junction • sternoclavicular joint

SCK serum creatine kinase

SCL scleroderma *also* SD • serum copper level • sinus cycle length • skin conductance level • soft contact lens • spinocervicolemniscal • symptom checklist • syndrome checklist

Scl, scl sclerosis/sclerotic

ScLA [L. *scapulolaeva anterior*] left scapuloposterior (fetal position)

SCLAX subcostal long axis

SCLC small cell lung cancer

SCLE subcutaneous lupus erythematosis

ScLP [L. *scapulolaeva posterior*] left scapuloposterior (fetal position)

SCM Schwann cell membrane • sensation, circulation, and motion • soluble cytotoxic medium • spleen cell–conditioned medium • spondylotic caudal myelopathy • State Certified Midwife • steatocystoma multiplex • sternocleidomastoid • streptococcal cell membrane • structure of the cytoplasmic matrix • surface–connecting membrane

ScM scalene muscle

SCMC sodium carboxymethyl-cellulose • spontaneous cell–mediated cytotoxicity

SCMD senile choroidal macular degeneration

SCMO Senior Clerical Medical Officer

SCN serum thiocyanate • sodium thiocyanate • special care nursery • suprachiasmatic nucleus

SC$_{Na}$ sieving coefficient for sodium

SCNS subcutaneous nerve stimulation

SCO somatic crossing–over • subcommissural organ

SCOP scopolamine

SCP single–celled protein • sodium cellulose phosphate • soluble cytoplasmic protein • Standardized Care Plan • submucous cleft palate • superior cerebellar peduncle

scp spherical candle power

SCPK, S–CPK serum creatine phosphokinase

SCPN serum carboxypeptidase N

SCPNT Southern California Postrotary Nystagmus Test

SCR silicon–controlled rectifier • skin conductance response • special care room • spondylotic caudal radiculopathy

SCr serum creatinine *also* SC

scr scruple *also* SC

SCRAM speech–controlled respirometer (for) ambulation measurement

SCRAP Simple–Complex Reaction–Time Apparatus

SCRS Short Clinical Rating Scale

SCS Saethre–Chotzen syndrome • silicon–controlled switch

SCSAX subcostal short axis

SCSP supracondylar • suprapatellar

SCT salmon calcitonin • Sentence Completion Test • sex chromatin test • sickle–cell trait • sperm

cytotoxic • spinal computed tomography • spinocervicothalamic • staphylococcal clumping test • sugar–coated tablet

SCTAT sex cord tumor (with) anular tubules

SCU self–care unit • special care unit

SCUBA self–contained under-water breathing apparatus

SCUD septicemic cutaneous ulcerative disease

SCUF slow continuous ultrafiltration

SCUM secondary carcinoma (of the) upper mediastinum

SCUT schizophrenia, chronic undifferentiated type

SCV sensory conduction velocity • smooth, cap-sulated, virulent (bacteria) • squamous cell carcinoma (of) vulva • subclavian vein • subcutaneous vaginal (block)

SCV–CPR simultaneous compression ventilation–cardiopulmonary resuscitation

SD sagittal depth (of cornea) • Sandhoff disease • scleroderma *also* SCL • secretion droplet • senile dementia • septal defect • serologically defined • serologically detectable • serologically determined • serum defect • severely disabled • shoulder disar-ticulation • shoulder dislocation • Shy–Drager • skin destruction • skin

dose • socialized delin-
quency • somadendritic •
spontaneous delivery •
sporadic depression •
Sprague–Dawley (rat) •
spreading depression •
standard deviation •
standard diet • statistical
documentation • Stensen
duct • sterile dressing •
Still disease • stimulus
drive *also* Sd • stone
disintegration • straight
drainage • streptodornase •
streptozocin (and) doxorubicin • succinate dehydrogenase *also* SDG • sudden
death • sulfadiazine •
superoxide dismutase •
surgical drain • systolic
discharge

S–D sickle cell–(hemoglobin)
D (disease) • strength–
duration (curve)

S/D sharp/dull • systolic/
diastolic (ratio)

S&D stomach and duodenum

Sd stimulus drive *also* SD

S^d stimulus, discriminative

SDA [L. *sacrodextra anterior*]
right sacroanterior (fetal
position) • Sabouraud
dextrose agar • salt–
dependent agglutinin •
Seventh–Day Adventist •
sialodacryoadenitis (virus) •
specific dynamic action •
steroid–dependent asth-
matic • succinic dehydro-
genase activity • super-
ficial distal axillary (node)

SDAT senile dementia,
Alzheimer type

SDB sleep–disordered
breathing

SDBP seated diastolic blood
pressure • standing
diastolic blood pressure •
supine diastolic blood
pressure

SDC sensitivity depth
compensation (ramp) •
serum digoxin
concentration • size/date
consistency • sodium
deoxycholate • subacute
combined degeneration •
succinyldicholine •
sulfodeoxycholate

SD&C suction, dilation, and
curettage

SDCL symptom distress check
list

SDD selective digestive (tract)
decontamination • sporadic
depressive disease • sterile
dry dressing

SDE specific dynamic effect

SDEEG stereotactic depth
electroencephalogram

SDES symptomatic diffuse
esophageal spasm

SDF slow death factor •
stream dilution factor •
stress distribution factor

SDFP single–donor frozen
plasma

SDG short distance group •
succinate dehydrogenase
also SD • sucrose density
gradient

SDGC sucrose density gradient
centrifugation

SDGU sucrose density gradient
ultracentrifugation

SDH serine dehydrase •
sorbitol dehydrogenase •

spinal dorsal horn • subdural hematoma • subjacent dorsal horn • succinate dehydrogenase

SDHD sudden death heart disease

SDI size/date inconsistency • standard deviation interval • Surtees Difficulties Index

SDIHD sudden death ischemic heart disease

SDL self–directed learning • serum digoxin level • serum drug level • speech discrimination loss

SDLRS self–directed–learning readiness scale

sdly sidelying

SDM sensory detection method • single, divorced, married • standard deviation (of) mean • sulfadimidine

SDMT Symbol Digit Modalities Test

SDN sexually dimorphic nucleus

SDNA single–strand deoxyribonucleic acid

SDO sudden–dosage onset

SDP [L. *sacrodextra posterior*] right sacroposterior (fetal position) • single–donor platelets • stomach, duodenum, and pancreas

SDPH sodium diphenylhydantoin

SDR spontaneously diabetic rat • surgical dressing room

SDRT Stanford Diagnostic Reading Test

SDS same day surgery • school dental service • Self–Rating Depression Scale • sensory deprivation syndrome • sexual differentiation scale • Shy–Drager syndrome • simple descriptive scale • single dose suppression • sodium dodecyl sulfate • specific diagnosis service • speech discrimination score • standard deviation score • sulfadiazine silver • sudden death syndrome • sustained depolarizing shift

Sds, sds sounds

SD–SK streptodornase–streptokinase

SDS/PAGE, SDS–PGE sodium dodecyl sulfate–polyacrylamide gel electrophoresis

SDT [L. *sacrodextra transversa*] right sacrotransverse (fetal position) • sensory decision theory • single–donor transfusion • speech detection threshold

SDU short double upright • Standard Deviation Unit • step–down unit

SDW separated, divorced, widowed

SE saline enema • sanitary engineering • Seeing Eye • self–explanatory • sheep erythrocyte • side effect • smoke exposure • smoke extract • soft exudate • solid extract • spheno-ethmoidal • spherical equivalent • spin–echo • spongiform encephalopathy • squamous epithelium • standard error • Starr–Edwards (prosthesis) *also* S–E • starch equivalent • status epilepticus • sterol ester • subendocardial • subendothelial • supernormal excitability • sustained engraftment

S–E Starr–Edwards (prosthesis) *also* SE

S&E safety and efficiency

Se selenium

SEA sheep erythrocyte agglutination • shock–elicited aggression • soluble egg antigen • Southeast Asia • spontaneous electrical activity • staphylococcal enterotoxin A

SEAR Southeast Asia refugee

SEAT sheep erythrocyte agglutination test

SEB Scale for Emotional Blunting • staphylococcal enterotoxin B

SEBA staphylococcal enterotoxin B antiserum

seb derm seborrheic dermatitis

seb ker seborrheic keratosis *also* SK

SEBL self–emptying blind loop

SEC [L. *secundum*] according to • secondary *also* sec • secretin • secretion • section *also* S, s, sec, sect • series elastic component (of

muscles) • Singapore epidemic conjunctivitis • size exclusion chromatography • soft elastic capsule • squamous epithelial cell • strong exchange capacity (re: resin)

Sec Seconal

sec second *also* S • secondary *also* sec • secretary • section *also* S, s, SEC, sect

sec a [L. *secundum artem* according to art] by skill *also* sa

SECG stress electrocardiography

SECPR standard external cardiopulmonary resuscitation

SECSY spin–echo correlated spectroscopy

sect section *also* S, s, SEC, sec

SED sedimentation (rate) • skin erythema dose • spondyloepiphyseal dysplasia • standard error of difference • staphylococcal enterotoxin D • strain energy density • suberythemal dose • surgeon, emergency department

sed sedate • sedative • sedimentation • [L. *sedes*] stool

SEDD Szondi's Experimental Diagnostics of Drives

sed rt sedimentation rate

SEE scopolamine–Eukodal–Ephetonin • series elastic element • standard error of estimate

SEEP small end–expiratory pressure

SEER Surveillance, Epidemiology, and End Results (Program)

SEF somatically evoked field • staphylococcal enterotoxin F

SEG segment • soft elastic gelatin (capsule) • sonoencephalogram

segm segment/segmented

SEGS, segs segmented neutrophils (polymorpho-nuclear leukocytes)

SEH subependymal hemorrhage

SEI Self–Esteem Inventory • subepithelial (corneal) infiltrate • Suretee's Events Index

SELFVD sterile elective low forceps vaginal delivery

SEM (verbal) sample evaluation method • scanning electron microscopy • secondary enrichment medium • semen *also* sem • serum methylguanidine • smoke exposure machine • standard error of mean • systolic ejection murmur

sem [L. *semis*] half *also* S, s, semi, ss • semen *also* SEM • seminal

SEMDJL spondyloepi-metaphyseal dysplasia (with) joint laxity

SEMI subendocardial myocardial infarction/injury

semi [L. *semis*] half *also* S, s, sem, ss

semid half a dram

semih [L. *semihora*] half an hour

sem in d [L. *semil in die*] once a day

SEN State Enrolled Nurse

sen sensitive/sensitivity

SENA sympathetic efferent nerve activity

sens sensation • sensorium • sensory • sensitivity

SEO surgical emergency officer

SEP sensory evoked potential • separate • serum electrophoresis • somatosensory evoked potential *also* SSEP • sperm entry point • spinal evoked potential • surface epithelium • systolic ejection period

separ separately • separation

sept septum • [L. *septem*] seven

SEQ side–effects questionnaire • simultaneous equation

seq sequence • sequel/sequela/sequelae • sequestrum

seq dev ex sequential developmental exercises

seq luce [L. *sequenti luce*] the following day

SER scanning equalization radiography • sebum excretion rate • sensory evoked response • service *also* serv • smooth endoplasmic reticulum *also*

sER • somatosensory evoked response *also* SSER • supination external rotation (type of fracture) • systolic ejection rate

Ser serine *also* S

sER smooth endoplasmic reticulum *also* SER

ser serial • series *also* S, s

SERHOLD National Biomedical Serials Holding Database

SERI Spondee Error Index

ser ind serum index

SERLINE Serials on Line

sero, serol serologic • serology

ser sect serial sections

SERT sustained ethanol release tube

serv [L. *serva*] keep, preserve • service *also* SER

SERVHEL Service and Health (Records)

SES socioeconomic status • spatial emotional stimuli • subendothelial space

SESAP Surgical Education and Self–Assessment Program

sesquih [L. *sesquihora*] an hour and a half

sesquiunc [L. *sesquiuncia*] an ounce and a half

Sess sessile

SET skin endpoint titration • systolic ejection time

sev sever • several • severe • severed

SEWHO shoulder–elbow–wrist–hand orthosis

SEXAF surface extended x-ray absorption fine (structure)

SeXO serum xanthine oxidase

s expr [L. *sine expressioe*] without pressing

SF Sabin–Feldman (dye test) • safety factor • salt free • saturated fat • scarlet fever • Schilder–Foix (disease) • seizure frequency • seminal fluid • serosal fluid • serum factor • serum ferritin • serum fibrinogen • sham feeding • shell fragment • shrapnel fragment • shunt flow • sickle (cell–hemoglobin) F (disease) • simian foam–virus • skin fibroblast • skin fluorescence • slow function • slow (initial) function • snack food • sodium azide, fecal (medium) • soft feces • spinal fluid *also* sp fl • spontaneous fibrillation • spontaneous fission (radioactive isotopes) • spontaneous fluctuation • spontaneous fracture • stable factor • sterile female • stress formula • sugar free • sulfation factor (of blood serum) • superior facet • suppressor factor • suprasternal fossa • survival fraction • Svedberg flotation (unit) • symptom free • synovial fluid *also* syn fl

SF% shortening fraction percentage

S&F soft and flat

S_f negative sedimentation Svedberg unit

SFA saturated fatty acid • seminal fluid assay • serum folic acid • stimulated fibrinolytic activity • superficial femoral angioplasty • superficial femoral artery

SFB Sanfilippo (syndrome type) B • surgical foreign body

SFBL self–filling blind loop

SFC serum fungicidal • soluble fibrin–fibrinogen complex • spinal fluid count

SFD sheep factor delta • short foot drape • skin–film distance • small for dates (gestational age) • soy–free diet • spectral frequency distribution

SFEMG single–fiber electromyography

SFF speaking fundamental frequency

SFFA serum–free fatty acid

SFFF sedimentation field flow fractionation

SFFV spleen focus–forming virus • spleen focus Friend virus

SFG spotted fever group

SFH schizophrenia family history • serum–free hemoglobin • stroma–free hemoglobin

SFHb stroma–free hemoglobin

SFI Sexual Functioning Index • Social Function Index

SFL synovial fluid lymphocyte

SFLE Stress From Life Experience

SFM soluble fibrin monomer

SFMC soluble fibrin monomer complex

SFO subfornical organ

SFP screen filtration pressure • simultaneous foveal perception • spinal fluid pressure • stopped flow pressure

SFPT standard fixation preference test

SFR screen–filtration resistance • stroke with full recovery

SFS serial focus seizures • serum fungistatic • skin (and) fascia stapler • split function study

SFT sensory feedback therapy • serum–free thyroxin • skinfold thickness

SFTR sagittal, frontal, transverse, rotation

SFV Semliki Forest virus • shipping fever virus • Shope fibroma virus • squirrel fibroma virus • superficial femoral vein

SFW sexual function of women • shell fragment wound • shrapnel fragment wound • slow filling wave

SG Sachs–Georgi (test) *also* S-G, S–Gt • salivary gland • secretory granule • serous granule • serum globulin • serum glucose • sign(s) • skin graft • soluble gelatin • specific gravity *also* SPG, SpG, sp gr • substantia gelatinosa • Surgeon General • Swan–Ganz (catheter) *also* S–G, SGC

S–G Sachs–Georgi (test) *also* SG, S–Gt • Swan–Ganz (catheter) *also* SG

SGA small for gestational age

SGAW, SG$_{AW}$ specific airway conductance

SGC spermicide–germicide compound • Swan–Ganz catheter *also* SG, S–G

SG–C serum gentamicin concentration

SGc specific conductance

SGD straight gravity drainage

SGE secondary generalized epilepsy • significant glandular enlargement

SGF sarcoma growth factor • silica gel filtered • skeletal growth factor

SGFR single–nephron glomerular filtration rate *also* SNGFR

SGGT serum γ–glutamyl-transferase

SGH subgaleal hematoma

s̄ gl without correction/ without glasses *also* SC

SGL salivary gland lymphocyte

SGO Surgeon General's Office • surgery, gynecology, and obstetrics

SGOT serum glutamic–oxaloacetic transaminase (aspartate aminotransferase)

SGP serine glycerophos-phatide • sialoglycopro-tein • soluble glycoprotein

SGPT serum glutamic–pyruvic transaminase (alanine aminotransferase)

SGR Sachs–Georgi reaction • Shwartzman generalized reaction • submandibular gland renin

SGS second generation sulfonylurea • subglottic stenosis

S–Gt Sachs–Georgi test

SGTT standard glucose tolerance test

SGV salivary gland virus • selective gastric vagotomy • small granular vesicle

SH Salter–Harris (fracture) • Schönlein–Henoch (purpura) *also* SHP • serum hepatitis • service hours • sexual harassment • sex hormone • sham operated • shared haplotypes • Sherman (rat) • short • shoulder *also* Sh, sh, SHLD • shower • sick (in) hospital • sinus histiocytosis • social history • somatotropic hormone *also* STH • spontaneously hypertensive (rat) • sulfhydryl • surgical history • symp-tomatic hypoglycemia • systemic hyperthermia

S/H sample and hold • suicidal/homicidal ideation

S&H speech and hearing

Sh sheep • short *also* sh • shoulder *also* SH, sh, SHLD

sh short *also* Sh • shoulder *also* SH, Sh, SHLD

SHA soluble HLA antigen • staphylococcal hemagglutinating antibody • super–heated aerosol

SHAA serum hepatitis–associated antigen

SHAA–Ab serum hepatitis–associated antigen antibody

SHARP School Health Additional Referral Program

SHAV superior hemiazygos vein

SHB sequential hemibody (irradiation) • subacute hepatitis (with) bridging • sulfhemoglobin *also* S–Hb

S Hb sickle hemoglobin (screen)

S–Hb sulfhemoglobin *also* SHB

SHBD serum hydroxybutyric dehydrogenase

SHBG sex hormone–binding globulin

SHCO sulfated hydrogenated caster oil

SHDI supraoptical hypophysial diabetes insipidus

SHE Syrian hamster embryo

SHEENT skin, head, eyes, ears, nose, throat

SHF simian hemorrhagic fever

shf super high frequency

SHG synthetic human gastrin

SHHP semihorizontal heart position

SHL sensorineural hearing loss

also SNHL • supraglottic horizontal laryngectomy

SHLD shoulder *also* SH, Sh, sh

SHML sinus histiocytosis (with) massive lymphadenopathy

SHMO Senior Hospital Medical Officer

SHMT serine hydroxymethyl-transferase

SHN spontaneous hemorrhagic necrosis • subacute hepatic necrosis

SHO secondary hypertrophic osteoarthropathy • Senior House Officer

SHORT, S–H–O–R–T short (stature), hyperextensibility (of joints or) hernia (or both), ocular (depression), Rieger (anomaly), teething (delayed)

SHP Schönlein–Henoch purpura *also* SH • secondary hyperpara-thyroidism • state health plan • surgical hypo-parathyroidism

SHPDA State Health Planning and Development Agency

sHPT secondary hyperpara-thyroidism

SHR spontaneously hypertensive rat

SHRC shortened, held, resisted, contracted

SHS Sayre head sling • sheep hemolysate supernatant • Shipley–Hartford Scale • student health service • super high speed

SHSP spontaneously hypertensive stroke–prone (rat)

SHSS Stanford Hypnotic Susceptibility Scale

SHT simple hypocalcemic tetany • subcutaneous histamine test

SHUR System for Hospital Uniform Reporting

SHV simian herpesvirus

SHx social history

SI [Fr. *Système International d'Unites*] International System of Units • sacroiliac *also* sac–il • saline infusion • saline injection • saturation index • self–inflicted • sensitive index • serious illness • serum insulin • serum iron • service index • severity index • sex inventory • Singh Index • single injection • small intestine • social introversion • soluble insulin • special intervention • spirochetosis icterohaemorrhagica • stimulation index • streptozotocin induced • stress incontinence • strict isolation • stroke index • suicidal ideation • sulfated insulin • suppression index • systolic index

S/I sucrose to isomaltase (ratio)

S&I suction and irrigation

SI most anterior point on lower contour of sella turcica (point) • silicon • (venous) sinus

SIA serum inhibitory activity • stimulation–induced analgesia • stress–induced analgesia • stress–induced

anesthesia • subacute infectious arthritis • synalbumin–insulin antagonism • syncytia induction assay

SIADH syndrome (of) inappropriate (secretion of) antidiuretic hormone

SIB self–injurious behavior

sib sibling

sibs siblings

SIC [L. *siccus*] dry *also* sic • serum inhibitory concentration • serum insulin concentration

sic [L. *siccus*] dry *also* SIC

SICD Sequenced Inventory of Communication Development • serum isocitrate dehydrogenase

SICSVA sequential impaction cascade sieve volumetric air (sampler)

SICT selective intracoronary thrombolysis

SICU spinal intensive care unit • surgical intensive care unit

SID sucrase–isomaltase deficiency • sudden inexplicable death • sudden infant death • suggested indication of diagnosis • systemic inflammatory disease

sid [L. *semel in die*] once a day

SIDER siderocyte

SIDS sudden infant death syndrome

SIE stroke in evolution

SIECUS Sex Information and Educational Council of the United States

SIF serum inhibitory factor • small, intensely fluorescent (ganglia)

SIf segment inferior

SIFT selected ion flow tube

SIG sigmoidoscope • special interest group

SIg serum immune globulin • surface immunoglobulin *also* sIg

Sig signature • signed

sIg surface immunoglobulin *also* SIg

sig [L. *signa*] label, write *also* S, s • [L. *signetur*] let it be written, labeled • sigmoidoscopy • signal • significant

SIgA surface immunoglobulin A

S–IgA secretory immunoglobulin A

sigma (Σ, σ) eighteenth letter of Greek alphabet

Σ foaminess • sum • summation of all quantities following the symbol • syphilis

σ conductivity *also* cond • cross–section • millisecond *also* msec, ms • population standard deviation • Stefan–Boltzmann constant • stress • surface tension *also* ST • type of molecular bond • wavenumber

sig n pro [L. *signa nomine proprio*] label with proper name

SIH stimulation–induced hypalgesia

SIhPTH serum immunoreactive human parathyroid hormone

SIJ, SI jt sacroiliac joint

SIL seriously ill list • speech interference level

SILD Sequenced Inventory of Language Development

SILFVD sterile indicated low forceps vaginal delivery

SILS Shipley Institute of Living Scale

SIM selected ion monitoring • Similac • sucrose–isomaltose • sulfide, indole, motility (medium)

Simkin simulation kinetics (analysis)

simp [L. *simplex*] simple

SIMS secondary ion mass spectroscopy

simul simultaneously

SIMV synchronized intermittent mandatory ventilation

sin. [L. *sex in nocte*] six times a night • [L. *sine*] without

sing. [L. *singulorum*] of each • singular

sing. aur [L. *singulis auroris*] every morning

sing. hor quad [L. *singulis horae quadrantibus*] every quarter of an hour

si non val [L. *si non valeat*] if it is not enough

si op sit [L. *si opus sit*] if it is necessary

SIP segment inertial properties • Sickness Impact Profile • slow inhibitory potential • surface inductive plethysmography

sIPTH serum immunoreactive parathyroid hormone

SIQ sick in quarters (military)

SIR single isomorphous replacement • specific immune release • standardized incidence ratio

SIREF specific immune-response–enhancing factor

SIRF severely impaired renal function

SIRS soluble immune response suppressor

SIS sisomicin • sister • social information system • spontaneous interictal spike • sterile injectable solution • sterile injectable suspension

SISI short–increment sensitivity index

SISS serum inhibitor (of) streptolysin S

SISV, SISV simian sarcoma virus *also* SSV

SIT serum inhibiting titer • Slosson Intelligence Test • sperm immobilization test

SIT BAL sitting balance

SIT–F Sperm Immobilization Test–Fjabrant

SIT–I Sperm Immobilization Test–Isojima

SIT TOL sitting tolerance

SIV simian immunodeficiency virus • Sprague–Dawley–Ivanovas (rat)

si vir perm [L. *si vires permitant*] if strength will permit

SIVP slow intravenous push

SIW self–inflicted wound

SIWIP self–induced water intoxication (and) psychosis

SJ, S–J Stevens–Johnson (syndrome) *also* SJS

SJR Shinowara–Jones–Reinhart (unit)

SJS Stevens–Johnson syndrome *also* SJ, S–J • Swyer–James syndrome

SjS Sjögren syndrome

SK seborrheic keratosis *also* seb ker • senile keratosis • skin *also* Sk, SKI • Sloan–Kettering (Institute) *also* SKI • solar keratosis • spontaneous killer (cell) • streptokinase • striae keratopathy • swine kidney

Sk skin *also* SK, SKI

sk skeletal *also* skel • skimmed

SKA supracondylar knee–ankle (orthosis)

SKAB skeletal antibody

SKAO supracondylar knee–ankle orthosis

SKAT Sex Knowledge and Attitude Test

skel skeletal *also* sk • skeleton

SKI skin *also* SK, Sk • Sloan–Kettering Institute *also* SK

SKL serum–killing level

SKSD, SK–SD streptokinase-streptodornase

sk tr skeletal traction

SKW Sturge–Kalischer–Weber (syndrome)

SL [L. *secundum legem*] according to rules *also* sl • salt loser • sarcolemma • satellite–like • sclerosing leukoencephalopathy • sensation level (of hearing) • sensory latency • serious list • short–leg (cast) *also* SLC • Sibley–Lehninger (unit) • signal level • Sinding Larsen (disease) • Sjögren–Larsson (syndrome) • slight • slit lamp • small leukocyte • small lymphocyte • soda lime • sodium lactate • solidified liquid • sound level • Stein–Leventhal (syndrome) • streptolysin • Strümpell–Lorrain (disease) • sublingual(ly)

S/L slit lamp (examination) • sucrase to lactase (ratio) *also* S:L

S:L sucrase to lactase (ratio) *also* S/L

Sl slight • Steel (mouse)

sl [L. *secundum legem*] according to rules *also* SL • slice • slight • slow • slyke (unit of buffer value) • sublingual

SLA [L. *sacrolaeva anterior*] left sacroanterior (fetal position) • single–cell liquid cytotoxic assay • slide latex agglutination • surfactant–like activity

SLAM scanning laser acoustic microscope

SLAP serum leucine aminopeptidase

SLB short–leg brace

SLC short–leg cast *also* SL • Sociopolitical Locus of Control • sodium lithium countertransport

SLCC short–leg cylinder cast • sulfated lithocholic conjugate

SLCG sulfolithocholylglycine

SLD, SLDH serum lactate dehydrogenase

SLE slit–lamp examination • St. Louis encephalitis • systemic lupus erythematosus

SLEA sheep erythrocyte antibody • sheep erythrocyte antigen

SLEP short latent–evoked potential

SLEV St. Louis encephalitis virus

SLFIA substrate–labeled fluorescent immunoassay • substrate–linked fluorescent immunoassay

SLFVD sterile low forceps vaginal delivery

SLGXT symptom–limited graded exercise test

SLHR sex–linked hypophosphatemic rickets

SLI secretin–like immunoreactivity • selective lymphoid irradiation • somatostatin–like immunoreactivity • speech (and) language impaired • splenic localization index

SLIP Singer–Loomis Inventory of Personality

SLIR somatostatin–like immunoreactivity

SLK, SLKC superior limbic keratoconjunctivitis

SLM sound level meter

SLMC spontaneous lymphocyte–mediated cytotoxicity

SLMFD sterile low midforceps (vaginal) delivery

SLMP since last menstrual period

SLN sublentiform nucleus • superior laryngeal nerve

SLNTG sublingual nitroglycerin

SLNWBC short leg non–weight–bearing cast

SLNWC short–leg nonwalking cast

SLO streptolysin O

SLP [L. *sacrolaeva posterior*] left sacroposterior (fetal position) • segmental limb (systolic) pressure • sex–limited protein • short luteal phase • speech–language pathologist • subluxation (of) patella

SLPP serum lipophosphoprotein

SLPMS short–leg posterior–molded splint

SLR Shwartzman local reaction • single lens reflex • straight leg raising

SLRT straight leg–raising tenderness • straight leg–raising test

SLS segment long–spacing (collagen fibers) • short–leg splint • single limb support • Sjögren–Larsson

syndrome • Stein–Leventhal syndrome

SLSQ Speech and Language Screening Questionnaire

SLT [L. *sacrolaeva transversa*] left sacrotransverse (fetal position) • swing light test

SlTr silent treatment

SLUD salivation, lacrimation, urination, defecation

SLWC short–leg walking cast

SLZ serum lysozyme

SM sadomasochism • self–monitoring • semimembranous • Sexual Myths (Scale) • Shigella mutant • simple mastectomy • skim milk • small • smoker • smooth muscle • somatomedin • space medicine • sphingomyelin • splenic macrophage • sports medicine • stapedius muscle • staphylococcus medium • streptomycin *also* S • StrHmpell–Marie (disease) • submandibular • submucosal • submucous • substituted metabolite • substitute (for) morphine • suckling mouse *also* sM • sucrose medium • suction method • sulfamerazine • superior mesenteric • supramamillary (nucleus) • sustained medication • symptoms • synaptic membrane • synovial membrane • systolic mean (pressure) • systolic motion • systolic murmur

S/M sadism/masochism

Sm samarium • small *also* S, sm • Smith (antigen) • symptom

sM suckling mouse *also* SM

sm small *also* S, Sm

SMA schedule (of) maximal allowance • sequential multichannel autoanalyzer • sequential/serial multiple analysis • serum muramidase activity • simultaneous multichannel autoanalyzer • smooth muscle antibody/autoantibody • spinal muscular atrophy • spontaneous motor activity • standard method agar • superior mesenteric artery • supplementary motor area

SM–A somatomedin A

SMA–6 Sequential Multiple Analysis—six different serum tests

SMA 6/60 Sequential Multiple Analysis—six tests in sixty minutes

SMA–12 Sequential Multiple Analysis—twelve–channel biochemical profile

SMA 12/60 Sequential Multiple Analysis—twelve different serum tests in sixty minutes

SMA–20 Sequential Multiple Analysis of twenty chemical constituents

SMA–60 Sequential Multiple Analysis of sixty chemical constituents

SMABF superior mesenteric artery blood flow

SMABV superior mesenteric artery blood velocity

SMAC Sequential Multiple Analyzer Computer

SMAE superior mesenteric artery embolus

SMAF smooth muscle activating factor • specific macrophage–arming factor • superior mesenteric artery (blood) flow

SMAL serum methyl alcohol level

sm an small animal

SMAO superior mesenteric artery occlusion

SMART simultaneous multiple–angle reconstruction technique

SMAS submucosal aponeurotic system (flap) • superior mesenteric artery syndrome

SMAST Short Michigan Alcoholism Screening Test

SMAT School Motivation Analysis Test

SMB selected mucosal biopsy • standard mineral base

sMB suckling mouse brain

SMBFT small bowel follow–through *also* SBFT

SMBG self–monitored blood glucose

SMBP serum myelin basic protein

SMC smooth muscle cell • special monthly compensation • special mouth care • succinylmonocholine

SM–C, Sm–C somatomedin C

SMCA smooth muscle contracting agent

SMCD senile macular chorioretinal degeneration

SM–C/IGF somatomedin C/insulin–like growth factor

SMD senile macular degeneration • sternocleidomastoid diameter • submanubrial dullness

SMDA starch methylenedianiline

SMEDI stillbirth, mummification, embryonic death, infertility (syndrome)

SMEM supplemented Eagle minimal essential medium

SMEPP subminiature end–plate potential

sm–FeSV McDonough feline sarcoma virus

SMFP state medical facilities plan

SMFVD sterile midforceps vaginal delivery

SMG submandibular gland

SMH state mental hospital • strongyloidiasis with massive hyperinfection

SMI senior medical investigator • sensory motor integration • severely mentally impaired • stress myocardial image • Style of Mind Inventory • supplementary medical insurance • sustained maximal inspiration

SmIg surface membrane immunoglobulin

SMILE sustained maximal inspiratory lung exercises

SML single major locus

SMMD specimen mass measurement device

SMN second malignant neoplasm

SMNB submaximal neuromuscular block

SMO Senior Medical Officer • serum monoamine oxidase • slip made out

SMOH Senior Medical Officer of Health

SMON subacute myelo–opticoneuropathy

SMP self–management program • slowest moving protease • special monthly pension • standard medical practice • standard medical procedure • submitochondrial particle

SMR senior medical resident • sensorimotor rhythm • severe mental retardation • skeletal muscle relaxant • somnolent metabolic rate • standard metabolic rate • standardized mortality ratio • stroke (with) minimal residuum • submucous resection

SMRR submucous resection (and) rhinoplasty

SMRV squirrel monkey retrovirus

SMS senior medical student • somatostatin *also* SS • stiff–man syndrome • supplemental minimal sodium

SMSA standard metropolitan statistical area

SMSV San Miguel sea–lion virus

SMT Sertoli cell/mesenchyme tumor • Snider Match

Test • spindle microtubule • spontaneous mammary tumor

SMuLV Scripps murine leukemia virus

SMV slow–moving vehicle • small volume • submental vertex (view) • submentovertical • superior mesenteric vein

SMVT sustained monomorphic ventricular tachycardia

SMX, SMZ sulfamethoxazole

SMZ sulfamethazine

SN sciatic notch • school (of) nursing • sclerema neonatorum • scrub nurse • sensorineural • sensory neuron • seronegative • serum neutralizing/neutralization • single nephron • sinus node • spinal needle • spontaneous nystagmus • staff nurse • standard nomenclature • streptonigrin • student nurse • subnormal • substantia nigra • supernatant • supernormal • suprasternal notch *also* SSN

S–N sella to nasion (cephalometrics)

S/N sample to negative control (ratio) • signal to noise (ratio) • speech to noise (ratio)

Sn subnasale • [L. *stannum*] tin

sn [L. *secundum naturam*] according to nature

SNA specimen not available • superior nasal artery • systems network architecture

S–N–A sella–nasion–subspinale (–point A, in cephalometrics)

SNa serum sodium (concentration)

SNagg serum normal agglutinator

SNAI Standard Nomenclature (of) Athletic Injuries

SNAP sensory nerve action potential

SNAT suspected nonaccidental trauma

SNB scalene node biopsy • Silverman needle biopsy

S–N–B sella–nasion–supramentale (–point B, in cephalometrics)

SNC [L. *sistema nervosum centrale*] central nervous system • skilled nursing care • spontaneous neonatal chylothorax

SNCL sinus node cycle length

SNCV sensory nerve conduction velocity

SND single needle device • sinus node dysfunction • striatonigral degeneration

SNDO Standard Nomenclature of Diseases and Operations

SNE sinus node electrogram • spatial nonemotional (stimuli) • subacute necrotizing encephalomyelopathy

SNEF skilled nursing extended (care) facility

SNF sinus node formation • skilled nursing facility

SNFH schizophrenia nonfamily history

SNGBF single nephron glomerular blood flow

SNGFR single nephron glomerular filtration rate *also* SGFR

SNGPF single nephron glomerular plasma flow

SNHL sensorineural hearing loss *also* SHL

SNM sulfanilamide

SNOBOL String–Oriented Symbolic Language

SNODO Standard Nomenclature of Diseases and Operations

SNOMED Standardized Nomenclature of Medicine

SNOOP Systematic Nursing Observation of Psychopathology

SNOP Systematized Nomenclature of Pathology

SNP School Nurse Practitioner • sinus node potential • sodium nitroprusside

SNQ superior nasal quadrant

SNR signal–to–noise ratio

snRNA small nuclear ribonucleic acid

snRNP small nuclear ribonucleoprotein

SNRT sinus node recovery time *also* SRT

SNRTd sinus node recovery time, direct (measuring)

SNS sterile normal saline • sympathetic nervous system

SNSA seronegative spondyloarthropathy

SNT sinuses, nose, throat

SNV spleen necrosis virus • superior nasal vein

SO salpingo–oophorectomy *also* S&O, S–O • second opinion • sex offender • shoulder orthosis • significant other *also* S/O • slow oxidative • spheno–occipital (synchondrosis) • sphincter of Oddi • standing orders • superior oblique • supraoptic • supraorbital • suboccipital • sutures out

S/O significant other *also* SO

S&O, S–O salpingo–oophorectomy *also* SO

SO$_2$ oxygen saturation *also* OS, O$_2$ sat., SaO$_2$, S$_{AO2}$

So socialization

SOA serum opsonic activity • spinal opioid analgesia • supraorbital artery • swelling of ankles

SOAA signed out against (medical) advice *also* SOAMA

SOAM stitches/sutures out in morning

SOAMA signed out against medical advice *also* SOAA

SOA–MCA superficial occipital artery to middle cerebral artery

SOAP subjective (data), objective (data), assessment, (and) plan (problem–oriented record)

SOAPIE subjective (data), objective (data), assessment,

plan, implementation, (and) evaluation (problem–oriented record)

SOAPS suction, oxygen, apparatus, pharmaceuticals, saline (anesthetia equipment)

SOB see order blank • see order book • shortness of breath • side of bed • suboccipitobregmatic

SOBOE shortness of breath on exertion

SOC sequential oral contraceptive • socialization *also* So • standard of care • state of consciousness • syphilitic osteochondritis

S&OC signed and on chart

SoC state of consciousness

soc social • society

SOCD Separation of Circle–Diamond

SocSec Social Security

S–OCT serum ornithine carbamoyltransferase

SOD sinovenous occlusive disease • spike occurrence density • superoxide dismutase • surgical officer of the day

sod sodium

sod bicarb sodium bicarbonate

SOFS spontaneous osteoporotic fracture (of) sacrum

SOFT Sorting of Figures Test

SOG suggestive of good

SOH sympathetic orthostatic hypotension

SOHN supraoptic hypothalamic nucleus

SOL solution *also* sol, soln • space–occupying lesion

sol solution *also* SOL, soln • soluble

SOLER squarely (face person), open (posture), lean (toward person), eye (contact) • relaxed

soln solution *also* SOL, sol

SOLST Stephens Oral Language Screening Test

solu solute

solv [L. *solve*] dissolve • solvent

SOM secretory otitis media • sensitivity of method • serous otitis media • somatotropin • somnolent • sulformethoxine

somat somatic

SOMI sternal occipital mandibular immobilization

SON supraoptic nucleus

SONK spontaneous osteonecrosis of knee

sono sonogram/sonography

SONP soft/solid organs not palpable

SOP standard operating procedure

SOPA syndrome of primary aldosteronism

SOPM stitches out in afternoon

SOPP splanchnic occluded portal pressure

s op s, s op sit [L. *si opus sit*] if it is necessary *also* SOS

SOQ Suicide Opinion Questionnaire

SOR sign own release • stimulus–organism response

SOr supraorbitale

Sorb, sorb sorbitol

SOREMP sleep–onset rapid eye movement period

SOS [L. *si opus sit*] if it is necessary *also* s op s, s op sit, sos • self–obtained smear • stimulation of senses • supplemental oxygen system

sos [L. *si opus sit*] if it is necessary *also* s op s, s op sit, SOS

SOT something other than • stream of thought • systemic oxygen transport

SOTT synthetic (medium) old tuberculin trichloroacetic (acid precipitated)

SP sacral promontory • sacrum posterior • sacrum (to) pubis • salivary progesterone • schizotypal personality • secretory piece • semiprivate *also* S/P • senile plaque • septal pore • septum pellucidum • sequential pulse • serine proteinase • seropositive • serum protein *also* S/P • shunt pressure • shunt procedure • silent period • skin potential • sleep deprivation • small protein • soft palate • solid phase • spatial peak • speech • speech pathology • spike potential • spine/spinal *also* S/P • spiramycin • spirometry •

spleen • spouse • standard (of) performance • standard practice • standard procedure • stand (and) pivot *also* S/P • staphylococcal protease • status post *also* S/P • steady potential • stool preservative • subliminal perception • substance • subtilopeptidase • suicide precautions *also* S/P • sulfapyridine • summating potential • suprapatellar pouch • suprapubic *also* S/P • suprapubic puncture • symphisis pubis • synthase phosphatase • systolic pressure *also* S/P

S/P semiprivate *also* SP • serum protein *also* SP • spinal *also* SP • stand (and) pivot *also* SP • status post *also* SP • suicide precautions *also* SP • suprapubic *also* SP • systolic pressure *also* SP

Sp most posterior point on posterior contour of sella turcica • sacropubic • species • speech • spine • summation potential

sP senile parkinsonism

sp space • species • specific • spine/spinal • [L. *spiritus*] spirit, alcohol *also* spir, Spt

SPA salt–poor albumin • schizophrenia with premorbid asociality • serum prothrombin activity • sheep pulmonary adenomatosis • sperm penetration assay • spinal progressive amyotrophy • spondyloarthropathy • spontaneous platelet aggregation • staphylococcal protein A • stimulation–produced analgesia • suprapatellar amputation • suprapubic aspiration

SPAC sectionally processed antibody coated

SPAD stenosing peripheral arterial disease • subcutaneous peritoneal administration device

SPAG small particle aerosol generator

SPAI steroid protein activity index

SPAM scanning photoacoustic microscopy

SPAMM spatial modulation of magnetization

span. spansule

SPAR sensitivity prediction (by) acoustic reflex

SPAT slow paroxysmal atrial tachycardia

SPBI serum protein–bound iodine

S–PBIgG serum–platelet bindable immunoglobulin G

SPBT suprapubic bladder tap

SPC salicylamide, phenacetin, caffeine • serum phenyl-alanine concentration • sickle–shaped particle cell • single palmar crease • single photoelectron counting • single proton counting • small pyramidal cell • spike–processed contraction • spleen cell *also* SC • standard plate count • synthesizing protein complex

SPCA serum prothrombin conversion accelerator (factor VII)

sp cd spinal cord

SPCK serum creatinine phosphokinase

SPD salmon–poisoning disease • silicon photodiode • sociopathic personality disorder • specific paroxysmal discharge • spectral power distribution • spermidine • standard peak dilution • subcorneal pustular dermatosis

Spd spermidine

SPDC striopallidodentate calcinosis

SPDT single–pole, double–throw (switch)

SPE septic pulmonary edema • serum protein electrolyte • serum protein electrophoresis • strepto-coccal pyrogenic exotoxin • subjective paranormal ex-perience • sucrose polyester

Spec specialist/specialty

spec special • specific • specimen

Spec Ed special education

SPECT single photon emission computed tomography

SPEG serum protein electrophoretogram

SPEM smooth pursuit eye movement

SPEP serum protein electrophoresis

SPET single photon emission tomography

SPF skin protection factor · specific–pathogen free · spectrophotofluorometer · split products (of) fibrin · standard perfusion fluid · streptococcal proliferative factor · Stuart–Prower factor · sun protective factor · suntan photoprotection factor

sp fl spinal fluid *also* SF

SPFT Sixteen Personality Factors Test

SPG serine phosphogly-ceride · specific gravity *also* SG, SpG, sp gr · sphenopalatine ganglion · sucrose–phosphate–glutamate · symmetrical peripheral gangrene

SpG specific gravity *also* SG, SPG, sp gr

spg sponge

sp gr specific gravity *also* SG, SPG, SpG

SPH secondary pulmonary hemosiderosis · severely (and) profoundly handi-capped · spherocyte · sphingomyelin *also* Sph

Sph sphenoidale · spherical · spherical (lens) · sphero-cytosis · sphingomyelin *also* SPH

sph spherical · spherical (lens) · spheroid

SPHE, SPHER spherocytes

sp ht specific heat

SPI selective protein index · serum precipitable iodine · Shipley Personal Inventory · somatotyping ponderal index · speech processor

interface · subclinical papillomavirus infection

SPIA solid–phase immunoabsorbent assay · solid–phase immunoassay

SPID summed pain intensity difference

SPIF solid–phase immunoassay fluorescence · spontaneous peak inspiratory force

SPIH superimposed pregnancy–induced hypertension

spln spine/spinal

spir spiral · [L. *spiritus*] spirit, alcohol *also* sp, Spt

spiss [L. *spissus*] dried · [L. *spissatus*] inspissated, thickened by evaporation

SPK serum pyruvate kinase · spinnbarkeit · superficial punctate keratitis

spkr speaker

SPL skin potential level · sound pressure level · spontaneous lesion · staphylococcal phage lysate

SPLATT split anterior tibial tendon (transfer)

SPLV serum parvovirus–like virus

SPM self–phase modulation · shocks per minute · significance probability mapping · spectinomycin · spermine · subhuman primate model · suspended particulate matter · syllables per minute · synaptic plasma membrane

SpM spiriformis medialis (nucleus)

SPMA spinal progressive muscular atrophy

SPMB strong partial maternal behavior

SPMI status post myocardial infarction

SPMR standardized proportionate mortality

SPN solitary pulmonary nodule • student practical nurse • supplementary parenteral nutrition • sympathetic preganglionic neuron

sp n [L. *species novum*] new species

SPO status post–operative

SPOD spouse's perception of disease

spon, spont spontaneous

SPOOL simultaneous peripheral operation on–line

SPORO sporatrichosis

SPP Sexuality Preference Profile • skin perfusion pressure • suprapubic prostatectomy

Spp, spp species (plural)

SPPS solid phase peptide synthesis • stable plasma protein solution

SPPT superprecipitation (response)

SPR scan projection radiography • serial probe recognition • skin potential reflex • solid phase radioimmunoassay *also* SPRIA • solid phase receptacle

SPRIA solid phase radio-immunoassay *also* SPR

SPROM spontaneous premature rupture of membranes

SPRT sequential probability ratio test

SPS shoulder pain (and) stiffness • simple partial seizure • slow–progressive schizophrenia • sodium polyanetholesulfonate • sodium polyethylene sulfonate • sound production sample • special Pap smear • status postsurgery • stimulated protein synthesis • sulfite polymyxin sulfadiazine (agar) • Symonds Picture–Story (Test) *also* SPST • systemic progressive sclerosis

SpS sphenoid sinus

spSHR stroke–prone spontaneous hypertensive

SPST single–pole, single–throw (switch) • Symonds Picture–Story Test *also* SPS

SPT skin prick test • slow pull–through • sound production tasks • spectinomycin • spinal tap • Spondee Picture Test • standing pivotal transfer • Supervisory Practices Test • Symbolic Play Test

Spt [L. *spiritus*] spirit, alcohol *also* sp, spir

SPTA spacial peak temporal average

Sp tap spinal tap

SPTI systolic pressure time index

SPTP spatial peak temporal peak

SPTS subjective posttraumatic syndrome

SPTURP status post–transurethral resection of prostate

SPTx static pelvic traction

SPU short procedure unit

SPUT sputum

SPV Shope papilloma virus • slow–phase velocity • sulfophosphovanillin

SPVR systemic peripheral vascular resistance

SPZ secretin pancreozymin • sulfinpyrazone

SQ social quotient • squalene • square *also* sq • status quo • subcutaneous *also* SC, sc, subcu, subcut, subq • survey question • symptom questionnaire

Sq, sq squamous

sq square *also* SQ

SQC semiquantitative culture

SqCCA squamous cell carcinoma *also* SCC, SCCA, sq cell ca

sq cell ca squamous cell carcinoma *also* SCC, SCCA, SqCCA

sqq [L. *sequentia*] and following

SQUID superconducting quantum interference device

SR sarcoplasmic reticulum • saturation–recovery • scanning radiometer • screen • secretion rate •

sedimentation rate • see report • seizure resistant • self–recording • senior • sensitivity response • sensitization response (cell) • sentence repetition • service record • sex ratio • short hair (guinea pig) • side rails • sigma reaction • silicone rubber • sinus rhythm • skin resistance • slow release • smooth–rough (bacterial colony) *also* S–R • soluble repository • specific release • specific resistance • specific response • stage (of) resistance • stimulus response • stress relaxation • stretch reflex • sulfonamide–resistant • superior rectus • supply room • sustained release • systemic reaction • systemic resistance • systems research • systems review

S–R smooth–rough (bacterial colony) *also* SR

S&R seclusion and restraint(s)

Sr strontium

sr steradian (unit of three–dimensional measure)

SRA segmented renal artery • spleen repopulating activity

SRAM static random access memory

STRAN surgical resident's admission note

SR$_{AW}$ specific airway resistance

SRBC sheep red blood cell *also* SRC • sickle red blood cell

SRBOW spontaneous rupture (of) bag of waters

SRC sedimented red cell • sheep red cell *also* SRBC

SRCA specific red cell adherence

SRCBC serum reserve cholesterol binding capacity

SRD service–related disability • sodium–restricted diet • specific reading disability

SRDT single radial diffusion test

SRE Schedule of Recent Experiences

SRF severe renal failure • skin reactive factor • slow–reacting factor • somatotropin–releasing factor • split renal function • subretinal fluid

SRF–A slow–reacting factor (of) anaphylaxis *also* SRFOA

SRFC sheep (red cell) rosette–forming cell

SRFOA slow–reacting factor of anaphylaxis *also* SRF–A

SRFS split renal function study

SRH signs (of) recent hemorrhage • single radial hemolysis • somatotropin–releasing hormone • spontaneously responding hyperthyroidism • stigmata (of) recent hemorrhage

SRI severe renal insufficiency

SRID single radial immunodiffusion

SRIF somatotropin–release inhibiting factor

SRM Standard Reference Material • superior rectus muscle

SMRD stress–related mucosal damage

SRN subretinal neovascularization *also* SRNV

sRNA soluble ribonucleic acid

SR/NE sinus rhythm, no ectopy

SRNG sustained release nitroglycerin

SRNP soluble ribonuclear protein

SRNS steroid–responsive nephrotic syndrome

SRNV subretinal neovascularization *also* SRN

SRNVM senile retinal neovascular membrane • subretinal neovascular membrane

SRO single room occupancy

SROM spontaneous rupture of membranes

SRP short rib–polydactyly (syndrome) • signal recognition protein • simple response paradigm • stapes replacement prosthesis • State Registered Physiotherapist

SRPS short rib–polydactyly syndrome

SRR slow rotation room • stabilized relative response • standardized rate ratio • surgical recovery room

SRRS Social Readjustment
Rating Scale

SR–RSV Schmidt–Ruppin
(strain) Rous sarcoma virus

SRS schizophrenic residual
state • sex reassignment
surgery • Silver–Russell
syndrome • slow–reacting
substance • Social and
Rehabilitation Service •
Symptom Rating Scale

SRSA, SRS–A slow–reacting
substance (of) anaphylaxis

SRT sedimentation rate test •
sick role tendency • simple
reaction time • sinus (node)
recovery time *also* SNRT •
speech reception test •
speech reception threshold •
spontaneously resolving
thyrotoxicosis • sustained
release theophylline •
Symptom Rating Test

SRU side rails up • solitary
rectal ulcer • structural
repeating unit

SRUS solitary rectal ulcer
syndrome

SRV Schmidt–Ruppin virus •
superior radicular vein

S–R variation smooth–rough
variation

SRVT sustained re–entrant
ventricular tachyarrhythmia

SRW short ragweed (test)

SS sacrosciatic • saline
soak • saline solution •
saliva sample • saliva
substitute • *Salmonella–
Shigella* (agar) • salt
substitute • saturated
solution • schizophrenia
spectrum • Schizophrenia

Subscale • seizure sensi-
tive • serum sickness •
Sézary syndrome •
siblings • sickle cell
(anemia) • side–to–side •
signs (and) symptoms •
single stranded *also* ss •
Sjögren syndrome • sliding
scale • slip sent • slow–
wave sleep • soap suds
also ss • Social Security •
social services • somato-
statin *also* SMS • sparingly
soluble • special service •
stable sarcoidosis • staccato
syndrome • standard
score • statistically
significant • steady state
also ss • sterile solution •
steroid sensitivity • steroid
sulfurylation • Stickler
syndrome • Strachan–Scott
(syndrome) • subaortic
stenosis • subscapularis •
subsegmental • subsequent
sibling • substernal •
suction socket •
sulfasalazine • sum (of)
squares • supersaturated •
support (and) stimulation •
susceptible • Sweet
syndrome • symmetrical
strength • systemic sclerosis

S&S shower and shampoo •
signs and symptoms *also*
S/S • support and
stimulation

S/S signs and symptoms *also*
S&S

Ss serum soluble (antigen) •
subjects

ss [L. *semis*] half *also* S, s,
sem, semi • single stranded
also SS • soap suds *also*
SS • steady state *also* SS •
subspinale

SSA sagittal split advancement • salicylsalicylic acid • *Salmonella–Shigella* agar • sickle cell anemia • Sjören syndrome antigen A • skin–sensitizing antibody • skin sympathetic activity • Smith surface antigen • Social Security Administration • special somatic afferent • sperm–specific antigen • sperm–specific antiserum • subsegmental airway • subsegmental atelectasis • sulfosalicylic acid

SS–A Sjögren syndrome A (antibody)

SSAV simian sarcoma–associated virus

SSB short spike burst • stereospecific binding

SS–B Sjögren syndrome B (antibody)

SSBG sex steroid–binding globulin

SSBR see separate bacteriology report

SSC somatosensory cortex • standard saline citrate • Stein Sentence Completion (test) • superior semicircular canal • syngeneic spleen cell

SSc systemic sclerosis

SSCA sensitized sheep cell agglutination • single shoulder contrast arthrography • spontaneous suppressor cell activity

SSCCS slow spinal cord compression syndrome

SSCF sleep stage change frequency

SSCP substernal chest pain

SSCr stainless steel crown

SSCVD sterile spontaneous controlled vaginal delivery

SSD shock(–induced) suppression (of) drinking • sickle cell disease • silver sulfadiazine • single saturating dose • Social Security Disability • source–skin distance • source–surface distance • speech–sound discrimination • succinate semialdehyde dehydrogenase • sudden sniffing death • sum (of) square deviations • syndrome (of) sudden death

SSDI Social Security disability income

SS–DNA, ssDNA single–stranded deoxyribonucleic acid

SSE saline solution enema • skin self–examination • soapsuds enema • steady–state exercise • systemic side effects

SSEA stage–specific embryonic antigen

SSEP somatosensory evoked potential *also* SEP

SSER somatosensory evoked response *also* SER

SSF soluble suppressor factor • subscapular skinfold (thickness) • supplementary sensory feedback

SSFI social stress (and) functionability inventory

SSG sublabial salivary gland

SSHb homozygous for sickle cell hemoglobin

SSHL severe sensorineural hearing loss

SSI segmental sequential irradiation • small–scale integration • Social Security income • stuttering severity instrument • subshock insulin • Supplemental Security Income • synthetic sentence identification • System Sign Inventory

SSIAM Structured and Scaled Interview to Assess Maladjustment

SSIDS sibling of sudden infant death syndrome (victim)

SSIE Smithsonian Science Information Exchange

SSII Safran Student's Interest Inventory

SSIT subscapularis, supraspinatus, infraspinatus, teres minor (muscles)

SSKI saturated solution of potassium iodide

SSL skin surface lipid • synthetic sentence list

SSM subsynaptic membrane • superficial spreading melanoma

SSN severely subnormal • Social Security number • suprasternal notch *also* SN

SSNS steroid–sensitive nephrotic syndrome

SSO Spanish–speaking only • special sense organs

SSOP Second Surgical Opinion Program

SSP Sanarelli–Shwartzman phenomenon • small spherical particle • subacute sclerosing panencephalitis *also* SSPE • supersensitivity perception

Ssp, ssp subspecies *also* subsp

SSPE subacute sclerosing panencephalitis *also* SSP

SSPG steady–state plasma glucose

SSPI steady–state plasma insulin

SSPL saturation sound pressure level

SSPP subsynaptic plate perforation

SSPS side–to–side portacaval shunt

SS–PSE Schizophrenic Subscale of Present State Examination

SSPU surgical short procedure unit

SSR somatosensory response • steady–state rest • steroid–resistant rejection • surgical supply room

SSS [L. *stratum super stratum*] layer upon layer *also* sss • scalded skin syndrome • sensation–seeking scale • sick sinus syndrome • specific soluble substance • Stanford Sleepiness Scale • sterile saline soak • strong soap solution • structured sensory stimulation • systemic sicca syndrome

sss [L. *stratum super stratum*] layer upon layer *also* SSS

SSSB sagittal split setback

SSSS staphylococcal scalded skin syndrome

SSST superior sagittal sinus thrombosis

SSSV superior sagittal sinus velocity

SST sagittal sinus thrombosis • sodium sulfite titration • somatosensory thalamus • somatostatin

s str [L. *sensu stricto*] in the strict sense

SSU self–service unit • sterile supply unit

SSV Schoolman–Schwartz virus • sheep seminal vesicle • simian sarcoma virus *also* SISV, SiSV • [L. *sub signo veneni*] under a poison label

SSW staggered spondaic word (test)

SSX sulfisoxazole

S/SX signs/symptoms

ST electrocardiographic wave segment • esotropia • sacrum transverse • scala tympani • sclerotherapy • sedimentation time • semitendinosus • septal thickness • serum transferrin • shock therapy • siblings (raised) together • similarly tested • sinus tachycardia • sinus tympani • skin temperature • skin test • skin thickness • slight trace • slow twitch • speech therapist • sphincter tone • split thickness • (heat-)stable (entero)toxin •

standard test • starting time • sternothyroid • stimulus *also* R, S • stomach *also* St, st, stom • store *also* STO • straight • stress test • stretcher • striatum *also* Str • sublingual tablet • subtalar • subtotal • sulfathiozole • surface tension *also* σ • surgical therapy • survival time • systolic time

S–T sickle–cell thalassemia

St, st [L. *stet*] let it stand • [L. *stent*] let them stand • stage (of disease) • stere (measure of capacity) • stokes (unit of kinematic viscosity) • stomach *also* stom • stomion (median point of oral slit when lips are closed) • stone (unit) • straight • stroke • subtype

ST37 hexylresorcinol

STA second trimester abortion • serum thrombotic accelerator • serum tobramycin assay • superficial temporal artery • superior temporal artery

Sta staphylion • station

stab stabilization • "stabkernige" (staff or band neutrophils) • stabnuclear neutrophil

STACL Screening Test for Auditory Comprehension of Language

St AE standard above–elbow (cast)

STAG split thickness autogenous graft

S–TAG slow–binding target–attaching globulin

STAI State Trait Anxiety Inventory

STAI–I State–Trait–Anxiety Index–I

STA–MCA superficial temporal artery to middle cerebral artery

StanPsych standard psychiatric (nomenclature)

staph staphylococcus

STAT [L. *statim*] at once *also* stat • Suprathreshold Adaptation Test

stat [L. *statim*] at once *also* STAT • radiation emanation unit (German)

STB, Stb stillborn *also* SB, stillb

STBAL standing balance

ST BY stand by *also* SB

STC serum theophylline concentration • sexually transmitted condition • soft tissue calcification • stimulate to cry • Stroke Treatment Center • subtotal colectomy • sugar tongue cast

STD sexually transmitted disease • skin test done • skin test dose • skin–to–tumor distance • sodium tetradecyl (sulfate) • standard density (reference) • standard test dose

std saturated *also* sat'd • standardized

STDH skin test (for) delayed–type hypersensitivity

STDT standard tone–decay test

STD TF standard tube feeding

STEAM stimulated–echo acquisition mode

STEM scanning transmission electron microscope

sten stenosis/stenosed

STEPS sequential treatment employing pharmacologic support

stereo stereogram • stereophonic

STET submaximal treadmill exercise test

STETH stethoscope

STF serum thymus factor • slow twitch fiber • small third–trimester fetus • specialized treatment facility • special tube feeding • standard tube feeding • sudden transient freezing

ST–FeSv Synder–Thielen feline sarcoma virus

STG short–term goal • split–thickness graft

STGC syncytiotrophoblastic giant cell

STH soft tissue hemorrhage • somatotropic hormone *also* SH • subtotal hysterectomy • supplemental thyroid hormone

STh, S–Thal sickle cell thalassemia

STHB said to have been

STI scientific and technical information • serum trypsin inhibitor • soft tissue injury • soybean trypsin inhibitor *also* SBTI • systolic time interval

STIC serum trypsin inhibition capacity • solid–state transducer intracompartment

stillat [L. *stillatim*] drop by drop

stillb stillborn *also* SB, Stb

stim, stimn stimulation*also* stm, stmn

STIP (basophilic) stippling

STJ subtalar joint

STK streptokinase

STL serum theophylline level • status thymicolymphaticus • swelling, tenderness, limited (motion)

STLE St. Louis encephalitis

STLOM swelling, tenderness, limitation of motion

STLV simian T–cell lymphotropic virus

STM scanning tunneling microscope • short–term memory • streptomycin

stm, stmn stimulation *also* stim, stimn

StMPM syncytiotrophoblast microvillar plasma membrane

STN subthalamic nucleus • supratrochlear nucleus

STNR symmetric tonic neck reflex

STNS sham transcutaneous nerve stimulation

STNV satellite tobacco necrosis virus

STO store *also* ST

stom stomach *also* ST, St, st

STORCH syphilis, toxoplasmosis, rubella, cytomegalovirus, (and) herpesvirus

STP scientifically treated petroleum • serenity, tranquility, peace user's term for (dimethoxymethylamphetamine) • Sibling Training Program • sodium thiopental • standard temperature (and) pressure • standard temperature (and) pulse

STPD standard temperature (and) pressure, dry

STPI State–Trait Personality Inventory

STPP sodium tripolyphosphate

STPS specific thalamic projection system

STQ superior temporal quadrant

STR soft–tissue rheumatism • special treatment room

Str striatum *also* ST

strab strabismus *also* Sb

Strep streptomycin

STRESS subject's treatment–emergent symptom scale

STRT skin temperature recovery time

struct structure/structural

STS serologic test (for) syphilis • sexual tubal sterilization • short–term storage • sodium tetradecyl sulfate • sodium thiosulfate • soft tissue swelling • standard test (for) syphilis • sugar–tong splint

STSG split–thickness skin graft

STSS staphylococcal toxic shock syndrome

STT sensitization test • serial thrombin time • skin temperature test • standard triple therapy

STTOL standing tolerance

STU shock trauma unit • skin test unit

STV short–term variability • soft tissue view • superior temporal vein

STVA subtotal villous atrophy *also* SVA

STVS short–term visual storage

STX saxitoxin • structure

STYCAR Screening Tests for Young Children and Retardates

STZ streptozocin *also* SZ, Sz, SZN • streptozyme

SU salicyluric (acid) • sensation unit • sensory urgency • solar urticaria • Somogyi unit • sorbent unit • spectrophotometric unit • strontium unit • subunit • sulfonamide *also* Su • sulfonylurea • supine

S&U supine and upright

Su sulfonamide *also* SU

su [L. *sumat*] let him take

SUA serum uric acid • single umbilical artery • single unit activity

SUB Skene, urethral and Bartholin (glands)

subac subacute

subconj subconjunctival

subcu, subcut subcutaneous *also* SC, sc, SQ, subq

sub fin coct [L. *sub finem coctionis*] toward the end of boiling

subl, subling sublingual

submand submandibular

SubN subthalamic nucleus

subq subcutaneous *also* SC, sc, SQ, subcu, subcut

subsp subspecies *also* Ssp, ssp

substd substandard

suc [L. *succus*] juice

SUCC succinylcholine

Succ succinate/succinic

SUD skin unit dose • sudden unexpected death • sudden unexplained death

SUDS single–unit delivery system • Subjective Unit of Distress Scale

SUF sequential ultrafiltration

Suff sufficient

SUHT subject's height (in inches)

SUI stress urinary incontinence • suicide

SUID sudden unexpected/ unexplained infant death

sulf sulfate

sulfa sulfonamide

SULFHB sulfhemoglobin

SULF–PRIM sulfamethoxazole (and) trimethoprim

sum. [L. *sumat*] let him take • [L. *sumendum*] to be taken • summation

SUMIT streptokinase–urokinase myocardial infarction trial

sum. tal [L. *sumat talem*] let the person take one like this

SUN serum urea nitrogen • Standard Units and Nomenclature

SUO syncope (of) unknown origin

SUP superficial *also* sup. • superior *also* sup. • supination *also* supin • supinator (muscle) *also* sup. • symptomatic uterine prolapse

sup. [L. *supra*] above • superficial *also* SUP • superior *also* SUP • supervision/supervisor • supinator *also* SUP

supin supination *also* SUP

supp support • suppository

suppl supplement/supplementary

supp, suppos suppository

SURG, surg surgery/surgeon/surgical *also* S

SURS solitary ulcer of rectum syndrome

SUS solitary ulcer syndrome • stained urinary sediment • suppressor sensitive

susp suspension/suspended

SUTI symptomatic urinary tract infection

SUUD sudden unexpected unexplained death

SUX succinylcholine • suction

SV saphenous vein • sarcoma

virus • satellite virus • selective vagotomy • semilunar valve • seminal vesicle • Sendai virus • severe • sigmoid volvulus • simian virus • single ventricle • sinus venosus • snake venom • splenic vein • spoken voice • spontaneous ventilation • stroke volume • subclavian vein • subventricular • supravital

S/V surface/volume (ratio)

SV40 simian vacuolating virus 40

Sv sievert (unit) *also* sv

sv sievert *also* Sv • single vibration • [L. *spiritus vini*] spirit of wine

SVA selective vagotomy (with) antrectomy • selective visceral angiography • sequential ventriculoatrial (pacing) • spatial voltage (at maximal) anterior (force) • special visceral afferent • subtotal villous atrophy *also* STVA

SVAS subvalvular aortic stenosis • supravalvular aortic stenosis

SVB saphenous vein bypass

SVBG saphenous vein bypass graft

SVC segmental venous capacitance • slow vital capacity • subclavian vein catheterization • superior vena cava • suprahepatic vena cava

SVCG spatial vector-cardiogram

SVCO superior vena cava obstruction

SVCP Special Virus Cancer Program

SVC–PA superior vena cava–pulmonary artery (shunt)

SVCR segmented venous capacitance ratio

SVC–RPA superior vena cava–right pulmonary artery (shunt)

SVCS superior vena cava syndrome

SVD single vessel disease • singular value decomposition • small vessel disease • spontaneous vaginal delivery • spontaneous vertex delivery • swine vesicular disease

SVE slow volume encephalography • soluble viral extract • special visceral efferent • sterile vaginal examination • *Streptococcus viridans* endocarditis • supraventricular ectopy

SVG saphenous vein graft

SVI stroke volume index • systolic velocity integral (Doppler)

SVL severe visual loss • superficial vastus lateralis

SVM seminal vesicle microsome • spatial voltage (at) maximal (posterior force) • syncytiovascular membrane

SVN small volume nebulizer

SvO₂, S$_{VO2}$ venous oxygen saturation

SVOM sequential volitional oral movement

SVP selective vagotomy (with) pyloroplasty • small volume parenteral (infusion) • spatial voltage (at maximal) posterior (force) • spontaneous venous pulse • standing venous pressure • static volume pressure • superficial vascular plexus

SVPB supraventricular premature beat

SVPC supraventricular premature contraction

SVR sequential vascular response • supraventricular rhythm • systemic vascular resistance

svr [L. *spiritus vini rectificatus*] rectified spirit of wine (distilled)

SVRI systemic vascular resistance index

SVS slit ventricle syndrome

SVSe supravaginal septum

SVT sinoventricular tachyarrhythmia • subclavian vein thrombosis • supraventricular tachyarrhythemia • supraventricular tachycardia

svt [L. *spiritus vini tenuis*] thin spirit of wine (diluted)

SW Schwartz–Watson (test) • seriously wounded • short wave • slow wave • social worker • spherule wall • spike wave • spiral wound • stab wound • sterile water • stroke work • Sturge–Weber (syndrome) • Swiss Webster (mouse)

Sw swine

sw switch

SWAMP swine–associated mucoprotein

SWC submaximal working capacity

SWD short wave diathermy

SWFI sterile water for injection *also* SWI

SWG standard wire gauge

SWI skin (and) wound isolation • sterile water (for) injection *also* SWFI • stroke work index • surgical wound infection

SWIM sperm–washing insemination method

SWM segmental wall motion

SWO superficial white onychomycosis

SWP small whirlpool

SWR serum Wassermann reaction

SWS slow–wave sleep • spike–wave stupor • Sturge–Weber syndrome

SWT sine–wave threshold • Speech Weber Test • stab wound (of) throat

SWU septic work–up

SX sulfamethoxypyridazine

Sx, S$_x$ signs • surgery • symptoms

SXR skull x–ray

SXT sulfamethoxazole/ trimethoprim

SY syphilis/syphilitic *also* syph

SYA subacute yellow atrophy

SYC small, yellow, constipated (stool)

sym symmetrical • symptom *also* symp, sympt

symb symbol • symbolic

sympath sympathetic

symph symphysis

symp, sympt symptom *also* sym

syn synonym • synovial

syn, synd syndrome

sync synchronous

syn fl synovial fluid *also* SF

synth synthetic

syph syphilis/syphilitic *also* SY

SYR Syrian (hamster)

Syr [L. *syrupus*] syrup *also* syr

syr syringe • [L. *syrupus*] syrup *also* Syr

SYS stretching–yawning syndrome

sys system/systemic *also* syst

SYS BP systolic blood pressure *also* SBP

syst system/systemic *also* sys • systole/systolic

SZ schizophrenic • seizure *also* Sz • Skevas–Zerfus (disease) • streptozocin *also* STZ, Sz, SZN • suction • sulfamethizole

Sz seizure *also* SZ • schizophrenia • skin impedance • streptozocin *also* STZ, SZ, SZN

SZD streptozocin diabetes

SZN streptozocin *also* STZ, SZ, Sz

T electrocardiographic wave corresponding to repolarization of ventricles • life(time) *also* t • obtained under test conditions • period (time) • ribosylthymine • ribothymidine • tablespoonful *also* tbsp • tamoxifen *also* TAM, TMX • tanycyte (ependymal cell) • T–bandage • T–bar • telomere or terminal banding • temperature *also* temp • temporal electrode placement in electroencephalography • temporary *also* temp • tender • tension (intraocular) *also* TEM • tera– • tertiary *also* t, ter, tert • tesla • testicle • testosterone • tetra • tetracycline *also* TC, TCN, TCNE, TE • T-fiber • theophylline • thoracic *also* thor • thoracoabdominal (stapler) • thorax *also* th, Th, thor • threatened (animal) • threonine • thrombus *also* throm, thromb • thymidine *also* TdR • thymine *also* Thy • thymus (cell) *also* thy. • thymus–derived (lymphocyte) • thyroid • tidal gas • tidal volume (subscript) • time • timolol • tincture *also* TR, Tr, tr • tocopherol • tone • tonometer reading • topical *also* top. • torque • total • toxicity *also* Tox, tox • trace *also* TR • training (group) • transition (point) *also* TP • transmittance • transverse *also* trans • tray • triangulation • triggered • tritium • tuberculin •

T

tuberculosis *also* TB, Tb, tb, TBC, Tbc, tuberc • tuberculum • tuberosity • tumor • turnkey system • type

T– decreased tension (pressure)

T+ increased tension (pressure)

T$\frac{1}{2}$ (mitral) pressure half–time (Doppler) • terminal half–life (of isotopes)

T$_1$ monoiodotyrosine • tricuspid first heart sound

T1 spin–lattice or longitudinal relaxation time (MRI scan)

T1–T12 first to twelfth thoracic vertebrae or nerves

T+1, T+2, T+3 first, second, and third stages of increased intraocular tension

T–1, T–2, T–3 first, second, and third stages of decreased intraocular tension

T$_2$ diiodothyronine • tricuspid second heart sound

T2 spin–spin or transverse relaxation time (MRI scan)

T$_3$ triiodothyronine *also* TIT, TITh, TRIT

T3 Tylenol with codeine (30 mg)

T$_4$ levothyroxine • tetraiodothyronine (thyroxine)

T–7 free thyroxin factor

2,4,5–T 2,4,5–trichlorophenoxyacetic acid

T–1824 Evans blue (dye)

T absolute temperature (Kelvin)

t duration • life(time) *also* T • Student test variable • teaspoonful • temperature (Celsius, Fahrenheit) • temporal • terminal • tertiary *also* T, ter, tert • [L. *ter*] three times • test of significance • ton (metric) • tonne • translocation • tritium

t½ reaction half–time • time taken for half of initial concentration of deoxyribonucleic acid to renature

TA tactile afferent • Takayasu arteritis • technical assistance • teichoic acid • temperature, axillary *also* T(A) • temporal arteritis • temporal average • tendon (of) Achilles • tension (by) applanation *also* Ta • tension, arterial • terminal antrum • test age • therapeutic abortion *also* TAB • thermophilic *Actinomyces* • thymocytotoxic autoantibody • thyroglobulin autoprecipitation • thyroglobulin autoprecipitin • thyroid antibody • thyroid autoantibody • tibialis anterior • titratable acid • total alkaloids • toxic adenoma • toxin–antitoxin *also* T–A, TAT • tracheal aspirate • traffic accident *also* T/A • transactional analysis • transaldolase • transantral • transplantation antigen • trapped air • treatment assignment • triamcinolone acetonide *also* TAA • tricholomic acid • tricuspid

annuloplasty • tricuspid atresia • trophoblast antigen • true anomaly • truncus arteriosus • tryptamine • tryptophan–acid (reaction) • tryptose agar • tube agglutination • tuberculin, alkaline • tumor antigen • tumor associated

T–A toxin–antitoxin *also* TA

T/A time (and) amount • traffic accident *also* TA, TAT

T&A tonsillectomy and adenoidectomy • tonsils and adenoids

T(A) temperature, axillary *also* TA

TA₄ tetraiodothyroacetic acid

Ta T–amplifier • tantalum • tension (by) applanation *also* TA • tonometry applanation

TAA thoracic aortic aneurysm • total ankle arthroplasty • transverse aortic arch • triamcinolone acetonide *also* TA • tumor–associated antigen

TAAF thromblastic activity (of) amniotic fluid

TAB tablet *also* tab. • therapeutic abortion *also* TA • triple antibiotic • typhoid, paratyphoid A, and paratyphoid B (vaccine)

TAb therapeutic abortion

tab. tablet *also* TAB

TABC total aerobic bacteria count • typhoid, paratyphoid A, paratyphoid B, and paratyphoid C (vaccine)

TABTD typhoid, paratyphoid A, paratyphoid B, tetanus toxoid, and diphtheria toxoid (vaccine)

TAC terminal antrum contraction • tetracaine, Adrenalin (epinephrine), and cocaine • time–activity curve • total aganglionosis coli • Toxicant Analysis Center • triamcinolone acetonide cream

TACE teichoic acid crude extract • trianisylchloro-ethylene

tach, tachy tachycardia

TACL Test for Auditory Comprehension of Language

TAD thoracic asphyxiant dystrophy • total administered dose • transverse abdominal diameter • tricyclic antidepressant drug

TADAC therapeutic abortion, dilation, aspiration, curettage

TAE transcatheter arterial embolization

TAF [Ger. *Tuberculin Albumose frei*] albumose–free tuberculin • tissue angiogenesis factor • toxoid–antitoxin floccule • trypsin–aldehyde–fuchsin • tumor angiogenesis factor

TAG target–attaching globulin • thymine, adenine, guanine • triacylglycerol

TAGH triiodothyronine, amino acids, glucagon, heparin

TAH total abdominal hysterec-tomy • total artificial

heart • transabdominal hysterectomy

TAHBSO total abdominal hysterectomy and bilateral salpingo–oophorectomy

TAI tissue antagonist (of) interferon

TAL tendo Achillis lengthen-ing • thymic alympho-plasia • total arm length

tal [L. *talis*] such a one

tal dos such doses

talc talcum

TALH thick ascending limb (of) Henle's (loop)

TALL, T–ALL T–cell acute lymphoblastic leukemia

TALTFR tendo Achillis lengthening and toe flexor release

TAM tamoxifen *also* T, TMX • teenage mother • thermoacidurans agar modified • total active motion • toxoid–antitoxoid mixture • transient abnormal myelopoiesis

TAMe toxoid–antitoxoid mixture esterase

TAMIS Telemetric Automated Microbial Identification System

TAML, t–AML therapy-related acute myeloid leukemia

TAN total adenine nucleotide • total ammonia nitrogen

tan. tandem translocation • tangent

TANI total axial (lymph) node irradiation

TAO thromboangiitis obliterans · triacetyl-oleandomycin · turning against object

TAP tension (by) applanation · tonometry (by) applanation

TAPS training and placement service · trial assessment procedure scale

TAPVC total anomalous pulmonary venous connection

TAPVD total anomalous pulmonary venous drainage

TAPVR total anomalous pulmonary venous return

TAQW transient abnormal Q wave

TAR thrombocytopenia (with) absent radii (syndrome) · tissue–air ratio · total abortion rate · total ankle replacement · Treatment Authorization Request

TARA total articular replacement arthroplasty · tumor–associated rejection antigen

TAS test (for) ascendance-submission · tetanus antitoxic serum · Therapeutic Activities Specialist · turning against self · typical absence seizure

TASA tumor–associated surface antigen

T'ase, Tase tryptophan synthetase

TAT Tell a Tale (psychiatry) · tetanus antitoxin · thematic apperception test · thematic aptitude test · thromboplastin activation test · till all taken · total antitryptic

activity · toxin–antitoxin *also* TA, T–A · transaxial tomogram · transverse axial tomography · tray agglutination test · tumor activity test · turnaround time · tyrosine aminotransferase

TATA tumor–associated transplantation antigen

TATBA triamcinolone acetomide *tert*–butyl acetate

TATR tyrosine aminotransferase regulator

TATST tetanus antitoxin skin test

tau (T, τ) nineteenth letter of Greek alphabet

τ life (of radioisotope) · relaxation time · shear stress · spectral transmittance · transmission coefficient

$\tau_{\frac{1}{2}}$ half–life (of radioactive isotopes)

TAV trapped air volume

TB Tapes for the Blind · terminal bronchiole · thromboxane B · thymol blue · toluidine blue · total base · total bilirubin · total body · tracheal bronchiolar (region) · tracheobronchitis · trapezoid body · tub bath · tubercle bacillus *also* Tb, TBA · tuberculin · tuberculosis *also* T, Tb, tb, TBC, Tbc, tuberc · tumor bearing

T–B Thomas–Binetti (test)

Tb terbium · tubercle bacillus *also* TB, TBA · tuberculosis *also* T, TB, tb, TBC, Tbc, tuberc

T$_b$ temperature, body

tb biologic half–life • tuberculosis *also* T, TB, Tb

TBA tertiary butyl acetate • testosterone–binding affinity • thiobarbituric acid • thyroxin–binding albumin • to be absorbed • to be added • to be administered • to be admitted • total bile acid • total body (surface) area • traditional birth attendant • trypsin–binding activity • tubercle bacillus *also* TB, Tb • tumor–bearing animal

TBAB tryptose/blood/agar base

T banding telomere/terminal banding (of chromosomes)

TBB transbronchial biopsy

TBBC total (vitamin) B$_{12}$ binding capacity

TBBM total body bone mineral

TBC thyroxin–binding coagulin • total body calcium • total body clearance *also* Q$_B$ • total body counting • tubercidin • tuberculosis/ tuberculous *also* T, TB, Tb, tb, Tbc, tuberc

Tbc tuberculosis *also* T, TB, Tb, tb, TBC, tuberc

TBD total body density • Toxicology Data Base

TBE tick–borne encephalitis • tuberculin bacillary emulsion

TBF total body fat

TBFB tracheobronchial foreign body

TBG testosterone–binding globulin • thyroxin–binding globulin • tracheobronchogram • tris–buffered Grey (solution)

TBGE thyroxin–binding globulin, estimated

TBGI thyroid–binding globulin index • thyroxin–binding globulin index

TBGP total blood granulocyte pool

TBH total–body hematocrit

TBHT total–body hyperthermia

TBI thyroid–binding index • thyroxin–binding index • tooth–brushing instruction • total–body irradiation *also* TBX • traumatic brain injury

TBII thyroid–stimulating hormone (TSH)–binding inhibitory immunoglobulin

TBIL, T BIll total bilirubin (assay)

TBK total body kalium (potassium)

TBLB transbronchial lung biopsy

TBLC term birth, living child

TBLF term birth, living female

TBLI term birth, living infant

TBLM term birth, living male

TBM thyroxin–binding meningitis • total body mass • tracheobronchomalacia • tuberculous meningitis • tubular basement membrane

TBN bacillus emulsion • total body nitrogen

TBNA total–body neutron activation • total–body sodium • transbronchial needle aspiration • treated but not admitted

TBNAA total–body neutron activation analysis

TBP testosterone–binding protein • thiobisdichlorophenol (bithionol) • thyroxin–binding protein • total–body photograph • total bypass • tributyl phosphate • tuberculous peritonitis

TBPA thyroxin–binding prealbumin

TBPT total–body protein turnover

TBR total bed rest • tumor–bearing rabbit

TB–RD tuberculosis–respiratory disease

TBRS Timed Behavioral Rating Sheet

TBS total body solids • total body solute • total body surface • total burn size • tracheal bronchial submucosa • tracheobronchoscopy • tribromsalan (tribromosalicylanilide) • triethanolamine–buffered saline

tbs tablespoon

TBSA total body surface area • total burn surface area

tbsp tablespoonful *also* T

TbT, TBT tolbutamide test • tracheobronchial toilet • tracheobronchial tree

TBTNR Toronto Biculture Test of Nonverbal Reasoning

TBTT tuberculin tine test

TBUT tear break–up time

TBV total blood volume • transluminal balloon valvuloplasty

TBV$_p$ total blood volume predicted (from body surface)

TBW total body washout • total body water *also* TBWA • total body weight

TBWA total body water *also* TBW

TBX total body irradiation *also* TBI • thromboxane *also* Thx, TX

TBZ tetrabenazine • thiabendazole

TC target cell • taurocholate • taurocholic (acid) • telephone call *also* T/C • temperature compensation • teratocarcinoma • tertiary cleavage • tetracycline *also* T, TCN, TCNE, TE • therapeutic community • therapeutic concentrate • thermal conductivity *also* λ • thermal conductivity (detector) • thoracic cage • throat culture *also* TH–CULT • thyrocalcitonin *also* TC • tissue culture • to contain • total calcium • total capacity • total cholesterol • total colonoscopy • total correction • transcobalamin • transcutaneous *also* tc • transplant center • transverse colon • trauma center • Treacher Collins (syndrome) • treatment completed • true conjugate • tuberculin, contagious • tuberculosis, contagious • tubocurarine • tumor cell • type (and) cross–match *also* T&C, T&M

T/C telephone call *also* TC • to consider

T&C test and cross–match • turn and cough • type and cross–match *also* TC, T&M

TC I, TC II transcobalamin I, transcobalamin II

TC$_{50}$ median toxic concentration

T$_4$(C) serum thyroxin measured by column chromatography

Tc core temperature • T (cell) cytolytic • T (cell) cytotoxic • technetium • temporal complex • tetracycline • transcobalamin

T$_c$ generation time of cell cycle

tc transcutaneous *also* TC • translational control

TCA terminal cancer/carcinoma • tetracyclic antidepressant • thioguanine (and) cytarabine • thyrocalcitonin • total cholic acid • total circulating albumin • total circulatory arrest • transluminal coronary angioplasty • tricalcium aluminate • tricarboxylic acid • trichloroacetate • trichloracetic acid • tricuspid atresia • tricyclic amine • tricyclic antidepressant *also* TCAD

TCABG triple coronary artery bypass graft *also* TCAG

TCAD tricyclic antidepressant *also* TCA

TCAG triple coronary artery (bypass) graft *also* TCABG

TCB tetrachlorobiphenyl • to call back • total cardiopulmonary bypass • transcatheter biopsy • tumor cell burden

TCBS triosulfate–citrate–bile salts–sucrose (agar)

TCC thromboplastic cell component • toroidal coil chromatography • transitional cell carcinoma • trichlocarban *also* Tcc • trichlorocarbanilide

Tcc triclocarban *also* TCC

TCCA transitional cell cancer–associated (virus)

TCCB transitional cell carcinoma (of) bladder

TCCL T–cell chronic lymphocytic (leukemia)

TC CO$_2$ transcutaneous carbon dioxide (monitor)

TCD thermal conductivity detector • tissue culture dose • transverse cardiac diameter

TCD$_{50}$ median tissue culture dose

TCDB, TC&DB turn, cough, deep breath

TCDC taurochenodeoxycholate

TcDISIDA technetium diisopropyliminodiacetic acid (scan)

TCE T cell enriched • tetrachlorodiphenyl ethane •

trichloroethylene · trichloroethanol

TCES transcutaneous cranial electrical stimulation

TCESOM trichloroethylene–extracted soybean–oil meal

TCET transcerebral electrotherapy

TCF tissue–coding factor *also* TSF · total coronary flow · Treacher–Collins–Franceschetti syndrome

TCFU tumor colony–forming unit

TCG time compensation gain

TCGF thymus cell growth factor

TCH tanned cell hemagglutination · total circulating hemoglobin · turn, cough, hyperventilate

TChE total cholinesterase

TcHIDA technetium hepato-iminodiacetic acid (scan)

TCI to come in (to hospital) · total cerebral ischemia · transient cerebral ischemia · tricuspid insufficiency · Totman's Change Index

TCi teracurie

TCID tissue culture infective dose · tissue culture inoculated dose

TCID$_{50}$ median tissue culture infective dose

TcIDA technetium iminodiacetic acid

TCIE transient cerebral ischemic episode

TCIPA tumor–cell–induced platelet aggregation

TCL triazine chlorguanide · thermochemiluminescence · total capacity (of) lung

T–CLL T–cell chronic lymphatic leukemia

TCM tissue culture medium · traditional Chinese medicine · transcutaneous monitor

TCMA transcortical motor aphasia

TCMH tumor–direct cell–mediated hypersensitivity

TCMP thematic content modification program

TCMZ trichloromethiazide

TCN, TCNE tetracycline *also* T, TC, TE

TCNS transcutaneous nerve stimulator/stimulation *also* TNS

TCOM transcutaneous oxygen monitor *also* TOM

TCP teacher–child–parent · therapeutic class profile · therapeutic continuous penicillin · total circulating protein · tranylcypromine · tricalcium phosphate · trichlorophenol · tricresyl phosphate

TCPA tetrachlorophthalic anhydride

TCPCO$_2$, tcPCO$_2$ trans-cutaneous carbon dioxide pressure

TCPE trichlorophenoxyethanol

TCPO$_2$, tcPO$_2$ transcutaneous (partial) pressure of oxygen

TCR T–cell reactivity · T–cell rosette · thalamocortical relay · total cytoplasmic ribosome

tcRNA translational control ribonucleic acid

TCRP total cellular receptor pool

TCRV total red cell volume

TCS T–cell supernatant · total cellular score · total coronary score

Tcs T–cell–mediating contact sensitivity

TCSA tetrachlorosalicylanilide

TCT thrombin clotting time · thyrocalcitonin *also* TC

TCV thoracic cage volume · three concept view

TCVA thromboembolic cerebral vascular accident

TD Takayasu disease · tardive dyskinesia *also* TDK · T-cell dependent · temporary disability · teratoma differentiated · terminal device · tetanus and diphtheria (toxoid) · tetrodotoxin · therapeutic dietitian · therapy discontinued · thermal dilution · thoracic duct · three times per day · threshold of detectability · threshold of discomfort · threshold dose · thymus–dependent · tidal volume · timed disintegration · tocopherol deficient · to deliver · tolerance dose · tone decay · torsion dystonia · total disability · total dose · totally disabled · toxic dose · tracheal diameter · tracking dye ·

transdermal · transverse diameter *also* trans D · traveler's diarrhea · treatment discontinued · tuberoinfundibular dopaminergic · typhoid dysentery

T$_D$ time required to double number of cells in given population

T$_4$(D) serum thyroxin measured by displacement analysis

TD$_{50}$ median toxic dose

Td tetanus–diphtheria toxoid (adult type)

td [L. *ter die*] three times daily

TDA therapeutic drug assay · thyroid–stimulating–hormone displacing antibody · thyrotropin–displacing activity · tryptophan deaminase agar

TDB Toxicology Data Bank

TDC taurodeoxycholate · taurodeoxycholic (acid) · total dietary calories

TDD telecommunication device (for the) deaf · tetradecadiene · thoracic duct drainage · total digitalizing dose

tdd [L. *ter de die*] three times a day

TDDA tetradecadiene acetate

TDE tetrachlorodiphenyl-ethane · time–delayed exponential · total daily energy (requirement) · total digestible energy · triethylene glycol diglycidyl ether

TDEC test declined (no longer offered)

TDF testis–determining factor • Thinking Disturbance Factor • thoracic duct fistula • thoracic duct flow • time–dose fractionation (factor) • tissue–damaging factor *also* TF • tumor dose fractionation

TDH threonine dehydrogenase • total decreased histamine • toxic dose, high

TDI temperature difference integrator • total dose infusion

TDK tardive dyskinesia *also* TD

TDL thoracic duct lymph • thoracic duct lymphocyte • thymus–dependent lymphocyte • toxic dose, low

TDM tartaric dimalonate • therapeutic drug monitoring • trehalose dimycolate

TDN total digestible nutrients • transdermal nitroglycerin *also* TDNTG

tDNA transfer deoxyribonucleic acid

TDNTG transdermal nitroglycerin *also* TDN

TDO trichodento–osseous (syndrome)

TDP thermal death point • thoracic duct pressure • thymidine diphosphate

TdP torsade des pointes

TdR thymidine *also* T

TDS temperature, depth, salinity

tds [L. *ter die sumendum*] to be taken three times a day

TDT tentative discharge tomorrow • terminal deoxynucleotidyl transferase *also* TdT • thermal death time • tone decay test • tumor doubling time

TdT terminal deoxynucleotidyl tansferase *also* TDT

TDWB touch down weight–bearing

TDZ thymus–dependent zone (of lymph node)

TE echo–time • tennis elbow • test ear • tetanus *also* Te, tet • tetracycline *also* T, TC, TCN, TCNE • threshold energy • thromboembolism • thymus epithelium • thyrotoxic exophthalmos • time estimation • tissue–equivalent • tooth extracted • total estrogen • *Toxoplasma* encephalitis • trace element • tracheo–esophageal • transepithelial elimination (terminated) • treadmill exercise • trial (and) error *also* T&E

T&E testing and evaluation • training and experience • trial and error *also* TE

Te tellurium • tetanic (contraction) • tetanus *also* TE, tet

te effective half–life *also* teff

TEA temporal external artery • tetraethylammonium • thermal energy analyzer • thromboendarterectomy • total elbow arthroplasty • transient emboligenic aortoarteritis • transversely excited atmospheric (pressure) • triethanolamine

TEAB tetraethylammonium bromide

TEAC tetraethylammonium chloride

TEAE triethylaminoethyl

TEAM Training in Expanded Auxiliary Management

TEB tris–ethylenediamine-tetraacetate borate

TEBG, TeBG testosterone–estradiol–binding globulin

TEC total eosinophil count • total exchange capacity • transient erythroblastopenia (of) childhood

T&EC trauma and emergency center

TECA technetium albumin (study)

tech technical • technique

TECV traumatic epiphyseal coxa vara

TED Tasks of Emotional Development • threshold erythema dose • thromboembolic disease (hose, stockings) • tracheoesophageal dysraphism • tris–ethylenediamine-tetraacetate dithiothreitol

TEDP tetraethyl dithionopyrophosphate

TEE thermal effect (of) exercise • transesophageal echocardiography • tyrosine ethyl ester

TEEM tanned erythrocyte electrophoretic mobility

TEEP tetraethyl pyrophosphate

TEF thermal effect (of) food • tracheoesophageal fistula • trunk extension–flexion (unit)

teff effective half–life *also* te

TEFS transmural electrical field stimulation

TEG thromboelastogram

TEGDMA tetraethylene glycol dimethacrylate

TEI transesophageal imaging

TEIB triethyleneimino-benzoquinone

TEL telemetry *also* tele • tetraethyl lead

tele telemetry *also* TEL

TEM transmission electron microscope/microscopy • transverse electromagnetic • triethylenemelamine

temp temperature *also* T • temple • temporal • temporary *also* T

temp dext [L. *tempori dextro*] to the right temple

temp sinist [L. *tempori sinistro*] to the left temple

TEN tension (intraocular pressure) *also* T • total enteral nutrition • total epidermal necrolysis • total excretory nitrogen • toxic epidermal necrolysis • toxic epidermal necrosis

tenac tenaculum

TENS transcutaneous electrical nerve stimulation • transelectrical nerve stimulator

TEP thromboendo-
phlebectomy · tracheo-
esophageal puncture ·
tubal ectopic pregnancy

TEPA triethylenephos-
phoramide

TEPG triethylphosphine gold

TEPP tetraethylpyrophosphate

TEQU test equivocal (possible
low titer)

TER total elbow replacement ·
total endoplasmic
reticulum · transcapillary
escape rate

ter [L. *tere*] rub · terminal or
end *also* term., TRML,
Trml · ternary · tertiary
also T, t, tert · three
times · threefold

Terb terbutaline

term. full term (infant) · terminal *also* ter, TRML, Trml

ter sim [L. *tere simul*] rub
together

tert tertiary *also* T, t, ter

TES tetradecyl sulfate, ethanol,
saline · thymic epithelial
supernatant · toxic
epidemic syndrome ·
transcutaneous electrical
stimulation · transmural
electrical stimulation ·
treatment (of) emergent
symptom

TESPA triethylenethio-
phosphoramide (thiotepa)

testos testosterone

TET tetanus *also* TE, Te, tet ·
tetralogy (of Fallot) *also*
Tet, TF, TOF · tetroxi-
prim · total exchangeable

thyroxin · transcranial
electrostimulation therapy ·
treadmill exercise test ·
triethyltryptamine

Tet tetralogy of Fallot *also*
TET, TF, TOF

tet tetanus *also* TE, Te, TET

TETA test–estrin timed
action · triethylenetetra-
mine

TETCYC tetracycline

TETD tetraethylthiuram
disulfide (disulfiram)

TETRAC tetraiodothyroacetic
acid

tet tox tetanus toxoid *also* TT

TEV talipes equinovarus

TEWL transepidermal water
loss *also* TWL

TF tactile fremitus · tail flick
(reflex) · temperature
factor · testicular feminization · tetralogy (of) Fallot
also TET, Tet, TOF ·
thymol flocculation ·
thymus factor · thymus
(tolerance) factor · thymus
(transfer) factor · tissue–
damaging factor *also* TDF ·
tissue factor · to follow ·
total flow · transfer
factor · transferrin *also* Tf,
TFN · transformation
frequency · transfrontal ·
tube feeding · tuberculin
filtrate · tubular fluid ·
tuning fork

Tf transferrin *also* TF, TFN

T$_f$ temperature, freezing

TFA total fatty acids ·
transverse fascicular area ·
trifluoroacetic acid

TFB trifascicular block

TFd transfer factor, dialyzable

TFE polytetrafluoroethylene (Teflon)

TFEV timed forced expiratory volume

TFF tube–fed food

Tf–Fe transferrin–bound iron

TFL tensor fascia lata

TFM testicular feminization mutation • total fluid movement • transmission electron microscopy • trifluoromethyl nitrophenol

Tfm testicular feminization (syndrome) *also* TFS

TFN total fecal nitrogen • totally functional neutrophil • transferrin *also* TF, Tf

TFP treponemal false positive • trifluoperazine *also* TFZ

TF/P tubule fluid to plasma (ratio)

(TF/P) In tubule fluid to plasma inulin (ratio)

TFR total fertility rate • total flow resistance

TFS testicular feminization syndrome *also* Tfm • tube–fed saline

TFT thrombus formation time • thyroid function test • tight filum terminale • transfer factor test • trifluorothymidine

TFZ trifluoperazine *also* TFP

TG tendon graft • testosterone glucuronide • tetraglycine •

theophylline–guaifenesin • thioglucose • thioglycolate (broth) *also* THIO • thioguanine • thyroglobulin *also* Thg • toxic goiter • transglutaminase • transmissible gastroenteritis *also* TGE • treated group • triacylglycerol • trigeminal (neuralgia) • triglyceride *also* TRIG, trig • tumor growth • type genus *also* tg

Tg generation time *also* GT • thyroglobulin

T$_g$ glass transition temperature

tg type genus *also* TG

tG$_1$ time required to complete G$_1$ phase of cell cycle

tG$_2$ time required to complete G$_2$ phase of cell cycle

TGA taurocholate gelatin agar • thyroglobulin antibody *also* TgAb • total glycoalkaloids • transient global amnesia • transposition (of) great arteries • tumor glycoprotein assay

TgAb thyroglobulin antibody *also* TGA

TGAR total graft area rejected

TGB thyroid–binding globulin

TGC time–gain compensator

TGD thermal green dye

TGE theoretical growth evaluation • transmissible gastroenteritis (virus) *also* TG • tryptone glucose extract

TGF T–cell growth factor • transforming growth factor • tubuloglomerular feedback • tumor growth factor

TGFA triglyceride fatty acid

TGG turkey gamma globulin

TGL triglyceride • triglyceride lipase

TGP tobacco glycoprotein

TGR tenderness, guarding, rigidity (abdominal exam) • thioguanosine

T–group training group

TGS tincture (of) green soap • triglycine sulfate

TGT thromboplastin generation test/time • tolbutamide–glucagon test

TGV thoracic gas volume • transposition (of) great vessels

TGXT thallium–graded exercise test

TGY tryptone glucose yeast (agar)

TGYA tryptone glucose yeast agar

TH tetrahydrocortisol • T helper (cell) • theophyl-line • thrill • thyrohyoid • thyroid hormone • thyro-tropic hormone *also* TTH • topical hypothermia • torcular herophili • total hysterectomy • tube holder • tyrosine hydroxylase

T&H type and hold

Th thenar • thoracic/thorax *also* T, th, thor • thorium • throat

th thoracic *also* T, Th, thor

THA tetrahydroaminoacridine (tacrine) • total hip arthroplasty • total hydroxyapatite • transient hemispheric attack • *Treponema* hemagglutination

ThA thoracic aorta

THAM tris(hydroxymethyl)-aminomethane (tromethamine) *also* TRIS

THAN transient hyper-ammonemia of newborn

THARIES total hip arthroplasty (with) internal eccentric shells

THb total hemoglobin

THC tetrahydrocannabinol • tetrahydrocortisol • thio-carbanidin • transhepatic cholangiogram • transplantable hepatocellular carcinoma

THCA trihydroxycoprostanoic acid

THCCRC tetrahydro-cannabinol cross–reacting cannabinoids

TH–CULT throat culture *also* TC

THD thioridazine • transverse heart diameter

Thd ribothymidine

THDOC tetrahydrodeoxy-corticosterone

THE tetrahydrocortisone E • tonic hind (limb) extension • transhepatic embolization • tropical hypereosinophilia

theor theory/theoretical

ther therapy/therapeutic *also* therap • thermometer *also* therm

therap therapy/therapeutic *also* ther

Ther Ex, ther ex therapeutic exercise

therm thermometer *also* ther

theta (Θ, θ) eighth letter of Greek alphabet

Θ thermodynamic temperature

θ angular coordinate variable • customary temperature • latent trait (statistics) • temperature interval

THF tetrahydrocortisone F • tetrahydrofolate • tetrahydrofolic • tetrahydrofuran • tetrahydrofluorenone • thymic humoral factor

THFA tetrahydrofolic acid • tetrahydrofurfuryl alcohol

Thg thyroglobulin *also* TG

THH telangiectasia hereditaria haemorrhagica

THI transient hypogamma-globinemia (of) infancy • trihydroxyindole

THIO thioglycolate *also* TG

Thio–T, Thio–TEPA thio-triethylene phosphoramide

THIP tetrahydroisoxazolo-pyridinol

THIQ tetrahydraisoquinolon

THKAFO trunk–hip–knee–ankle–foot orthosis

THM total heme mass

THO, TH$_2$O titrated water

THOR thoracentesis (fluid)

thor thorax/thoracic *also* T, Th, th

thou thousandth

THP take home pack • tetrahydropapaveroline • tissue hydrostatic pressure • total hip replacement • total hydroxyproline • transhepatic portography • trihexphenidyl

THPA tetrahydropteric acid

THPC tetrabis(hydroxymethyl) phosphonium chloride

tHPT tertiary hyperparathyroidism

THPV transhepatic portal vein

THQ tetroquinone

THR targeted heart rate • total hip replacement • training heart rate • transhepatic resistance

Thr threonine

thr thyroid/thyroidectomy

THR–CT thrombin control

THRF thyrotropic hormone–releasing factor

throm, thromb thrombosis • thrombus *also* T

THS tetrahydro–compound S • tetrahydrodeoxycortisol

THSC totipotent hematopoietic stem cell

THU tetrahydrouridine

THUG thyroid uptake gradient

THVO terminal hepatic vein obliteration

Thx thromboxane *also* TBX, TX

Thy thymine *also* T

thy. thymectomy • thymus *also* T

THz terahertz

TI inversion time • temporal integration • terminal ileum • thalassemia intermedia • therapeutic index • thoracic index • thymus independent • thyroxin iodine • threshold (of) intelligibility • time information • time interval • tonic immobility • total iron • translational inhibition • transverse (diameter between) ischia • transverse inlet • tricuspid incompetence • tricuspid insufficiency • trunk index • tumor inducing • tumor induction

Ti titanium

TIA transient ischemic attack • tumor–induced angiogenesis

TIA–IR transient ischemic attack, incomplete recovery

TIB tumor immunology bank

Tib, tib tibia

TIBC total iron–binding capacity

tib–fib tibia (and) fibula

TIC ticarcillin • Toxicology Information Center • trypsin inhibitory capability • tumor–inducing complex

tic diverticulum

TICCC time interval (between) cessation (of) contraception (and) conception

TID [L. *ter in die*] three times a day *also* tid • time interval difference • titrated initial dose

tid [L. *ter in die*] three times a day *also* TID

TIDA tuberoinfundibular dopamine • tuberoinfundibular dopaminergic (system)

TIE transient ischemic episode

TIF tumor–inducing factor • tumor–inhibiting factor

TIFB thrombin–increasing fibrinopeptide B

TIG, TIg tetanus immunoglobulin

TIH time interval histogram

TIL tumor–infiltrating lymphocyte

TIM transthoracic intracardiac monitoring • triose isomerase

TIMC tumor–induced marrow cytotoxicity

TIN three times a night *also* t.i.n. • tubulointerstitial nephropathy

t.i.n. [L. *ter in nocte*] three times a night *also* TIN

tinc, tinct tincture

TIP thermal inactivation point • Toxicology Information Program • translation–inhibiting protein • tumor–inhibiting principle

TIPPS tetraiodophenolphthalein sodium

TIQ tetrahydroisoquinoline

TIR terminal innervation ratio • total immunoreactive

TIS tetracycline–induced stentosis • transdermal infusion system • trypsin–insoluble segment • tumor in situ

TISP total immunoreactive serum pepsinogen

TISS Therapeutic Intervention Scoring System

TIT *Treponema (pallidum)* immobilization test

TIT, TITh triiodothyronine *also* T$_3$, TRIT

TIU trypsin–inhibiting unit

TIUP term intrauterine pregnancy

TIUV total intrauterine volume

TIVC thoracic inferior vena cava

TIW, tiw, tiwk three times a week

TJ tendon jerk • tetrajoule • tight junction • triceps jerk • Troell–Junet (syndrome)

TJA total joint arthroplasty

TJN twin jet nebulizer

TJR total joint replacement

TK through (the) knee • thymidine kinase • tourniquet *also* TQ • transketolase • triose–kinase

TKA total knee arthroplasty • transketolase activity

TKD thymidine kinase deficiency • tokodyna-mometer

TKG tokodynagraph

TKLI tachykinin–like immunoreactivity

TKM thymidine kinase, mitochondrial

TKNO to keep needle open

TKO to keep open (vein for IV)

TKP thermokeratoplasty

TKR total knee replacement

TKS thymidine kinase, soluble

TKVO to keep vein open

TL team leader • temporal lobe • terminal limen • theophylline • thermolabile • thermoluminescence • Thorndike–Lorge • threat (to) life • thymic lymphocyte • thymus leukemia (antigen) • thymus(-dependent) lymphocyte *also* T–L • thymus lymphoma • time lapse • time limited • tolerance level • total lipids • transverse line • trial leave • tubal ligation

T–L thymus(–dependent) lymphocyte *also* TL

T/L terminal latency (electromyography)

Tl thallium

TLA tissue lactase activity • translaryngeal aspiration • translumbar aortogram • transluminal angioplasty • trypsin–like amidase

TLAA T–lymphocyte-associated antigen

TLC tender loving care • thin–layer chromatography • total L–chain concentration • total lung capacity •

total lung compliance • total lymphocyte count • triple–lumen catheter

²⁰¹TlCl thallium chloride (radioisotope)

TLD thermoluminescent dosimeter • thoracic lymphatic duct • trans-luminescent dosimeter • tumor lethal dose

T/LD₁₀₀ minimal dose causing 100% death or malformation

TLE temporal lobe epilepsy • thin–layer electrophoresis • total lipid extract

TLI thymidine labeling index • tonic labyrinthine inverted • total lymphoid irradiation • Totman's Loss Index • translaryngeal intubation • trypsin–like immunoactivity

TLNB term living newborn

TLP transitional living program

TLQ total living quotient

TLR tonic labyrinthine reflex

TLS tumor lysis syndrome

TLSO thoracic lumbar sacral orthosis • thoracolumbar spinal orthosis • thoracolumbosacral spinal orthosis *also* TLSSO

TLSSO thoracolumbosacral spinal orthosis *also* TLSO

TLT tryptophan load test

TLV threshold limit value • total lung volume

TLW total lung water

TLX trophoblast–lymphocyte cross–reactivity

TM tectorial membrane • temperature (by) mouth • temporalis muscle • tem-poromandibular (joint) • teres major (muscle) • term milk • thalassemia major • Thayer–Martin (medium) *also* T–M • time (and) modifying • time–motion • tobramycin *also* TOB • trabecular mesh-work • Transcendental Meditation • transitional mucosa • transmediastinal • transmetatarsal • transport maximum • transport mechanism • transport medium • transverse myelitis • trimester *also* TRI • Tropical Medicine • tubular myelin • tumor • tympanic membrane • tympanometric

T&M type and cross–match *also* TC, T&C

T–M Thayer–Martin (medium) *also* TM

Tm temperature, muscle • thulium • tubular maximal (excretory capacity of kidneys) *also* T_m • tumor–bearing mice

T_m temperature midpoint (Kelvin) • tubular maximal (excretory capacity of kidneys) *also* Tm

tM time required to complete M phase of cell cycle

t_m temperature midpoint (Celsius)

TMA tetramethylammonium • thrombotic microangiopathy • thyroid microsomal antibody *also*

TMAb • transmetatarsal amputation • trimethoxyamphetamine • trimethoxyphenyl aminopropane • trimethylamine • trimethylxanthine amphetamine

TMAb thyroid microsomal antibody *also* TMA

TMAH trimethylphenyl-ammonium (anilinium) hydroxide

TMAI trimethylphenyl-ammonium (anilinium) iodide

TMAO trimethylamine oxide

TMAS Taylor Manifest Anxiety Scale

T–MAX time of maximal concentration *also* T$_{max}$

T$_{max}$ highest temperature • time of maximal concentra-tion *also* T–MAX

TMB tetramethyl benzidine • transient monocular blindness • trimethoxy-benzoate • tris–maleate buffer

TMBA trimethoxybenz-aldehyde • trimethylbenz-anthracene

TMC transmural colitis • triamcinolone (and terra)mycin capsule

TMCA trimethylcolchicinic acid

TMD trimethadione *also* TMO

TMDS, t–MDS therapy-related myelodysplasia

TME thermolysin–like

metalleondopeptidase • total metabolizable energy • transmissible mink encephalopathy • transmural enteritis

TMET treadmill exercise test

TMF transformed mink fibroblast

TmG,TM$_G$ maximal tubular reabsorption rate for glucose

TMH tetramethylammonium hydroxide

TMI threatened myocardial infarction • transmural infarction

TMIC Toxic Materials Information Center

TMIF tumor–cell migratory inhibition factor

TMIS Technicon Medical Information System

TMJ temporomandibular joint

TMJ–PDS temporomandibular joint–pain dysfunction syndrome

TMJS temporomandibular joint syndrome

TML terminal motor latency • tetramethyl lead

TMM torn medial meniscus

Tmm McKay–Marg tension

TMNG toxic multinodular goiter

TMO trimethadione *also* TMD

T–MOP 6–thioguanine, methotrexate, Oncovin (vincristine), and prednisone

TMP thallium myocardial

perfusion • thymidine monophosphate • thymolphthalein • transmembrane potential • transmembrane (hydrostatic) pressure • trimethoprim • trimethylpsoralen

TM$_{PAH}$ maximal tubular (excretory capacity for) *para*–aminohippuric acid

TMPD tetramethylparaphenyl-inediamine

TMPDS temporomandibular pain (and) dysfunction syndrome

TMP–SMX, TMP–SMZ tri-methoprim–sulfa-methoxazole

TMR tetramethylrhodamine • tissue maximal ratio • topical magnetic resonance • trainable mentally retarded

TMRI tetramethylrhodamine isothiocyanate

TMS tetramethylsilane • thallium myocardial scintigraphy • thread mate system • trimethylsilane • trimethylsilyl *also* TMSi

TMSI trimethylsilylimidazole

TMSi trimethylsilyl *also* TMS

TMST treadmill stress test *also* TST

TMT Trail–Making Test (psychiatry) • treadmill test

TMTC too many to count

TMTD tetramethylthiuram disulfide

TMTX trimethexate

TMU tetramethylurea

TMV tobacco mosaic virus • tracheal mucous velocity

TMX tamoxifen *also* T, TAM • trimazosin

TMZ temazepam • transformation zone

TN talonavicular • team nursing • temperature normal • (intraocular) tension, normal *also* Tn • tiodazosin • total negatives • trigeminal nucleus • trochlear nucleus • true negative

T/N tar (and) nicotine

T&N tension and nervousness

T$_4$N normal serum thyroxin

Tn (intraocular) tension, normal *also* TN • thoron • transposon

TNA total nutrient admixture

TNB term newborn • Tru–Cut needle biopsy

TNC turbid, no creamy (layer)

TNCB trinitrochlorobenzene

TND term normal delivery

TNEE titrated norepinephrine excretion

TNF trinitrofluorenone • true negative fraction • tumor necrosis factor

TNG trinitroglycerol (nitro-glycerin) • toxic nodular goiter

Tng training

tng tongue

TNH transient neonatal hyperammonemia

TNI total nodal irradiation

TNM tumor, node, metastasis (tumor staging) • thyroid node metastasis

TNMR tritium nuclear magnetic resonance

TNP total net positive • trinitrophenyl

TNPM transient neonatal pustular melanosis

TNR tonic neck reflex • true negative rate

TNS total nuclear score • transcutaneous nerve stimulation *also* TCNS • tumor necrosis serum

TNT tramcinolone (and) nystatin

TNTC too numerous to count

TNV tobacco necrosis virus

TO old tuberculin • original tuberculin • target organ • telephone order • temperature, oral *also* T(O) • Theiler's Original (mouse encephalomyelitis virus) • tincture (of) opium *also* t.o. • total obstruction • tracheoesophageal • transfer out • tubo–ovarian • turned on • turnover

T(O) oral temperature *also* TO

T&O tandem and ovoids • tubes and ovaries

TO₂ oxygen transport rate

t.o. tincture (of) opium *also* TO

TOA time of arrival • tubo–ovarian abscess

TOAP thioguanine, Oncovin (vincristine), araC (cytarabine), and prednisone

TOB tobramycin *also* TM

TOBP tobranycin, peak

TobRV tobacco ringspot virus *also* TRSV

TOC test of cure • total organic carbon • tubo–ovarian complex

TOCE transcatheter oily chemoembolization

TOCO tocodynamometer

TOCP triorthocresyl phosphate

TOD tension of oculus dexter (right eye) • tail on detector • Time–oriented Data (Bank)

TOE tracheo(o)esophageal

TOES toxic oil epidemic syndrome

TOF tetralogy of Fallot *also* TET, Tet, TF • total of four • tracheo(o)esophageal fistula

T of A transposition of aorta

TOGV transposition of great vessels

TOH throughout hospitalization • transient osteoporosis (of) hip

TOL trial of labor

tol tolerance • tolerated

tolb tolbutamide

TOM tomorrow • transcutaneous oxygen monitor *also* TCOM

tomo tomogram/tomography

TON tonight *also* tonoc

TONAR the oral–nasal acoustic ratio

tonoc [to + L. *nocte*] tonight *also* TON

TOP temporal, occipital, parietal • termination of pregnancy • tissue oncotic pressure

top. topical *also* T

TOPS Take Off Pounds Sensibly

TOPV trivalent oral polio vaccine

TORCH toxoplasmosis, rubella, cytomegalovirus, and herpes simplex (titer)

TORP total ossicular (chain) replacement prosthesis

TOS tension of oculus sinister (left eye) • thoracic outlet syndrome

TOT "tincture of time" • total operating time

TOTAL–C total cholesterol

TOTP triorthotolyl phosphate

TOTPAR total pain relief

Tot prot total protein *also* TP, T PROT

TOV thrombosed oral varix • trial of void

TOWER testing, orientation, work, evaluation, rehabilitation

Tox toxicity *also* T, tox

tox toxic • toxicity *also* T, Tox • toxoid

TOXGR toxic granulation (differential)

TOXICON Toxicology

Information Conversational On–Line Network

TOXLINE Toxicology Information On–Line

TOXO, Toxo toxoplasmosis

TP posterior tibial *also* PT • tail pinch • temperature (and) pressure • temporal peak • temporoparietal • terminal phalanx • testosterone propionate • tetanus–pertussis • therapeutic pass • thickly padded • threshold potential • thrombocytopenic purpura • thrombophlebitis • thymic polypeptide • thymidine phosphorylase • thymus protein • tissue pressure • Todd paralysis • toilet paper • total population • total positives • total protein *also* Tot prot, T PROT • trailing pole • transforming principle • transition point *also* T • transpyloric • transverse polarization • treating physician • treatment period • triamphenicol • triazolophthalazine • trigger point • triphosphate • true positive • tryptophan *also* Tp, Trp, Try, Tryp • tryptophan pyrrolase • tube precipitin • tuberculin precipitate

TP5 thymopoietin pentapeptide

T&P, T+P temperature and pulse • turn and position

Tp tampon • tryptophan *also* TP, Trp, Try, Tryp

tp physical half–life

TPA tannic acid, polyphospho-molybdic acid, and amido acid (staining technique) • tissue plasminogen activator • tissue polypeptide antigen • total parenteral alimentation • total phobic anxiety • *Treponema pallidum* agglutination • tumor polypeptide antigen

t–PA tissue–type plasminogen activator

TPAL term infants, premature infants, abortions, living children (obstetric history)

TPB tryptone phosphate broth

TPBF total pulmonary blood flow

TPBS three–phase (radio-nuclide) bone scanning

TPC telescoping plugged catheter • telopeptide–poor collagen • thromboplastic plasma component • time–to–pulse–height converter • total patient care • total plasma catecholamines • total plasma cholesterol • treatment planning conference • *Treponema pallidum* complement

TPCC *Treponema pallidum* cryolysis complement

TPCF *Treponema pallidum* complement fixation

TPCV total packed cell volume

TPD temporary partial disability • thiamine propyl disulfide • tropical pancreatic diabetes • tumor–producing dose

TPE therapeutic plasma exchange • total protective environment

TPEY tellurite polymyxin egg yolk (agar)

TPF thymus permeability factor • trained participating father • true positive fraction

TPG therapeutic play group • transmembrane potential gradient • transplacental gradient • tryptophan peptone glucose (broth)

TPGYT trypticase–peptone–glucose–yeast extract–trypsin (medium)

TPH thromboembolic pulmonary hypertension • trained participating husband • transplacental hemorrhage • tryptophan hydroxylase

TPHA *Treponema pallidum* hemagglutination

TPHOS triple phosphate (crystal)

TPI *Treponema pallidum* immobilization (test) • triose phosphate isomerase

TPIA *Treponema pallidum* immune adherence

TPL triphosphate (of) lime • tyrosine phenol–lyase

T plasty tympanoplasty

TPM temporary pacemaker • thrombophlebitis migrans • total particulate matter • total passive motion • triphenylmethane

TPMT thiopurine methyltransferase

TPN thalamic projection neuron • total parenteral nutrition • triphospho-pyridine nucleotide

TPNH triphosphopyridine nucleotide, reduced

TPO thrombopoietin · thyroid peroxidase · trial prescription order · tryptophan peroxidase

TPP tetraphenylporphyrin · thiamine pyrophosphate · transpulmonary pressure

TP&P time, place, and person

TPPase thiamine pyrophosphatase

TPPN total peripheral parenteral nutrition · trans pars plana vitrectomy

TPR temperature · temperature, pulse, (and) respiration · testosterone production rate · total peripheral resistance · total pulmonary resistance · true positive rate

TPRI total peripheral resistance index

T PROT total protein *also* Tot prot, TP

TPS trypsin · tumor polysaccharide substance

TPST true positive stress test

TPT tetraphenyl tetrazolium · time (to) peak tension · total protein tuberculin · treadmill performance test · typhoid–paratyphoid (vaccine)

TPTHS total parathyroid hormone secretion

TPTX thyroid–parathyroidectomy

TPTZ tripyridyltriazine

TPUR transperineal uretheral resection

TPV tetanus–pertussis vaccine

TPVR total peripheral vascular resistance · total pulmonary vascular resistance

TQ time questionnaire · tocopherolquinone · tourniquet *also* TK

TR recovery time · rectal temperature *also* T(R) · repetition time · residual tuberculin · tetrazolium reduction · therapeutic radiology · therapeutic recreation · timed release · tincture *also* T, Tr, tr · to return · total repair · total resistance · total response *also* R · trace *also* T, Tr, tr · trachea · transfusion reaction · transplant recipient · treatment *also* Tr, tr, treat., TX, Tx, T_x · tremor · tricuspid regurgitation · triradial · tuberculin Ruckland (new tuberculin) · tuberculin residue · tubular reabsorption · tumor registry · turbidity reducing · turnover rate

T(°R) absolute temperature on the Rankine scale

T(R) rectal temperature *also* TR

T&R tenderness and rebound

Tr tincture *also* T, TR, tr · trace *also* T, TR, tr · tragion · treatment *also* TR, tr, treat., TX, Tx, T_x · trypsin

T_r radiologic half–life · retention time

tr tincture *also* T, TR, Tr, tr · trace *also* T, TR, Tr, tr ·

traction *also* Tr • treatment *also* TR, Tr, tr, treat., TX, Tx, T_x • tremor

TRA therapeutic recreation associate • to run at • total renin activity • transaldolase • tumor–resistant antigen

tra transfer

TRAb thyrotrophin receptor antibody

trach trachea/tracheal • tracheostomy • tracheotomy

TRAJ timed repetitive ankle jerk

TRAM transverse rectus abdominus myocutaneous (breast reconstruction) • Treatment Rating Assessment Matrix • Treatment Response Assessment Method

TRAN transfusion

trans transference • transverse *also* T

trans D transverse diameter *also* TD

transm transmission • transmitted

transpl transplantation/ transplanted *also* TX

trans sect transverse section *also* TS, T sect

transsex transsexual

TRAP tartrate–resistant (leukocyte) acid phosphatase • thioguanine, rubidomycin, ara–C, and prednisone

TRAS transplant renal artery stenosis

tran, traum trauma/traumatic

TRB terbutaline

TRBF total renal blood flow

TRC tanned red cell • total renin concentration • total respiratory conductance • total ridge count

TRCA tanned red cell agglutination

TRCH tanned red cell hemagglutination

TRCHI tanned red cell hemagglutination inhibition

TRCV total red cell volume

TRD tongue–retaining device • traction retinal detachment

TRE true radiation emission

TREA thoroughness, reliability, efficiency, analytic (ability) • triethanolamine

treat. treatment *also* TR, Tr, tr, TX, Tx, T_x

Tren, TREND Trendelenburg (position) *also* TRND

TRF T–cell replacing factor • thyrotropin–releasing factor

trf transfer

TRFC total rosette–forming cell

trg, trng training

TRGI triglycerides incalculable

TRH tension–reducing hypo-thesis • thyroid–releasing hormone • thyrotropin–releasing hormone

TRH–ST thyrotropin–releasing hormone stimulation test

TRI tetrazolium reduction inhibition • Thyroid

Research Institute • total response index • trifocal • trimester *also* TM • tubuloreticular inclusion

trl tricentric

T₃RIA, T₃(RIA) triiodothyronine radioimmunoassay

T₄RIA, T₄(RIA) tetraiodothyronine (thyroxine) radioimmunoassay

TRIAC, Triac triiodothyroacetic acid

TRIC trachoma inclusion conjunctivitis (organism)

TRICB trichlorobiphenyl

TRICH, Trich trichinosis

Trid, trid [L. *triduum*] three days

TRIG, trig triglyceride *also* TG

TRIMIS Tri–Service Medical Information System

TRIS tris(hydroxymethyl)-aminomethane *also* THAM

TRISS Trauma and Injury Severity Score

TRIT triiodothyronine *also* T₃, TIT, TITh

Trit, trit triturate

TRITC tetrarhodamine isothiocyanate

TRK transketolase

TRML, Trml terminal *also* ter, term.

tRNA transfer ribonucleic acid

TRND Trendelenburg (position) *also* Tren, TREND

TRO tissue reflectance oximeter • to return (to) office

TROCA tangible reinforcement operant conditioning audiometry

TROCH, Troch troche (lozenge)

Trop tropical

TRP Tactical Reproduction Pegboard • total refractory period • trichorhinophalangeal (syndrome) • tubular reabsorption (of) phosphate

Trp tryptophan *also* TP, Tp, Try, Tryp

TRPA tryptophan–rich prealbumin

TrPl treatment plan

TRPS trichorhinophalangeal syndrome

TRPT theoretical renal phosphorus threshold

TRR total respiratory resistance

TRS Therapeutic Recreation Specialist • total reducing sugars • tubuloreticular structure

TrS traumatic surgery

TRSV tobacco ringspot virus *also* TobRV

TRT thermoradiotherapy • total reading time

trt treatment

TRU turbidity–reducing unit

T₃RU triiodothyronine resin uptake

TRUS transrectal ultrasound

TRUSP transrectal ultrasound of prostate

TRV tobacco rattle virus

Try, Tryp tryptophan *also* TP, Tp, Trp

TRZ tartrozine • triazolam

TS Tay–Sachs • temperature sensitivity • temporal stem • terminal sensation • testosterone sulfate • test solution • thermostable • thiosporin • thoracic surgery • tissue space • tocopherol supplemented • toe sign • total solids (in urine) • Tourette syndrome • toxic substance • toxic syndrome • tracheal sound • trachael spiral • transitional sleep • transsexual • transverse section *also* trans sect, T sect • transverse sinus • Trauma Score • treadmill score • trichostasis spinulosa • tricuspid stenosis • triple strength • tropical sprue • trypticase soy (plate) • T suppressor (cell) • tuberous sclerosis • tubular sound • tumor specific • Turner syndrome • type specific

T+S type and screen

T/S thyroid–serum (iodide ratio) • thyroid to serum (ratio)

Ts skin temperature • tension by Schiotz tonometer • tosylate • T suppressor

tS time required to complete S phase of cell cycle

ts, tsp teaspoon

TSA technical surgical assistance • Test of Syntactic Ability • tissue–

specific antigens • toluene sulfonic acid • Total Severity Assessment • total shoulder arthroplasty • total solute absorption • toxic shock antigen • trypticase–soy agar • tumor–specific antigen • tumor surface antigen • tumor–susceptible antigen • type–specific antibody

T$_4$SA thyroxin–specific activity

TSAb thyroid–stimulating antibody

TSAP toxic shock–associated protein

Tsaph temperature (in) saphenous (vein)

TSAS total severity assessment score

TSAT tube slide agglutination test

TSB total serum bilirubin • trypticase soy broth • tryptone soy broth

TSBA total serum bile acids

TSBB transtracheal selective bronchial brushing

TSBC Time–Sample Behavioral Checklist

TSC technetium sulfur colloid • theophylline serum concentration • thiosemicarbazide • total static compliance • transverse spinal sclerosis

TSCA Toxic Substance Control Act

TSCS Tennessee Self–Concept Scale

TSD target–skin distance · Tay–Sachs disease · theory (of) signal detectability · transfer summary dictated

TSE testicular self–examination · total skin examination · trisodium edetate

TSEB total skin electron beam

T sect transverse section *also* trans sect, TS

TSEM transmission scanning electron microscopy

T set tracheotomy set

TSF thrombopoiesis–stimulating factor · tissue–(coding) factor *also* TCF · total systemic flow · triceps skinfold · T–suppressor factor

TSG tumor–specific glycoprotein

TSH thyroid–stimulating hormone

TSH–RF thyroid–stimulating hormone–releasing factor

TSH–RH thyroid–stimulating hormone–releasing hormone

TSI thyroid–stimulating immunoglobulin · triple sugar iron (agar) *also* TSIA

TSIA total small intestinal allotransplantation · triple sugar iron agar *also* TSI

TSL terminal sensory latency

TSM type–specific M protein

TSN tryptophan peptone sulfide neomycin (agar)

TSP total serum protein · total suspended

particulate · tribasic sodium phosphate · trisodium phosphate

tsp teaspoon

TSPA thiophosphoramide (Thiotepa)

TSPAP total serum prostatic acid phosphatase

T–spica thumb spica (bandage)

T–spine, T/spine thoracic spine

TSPP tetrasodium pyrophosphate

TSR testosterone–sterilized (female) rat · theophylline–sustained release · thyroid–serum ratio · total shoulder replacement · total systemic resistance · transfer · transient situational reaction

TSRBC trypsinized sheep red blood cell

TSS toxic shock syndrome · tropical splenomegaly syndrome

TSSA tumor–specific (cell) surface antigen

TSSE toxic shock syndrome exoprotein · toxic shock syndrome exotoxin

TSST toxic shock syndrome toxin

TSSU (operating) theater sterile supply unit

TST thromboplastin screening test · total sleep time · transition state theory · transscrotal testosterone · treadmill stress test *also* TMST · tumor skin test

TSTA toxoplasmin skin test antigen • tumor–specific tissue antigen • tumor–specific transplantation antigen

TSU triple sugar urea (agar)

TSV total stomach volume

TSY trypticase soy yeast

TT tablet triturate • tactile tension • talking task • terminal transferase • tetanus toxin • tetanus toxoid *also* tet tox • tetrathionate (broth) • tetrazol • thrombin time • thymol turbidity • tibial tubercle • tibial tuberosity • tilt table • tine test • token test • tooth treatment • total thyroxin • total time • transferred to • transient tachypnea • transit time • transthoracic • transtracheal • tube thoracostomy • tuberculin test • tumor thrombus • turnover time • tyrosine transaminase

TT$_4$ total thyroxine

T/T trace of/trace of (different substances on tests)

T&T time and temperature • tobramycin and ticarcillin • touch and tone

TTA tetanus toxoid antibody • timed therapeutic absence • total toe arthroplasty • transtracheal aspiration

TTBV total trabecular bone volume

TTC triphenyltetrazolium chloride

TTD temporary total disability • tetraethyl-thiuram disulfide • tissue tolerance dose • total temporary disability • transient tic disorder • transverse thoracic diameter

TTFD thiamine tetrahydro-furfuryl disulfide

TTG tellurite, taurocholate, gelatin

TTGA tellurite, taurocholate, (and) gelatin agar

TTH thyrotropic hormone *also* TH • tritiated thymidine

TTI tension–time index • time–tension index • tissue thromboplastin inhibition (test) • transtracheal insufflation

TTIB tension–time index per beat

TTL training and test lung

TTLC true total lung capacity

TTM transtelephonic (electrocardiographic) monitoring

TTN transient tachypnea (of) newborn *also* TTNB

TTNA transthoracic needle aspiration

TTNB transient tachypnea (of) newborn *also* TTN • transthoracic needle (aspiration) biopsy

TTO to take out • transtracheal oxygen

TTOD tetanus toxoid outdated

TTOT transtracheal oxygen therapy

TTP Testicular Tumour

Panel • thrombotic thrombocytopenic purpura • thymidine triphosphate • time to peak

TTPA triethylene thiophosphoramide

TTP–HUS thrombotic thrombocytopenic purpura–hemolytic uremic syndrome

TTR transthoracic resistance • triceps tendon reflex • type to token ratio

TTS tarsal tunnel syndrome • temporary threshold shift • through the skin • transdermal therapeutic system

TTT thymol turbidity test • tolbutamide tolerance test • total twitch time

TTTT test tube turbidity test

TTUTD tetanus toxoid up–to–date

TTV tracheal transport velocity • transfusion transmitted virus

TTVP temporary transvenous pacemaker

TTWB touch–toe weight–bearing

TTX tetrodotoxin

TU thiouracil • thiourea • thyroidal uptake • Todd unit • toxic unit • transmission unit • transurethral • tuberculin unit • turbidity unit

T₃U triiodothyronine uptake *also* T_3UP

TUB tubouterine (junction)

tuberc tuberculosis *also* T, TB, Tb, tb, TBC, Tbc

TUD total urethral discharge

TUDC tauroursodeoxycholate

TUDCA tauroursodeoxycholic acid

TUF total ultrafiltration

TUG total urinary gonadotropin

TUI transurethral incision

TUN total urinary nitrogen

T₃UP triiodothyronine uptake *also* T_3U

TUPR transurethral prostatic resection

TUR transurethral resection

T₃UR triiodothyronine uptake ratio

TURB transurethral resection (of) bladder (tumor)

turb turbid • turbidity

TURBN transurethral resection (of) bladder neck

TURBT transurethral resection (of) bladder tumor

TURP transurethral prostatec-tomy • transurethral resection of prostate

TURV transurethral resection (of) valves

tus [L. *tussis*] cough

TUU transureteroureterostomy

TV talipes varus • temporary visit • tetrazolium violet • thoracic vertebra • tick-borne virus • tidal volúme • total volume • toxic vertigo • transfer vesicle • transvenous • trial visit • tricuspid valve • trivalent • true vertebra • truncal vagotomy • tuberculin volutin • tubulovesicular

T/V touch/verbal

TVA truncal vagotomy (plus) antrectomy

TVC third–ventricle cyst • timed ventilatory capacity • timed vital capacity • total viable cells • total volume capacity • transvaginal cone • triple voiding cystogram • true vocal cord

TVD transmissible virus dementia • triple vessel disease

TVDALV triple vessel disease (with) abnormal left ventricle

TVF tactile vocal fremitus

TVG time–varied gain (control)

TVH total vaginal hysterectomy • turkey virus hepatitis

TVL tenth value layer (radiation)

TVP tensor veli palatini • textured vegetable protein • transvenous pacemaker • transvesicle prostatectomy • tricuspid valve prolapse • truncal vagotomy (plus) pyloroplasty

TVR total vascular resistance • total vibration reflex • tricuspid valve replacement

TVSC transvaginal (sector) scan

TVT transmissible venereal tumor • tunica vaginalis testis

TVU total volume (of) urine

TVUS transvaginal ultrasound

TW tap water • terminal web • test weight •

thymic weight • total (body) water

TWA time–weighted average

Twb wet bulb temperature

TWBC total white blood cells

TWD total white (and) differential (cell count)

TWE tap water enema • tepid water enema

TWETC tap water enema til clear

TWG total weight gain

TWHW toe walking (and) heel walking

TWL transepidermal water loss *also* TEWL

TWN twin

TWR total wrist replacement

TWWD tap water wet dressing

TX derivative of contagious tuberculin • thromboxane *also* TBX, Thx • thyroidectomized • transplantation *also* transpl • treatment *also* TR, Tr, tr, treat., Tx, T_x

T&X type and cross–match *also* TXM

Tx, T_x therapy • traction • transfuse • transplant • treatment *also* TR, Tr, tr, treat., TX • tympanostomy

TXA, TxA thromboxane A

TXA2, TXA_2 thromboxane A2 (A_2)

TXB2, TXB_2 thromboxane B2 (B_2)

TXM T–cell cross–match • type and cross–match *also* T&X

Txn transplant

Ty thyroxine • type •
    typhoid • tyrosine *also* Tyr

TYCO Tylenol with Codeine

Tyl Tylenol • tyloma

TYMP tympanogram

Tymp tympanic • tympanicity
    (auscultation of chest) •
    tympanostomy •
    tympanium

typ typical

TYR tyramine • tyrode

Tyr tyrosine *also* Ty

TyRIA thyroid
    radioimmunoassay

TZ transition zone •
    triazolam • [Ger.
    Tuberculin zymoplastische]
    zymoplastic tuberculin

U internal energy • International Unit (of enzyme activity) • kilurane (radioactivity unit) • Mann–Whitney rank sum statistic • potential difference (in volts) • ulna • ultralente (insulin) • unerupted • uncertain • unit • unknown *also* UK • upper • uracil *also* URA, Ura • uranium • urethra *also* UA, ureth • uridine *also* Urd • uridylic acid *also* UA • urinary (concentration) • urine *also* UR, Ur, ur • urology *also* Urol • uvula • wave on electrocardiogram

U100 100 units per milliliter

U/1 one fingerbreadth below umbilicus

1/U one fingerbreadth above umbilicus

U/3 upper third (of long bone)

u [L. *utendus*] to be used • unified atomic mass unit

UA Ulex agglutinin • ultra–audible (sound) • ultrasonic arteriogram • umbilical artery • unaggregated • uncertain about • unit (of) analysis • unauthorized absence • unrelated (children raised) apart • unstable angina • upper airway • upper arm • urethra *also* U, ureth • uric acid *also* U/A • uridylic acid *also* U • urinalysis *also* U/A • urinary aldosterone • urine aliquot • urocanic acid • uronic acid • uterine aspiration

U/A uric acid *also* UA • urinalysis *also* UA • uterine activity

ua [L. *usque ad*] as far as • up to

UAC umbilical artery catheter • underactive • upper airway congestion

UA/C uric acid–creatinine (ratio)

UAD upper airway disease

UAE unilateral absence (of) excretion

UAG uracil–adenine–guanine

UAI uterine activity integral

UAL [up + L. *ad libitum*] up (out of bed) as desired *also* up ad lib • umbilical artery line

UA&M urinalysis and microscopy

U–AMY urinary amylase

UAN uric acid nitrogen

UAO upper airway obstruction

UAP unstable angina pectoris *also* USAP

UAPF upon arrival patient found

UAR upper airway resistance

UAS upper abdominal surgery

UASA upper airway sleep apnea

UAT up (out of bed) as tolerated

UAU uterine activity unit

UAVC univentricular atrioventricular connection

UB ultimobranchial body • Unna boot • urinary bladder

UBA undenatured bacterial antigen

UBBC unsaturated (vitamin) B_{12}–binding capacity

UBC University of British Columbia (Brace) • unsaturated binding capacity

UBF unknown black female • uterine blood flow

UBG ultimobranchial gland(s) • urobilinogen

UBI ultraviolet blood irradiation

UBL undifferentiated B–cell lymphoma

UBM unknown black male

UBO unidentified bright object

UBP ureteral back pressure

UBW usual body weight

UC ulcerative colitis • Uldall catheter • ultracentrifugal • umbilical cholesterol • umbilical cord • un-changed • unclassifiable • unconscious *also* UCS, Ucs • unfixed cryostat • unit clerk • unit coordinator • unsatisfactory condition • untreated cell • urea clearance *also* UCL • urethral catheterization • urinary catheter • urine concentrate • urine culture

also U/C, UCX • usual care • uterine contraction

U/C urine culture *also* UC

U&C urethral and cervical (cultures) • usual and customary

U$_{Ca}$V urinary calcium volume (excretion rate)

UCB unconjugated bilirubin *also* UCBR

UCBC umbilical cord blood culture

UCBR unconjugated bilirubin *also* UCB

UCC urgent care center

UCD urine collection device • usual childhood diseases *also* UCHD, UDC

UCE urea cycle enzymopathy

UCG ultrasonic cardiogram/ cardiography • urinary chorionic gonadotropin

UCHD usual childhood diseases *also* UCD, UDC

UCHI usual childhood illnesses *also* UCI

UCHS uncontrolled hemorrhagic shock

UCI urethral catheter in • urinary catheter in • usual childhood illnesses *also* UCHI

UCL ulna collateral ligament • uncomfortable listening level • uncomfortable loudness level *also* ULL • upper confidence limit • urea clearance *also* UC

UCLP unilateral cleft (of) lip (and) palate

UCO urethral catheter out •
urinary catheter out

UCP urethral closure pressure •
urinary coproporphyrin •
urinary C– peptide

UCPP urethral closure
pressure profile

UCPT urinary coproporphyrin
test

UCR unconditioned reflex *also*
UR • unconditioned
response *also* UR • usual,
customary, (and) reasonable
(fees)

UCRE urine creatinine

UCRP Universal Control
Reference Plasma

UCS unconditioned stimulus
also UDS, US •
unconscious *also* UC, Ucs

Ucs unconscious *also* UC,
UCS

UCT unchanged conventional
treatment

UCTD unclassifiable
connective tissue disease

UCU urinary care unit

UCV uncontrolled variable

UCX urine culture *also* UC

UD ulcerative dermatosis •
ulnar deviation •
underdeveloped •
undesirable discharge •
unipolar depression • unit
dose • urethral discharge •
uridine diphosphate •
uroporphyrinogen
decarboxylase • uterine
distention • uterus delivery

ud [L. *ud dictum*] as directed

UDA under direct vision

UDC ursodeoxycholate •
usual diseases of childhood
also UCD, UCHD

UDCA ursodeoxycholic acid

UDE undetermined etiology

UDN updraft nebulizer

UDO undetermined origin

UDP uridine diphosphate

UDPG uridinediphospho-
glucose *also* UDPG

UDPGA uridinediphospho-
glucuronic acid *also*
UDP-GlcUA

UDPGal uridinediphospho-
galactose

UDPGlc uridinediphospho-
glucose *also* UDPG

UDP–GlcUA uridinedephos-
phoglucronic acid *also*
UDPGA

UDPGT uridinediphospho-
glucuronyl transferase

UdR uracil deoxyriboside
(deoxyuridine)

UDRP urine diribose phosphate

UDS ultra–Doppler
sonography •
unconditioned stimulus *also*
UCS, US • unscheduled
deoxynucleic acid
synthesis • unscheduled
deoxyribonucleic acid
synthesis

UE uncertain etiology • under
elbow • undetermined
etiology • uninvolved
epidermis • upper
esophagus • upper
extremity *also* U/E

U/E upper extremity *also* UE

UEA upper extremity arterial

UEG unifocal eosinophilic granuloma

UEM universal electron microscope

UEMC unidentified endosteal marrow cell

UER unaided equalization reference

UES upper esophageal sphincter

UESP upper esophageal sphincter pressure

u/ext upper extremity

UF ultrafiltrable · ultrafiltrate · ultrafiltration · ultrafine · ultrasonic frequency · unflexed · universal feeder · unknown factor · until finished · urea formaldehyde

UFA unesterified fatty acid

UFC urinary free cortisol

UFD ultrasonic flow detector

UFE uniform food encoding

UFF unusual facial features

UFFI urea formaldehyde foam insulation

UFN until further notice

UFO unflagged order · unidentified foreign object

UFR ultrafiltration rate · urine filtration rate

uFSH urinary follicle–stimulating hormone

UFV unclassified fecal virus

UG until gone · urinary glucose · urogastrone · urogenital · uteroglobulin

UGA under general anesthesia

UGD urogenital diaphragm

UGDP University Group Diabetes Project

UGF unidentified growth factor

UGH uveitis–glaucoma–hyphema (syndrome)

UGH+ uveitis–glaucoma–hyphema plus (vitreous hemorrhage, syndrome)

UGI upper gastrointestinal (tract) *also* UGIT

UGIH upper gastrointestinal (tract) hemorrhage

UGIS upper gastrointestinal series

UGIT upper gastrointestinal tract *also* UGI

UGK urine glucose ketone

UGPP uridyl diphosphate glucose pyrophosphorylase

UGS urogenital sinus

UH umbilical hernia · upper half

UHBI upper hemibody irradiation

UHC ultrahigh carbon

UHD unstable hemoglobin disease

UHDDS Uniform Hospital Discharge Data Set

UHF ultrahigh frequency

UHL universal hypertrichosis lanuginosa

UHMW ultrahigh molecular weight

UHR underlying heart rhythm

UHSC university health services clinic

UHT ultrahigh temperature

UHV ultrahigh vacuum • ultrahigh voltage

UI Ulcer Index • urinary incontinence • uroporphyrin isomerase

U/I unidentified

UIBC unbound iron–binding capacity • unsaturated iron–binding capacity

UID [L. *uno in die*] once daily

UIF undegraded insulin factor

UIP unusual interstitial pneumonitis • usual interstitial pneumonia • usual interstitial pneumonitis

UIQ upper inner quadrant

UIS Utilization Information Service

UJT unijunction transistor

UK unknown *also* U • urinary kallikrein *also* UKa • urine potassium • urokinase

UKA unicompartmental knee arthroplasty

UKa urinary kallikrein *also* UK

U$_k$V urinary potassium volume (excretion rate)

UL unauthorized leave • Underwriters' Laboratories • undifferentiated lymphoma • upper limb • upper limit • upper lobe • utterance length

U/L, U&L upper and lower

U/L, U/l unit per liter

ULA undedicated logic array

ULBW ultralow birth weight

ULL uncomfortable loudness level *also* UCL

ULLE upper lid, left eye

ULN upper limits (of) normal

uln ulna/ulnar

ULPE upper lobe pulmonary edema

ULQ upper left quadrant

ULRE upper lid, right eye

ULT ultralow temperature

ult ultimate/ultimately

ult praes [L. *ultimum praescriptus*] last prescribed

ULV ultralow volume

ULYTES urine electrolytes

UM unmarried • upper motor (neuron) • uracil mustard • Utilization Management

UMA urinary muramidase activity

Umax maximal urinary osmolality

UMB, umb umbilicus/umbilical

U$_{Mg}$V urinary magnesium volume (excretion rate)

UMN upper motor neuron

UMNB upper motor neurogenic bladder

UMNL upper motor neuron lesion

UMP uridine monophosphate (uridylic acid)

UMPK uridine monophosphate kinase

UMS urethral manipulation syndrome

UMT unit (of) medical time

UN ulnar nerve • undernourished • unilateral neglect • urea nitrogen • urinary nitrogen

UNA urinary nitrogen appearance

UNa urinary sodium

U$_{Na}$ urinary concentration of sodium

uncomp uncompensated

uncond unconditioned

uncor uncorrected

UnCS, unCS unconditioned stimulus *also* UnS

unct [L. *unctus*] smeared

UNCV ulnar nerve conduction velocity

undet undetermined

UNE urinary norepinephrine

Ung, ung [L. *unguentum*] ointment

U$_{NH4}$+ urinary ammonium

UNID unidentified

unilat unilateral

univ universal

unk, unkn unknown

UNL upper normal limit

UNOS United Network of Organ Sharing

UNS, uns unsatisfactory *also* unsat • unsymmetrical

UnS unconditioned stimulus *also* UnCS, unCS

unsat unsatisfactory *also* UNS, uns • unsaturated

unsym unsymmetrical

UNTS unilateral nevoid telangiectasia syndrome

UO under observation *also* U/O, u/o • undetermined origin • ureteral orifice • urinary output *also* UOP

U/O, u/o under observation *also* UO

UOP urinary output *also* UO

UOQ upper outer quadrant

UOsm urinary osmolality

UOV unit of variance

UOZ upper outer zone (quadrant)

UP ulcerative proctitis • ultrahigh purity • unipolar • Unna–Pappenheim (stain) • upright posture • ureteropelvic • uridine phosphorylase • uroporphyrin • uteroplacental

U/P urine–plasma (ratio)

up ad lib [up + L. *ad libitum*] up (out of bed) as desired *also* UAL

UPC usual provider continuity

UPD urinary production (rate)

UPEP urine protein electrophoresis

UPF universal proximal femur (prosthesis)

UPG uroporphyrinogen

UPI uteroplacental insufficiency • uteroplacental ischemia

UPJ ureteropelvic junction

UPL unusual position (of) limbs

UPN unique patient number

UPOR usual place of residence

UPP urethral pressure profile • urethral pressure profilometry • uvuloplatoplasty

UPPP uvulopalatopharyngoplasty

UPPRA upright peripheral plasma renin activity

UPS ultraviolet photoelectron spectroscopy • uninterruptible power supply • uroporphyrinogen synthase • uterine progesterone system

upsilon (U, υ) twentieth letter of Greek alphabet

UPT uptake • urine pregnancy test

UQ ubiquinone • upper quadrant

UR unconditioned reflex *also* UCR • unconditioned response *also* UCR • unrelated • upper respiratory • urinal • urine *also* U, Ur, ur • urology • utilization review

Ur, ur urine/urinary *also* U, UR

URA, Ura uracil *also* U

ur anal urine analysis • urinalysin

URC upper rib cage • utilization review committee

URC–A uric acid

URC SP uric acid (urine) spot (test)

URD undifferentiated respiratory disease • upper respiratory disease

Urd uridine *also* U

UREA–S urea nitrogen (urine) spot (test)

URED unable to read (lab result)

ureth urethra *also* U

URF uterine–relaxing factor

UR–FST urine–fasting

urg urgent

UR HR urine—number of hours glucose tolerance

URI upper respiratory illness • upper respiratory infection

URIN random urine

url unrelated

UR&M urinalysis, routine and microscopic

URO urology • uroporphyrin • uroporphyrinogen

UROB, UROBIL urobilinogen

UROD uroporphyrinogen decarboxylase

URO–GEN urogenital

URO–2H urobilinogen—2 hours

Urol urology/urologist *also* U

UROS uroporphyrinogen synthetase

URQ upper right quadrant (of abdomen)

URS ultrasonic renal scanning

URSO ursodeoxycholic acid

URT upper respiratory tract

URTI upper respiratory tract illness/infection

UR–TIM urine–time

URVD unilateral renovascular disease

UR VOL urine volume

US ultrasonic • ultrasonography • ultrasound *also* U/S • unconditioned stimulus *also* UCS, UDS • unit secretary • upper segment • Usher syndrome

U/S ultrasound *also* US

USA unit services assistant

USAFH United States Air Force Hospital

USAFRHL United States Air Force Radiological Health Laboratory

USAH United States Army Hospital

USAHC United States Army Health Clinic

USAIDR United States Army Institute of Dental Research

USAMEDS United States Army Medical Service

USAN United States Adopted Names (Council)

USAP unstable angina pectoris *also* UAP

USASI United States of America Standards Institute

USB upper sternal border

USBS United States Bureau of Standards

USCVD unsterile controlled vaginal delivery

USD United States Dispensary

USDA United States Department of Agriculture

USDHHS United States Department of Health and Human Services

USE ultrasonic echography (ultrasonography) *also* USG

USFMG United States foreign medical graduates

USG ultrasonogram/ ultrasonography *also* USE

USH usual state (of) health

USHL United States Hygienic Laboratory

USI urinary stress incontinence

USMG United States medical graduate

USMH Unites States Marine Hospital

USN ultrasonic nebulizer

USNH United States Naval Hospital

USO unilateral salpingo– oophorectomy

USOGH usual state of good health

USP United States Pharmacopeia • upper sternal border

USPDI United States Pharmacopeia Drug Information

USPET Urokinase–
Streptokinase Pulmonary
Embolism Trial

USPHS United States Public
Health Service

USR unheated serum reagin

USS ultrasound scanning

ust [L. *ustus*] burnt

USUCVD unsterile uncontrolled vaginal delivery

USVH United States Veterans
Hospital

USVMD urine specimen
volume measuring device

USVMS urine specimen
volume measuring system

USW ultrashort wave

UT unrelated (children raised)
together • untested •
untreated • urinary tract •
urticaria

uT unbound testosterone

ut uterus

U$_{TA}$ urinary titrable acidity

UTBG unbound thyroxin–
binding globulin

UTD up to date

ut dict [L. *ut dictum*] as
directed

utend [L. *utendus*] to be used

utend mor sol [L. *utendus
more solitus*] to be used in
the usual manner

UTF usual throat flora

UTI urinary tract infection •
urinary trypsin inhibitor

UTLD Utah Test of Language
Development

UTO unable to obtain • upper
tibial osteotomy

UTP unilateral tension
pneumothorax • uridine
triphosphate

UTS Ullrich–Turner
syndrome • ulnar tunnel
syndrome • ultimate tensile
strength • ultrasound *also*
UTZ

ut supr [L. *ut supre*] as above

UTZ ultrasound *also* UTS

UU urinary urea • urine
urobilinogen

UUN urinary urea nitrogen

UUO unilateral ureteral
occlusion

UUP urine uroporphyrin

U UREA urinary
(concentration of) urea

UV ultraviolet • umbilical
vein *also* uv • uretero-
vesical • urinary volume

U$_v$ Uppsala virus

uv umbilical vein *also* UV

UVA ultraviolet light, long
wavelength •
ureterovesical angle

UVB ultraviolet light •
midrange spectrum

UVC umbilical venous
catheter • urgent visit
center

UVER ultraviolet–enhanced
reactivation

UVI ultraviolet irradiation

UVJ ureterovesical junction

UVL ultraviolet light •
umbilical venous line

UVP ultraviolet photometry

UVR ultraviolet radiation

UW unilateral weakness

U/WB unit (of) whole blood

UWF unknown white female

UWL unstirred water layer

UWM unknown white male •
unwed mother

UX uranium X (proactinium)

ux [L. *uxor*] wife

UYP upper yield point

V coefficient of variation • electrical potential (in volts) • gas volume • logical binary relation that is true if any argument is true and false otherwise • luminous efficiency • minute volume (of air or blood) • potential energy (joules) • unipolar chest lead • vaccinated • vaccine • vagina *also* VAG, Vag, vag • valine • valve • vanadium (element) • variation/variable *also* Var, var • varnish • vector • vegetarian • vegetation • vein *also* v • velocity *also* v • ventilation • ventral • ventricle • ventricular (fibrillation) • venous (blood) • venule • verbal (comprehension factor) • vertebral • vertex sharp transient (electroencephalography) • violet • viral (antigen) • virulence • virus • vision • visual acuity *also* VA • visual capacity • voice • volt *also* v • voltage • volume (of gas) *also* q, vol • vomiting

V̇ gas volume per unit of time (gas flow) • ventilation

V₁—V₆ precordial chest leads

v rate of reaction catalyzed by an enzyme • [L. *vide*] see • specific volume • vein *also* V • velocity *also* V • venous (blood) *also* VB • versus *also* vs • very • virus • vitamin • volt *also* V

v̄ mixed venous (blood)

v– vicinal isomer

+v positive vertical divergence

VA vacuum aspiration • valeric acid • valproic acid • vancomycin • vasodilator agent • ventricular arrhythmia • ventriculoatrial • ventroanterior • vertebral artery • Veterans Administration • viral antigen • visual activity • visual acuity *also* V • visual aid • visual axis • volcanic ash • volt–ampere • volume, alveolar • volume averaging

V_A alveolar ventilation

V/A variety • volt/ampere

V&A vagotomy and antrectomy

Va arterial gas volume • visual acuity • volt ampere *also* va

va volt ampere *also* Va

VAB vincristine, actinomycin D, and bleomycin

VABP ventroarterial bypass pumping

VAC ventriculoarterial connection • ventriculoatrial condition • ventriculoatrial conduction • vincristine, Adriamycin (doxorubicin), and cyclophosphamide • virus capsid antigen

vac vaccine • vacuum

vacc vaccination

VACTERL vertebral (abnormalities), anal (atresia), cardiac (abnormalities), tracheosophageal (fistula and/or) esophageal (atresia), renal (agenesis and dysplasia) limb (defects)

VAD vascular (venous) access device • ventricular assist device • vincristine, Adriamycin (doxorubicin), and dexamethasone • virus–adjusting diluent • vitamin A deficiency

VADA vincristine, Adriamycin (doxorubicin), dexamethasone, and actinomycin D

VADR vincristine, Adriamycin (doxorubicin), and cyclophosphamide

V$_A$eff effective alveolar ventilation

VAER visual auditory evoked response

VAFAC vincristine, Adriamycin (doxorubicin), 5–fluorouracil, Amethopterine (methotrexate), and cyclophosphasmide

VAG, Vag, vag vagina/vaginal *also* V

VAG HYST vaginal hysterectomy *also* VH

VAH vertebral ankylosing hyperostosis • Veterans Administration Hospital • virilizing adrenal hyperplasia

VAHS virus–associated hemophagocytic syndrome

VAIN vaginal intraepithelial neoplasia

VAKT visual, association, kinesthetic, tactile (reading)

VAL, Val valine

val valve

VALE visual acuity, left eye

VAM ventricular arrhythmia monitor • VP–16 (etoposide), Adriamycin (doxorubicin), and methotrexate

VAMC Veterans Administration Medical Center

VAMP vincristine, actinomycin, methotrexate, and prednisone

VAMS Visual Analogue Mood Scale

VAN ventricular aneurysmectomy

VANCO/P vancomycin–peak

VANCO/T vancomycin–trough

VAP variant angina pectoris • venous access port • vincristine, Adriamycin (doxorubicin), and prednisone (or procarbazine)

vap vapor

V̇A/Q̇, V$_A$/Q$_C$ ventilation–perfusion quotient ratio *also* V̇/Q̇

VAR visual auditory range

Var, var variable *also* V • variant • variety/variation

VARE visual acuity, right eye

VAS vascular *also* vasc • vasectomy *also* vas. • vesicle attachment site • viral analog scale • Visual Analogue Scale (pain)

vas. vasectomy *also* VAS

VASC Verbal Auditory Screen for Children

vasc vascular *also* VAS

vasodil vasodilation *also* VD

VAS RAD vascular radiology

vas vit, vas vitr [L. *vas vitreum*] glass vessel

VAT variable antigen type • ventricular activation time • ventricular (pacing), atrial (sensing), triggered (mode, pacemaker) • visual action time • visual apperception test • vocational apperception test

VATER vertebral (defects), (imperforate) anus, tracheosophageal (fistula) radial and renal (dysplasia)

VATH vinblastine, Adriamycin (doxorubicin), thiotepa, and Halotestin (fluoxymesterone)

VATs variable antigen, surface

VAV VP–16 (etopside), Adriamycin (doxorubicin), and vincristine

VB valence bond • Van Buren (catheter) • vagina bulbi • venous blood *also* v • ventrobasal • Veronal buffer • viable birth • vinblastine and bleomycin • voided bladder

VB$_1$ first voided bladder specimen

VB$_2$ second midstream bladder specimen

VB$_3$ third midstream bladder specimen

VBAC vaginal birth after cesarean

VBAIN vertebrobasilar artery insufficiency

VBAP vincristine, BCNU (carmustine), Adriamycin (doxorubicin), and prednisone

VBC vincristine, bleomycin, and cisplatin

VBD Veronal–buffered diluent • vinblastine, bleomycin, and cisplatin

VBG venoaortocoronary artery bypass graft • venous blood gas • veronal–buffered (serum with) gelatin • vertical–banded gastroplasty

VBI vertebrobasilar insufficiency • vertebrobasilar ischemia

VBL vinblastine

VBM vinblastine, bleomycin, and methotrexate

VBMCP vincristine, BCNU (carmustine), melphalan, cyclophosphamide, and prednisone

VBOS Veronal–buffered oxalated saline

VBP ventricular premature beat • vinblastine, bleomycin, and Platinol (cisplastin)

VBR ventricular–brain ratio

VBS Veronal–buffered saline • vertebral–basilar (artery) system

VBS:FBS Veronal–buffered saline–fetal bovine serum

VBT vertebral body tenderness

VC VP–16 (etoposide) and carboplatin • vascular change • vasoconstriction • vena cava • venous capacitance • venous capillary • ventilatory capacity • ventral column • verbal comprehension • vertebral canal • Veterinary Corps • videocasette • vincristine • vinyl chloride • vision, color • visual capacity • visual cortex • vital capacity • vocal cord • volume, capillary • voluntary closing • vomiting center • vowel–consonant

V/C ventilation circulation (ratio)

V&C vertical and centric (bite)

Vc pulmonary capillary gas volume

V_c pulmonary capillary blood volume

VCA vancomycin, colistin, and anisomycin • viral capsid antigen

VCA–EB viral capsid antigen, Epstein–Barr

VCAP vincristine, cyclophosphamide, Adriamycin (doxorubicin), and prednisone

VCC vasoconstrictor center • ventral cell column

VCCA velocity, common carotid artery

VCD vibrational circular dichroism

VCDQ verbal comprehension deviation quotient

VCE vagina, ectocervix, and endocervix

V_{CE} velocity (of) contracile element

V_{CF} velocity (of) circumferential fiber (shortening)

VCG vectorcardiogram/vectorcardiography • voiding cystogram

VCI volatile corrosion inhibitor

V–Cillin penicillin V

VCIU voluntary control (of) involuntary utterances

VCM vinyl chloride monomer

VCMP vincristine, cyclophosphamide, melphalan, and prednisone

VCN vancomycin, colistomethane, and nystatin • vancomycin hydrochloride, colistimethate sodium, and nystatin (medium) • vibrio cholerae neuraminidase

VCO, V_{CO} carbon monoxide (endogenous production)

VCO_2, V_{CO2} carbon dioxide output • volume, carbon dioxide elimination

VCP vincristine, cyclophosphamide, and prednisone

VCR vasoconstriction rate • vincristine • vincristine (sulfate) • volume clearance rate

VCS vasoconstrictor substance • vesiocervical space • Vocabulary Comprehension Scale

VCSA viral cell surface antigen

VCSF ventricular cerebrospinal fluid

VCT venous clotting time

VCU videocystourethrogram/ videocystourethrography • voiding cystourethrogram *also* VCUG

VCUG vesicoureterogram • voiding cystourethrogram *also* VCU

VCV vowel–consonant–vowel

VD vapor density • vascular disease • vasodilation/ vasodilator *also* vasodil • venereal disease • ventricular dilator • vertical deviation • video disk • viral diarrhea • voided • volume (of) distribution

+VD positive vertical divergence

V&D vomitiing and diarrhea

V$_D$ dead space • ventilation per minute of dead space • volume of dead space *also* VDS

V$_d$ apparent volume of distribution

vd double vibrations

VDA venous digital angiogram • visual discriminatory acuity

V$_D$A ventilation of alveolar dead space • volume of alveolar dead space

VDAC vaginal delivery after cesarean • voltage– dependent anion channel

V$_D$an ventilation of anatomic dead space • volume of anatomic dead space

VDBR volume (of) distribution (of) bilirubin

VDC vasodilator center

VDDR vitamin D–dependent rickets

VDEL Venereal Disease Experimental Laboratory

VDEM vasodepressor material

VDF ventricular diastolic fragmentation

VDG, VD–G venereal disease, gonorrhea

Vdg, vdg voiding

VDH valvular disease/vascular disease (of) heart

VDL vasodepressor lipid • visual detection level

VDM vasodepressor material

V$_{DM}$ volume of mechanical dead space

VD or M venous distention or mass

VDP ventricular premature depolarization • vinblastine, decarbazine, and cisplatin • vincristine, daunorubicin, and prednisone

VDR venous diameter ratio

V$_D$rb rebreathing ventilation

VDRL Venereal Disease Research Laboratory (test)

VDRR vitamin D–resistant rickets

VDRS Verdun Depression Rating Scale

VDRT venereal disease reference test

VDS vasodilator substance · vindesine

VDS, VD–S venereal disease–syphilis

VDS volume of dead space *also* V_D

Vd shunt dead space effect of Qs/Qt

VDT visual display terminal · visual distortion test

VDU visual display unit

VDV ventricular (end-)diastolic volume

V_D/V_T, VD/VT dead–space gas volume to tidal gas volume (ratio)

VE vacuum extraction · vaginal examination · Venezuelan encephalitis · venous emptying · venous extension · ventilation · ventricular elasticity · ventricular escape · ventricular extrasystole · vertex · vesicular exanthema · viral encephalitis · visual efficiency · visual examination · vitamin E · vocational evaluation · volume ejection · voluntary effort

V_E (volume) airflow per unit of time · environmental variance · respiratory minute volume · volume of expired gas

V&E Vinethine and ether

Ve ventilation

VEA ventricular ectopic activity · ventricular ectopic arrhythmia · viral envelope antigen

VEB ventricular ectopic beat · ventricular extra beat

VEC vecuronium

VECG vector electrocardiogram

VECP visually evoked cortical potential

vect vector

VED ventricular ectopic depolarization · vital exhaustion (and) depression

VEDP ventricular end–diastolic pressure

VEE Venezuelan equine encephalitis · Venezuelan equine encephalomyelitis

V–EEG vigilance–controlled electroencephalogram

VEF ventricular ejection fraction

V_{EH} extrahepatic distribution

vehic vehicle

vel, veloc velocity

VEM vasoexcitor material

$V_{E\,max}$ maximal flow per unit of time

VEMP vincristine, Endaxan (cyclophosphamide), mercaptopurine, and prednisone

vent ventilation · ventilator · ventral · ventricular

vent fib ventricular fibrillation *also* VF, V fib

ventric ventricle

VEP visual evoked potential

VER ventricular escape rhythm • veratridine • visual evoked response

vert vertebra/vertebral • vertical

ves [L. *vesica*] bladder • vesicular • vessel

vesic [L. *vesicula*] blister

vesp [L. *vesper*] evening

ves ur [L. *vesica urinaria*] urinary bladder

VESV vesicular exanthema of swine virus

VET vestigial testis

Vet veteran • veterinary/ veterinarian

v.et. [L. *vide etiam*] see also

Vet Med veterinary medicine

VETS Veterans (Adjustment) Scale

Vet Sci veterinary science

VEWA Vocational Evaluation and Work Adjustment

VF left leg electrode for electrocardiogram • ventricular fibrillation *also* vent fib, V fib • ventricular fluid • ventricular flutter • ventricular fusion • video frequency • vigil, fatiguing • visual field • vitreous fluorophotometry • vocal fremitus

Vf, vf visual field

V$_f$ variant frequency

VFA volatile fatty acid

Vfactor verbal (comprehension) factor

VFAM vincristine, 5–fluoro-uracil, Adriamycin (doxorubicin), and mitomycin C

VFC ventricular function curve

VFD visual feedback display

VFDF very fast death factor

VFI visual field(s) intact *also* VFIT

V fib ventricular fibrillation *also* vent fib, VF

VFIT visual field(s) intact *also* VFI

VFL ventricular flutter

VFP ventricular filling pressure • ventricular fluid pressure • vitreous fluorophotometry

VFPN Volu–feed premie nipple

VFR voiding flow rate

VFRN Volu–feed regular nipple

VFT venous filling time • ventricular fibrillation threshold

VFW velocity waveform

VG vein graft • ventilated group • ventricular gallop • very good

V&G vagotomy and gastroenterotomy

V$_G$ genetic variance

VGH very good health • veterinary general hospital

VGP viral glycoprotein

VH vaginal hysterectomy *also* VAG HYST • venous

hematocrit • ventricular hypertrophy • veteran's hospital • viral hepatitis • vitreous hemorrhage

V_H hepatic distribution volume • variable domain of heavy chain immunoglobulin

VHD valvular heart disease • ventricular heart disease • viral hematodepressive disease

VHDL very–high–density lipoprotein

VHF very high frequency • viral hemorrhagic fever • visual half–field

VHN Vickers hardness number

VI [L. *virgo intacta*] untouched girl (virgin) • vaginal irrigation • variable interval • vastus intermedius • virulence/virulent • viscosity index • Visual Imagery • visual impairment • visual inspection • vitality index • volume index

V_I volume of inspired gas (per minute)

VI virulence/virulent

VIA virus inactivating agent • virus infection–associated antigen

vib vibration

VIBS vocabulary, information, block (design), similarities (psychology)

VIC vasoinhibitory center • vehicle for initial crawling • visual communication (therapy) • voice intensity controller

vic [L. *vices*] times

VICA velocity internal carotid artery

VID vaginal intrapithelial dysplasia • video-densitometry • visible iris diameter

vid [L. *vide*] see

VIF virus–induced interferon

VIG, VIg vaccinia immunoglobulin

vig vigorous

VIH violence–induced handicap

VIM video–intensification microscopy

VIN vaginal intraepitheal neoplasia • vinbarbital • vulvar intraepithelial neoplasia

vin [L. *vinum*] wine

VIP vasoactive intestinal peptide • vasoactive intestinal polypeptide • vasoactive intracorpeal pharmacotherapy • vasoinhibitory peptide • venous impedance plethysmography • very important patient • very important person • vinblastine, ifosfamide, and cisplatin • voluntary interruption (of) pregnancy

VIQ Verbal Intelligence Quotient

VIR virology

Vir virus/viral

vir [L. *viridis*] green • virulent

VIR AC viral antibody, acute

VIS vaginal irrigation smear • visible • visual information storage

vis vision/visual • visiting • visitor

VISC vitreous infusion suction cutter

visc viscera/visceral • viscosity • viscous

VIT venom immunotherapy • vital *also* vit • vitamin *also* Vit

Vit vitamin *also* VIT

vit vital *also* VIT • vitreous • vitrectomy • [L. *vitellus*] yolk *also* vitel

VIT CAP vital capacity *also* vit cap

vit cap vital capacity *also* VIT CAP • vitamin capsule

vitel [L. *vitellus*] yolk *also* vit

vit ov sol [L. *vitello ovis solutus*] dissolved in egg yolk *also* vos

vitr [L. *vitrum*] glass • vitreous

vits vitamins

viz [L. *videlicet*] that is, namely • visualized

VJ Vogel–Johnson (agar)

VK vervet (African green monkey) kidney (cell)

VKC vernal keratoconjunctivitis

VKH Vogt–Koyanagi–Harada (syndrome)

VL left arm electrode for electrocardiogram • vastus lateralis • ventralis

lateralis • ventrolateral • visceral leishmaniasis • vision, left (eye)

V$_L$ variable domain of light chain immunoglobulin • (actual) volume of lung

VLA vanillactic acid • virus–like agent

VLB vincaleukoblastine (vinblastine)

VLBR very low birth rate

VLBW very low birth weight

VLCD very–low–calorie diet

VLCFA very–long–chain fatty acid

VLD very low density

VLDL, VLDLP very–low–density lipoprotein

VLDL–TG very–low–density lipoprotein triglyceride

VLDS Verbal Language Development Scale

VLF very low frequency

VLG ventral (nucleus of) lateral geniculate (body)

VLH ventrolateral (nucleus of) hypothalamus

VLM visceral larval migrans

VLP ventriculolumbar perfusion • vincristine, L-asparaginase, and prednisone • virus–like particle

VLSI very–large–scale integration

VM vasomotor • vastus medialis • ventricular mass • ventromedial • vestibular membrane •

viomycin • viral
myocarditis • voltmeter

V/m volt per meter

VM–26 teniposide

VMA vanillylmandelic acid

V–Mask Venturi mask

V$_{max}$ maximal velocity • peak
flow velocity (Doppler)

VMC vasomotor center •
village malaria com-
municator • vinyl chloride
monomer • void metal
composite • Von
Meyenburg complex

VMCG vector magneto-
cardiogram

VMCP vincristine, melphalan,
cyclophosphamide, and
prednisone

VMD [L. *Veterinariae
Medicinne Doctor*] Doctor
of Veterinary Medicine

vMDV virulent Marek disease
virus

VMF vasomotor flushing

VMH ventromedial hypothalamic (neuron, nuclei)

VMI visual motor integration

VMIT visual–motor integration
test

VMN ventromedial nucleus

VMO vastus medialis oblique
(muscle)

VMR vasomotor rhinitis

VMS visual memory span

VMSC Vineland Measurement
of Social Competence

VMST Visual–Motor
Sequencing Test

VMT vasomotor tone •
ventilatory muscle
training • ventromedial
tegmentum

VN vesicle neck • vestibular
nucleus • virus
neutralization • visceral
nucleus • Visiting Nurse •
visual naming • Vocational
Nurse • vomeronasal

VNA Visiting Nurse
Association

VNC vesicle neck contracture

VNDPT Visual Numerical
Discrimination Pretest

VNE verbal nonemotional
stimuli

VNO vomeronasal organ

VNR ventral nerve root

VNS villonodular synovitis •
Visiting Nursing Service

VO verbal order • volume
overload

VO$_2$, VO$_2$ volume of oxygen
consumption per unit of
time

VO$_2$max, VO$_2$max maximum
oxygen consumption

voc vocational

vocab vocabulary

VOCTOR void on call to
operating room

VOD veno–occlusive disease •
[L. *visio, oculus dexter*]
vision, right eye

vol volar • volatile • volume
also q, V • volumetric •
voluntary • volunteer

vol % volume percent

vol adm voluntary admission

vol/vol volume per volume (ratio)

VOM vinyl chloride monomer • volt–ohm–milliammeter • vomited *also* vom

vom vomited *also* VOM

VOP venous occlusion plethysmography

VOR vestibulo–occular reflex

VOS [L. *visio, oculus sinister*] vision, left eye

vos [L. *vitello ovi solutus*] dissolved in egg yolk *also* vit ov sol

VOT Visual Organization Test • voice onset time

VOU [L. *visio oculus uterque*] vision, each eye

voxel volume element

VP etoposide *also* VP–16 • vapor pressure • variegate porphyria • vascular permeability • vasopressin • velopharyngeal • venipuncture • venous pressure *also* Pv • venous (volume) plethysmograph • ventricular pacing • ventricular premature (beat) • ventriculoperitoneal (shunt) • vertex potential • vincristine and prednisone • viral protein • virus protein • Voges–Proskauer (medium, test) • volume–pressure • vulnerable period

V–P, V/P ventilation and perfusion *also* V&P

V&P vagotomy and

pyloroplasty • ventilation and perfusion *also* V–P, V/P

Vp plasma volume

VP–16 etoposide *also* VP

vp vapor pressure

VPA valproic acid

VPB ventricular premature beat

VPC vapor–phase chromatography • ventricular premature complex • ventricular premature contraction • volume–packed cells • volume percentage

VPCMF vincristine, prednisone, cyclophosphamide, methodrexate, and 5-fluorouracil

VPCT ventricular premature contraction threshold

VPD ventricular premature depolarization

VPDF vegetable protein diet (plus) fiber

VPF vascular permeability factor

VPG velopharyngeal gap

VPI velopharyngeal insufficiency • ventral posterior inferior

VPL ventroposterolateral

VPM ventilator pressure manometer • ventroposteromedial

vpm vibration per minute

VPO velopharyngeal opening

VPP viral porcine pneumonia

VPR volume–pressure response

VPRBC volume (of) packed red blood cells

VPRC volume (of) packed red (blood) cells

VPS valvular pulmonic stenosis • visual pleural space

vps vibration per second

VQ voice quality

V̇/Q̇ ventilation–perfusion (–quotient) ratio *also* V̇A/Q̇

VQR ventilation–perfusion (-quotient) ratio

VR right arm electrode for electrocardiogram • valve replacement • variable rate • variable ratio • vascular resistance • venous reflux • venous return • ventilation rate • ventilation ratio • ventral root • ventricular rate • ventricular response • ventricular rhythm • verbal reprimand • vesicular rosette • vision, right (eye) • visual reproduction • vital record • vocal resonance • vocational rehabilitation

Vr ventral root *also* vr • volume (of) relaxation

vr ventral root *also* Vr

VRA visual reinforcement audiometry

VRBC volume (of) red blood cells

VRC venous renin concentration

VR CON viral antibody, convalescent

VRD ventricular radial dysplasia

VR&E vocational rehabilitation and education

VRI viral respiratory infection

VRL ventral root, lumbar • Virus Reference Laboratory

VRNA viral ribonucleic acid

VROM voluntary range of motion

VRP very reliable product

VRR ventral root reflex

VRT variance (of) resident time • ventral root, thoracic • Visual Retention Test

VRV ventricular residual volume

VS vaccination scar • vaccine serotype • vagal stimulation • vasospasm • venesection • ventral subiculum • ventricular sense • ventricular septum • verbal scale • versus • very sensitive • vesicular sound • vesicular stomatitis • veterinary surgeon • villonodular synovitis • visual storage • vital sign(s) *also* V/S • volumetric solution • voluntary sterilization

V/S vital sign(s) *also* VS

V·s vibration–second • volt–second

V x s volts by seconds

vs [L. *versus*] against • [L. *vide supra*] see above • single vibration • [L. *venae sectio* cutting of vein] to draw blood • versus *also* v • vibration–second • vital sign • voids

VSA variant–specific surface antigen

VsB, vsb [L. *venae sectio brachii*] drawing blood from a vessel in arm

VSBE very short below–elbow (cast)

VSC voluntary surgical contraception

VSCS ventricular specialized conduction system

VSD ventricular septal defect • virtually safe dose

VSFP venous stop flow pressure

VSG variant surface glyco-protein

VSHD ventricular septal heart defect

VSI visual motor integration

VSMS Vineland Social Maturity Scale

vsn vision

VSO vertical subcondylar oblique

VSOK vital signs okay (normal)

VSR venereal spirochetosis (of) rabbits • venous stasis retinopathy

VSS vital signs stable

VSULA vaccination scar upper left arm

VSV vesicular stomatitis virus

VSW ventricular stroke work

VT tetrazolium violet (stain) • tidal volume • total

ventilation • vacuum tube • vacuum tuberculin • vasotocin • vasotonin • venous thrombosis • ventricular tachycardia • ventricular tachyar-rhythmia • Vero cytotoxin

VT, V$_T$ tidal volume

V$_t$ pulmonary parenchymal tissue volume

V&T volume and tension

VTA ventral tegmental area

V$_T$A alveolar tidal volume

V–TACH, V tach ventricular tachycardia

VTE venous thrombo-embolism • ventricular tachycardia event • vicarious trial (and) error

VTEC verotoxin–producing *Escherichia coli*

V–test Voluter test (radiology)

VTG volume thoracic gas

VTI volume thickness index

VTM mechanical tidal volume • variegated translocation mosaicism • virus transport medium

VTS vesicular transport system

VTSRS Verdun Target Symptom Rating Scale

VTVM vacuum tube voltmeter

VTX, Vtx vertex

VU varicose ulcer • very urgent • volume unit

VUR vesicoureteral reflex • vesicoureteral regurgitation

VUV vacuum ultraviolet

VV varicose vein • vesico-vaginal (fistula) *also* V–V • viper venom • vulva (and) vagina *also* V&V

V/V volume to volume (ratio)

V–V vesicovaginal (fistula) *also* VV

V&V vulva and vagina *also* VV

vv veins

v/v vice versa • volume (of solute) per volume (of solvent)

VVC village voluntary collaborator

VVD vaginal vertex delivery • vascular volume (of) distribution

VVFR vesicovaginal fistula repair

V/VI grade 5 on a 6–grade basis (cardiac murmur)

vvI vocal velocity index

vvMDV very virulent Marek disease virus

VVOR visual vestibulo–ocular reflex

VVQ verbalizer–visualization questionnaire

VVS vesicovaginal space

VW vascular wall • vessel wall • von Willebrand (disease) *also* vW

vW von Willebrand (disease, syndrome) *also* VW

v/w volume per weight

vWD, vWd von Willebrand disease

VWF velocity waveform • vibration–induced white finger • von Willebrand factor *also* vWF, vWf

vWF, vWf von Willebrand factor *also* VWF

VWFT variable–width forms tractor

VWM ventricular wall motion

vWS, vWs von Willebrand syndrome

Vx vertex • vitrectomy

VY veal yeast

V–Y shape of incisions in V–Y procedure (plasty)

VZ, V–Z varicella–zoster (virus) *also* VZW

VZIG, VZIg varicella zoster immunoglobulin

VZL vinzolidine

VZV varicella–zoster virus *also* VZ, V–Z

W dominant spotting (mouse) • energy (work) • section modulus • shape of surgical incisions (plasty) • tryptophan • [Ger. *wolfram*] tungsten • water • watt • Weber (test) • week *also* w • wehnelt (x–ray hardness) • weight *also* w • west • wetting • white *also* w, Wh, wh, wt • white cell • whole (response) *also* WR • widowed • width • wife • Wilcoxon rank sum statistic • Wistar (rat) • with *also* w • word fluency • wolframium (tungsten) • work

W+ weakly positive

w velocity (m/s) • watt • week *also* W • weight *also* W • white *also* W, Wh, wh, wt • widowed • wife • with *also* W

w/, w̄ with

WA Wellness Associates • when awake • while awake *also* wa • wide awake *also* W/A

W/A watt/ampere • wide awake *also* WA

W or A weakness or atrophy

wa while awake *also* WA

WAB, WABT Western Aphasia Battery(Test)

WACH wedge adjustable cushioned heel (shoe)

WADAO weak and dizzy all over

WAF weakness, atrophy, (and) fasciculation • white adult female

W

WAGR Wilms (tumor), aniridia, genitourinary (abnormalities), and (mental) retardation

WAIS Wechsler Adult Intelligence Scale

WAIS–R Wechsler Adult Intelligence Scale, Revised

WAM white adult male

WAP wandering atrial pacemaker

WARDS Welfare of Animals Used for Research in Drugs and Therapy

WARF warfarin

WAS weekly activity summary • Wiskott–Aldrich syndrome • Ward Atmosphere Scale (psychology)

Wass Wasserman (reaction, test)

WAT Word Association Test

WB waist belt • washable base • washed bladder • water bottle • Wechsler–Bellevue (Scale) • weight bearing *also* Wb • well baby • Western blot • wet bulb • whole blood *also* QB, W Bld • whole body • Willowbrook (virus)

Wb weber • weight bearing *also* WB

WBA wax bean agglutinin • whole–body activity

Wb/A weber per ampere

WBAPTT whole–blood activated partial thromboplastin time

WBAT weight–bearing as tolerated

WBC weight–bearing with crutches • well baby clinic • white blood cell • white blood cell (count) • white blood corpuscle

WBC/hpf white blood cells per high power field

WBCT whole–blood clotting time

WBDS whole–body digital scanner

WBE whole–body extract

WBF whole–blood folate

WBH whole–blood hematocrit • whole–body hyperthermia

WBI will be in

W Bld whole blood *also* QB, WB

WBM whole boiled milk

Wb/m² weber per square meter

WBN wellborn nursery • wide band noise

WBPTT whole–blood partial thromboplastin time

WBQC wide–base quad cane

WBR whole–body radiation • whole–body retention

WBRS Ward Behavior Rating Scale

WBRT whole–blood recalcification time

WBS Wechsler–Bellevue Scale • whole–body scan •

whole body shower • withdrawal body shakes • wound–breaking strength

WBT wet bulb temperature

WBTF Waring Blender tube feeding

WBTT weight–bearing to tolerance

WBUS weeks by ultrasound

WC ward clerk • ward confinement • water closet • wet compress • wheelchair *also* W/C, wh ch • white cell • white (cell) cast • white (cell) count • whole complement • whooping cough • will call • work capacity • writer's cramp

WC′ whole complement

W/C wheelchair *also* WC, wh ch

WCB will call back

WCC Walker carcinoma cell • well–child care • white cell count

WCD Weber–Christian disease

WCE work capacity evaluation

WCL Wenckebach cycle length • whole–cell lysate

WCOT wall coated open tubular

WCR Walthard cell rest

WCST Wisconsin Card Sorting Test

WD wallerian degeneration • ward • warm and dry *also* W/D • well– developed agar *also* wd, w/d • well differentiated • wet dressing • Whitney Damon (dextrose) • Wilson disease • with disease • withdrawal dyskinesia • without dyskinesia • Wolman disease • word *also* Wd • wound *also* WND, wnd • wrist disarticulation

W/D warm (and) dry *also* WD • withdrawal • withdrawn

W→D wet to dry

Wd ward • word *also* WD

wd well–developed *also* WD, w/d • wound/wounded

w/d well developed *also* WD, wd, w/d

W4D Worth Four–Dot (test)

WDCC well–developed collateral circulation

WDF white divorced female

WDHA watery diarrhea, hypokalemia, achlorhydria (syndrome)

WDHH watery diarrhea, hypokalemia, (and) hypochlorhydria

WDI warfarin dose index

WDLL well–differentiated lymphatic lymphoma

WDM white divorced male

WDS watery diarrhea syndrome • wet dog shakes (syndrome) • wounds

wds wounds *also* WDS

WDWN well developed, well nourished

WE wage earner • wax ester • weekend *also* W/E •

western encephalitis • western encephalomyelitis • whiskey equivalent

W/E weekend *also* WE

WEE western equine encephalitis/ encephalomyelitis

WEG water–ethyleneglycol

WEP weekend pass

WEUP willful exposure (to) unwanted pregnancy

WF Weil–Felix (reaction, test) • white female *also* W/F, wf • Wistar–Furth (rat) • word fluency

W/F, wf white female *also* WF

WFE Williams flexion exercises

WFI water for injection

WFL within functional limits

WF–O will follow (in) office

WFR Weil–Felix reaction • wheal–and–flare reaction

WFSS Wolpe Fear Survey Schedule

WG water gauge • Wegener granulomatosis • Wright– Giemsa (stain)

WGA wheat germ agglutinin

WH walking heel (cast) • well– healed • well–hydrated • whole homogenate • wound healing

Wh white *also* W, w, wh, wt

wh whisper/whispered • white *also* W, w, Wh, wt

w·h, whr watt–hour

WHA warmed, humidified air

wh ch wheelchair *also* WC, W/C • white child

WHD Werdnig–Hoffmann disease

WHML Wellcome Historical Medical Library

WHO World Health Organization • wrist–hand orthosis

WHP, Whp, whp whirlpool

WHPB whirlpool bath *also* WPB

whr watt hour

WHS Werdnig–Hoffman syndrome

WHV woodchuck hepatic virus

WHVP wedged hepatic venous pressure

WI walk–in (patient) • wash–in • water ingestion • waviness index • Wistar (rat)

W/I within

W&I work and interest

WIA walking imagined analgesia • wounded in action

WIC women, infants, (and) children

wid widow/widowed/widower

WIPI Word Intelligibility by Picture Identification

WIQ Waring Intimacy Questionnaire

WIS Ward Initiation Scale • Wechsler Intelligence Scale

WISC Wechsler Intelligence Scale for Children

WISC–R Wechsler Intelligence Scale for Children, Revised

WIST Whitaker Index of Schizophrenic Thinking

WITT Wittenborn (Psychiatric Rating Scale)

W–J, WJPB Woodcock–Johnson (Psychoeducational Battery)

WK week *also* wk • Wernicke–Korsakoff (syndrome) • work *also* wk

wk weak • week *also* WK • work *also* WK

WKD Wilson–Kimmelstiel disease

WKF well–known fact

W/kg watt per kilogram

WKS Wernicke–Korsakoff syndrome

WKY Wistar–Kyoto (rat)

WL waiting list • waterload (test) • wavelength *also* λ • weight loss • workload

WLE wide local excision

WLF whole lymphocyte fraction

WLI weight–length index

WLM work–level month

WLS wet lung syndrome

WLT waterload test • whole–lung tomography

WM Waldenström macroglobulinemia • wall motion • ward manager • warm, moist • wet mount • white male *also* W/M, wm • whole milk *also* wm •

whole mount (microscopy) *also* wm • woman milk

W/M white male *also* WM, wm

wm white male *also* WM, W/M • whole milk *also* WM • whole mount (microscopy) *also* WM

w/m₂ watt per square meter

WMA wall–motion abnormality

WMC weight–matched control

WME Williams medium E

WMF white married female • white middle–aged female

WMM white married male • white middle–aged male

WMP weight management program

WMR work metabolic rate • World Medical Relief

WMS wall–motion study • Wechsler Memory Scale

WMX whirlpool, massage, exercise

WN, wn, w/n well nourished

WND, wnd wound *also* WD

WNE West Nile encephalitis

WNF well–nourished female

WNL within normal limits

WNLS weighted nonlinear least squares

WNM well–nourished male

WNV West Nile virus

WO wash–out • weeks old *also* wo • without *also* s, s̄, w/o • written order

W/O water (in) oil (emulsion)

w/o without *also* s, s̄, WO, wo

wo weeks old *also* WO • without *also* s, WO, w/o

WOB work of breathing

WOFL wound fluid

WOP without pain

WOR Weber–Osler–Rondu (syndrome)

WORM write once, read many

WOU women's outpatient unit

W/O/W water (in) oil (in) water

WOWS Weak Opiate Withdrawal Scale

WP water packed • weakly positive • wet pack *also* WPk • wettable powder • whirlpool *also* WHP, Whp, whp, W/P • white pulp • word processor • working point

W/P water/powder (ratio) • whirlpool *also* WHP, Whp, whp, WP

WPB whirlpool bath *also* WHPB

WPCU weighted patient care unit

WPFM Wright peak flowmeter

WPk Ward pack • wet pack *also* WP

WPN white (mucosa with) punctation

WPPSI Wechsler Preschool and Primary Scale of Intelligence

WPRS Wittenborn Psychiatric Rating Scale

WPSI Wittenborn Psychiatric Symptoms Inventory

WPT marbled pure tone

WPW Wolff–Parkinson–White (syndrome)

WR washroom • Wassermann reaction • water retention • weakly reactive • whole response *also* W • wiping reaction • work rate • wrist

W/R with respect (to)

Wr, wr wrist

WRAMC Walter Reed Army Medical Center

WRAT Wide Range Achievement Test

WRBC washed red blood cell

WRC washed red (blood) cell • water–retention coefficient

WRE whole ragweed extract

WRK Woodward reagent K

WRMT Woodcock Reading Mastery Test

WRST Wilcoxon rank sum test

WRVP wedged renal vein pressure

WS Wardenburg syndrome • ward secretory • Warthin–Starry (stain) • water soluble • water swallow • watt–second • Werner syndrome • West syndrome • wet swallow • whole (response plus white) space • Wilder silver (stain) • Williams syndrome • work simplification

W&S wound and skin

WS, W•s watt–second

WSA water–soluble antibiotic

WSB wheat soy blend

WSD water seal drainage

WSepF white separated female

WSepM white separated male

WSF white single female

WSL Wesselsbron (virus)

WSM white single male

WSP wearable speech processor

WSR Westergren sedimentation rate

W/sr watt per steradian

WT walking tank • wall thickness • water temperature • wild type (strain) • Wilms tumor • wisdom teeth • work therapy

wt weight • white *also* W, w, Wh, wh

WTD wet tail disease

WTE whole time equivalent

WTF weight transferral frequency

W/U, w/u workup

WV walking ventilation • whispered voice

W/V, w/v weight (of solute) per volume (of solution)

W$_v$ variable dominant spotting (mouse)

WV–MBC walking ventilation to maximal breathing capacity (ratio)

WW Weight Watchers • wet weight

WxP wax pattern

W/W, w/w weight (of solute) per weight (of solvent)

WWAC walk with aid (of) cane

WWIdF white widowed female

WWIdM white widowed male

WWTP wastewater treatment plant

WX wound (of) exit

WxB wax bite

WxP wax pattern

WY women years

WY /NRT Weidel Yes/No Reliability Test

WZa wide zone alpha (hemolysis)

X androgenic (zone) • break • cross • cross–bite • cross–section • crossed with • cross–match • decimal scale of potency or dilution • except • exophoria distance *also* x • exposure • extra • female sex chromosome • ionization exposure rate • Kienböck unit (of x–ray exposure) • magnification • multiplication sign • reactance (electric current) • removal of • respirations (anesthesia chart) • start of anesthesia • translocation between two X chromosomes • transverse • unknown quantity • xanthine • xanthosine • xerophthalmia • X unit

$\overline{X}$ except • sample mean

X+ xyphoid plus (number of fingerbreadths)

X′ exophoria, near viewing *also* x′

x axis of cylindrical lens • except • exophoria distance *also* X • sample mean • horizontal axis of rectangular coordinate system • mole fraction • multiplied by • roentgen (rays)

x′ exophoria, near viewing *also* X′

XA xanthurenic acid

X–A xylene–alcohol (mixture)

Xa chiasma

Xaa unknown amino acid

Xan xanthine

XANT xanthochromic

Xanth xanthomatosis

Xao xanthosine

XBT xylose breath test

XC, Xc excretory cystogram/cystography

XCCE extracapsular cataract extraction

XD times daily • X–linked dominant

X&D examination and diagnosis

XDH xanthine dehydrogenase

XDP xanthine diphosphate • xeroderma pigmentosum

XDR transducer

Xe xenon

XeCT xenon–enhanced computed tomography

X–ed crossed

XEF excess ejection fraction

XES x–ray energy spectrometry

XF xerophthalmic fundus

Xfmr transformer

XGP xanthogranulomatous pyelonephritis *also* XPN

XH extra high

xi (Ψ, ψ) fourteenth letter of Greek alphabet

XIP x–ray in plaster

XKO not knocked out

XL excess lactate • extra large • xylose–lysine (agar base)

X–LA X–linked agammaglobulinemia

XLD xylose–lysine–deoxycholate (agar)

X–leg cross leg

XLH X–linked hypophosphatemia

XLI X–linked ichthyosis

XLJR X–linked juvenile retinoschisis

XLMR X–linked mental retardation

XLP X–linked (lympho)proliferative (syndrome)

XLR X–linked recessive

XM cross–match *also* X–mat., X–match

X$_m$ magnetic susceptibility

X–mat., X–match cross–match *also* XM

XMM xeromammography

XMP xanthine monophosphate

XN night blindness

Xn Christian

XO gonadal dysgenesis of Turner type • presence of only one sex chromosome • xanthine oxidase

XOM extraocular movement

XOP x–ray out of plaster

XOR exclusive operating room

XP xeroderma pigmentosum

Xp short arm of chromosome X

Xp– deletion of short arm of chromosome X

XPA xeroderma pigmentosum (group) A

XPC xeroderma pigmentosum (group) C

XPN xanthogranulomatous pyelonephritis *also* XGP

X–Prep bowel evacuation prior to radiography

XPS x–ray photoemission spectroscopy

Xq long arm of chromosome X

Xq– deletion of long arm of chromosome X

XR x–ray • x–linked recessive

XRD x–ray diffraction

XRF x–ray fluorescence

XRT x–ray technician • x–ray therapy (radiotherapy)

XS corneal scar • cross–section • excessive • xiphisternum

XSA cross–sectional area • xenograph surface area

XS–LIM exceeds limits (of procedure)

XSLR crossed straight leg–raising (sign)

XSP xanthoma striatum palmare

XT, xT exotropia

X(T), x(T) intermittent exotropia

Xta chiasmata

Xtab cross–tabulating

XTE xeroderma, talipes, (and) enamel (defect)

XTM xanthoma tuberosum multiplex

XTP xanthosine triphosphate

XU excretory urogram/urography • X–unit *also* Xu

Xu X–unit *also* XU

XULN times upper limit of normal

XUV extreme ultraviolet

xvse transverse

XX double strength • normal female sex chromosome type

46, XX 46 chromosomes, 2 X chromosomes (normal female)

47, XXY 47 chromosomes, 2 X and 1 Y chromosomes (Klinefelter syndrome)

XX/XY sex karyotypes

49, XXXXY 49 chromosomes, 4 X and 1 Y chromosomes (XXXXY syndrome)

XY normal male sex chromosome type

46, XY 46 chromosomes, 1 X and 1 Y chromosome (normal male)

47, XY +21 47 chromosomes, male, additional chromosome 21 (Down syndrome, chromosome 21 trisomy)

XYL, XYLO Xylocaine

Xyl xylose

47, XYY 47 chromosomes, 1 X and 2 Y chromosomes (XYY syndrome)

Y coordinate axis in plane • male sex chromosome • ordinate • tyrosine • year *also* y • yellow • young • yttrium

y vertical axis of rectangular coordinate system • wave on phlebogram • year *also* Y • yield

YA *Yersinia* arthritis

YACP young adult chronic patient

YADH yeast alcohol dehydrogenase

YAG yttrium–argon–garnet (laser)

Y/B yellow/blue

Yb ytterbium

YBT Yerkes–Bridges Test (psychology)

YCB yeast carbon base

YCT Yvon coefficient test

yd yard

YE yeast extract • yellow enzyme

YEH$_2$ reduced yellow enzyme

YEI *Yersinia enterocolitica* infection

Yel, yel yellow

YET youth effectiveness training

YF yellow fever

YFI yellow fever immunization

YHMD yellow hyaline membrane disease

YHT Young–Helmholtz theory

YJV yellow jacket venom

Yk York (antibody)

YLC youngest living child

YLF yttrium lithium fluoride

YM yeast (and) mannitol

YMA yeast morphology agar

Y/N yes/no

YNB yeast nitrogen base

YNS yellow nail syndrome

Y/O, y/o years old

YOB year of birth

YORA younger–onset rheumatoid arthritis

YP yeast phase • yield point • yield pressure

YPA yeast, peptone, (and) adenine (sulfate)

YPLL years (of) potential life lost (before age 65)

yr year

YRD Yangtze River disease

YS yolk sac *also* ys • Yoshida sarcoma

ys yellow spot (on retina) • yolk sac *also* YS

YSC yolk sac carcinoma

YST yeast (cells) • yolk sac tumor

YT, yt yttrium

YTD year to date

YVS yellow vernix syndrome

Z atomic number symbol • benzyloxycarbonyl • [Ger. *Zuckung*] contraction • [Ger. *Zwischenscheibe* intermediate disk] disk (band, line) that separates sacromeres • glutamine • impedance • ionic charge number • point formed by line perpendicular to nasion–menton line through anterior nasal spine • no effect • proton number • section modulus • shape of surgical incision (–plasty) • standard score • standardized deviate • zero • zone

Z′, Z″ [Ger. *Zuckung*] increasing degrees of contraction

z algebraic unknown or space coordinate • axis of three–dimensional rectangular coordinate system • catalytic amount • standard normal deviate • standardized device

ZAP zymosan–activated plasma (rabbit)

ZAPF zinc adequate pair–fed

ZAS zymosan–activated autologous serum

ZB zebra body

ZC zona compacta

ZCP zinc chloride poisoning

ZD zero defect *also* Z/D • zero discharge • zinc deficient

Z/D zero defect *also* ZD

ZDDP zinc dialkyldithiophosphate

ZDO zero differential overlap

ZDS zinc depletion syndrome

ZE, Z–E Zollinger–Ellison (syndrome)

ZEEP zero end–expiratory pressure

ZES Zollinger–Ellison syndrome

Z–ESR zeta erythrocyte sedimentation rate

zeta (Z, ζ) sixth letter of Greek alphabet

ZF zero frequency • zona fasciculata

ZG zona glomerulosa

ZGM zinc glycinate marker

Z/G zoster (serum) immuno-globulin *also* ZIG, ZIg

ZI zona incerta

ZI^a isotope with atomic number Z and atomic weight A

ZIG, ZIg zoster (serum) immunoglobulin *also* Z/G

ZIM zimelidine

ZIP zoster immune plasma

Zm zygomaxillare

ZMA zinc meta–arsenite

ZMC zygomatic • zygormaxillary complex

ZN Ziehl–Neelsen (method, stain)

Zn zinc

Zn fl zinc flocculation (test)

ZnOE zinc oxide–eugenol (white zinc) *also* ZOE

ZNS Ziehl–Neelsen stain

ZOE zinc oxide–eugenol (white zinc) *also* ZnOE

Zool zoology

ZPA zone (of) polarizing activity

ZPC zero point (of) charge • zopiclone

ZPG zero population growth

ZPLS Zimmerman Preschool Language Scale

ZPO zinc peroxide

ZPP zinc protoporphyrin

ZPT zinc pyrithione

ZR zona reticularis

Zr zirconium

ZSB zero stool (since) birth

ZSO zinc suboptimal

ZSR zeta sedimentation ratio

ZT Ziehen test

ZTN zinc tannate (of) naloxone

ZTS zymosan–treated serum

Z–TSP zephiran–trisodium phosphate

ZTT zinc turbidity test

Zy zygion

Zylo Zyloprim

Zz [L. *zingiber*] ginger

S Y M B O L S

Angles, Triangles, and Circles

∧ above • diastolic blood pressure (anesthesia records) • elevated • enlarged • improved • increased • superior (position) • upper

∨ below • decreased • deficiency • deficit • depressed • deteriorated • diminished • down • inferior (position) • lower • systolic blood pressure (anesthesia records)

> causes • demonstrates • distal • followed by • derived from • greater than • indicates • larger than • leads to • more severe than • produces • radiates to • radiating to • results in • reveals • shows • to • toward • worse than • yields

< caused by • derived from • less severe than • less than • produced by • proximal • smaller than

∠ angle • flexion • flexor

∡ angle of entry

∡ angle of exit

∟ factorial product • right lower quadrant

⌐ right upper quadrant

⌐ left upper quadrant

⌐ left lower quadrant

Δ anion gap • centrad prism • change • delta gap • heat • increment • occipital traiangle • prism diopter • temperature (anesthesia records)

Δ+ time interval

Δ A change in absorbance

Δ dB difference in decibels

Δ P change in (intraocular) pressure

Δ pH change in pH

Δ t time interval

Δ H, H's Δ Hesselbach's triangle

○ respiration (anesthesia records)

♀ female • female sex

♂ male • male sex

Ⓐ , ⓐx axilla (temperature)

Ⓗ , ⓗ hypodermic • hypodermically

ⒾⓂ intramuscular • intramuscularly

ⒾⓋ intravenous • intravenously

Ⓛ left

Ⓜ	murmur		Ⓡ	rectal • rectally • rectum (temperature) • right
ⓜ	by mouth • mouth (temperature) • murmur		Ⓧ	end of anesthesia (anesthesia records) • end of operation
√ⓜ	factitial murmur			
Ⓞ	by mouth • oral • orally			

Arrows

↑ above • elevated • elevation • enlarged • gas • greater than • improved • increase • increased • increases • more than • rising • superior (position) • up • upper

↑g increasing • rising

↑V increase due to in vivo effect (lab)

↓ below • decrease • decreased • deficiency • deficit • depressed • depression • deteriorated • deteriorating • diminished • diminution • down • falling • inferior (position) • less than • low • lower • normal plantar reflex • precipitate • precipitates

↓g decreasing • diminishing • falling • lowering

↓V decrease due to in vivo effect (lab)

↗ deviated • displaced • increasing

↘ decreasing

→ approaches limit of • causes • demonstrates • direction of flow or reaction • distal • due to • followed by • indicates • leads to • produces • radiating to • results in • reveals • shows • to • to right • toward • yields

← caused by • derived from • direction of flow or reaction • due to • produced by • proximal • resulting from • secondary to • to left

↑↑ extensor response (Babinski sign) • positive Babinski • testes undescended

↓↓ down bilaterally • plantar response (Babinski sign) • testes descended

↑↓ reversible reaction • up and down

⇆ , ⇌ reversible (chemical) reaction

Genetic Symbols

□	male
○	female
◊	sex unspecified
□─○	mating
□═○	consanguinity
□┬○	illegitimacy
I □┬○ II	parents and offspring, in generations
⌃	dizgotic twins
⌃	monozygotic twins
4 ③	number of children of sex indicated
(□)(○)	adopted individuals
⊙	abortion or stillbirth, sex unspecified
□ ○	normal individuals
♙ ♀	individual died without leaving offspring
□┬○	no issue
■ ●	affected individuals
■ ●	proband or propositus
⊞	examined professionally • normal for trait
⊡	not examined • dubiously reported to have trait
◫	not examined • reliably reported to have trait
◧ ◑	heterozygotes for autosomal recessive
⊙	carrier of sex-linked recessive
⊘ ⊘	death

658

Numbers

0 completely absent (pulse) • no response (reflexes)

+1, 1+ markedly impaired (pulse)

1+ low normal or somwhat diminished (reflexes) • slight reaction or trace (lab tests)

+2, 2+ moderately impaired (pulse)

2+ average or normal (reflexes) • noticable reaction or trace (lab tests)

+3, 3+ slightly impaired (pulse)

3+ moderate reaction (lab tests) • more brisk than average (reflexes)

+4, 4+ normal (pulse)

4+ hyperactive (reflexes) • large amount (lab tests) • pronounced reaction (lab tests) • very brisk (reflexes)

$\frac{\bullet}{1}$ bowel movement (numeral indicates number of stools in a given period)

1x once • one time

2x, x2 twice • two times

3x etc. three times, etc.

Arabic	Roman
0	
1	I, i
2	II, ii
3	III, iii
4	IV, iv
5	V, v
6	VI, vi
7	VII, vii
8	VIII, viii
9	IX, ix
10	X, x
11	XI, xi
12	XII, xii
13	XIII, xiii
14	XIV, xiv
15	XV
16	XVI

Arabic	Roman
17	XVII
18	XVIII
19	XIX
20	XX
30	XXX
40	XL
50	L
60	LX
70	LXX
80	LXXX
90	XC
100	C
1,000	M
5,000	$\overline{V}$
10,000	$\overline{X}$
100,000	$\overline{C}$
1,000,000	$\overline{M}$

Plus, Minus, and Equivalencies

+   acid (reaction) • added to • convex lens • decreased or diminished (reflexes) • excess • less than 50% inhibition of hemolysis (Wassermann) • low normal (reflexes) • markedly impaired (pulse) • mild (severity) • plus • plus (slightly more than stated amount) • positive (lab tests) • present • slight reaction or trace (lab tests) • sluggish (reflexes) • somewhat diminished (reflexes)

(+)   significant • uncommon or uncertain mode of inheritance

(+)ive   positive

+ to ++   slight pain

++   average (reflexes) • 50% inhibition of hemolysis (Wassermann) • moderate (pain, severity) • moderately impaired (pulse) • normally active (reflexes) *also* ‡ • noticeable reaction or trace (lab tests)

+++   increased reflexes • 75% inhibition of hemolysis (Wassermann) • moderate amount • moderate reaction (lab tests) • moderately hyperative (reflexes) • moderately severe (pain, severity) • more brisk than averge (reflexes) • slightly impaired (pulse)

++++   complete inhibition of hemolysis (Wasserman) • large amount (lab tests) • markedly hyperactive (reflexes) • markedly severe (pain, severity) • normal (pulse) • pronounced reaction (lab tests) • very brisk (reflexes)

-    absent • alkaline (reaction) • concave lens • deficiency • deficient • minus • negative (lab test) • none • subtract • without

(-)   insignificant

±   doubtful • either positive or negative • equivocal (reflexes, qualitative tests) • flicker (reflexes) • indefinite • more or less • plus or minus • possibly significant • questionable • suggestive •

	variable • very slight (reaction, severity, trace) • with or without
(±)	possibly significant
± to +	minimal pain
∓	minus or plus
‡	moderate (severity) • normally active (reflexes) *also* ++
#	fracture • gauge • number • pound(s) • weight
~	about • approximate • approximately • proportionate to
≈	approximately equal • nearly equal to
=	equal • equals • equal to
≠	does not equal • not equal • not equal to • unequal

◡	combined with
⊖	equivalent
⊘	not equivalent to
≡	identical • identical with
≢	not identical • not identical with
≟	nearly equal to
≑	approximately equal
≅	approximately • approximately equals • congruent to
≐	approaches
⊥	equilateral
≙	equiangular
>	greater than
<	less than
≯	not greater than
≮	not less than
≥, ≧	greater than or equal to
≤, ≦	less than or equal to

Primes, Checks, and Dots

? doubtful • equivocal (reflexes) • flicker (reflexes) *also* ± • not tested (severity) • possible • questionable • question of • suggested • suggestive (severity) • unknown

! factorial product

† death • deceased

/ divided by • either meaning • extension • extensor • fraction • of • per • to

' foot • hour • univalent

" bivalent • ditto • inch • minute • second (1/60 degree)

''' line (1/12 inch) • trivalent

√ check • observe for • urine • voided (urine)

√· urine and defecation • voided and bowels moved

√τ check with

√d checked • observed

√g, √ing checking

√qs voided sufficient quantity

√‾ radical root

²√‾ square root

³√‾ cube root

* birth • multiplication sign (genetics) • not verified • presumed • supposed

° degree • measurement (1/260 of circle) • severity (burns, wounds) • temperature • time (hour)

: is to • ratio

... no data (in given category)

∴ therefore

∵ because • since

:: as • equality between ratios • proportion • porportionate to

Statistical Symbols

α probability of Type I error • significance level

β probability of Type II error

$1\text{-}\beta$ power of statistical test

$_nC_k; \left(\frac{n}{k}\right)$ binomial coefficient • number of combination of n things taken k at a time

χ^2 chi-squared statistic

E expected frequency in cell of contingency table

$E(X)$ expected value of random variable X

F F statistic (variance ratio)

f frequency

H_0 null hypothesis

H_1 alternative hypothesis

μ population mean

N population size

n sample size

$n!$ n factorial

O obersved frequency in a contingency table

ϕ ability continuum • phi coefficient

P probability

p probability of success in independent trials

$P(A)$ probability that event A occurs

$P(A\backslash B)$ conditional probability that A occurs given that B has occurred

r sample correlation coefficient, usually the Pearson product-moment correlation

r^2 coefficient of determination

r_s Spearman rank correlation coefficient

ρ population correlation coefficient

s sample standard deviation

s^2 sample variance

SE standard error of estimate

σ population standard deviation

σ^2 population variance

$\sigma_{diff.}$ standard error of difference between scores

$\sigma_{est.}$ standard error of estimate

$\sigma_{meas.}$ standard error of measurement

$\sum_{i=1}^{n} x_i, \; \Sigma_i \overset{n}{=} x_i$ $x_1 + x_2 + \ldots + x_n$

t Student's t statistic • Student's test variable

θ	latent trait	≠	not equal
U	Mann-Whitney rank sum statistic	≈	approximately equal
		>	greater than
W	Wilcoxson rank sum statistic	≯	not greater than
$\overline{X}$	sample mean	<	less than
		≮	not less than
$\lvert \mathbf{x} \rvert$	absolute value of x	≥, ⩾	greater than or equal to
$\sqrt{x}$	square root of x		
z	standard score	≤, ⩽	less than or equal to
=	equal	∞	infinity